ESSENTIALS OF HUMAN EMBRYOLOGY

Second Edition

ESSENTIALS OF HUMAN EMBRYOLOGY

Rose Xaviour

MBBS, MD (Anatomy), DNB, MNAMS

Assistant Professor, Department of Anatomy
Government Medical College, Thrissur, Kerala, India

President's NBEMS Gold Medal for Anatomy in Diplomate of National Board Examination (DNB) [2019]

ACME (Advanced Course in Medical Education) from MCI Nodal Centre, Kottayam, Kerala

Nodal Officer, Student Support and Guidance Programme (SSGP), Kerala University of Health Sciences

District coordinator of Indian Medical Association Medical Students Network (IMA MSN)

Resource Person, NPTEL Swayam Prabha Project
Government of India, Ministry of Human Resource Development

Life Member, The Society of Clinical Anatomists (SOCA), India

Member of American Association of Clinical Anatomists (AACA)

Member of National Academy of Medical Sciences

Editorial Board Member (2020) & Reviewer, *National Journal of Clinical Anatomy* by Society of Clinical Anatomists, India

Member of Executive Committee of Society of Clinical Anatomists (SOCA), India

Academic Youtube channel – "Life In The Womb by Dr Rose"

ELSEVIER

ELSEVIER

RELX India Pvt. Ltd.
Registered Office: 818, Indraprakash Building, 8th Floor, 21, Barakhamba Road, New Delhi-110001
Corporate Office: 14th Floor, Building No. 10B, DLF Cyber City, Phase II, Gurgaon-122002, Haryana, India

Essentials of Human Embryology, 2e, Rose Xaviour

ISBN: 978-81-312-6910-7
e-Book ISBN: 978-81-312-6911-4

Content Strategist: Chandan Kumar
Content Project Manager: Goldy Bhatnagar
Sr Production Executive: Dhan Singh
Sr Graphic Designer: Milind Majgaonkar

Typeset by GW Tech India

Printed in India by Rajkamal Electric Press, Kundli, Haryana.

Dedicated to

My Beloved Parents, Dr VM Xaviour & Lissy Xaviour
My In-laws TL Jacob & Kochala Jacob
My Best Half, Dr Jose T Jacob
My Precious Gems, Danny & Dennis
My Only ones, My siblings, My Guiding Teachers, Role Models
and My Treasured Bunches...

Introduction

I am delighted and honored to present the 2nd edition of the embryology textbook, "Essentials of Human Embryology," authored by my student, Dr Rose. This concise and accessible reference book caters to the needs of both undergraduates and postgraduates. Driven by dedication and enthusiasm, Dr Rose's professional commitment is commendable, making this work a valuable contribution to the medical community. The book, a manifestation of Dr Rose's academic passion and innovative thinking, encapsulates the entire concept succinctly. It serves as an invaluable resource for undergraduates preparing for university examinations and postgraduates seeking a swift review.

Notably, this book stands out for its alignment with the KUHS examination pattern and adherence to the latest curriculum outlined by NMC. I extend my best wishes to Dr Rose, anticipating continued success in all her future endeavours.

Dr Mohanan Kunnummal
Honorable Vice Chancellor
Kerala University of Health Sciences, India

Introduction

Understanding the in-utero development of organs and organ systems is crucial for comprehending congenital anomalies. Dr Rose Xaviour, through her video lectures in developmental anatomy for the NPTEL-Swayamprabha Project, an initiative by the Government of India's Ministry of Human Resource Development, showcases a profound understanding of developmental anatomy. I commend her for the clarity and wonderfully lucid teaching style demonstrated in these lectures.

Having reviewed several chapters from this book, I wholeheartedly endorse it for graduate medical students. I am confident that they will find this book to be an extremely valuable resource in their academic journey.

Dr (Lt Col) T Vijay Sagar
MBBS, MS (Anatomy)
Dean, Symbiosis Medical College for Women &
CEO, Symbiosis University Hospital and Research Centre, Pune, India

Preface to the Second Edition

Embryology, the fascinating study of the unborn, explores the details of gamete development, fertilization, embryo formation, and congenital disorders. Its roots extend back to the 18th century, with Aristotle envisioning a miniature infant, evolving over time to modern concepts like cell signalling, mutations, and stem cell research. However, the vastness of contemporary embryological knowledge can overwhelm the average medical student. This book aims to distil these complexities into a comprehensible format.

Essentials of Human Embryology offers a clear and concise exploration of all facets of embryology, facilitating better understanding, easy recollection, and swift review. To enhance accessibility, the content is presented in a point-wise format, with each topic accompanied by subheadings for quick reference. The inclusion of well-labelled diagrams and vibrant photographs, along with outstanding flowcharts, enhances comprehension and connects topics with relevant clinical conditions (heartfelt thanks to the contributors).

Noteworthy features include the incorporation of multiple-choice questions (MCQs), aiding undergraduate exams (in line with new NMC guidelines) and postgraduate entrance preparations. Each chapter concludes with "KLINISCHE PERLEN," an exciting feature inviting readers to unravel pearls of clinical wisdom. Aligning with the new NMC curriculum, competencies are outlined at the start of each chapter, ensuring comprehensive coverage for board exam preparation.

This book is meticulously designed to be handy, precise, and visually engaging, positioning it as the preferred choice for undergraduates. Additionally, the structured representation of topics and the inclusion of MCQs cater to the needs of postgraduate students. For an in-depth exploration of challenging topics, I invite you to subscribe to the YouTube channel LIFE IN THE WOMB by DR ROSE.

I earnestly hope that both students and educators find this book not only useful but also intriguing. I eagerly await your valuable suggestions for enhancing subsequent edition.

Rosemol Xaviour

Preface to the First Edition

Embryology, study of the unborn, encompasses the development of gametes, fertilization, development of embryo, and the congenital disorders. The idea of embryology dates back as early as 18th century, during the era of Aristotle, where it was the notion of miniature infant to the modern-day cell signaling, mutations, and stem cell research. But the modern-day treatment of this voluminous data is in a way much above the head of an average medical student. The idea of this book is to bring them all together into a nutshell.

"Essentials of Human Embryology" gives a clear and concise idea regarding all aspects of embryology. For the better understanding, easy recollection, and quick review. Paragraph writing has been purposefully avoided and the topics are depicted point wise. Subheadings are given for each topic for its quick review. Another quality is the outstanding illustrations and excellent flowcharts pertaining to each topic. Well labeled diagrams for easy comprehension and colorful photographs of the corresponding topics and related clinical conditions (A big thanks for the contributors) have also been added. The other exceptional feature of this book is the inclusion of more than 100 **MCQs** which will be of great help for the postgraduate entrance preparations. An exciting feature **"KLINSCHE PERLEN"** at the end of every chapter is left for the readers to unravel. According to the new MCI curriculum,the topics were distributed in the form of competencies. In this edition the competencies are mentioned in the beginning of each chapter and effort has been taken to cover all the competencies as per the new curriculum which will help the students prepare well for the board exams.

This book has particularly been designed in such a way that it is handy, precise, and picturesque so that it gets to be the book of choice for undergraduates. In addition, the topic wise representation and the MCQs will assist the postgraduate students as well.

Please subscribe to the You Tube channel **LIFE IN THE WOMB DR ROSE** for further understanding of the topics.

I hope that both students and teachers would find this book useful and interesting and I look forward for their valuable suggestions for the further improvement of next editions.

Rosemol Xaviour

Acknowledgements

I extend my heartfelt gratitude to Dr Mohanan Kunnummal, Honorable Vice-Chancellor of Kerala University of Health Sciences and Dr (Lt Col) T Vijay Sagar, Dean of Symbiosis Medical College for Women & CEO of Symbiosis University Hospital and Research Centre, Pune for their insightful forewords and continuous encouragement.

I also want to express my sincere appreciation for the valuable contributions made by my colleagues and friends, who have played an essential role in this endeavour.

Dr Nandagopalan PA, MBBS, MD, Professor, & HOD, Department of Anatomy, Jubilee Mission Medical college, Thrissur, Kerala.

Dr PK Ramakrishnan, MBBS, MD, Professor, & HOD, Department of Anatomy, PKDIMS, Vaniamkulam, Kerala.

Dr Arjun Ashokan, MS, DNB, Mch, MRCS, Consultant Plastic Surgeon, Renai Medicity.

Dr Suja Arjun, MBBS, MD, DM, DNB, MNAMS, Consultant Endocrinologist, Renai Medicity.

Dr Aswin Prabhakaran P, MBBS, MS, MCh, Assistant Professor, Department of Pediatric Surgery, Amritha Institute of Medical Sciences.

Dr Jeena KJ, DLO, DNB, MNAMS, Assistant Surgeon, CHC Puthenchira.

Dr Nithya Shyam, MBBS, MD, Assistant Professor, Department of Pediatrics, Government Medical College, Thrissur.

Dr Rema G, MBBS, DNB, Assistant Professor, Department of Pediatrics, AIMS, Kochi.

Dr Sanitha Sathyan, DNB, FAICO, Medical Director, Vettam Eye Hospital, Mulanthuruthy, Kochi.

I am immensely grateful to my cherished team at PKDIMS, with special thanks to Dr Sharon for providing the cover photo for the first edition, Dr Kevin K Joseph for proofreading the second edition, Dr Ciona, and Dr Nimitha for their unwavering motivation. Additionally, I would like to acknowledge Dr Anjali (Assistant Professor Junior Resident, GMC, Thrissur) for her invaluable assistance with the proofreading of the first edition.

My sincere appreciation goes out to all my teachers at Government Medical College, Thrissur, Kerala, as well as my friends, relatives, students at PKDIMS, Government Medical College Thrissur, and Government Dental College, Thrissur, along with well-wishers, for their continuous support and guidance.

I extend my thanks to RELX team, especially Arvind Koul (Head – Content Strategy, Education), Chandan Kumar (Content Strategist), and Goldy Bhatnagar (Content Project Manager), for their assistance and cooperation throughout the process.

I am profoundly thankful to my husband and my precious gems who stood by me throughout this journey. Lastly, I express my gratitude to the Almighty for making this dream a reality.

Contents

Competency Map

Competency Code	Competency	Core (Y/N)	Chapter Numbers	Page Numbers
9.3	Describe development of breast.	N	23	304
13.8	Describe development of Upper Limb.	N	24	313
20.10	Describe basic concept of development of Lower Limb.	N	24	313
25.2	Describe development of pleura and lung.	Y	16	195
25.2	Describe development of heart.	Y	15	170
25.3	Describe fetal circulation and changes occurring at birth.	Y	15	185
25.4	Describe embryological basis of tracheo-oesophageal fistula.	Y	16	200
25.4	Describe embryological basis of atrial septal defect.	Y	15	188
25.4	Describe embryological basis of ventricular septal defect.	Y	15	189
25.4	Describe embryological basis of Fallot's tetralogy.	Y	15	189
25.5	Describe developmental basis of coarctation of aorta.	Y	15	190
25.5	Describe developmental basis of transposition of great vessels.	Y	15	190
25.5	Describe developmental basis of dextrocardia.	Y	15	190
25.5	Describe developmental basis of patent ductus arteriosus.	Y	15	191
25.6	Mention development of SVC.	N	15	174
25.6	Mention development of IVC.	N	15	174
25.6	Mention development of coronary sinus.	N	15	174
25.6	Mention development of aortic arch arteries.	N	15	181
43.4	Describe the development of branchial apparatus.	Y	14	150
43.4	Describe the development of thyroid gland.	Y	14	156
43.4	Describe the development of tongue.	Y	14	158
43.4	Describe the development basis of congenital anomalies of branchial apparatus, tongue, and thyroid gland.	Y	14	161
43.4	Describe the development of Face.	Y	19	245
43.4	Describe the development of Palate.	Y	19	249
43.4	Describe the developmental basis of congenital anomalies of Face and Palate.	Y	19	251, 253
43.4	Describe the development of pituitary gland.	Y	20	270

Continued

Competency Code	Competency	Core (Y/N)	Chapter Numbers	Page Numbers
43.4	Describe the developmental basis of congenital anomalies of pituitary gland.	Y	20	271
43.4	Describe the development of eye.	Y	21	281
43.4	Describe the developmental basis of congenital anomalies of eye.	Y	21	287
52.4	Describe the development of anterior abdominal wall.	N	11	116
52.5	Describe the development and congenital anomalies of diaphragm.	Y	11	121, 124
52.6	Describe the development and congenital anomalies of foregut, midgut, and hindgut.	Y	11 17	116 205
52.7	Describe the development of urinary system.	Y	18	222
52.8	Describe the development of male and female reproductive system.	Y	18	228
64.2	Describe the development of neural tube, spinal cord, medulla oblongata, pons, midbrain, cerebral hemisphere, and cerebellum.	Y	20	260
64.3	Describe various types of open neural tube defects with its embryological basis.	N	20	276
73.1	Describe the structure of chromosomes with classification.	Y	28	370
73.2	Describe technique of karyotyping with its applications.	Y	28	371
73.3	Describe the Lyon's hypothesis.	Y	28	375
74.1	Describe the various modes of inheritance with examples.	Y	28	376
74.2	Draw pedigree charts for the various types of inheritance and give examples of diseases of each mode of inheritance.	Y	28	376
74.3	Describe multifactorial inheritance with examples.	Y	28	380
74.4	Describe the genetic basis and clinical features of achondroplasia, cystic fibrosis, vitamin D-resistant rickets, haemophilia, Duchenne's muscular dystrophy and sickle cell anaemia.	N	28	380
75.1	Describe the structural and numerical chromosomal aberrations.	Y	28	383
75.2	Explain the terms mosaics and chimeras with example.	N	28	386
75.3	Describe the genetic basis and clinical features of Prader-Willi syndrome, Edwards syndrome and Patau syndrome.	N	28	387, 388
75.4	Describe genetic basis of variation-polymorphism and mutation.	Y	28	388
75.5	Describe the principles of genetic counselling.	Y	28 30	374 370
76.1	Describe the stages of human life.	Y	2	11
76.2	Explain the terms-phylogeny and ontogeny.	Y	2	13
76.2	Explain the terms-trimester and viability.	Y	10	105

Competency Code	Competency	Core (Y/N)	Chapter Numbers	Page Numbers
77.1	Describe the uterine changes occurring during the menstrual cycle.	Y	4	40
77.2	Describe the synchrony between the ovarian and menstrual cycles.	Y	4	41
77.3	Describe spermatogenesis and oogenesis along with diagrams.	Y	3	21
77.4	Describe the stages and consequences of fertilization.	Y	5	46
77.5	Enumerate and describe the anatomical principles underlying contraception.	Y	5	54
77.6	Describe fertility and sterility, surrogate motherhood, social significance of “sex-ratio.”	N	5	52, 54
77.6	Describe teratogenic influences.	N	26	333
78.1	Describe cleavage and formation of blastocyst.	Y	6	61
78.2	Describe the development of trophoblast.	Y	6	63
78.3	Describe the process of implantation.	Y	6	64
78.3	Describe the common abnormal sites of implantation.	Y	6	66
78.4	Describe the formation of extraembryonic mesoderm and coelom, bilaminar disc.	Y	7	70
78.4	Describe the formation of prochordal plate.	Y	8	85
78.5	Describe in brief abortion, decidual reaction, and pregnancy test.	Y	7	74, 75
79.1	Describe the formation and fate of the primitive streak.	Y	8	80
79.2	Describe formation and fate of notochord.	Y	8	81
79.3	Describe the process of neurulation.	Y	9	94
79.4	Describe the development of somites and intraembryonic coelom.	Y	9	93
79.4	Describe the development of somites.	Y	25	321
79.5	Explain embryological basis of sacrococcygeal teratomas.	N	8	81
79.5	Explain embryological basis of nucleus pulposus.	N	8	83
79.5	Explain embryological basis of neural tube defects.	N	9	98
79.6	Describe the role of teratogens.	N	26	334
80.1	Describe formation, functions and fate of-chorion, amnion, yolk sac, and decidua.	Y	7	70, 74
80.1	Describe the formation of allantois.	Y	8	83
80.2	Describe the formation and structure of umbilical cord.	Y	12	133
80.3	Describe the formation of placenta, its physiological functions, fetomaternal circulation, and placental barrier.	Y	12	127

Continued

Competency Code	Competency	Core (Y/N)	Chapter Numbers	Page Numbers
80.4	Describe embryological basis of twinning in monozygotic and dizygotic twins.	Y	13	140
80.5	Describe role of placental hormones in uterine growth and parturition.	Y	12	138
80.6	Explain embryological basis of estimation of fetal age.	N	10	104
80.7	Describe various types of umbilical cord attachments.	N	12	133
81.1	Describe various methods of prenatal diagnosis.	Y	10	106
81.2	Describe indications, process, and disadvantages of amniocentesis.	Y	10	109
81.3	Describe indications, process, and disadvantages of chorionic villus biopsy.	Y	10	108

SECTION 1

INTRODUCTION TO EMBRYOLOGY

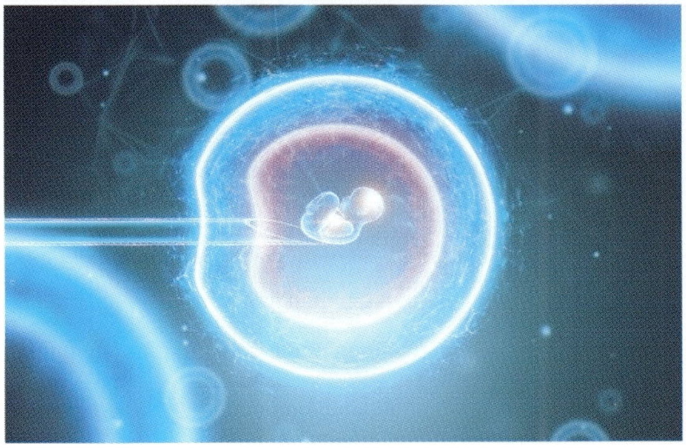

1 Understanding the Embryonic Coordinates

ANAMNESE

A 32-year-old expectant mother presents for a routine prenatal checkup and her ultrasound reveals a potential concern: the developing foetus exhibits a slightly smaller than expected crown–rump length for her gestational age, causing some initial worry. However, with a deep understanding of embryonic coordinates, the obstetrician is able to reassure the patient. She explains that early embryonic growth can vary and her understanding of the precise developmental milestones at various stages, including crown–rump length and gestational age in weeks postconception, allows her to accurately determine that the foetus is still within a normal range of development. By employing embryonic coordinates and a comprehensive knowledge of embryonic development, the obstetrician provides crucial reassurance to the mother and ensures that her pregnancy is progressing as expected. This case underscores the vital role of embryonic coordinates in accurately assessing and communicating the status of prenatal development, offering peace of mind to expectant parents.

HUMAN EMBRYONIC COORDINATES

In the context of human embryonic development, '***human embryonic coordinates***' typically refer to a system for describing the developmental stage of a human embryo. Following are some critical developmental milestones in human embryonic development:

- **Weeks postconception (WPC):** The age of the embryo is described in terms of weeks since fertilization. It is often used to track and describe the development of a human embryo. For example, at 4 WPC, significant milestones in early embryonic development occur, such as the formation of the neural tube.
- **Crown–rump length (CRL):** The CRL, which is the length from the top of the head (crown) to the base of the spine (rump), is another way to describe the developmental stage of a human embryo. CRL is often used in early pregnancy to estimate gestational age.
- **Trimesters:** Human pregnancy is often divided into trimesters, with each trimester lasting approximately 3 months. The first trimester covers the earliest stages of embryonic development, from conception to around 13 WPC. The second trimester extends from 14 to 27 weeks and the third trimester goes from 28 weeks until birth. These divisions help in tracking the progression of pregnancy.

These coordinates are essential in obstetrics and prenatal care to monitor the development of the embryo and foetus accurately. They are also used in research and medical practice to ensure that pregnancies are progressing as expected and to estimate due dates. Here are some key milestones and developmental stages in human embryonic coordinates:

Week 1 (0–7 days):

- Fertilization (conception) typically occurs around day 14 of a woman's menstrual cycle.
- The fertilized egg (zygote) undergoes several divisions, forming a blastocyst.

- Implantation of the blastocyst into the uterine wall usually occurs around day 6.

Week 2 (8–14 days):
- The blastocyst continues to implant and develop.
- The formation of the embryonic disc, which gives rise to the embryo, begins.

Week 3 (15–21 days):
- Gastrulation occurs, resulting in the formation of the three primary germ layers (ectoderm, mesoderm and endoderm).
- The neural tube begins to develop, which will eventually become the brain and the spinal cord.

Week 4 (22–28 days):
- The heart begins to form and beat.
- The notochord develops, contributing to the axial skeleton.
- The limb buds start to emerge.

Week 5 (29–35 days):
- Facial features begin to take shape.
- The placenta and umbilical cord continue to develop.
- The embryo undergoes rapid growth and differentiation.

Week 6 (36–42 days):
- Basic structures of the eyes, ears and nose become more apparent.
- Limb development progresses, with fingers and toes forming.
- The cardiovascular system continues to develop.

Week 7 (43–49 days):
- The developing embryo is referred to as a foetus by this stage.
- The brain undergoes significant development.
- External genitalia start to differentiate.

The terms used to describe the embryo are similar to anatomical terminology, but there are some common differences. Without knowing these distinctions, it is difficult to understand the structure of an embryo or foetus because they are three-dimensional objects that change their shape over time.

According to Larsen, ***if you do not know the co-ordinates, you will be like a person who reads a map without knowing its North, East, West and South directions.***

The *anatomical position* of an adult serves as a standard reference point in anatomy and medical practice.

It is defined as follows:

- The person is standing upright.
- The feet are together and flat on the floor.
- The arms hang naturally at the sides of the body with the palms facing forward.
- The head is facing forward with the eyes looking straight ahead.
- The body is in a straight line and all the body parts are in their neutral, unrotated positions.

This standard position is used to describe the location and orientation of various body structures, making it easier for healthcare professionals and anatomists to communicate and understand the human body's organization. It provides a consistent frame of reference for medical examinations, imaging and anatomical descriptions.

The anatomical position of an embryo is more challenging to define precisely than that of an adult because embryos and foetuses undergo significant morphological changes during development. However, in the early stages of embryonic development, there are some general principles that can be considered:

- **Axis alignment**: The embryo's main axis typically aligns from head to tail, with the head end containing the developing brain structures and the tail end forming the primitive beginnings of the spinal column.
- **Flexed position**: Early-stage embryos often exhibit a flexed or curved posture, with the limbs folded and the body bent forward, particularly in the early weeks of development.
- **Tail fold**: A notable feature is the presence of a tail fold, which is a natural, temporary structure at the caudal (tail) end. This fold recedes as development progresses.
- **Limbs**: Limb buds may be present but are often still in the early stages of development, tucked against the body.
- **Organ development**: Organogenesis is ongoing, and many organs are in the process of forming within the body.

It is important to note that as embryonic development progresses, the embryo gradually assumes a more stretched and less curved posture, with limbs becoming more apparent. Additionally, anatomical positions of various structures change as the embryo grows. Therefore, the precise anatomical position of an embryo depends on its developmental stage.

CRANIAL–CAUDAL AXIS

The cranial–caudal axis, often referred to as the '*cephalocaudal axis*', is a fundamental concept in embryology. It describes the longitudinal axis along which growth and development occur in embryos.

- **Cephalic (cranial/rostral) end**: This is the head end or the anterior part of the organism. In human embryos, the brain and head structures form at the cephalic end.
- **Caudal end**: This is the tail end or the posterior part of the organism. In human embryos, the spinal column and lower limbs develop along the caudal end (Fig. 1.1).

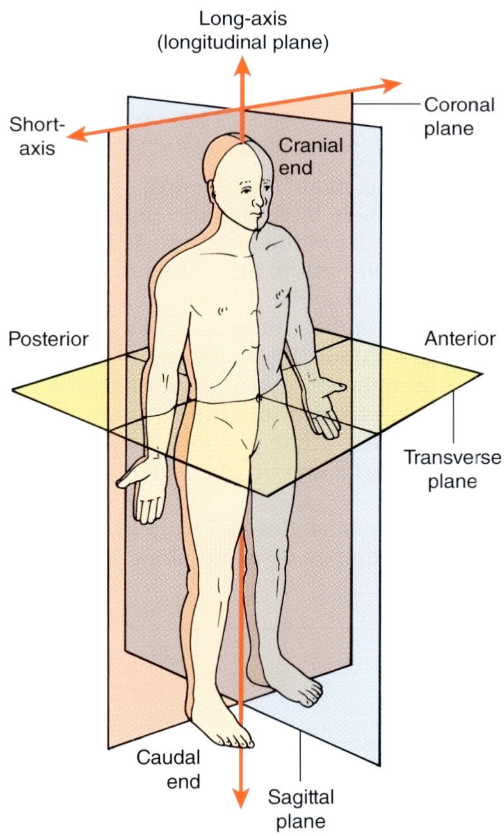

Fig. 1.1 Figure shows superior–inferior and anterior–posterior orientation. Ultrasound imaging planes. The sagittal and coronal planes are often referred to as longitudinal or long-axis planes and the transverse plane is often referred to as the short-axis plane. (Source: *Point-of-Care Ultrasound*, Second Edition, 2015.)

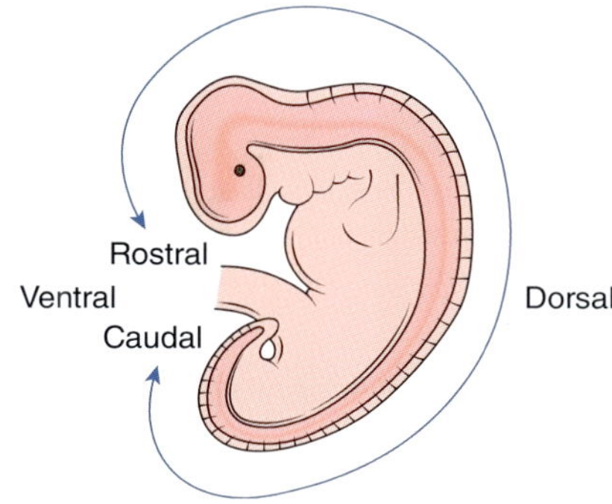

Fig. 1.2 Figure shows rostral–caudal and dorsal–ventral orientation in an embryo.

DORSAL–VENTRAL AXIS

The dorsal–ventral axis describes the longitudinal axis perpendicular to the cranial–caudal (cephalocaudal) axis, running from the back (dorsal) to the front (ventral) of the human embryo.

- **Dorsal side**: This is the back or posterior side of the embryo. Structures that develop along the dorsal side include the spinal cord and notochord, which play important roles in the development of the central nervous system and axial skeleton.
- **Ventral side**: This is the front or anterior side of the embryo. Structures that develop along the ventral side include the digestive system, heart and various ventral organs (Fig. 1.2).

MEDIAL–LATERAL

These terms help specify locations and orientations of structures during embryonic development:

- **Medial**: It refers to the direction or position closer to the midline of the body. The midline is an imaginary line that runs longitudinally down the centre of the body, dividing it into left and right halves. Structures that are closer to this midline are considered medial.
- **Lateral**: It refers to the direction or position farther away from the midline and closer to the sides of the body. Structures that are located away from the midline, towards the left or right sides, are considered lateral (Fig. 1.3).

PROXIMAL–DISTAL

The terms '*proximal*' and '*distal*' are used to describe the relative positions of structures in the developing human embryo, just as they are used in anatomical contexts for adults.

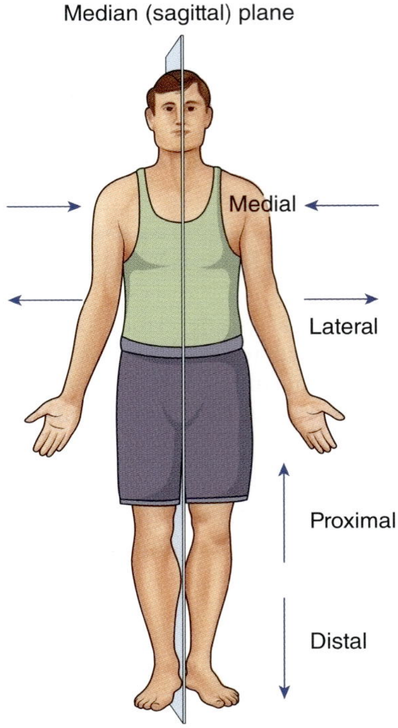

Fig. 1.3 Figure shows proximal–distal and medial–lateral orientation.

- **Proximal**: In the developing embryo, this often means structures that are closer to the centre of the body or a point of origin.
- **Distal**: In embryonic development, this typically denotes structures that are located farther from the centre of the body or the point of origin (Fig. 1.3).
  - Usually used to describe the limb structures. For example, the foot is distal to the knee joint.

SECTIONS

In embryology, various types of sections are used to study and analyse the development of embryos and foetuses. These sections are essential for understanding the intricate processes and structures that form during embryonic development.

Some common types of sections and techniques used in embryology include following:

- **Transverse sections**: Also known as cross-sections, these are made by cutting the embryo or tissue perpendicular to the long axis. Transverse sections provide information about the internal structures and the arrangement of tissues across the width of the embryo (Fig. 1.4).
- **Sagittal sections**: Sagittal sections are created by cutting the embryo or tissue along the sagittal plane, which divides the body into left and right halves. These sections are useful for studying structures in the anterior–posterior direction.
- **Coronal sections**: Coronal sections involve cutting the embryo or tissue along the coronal

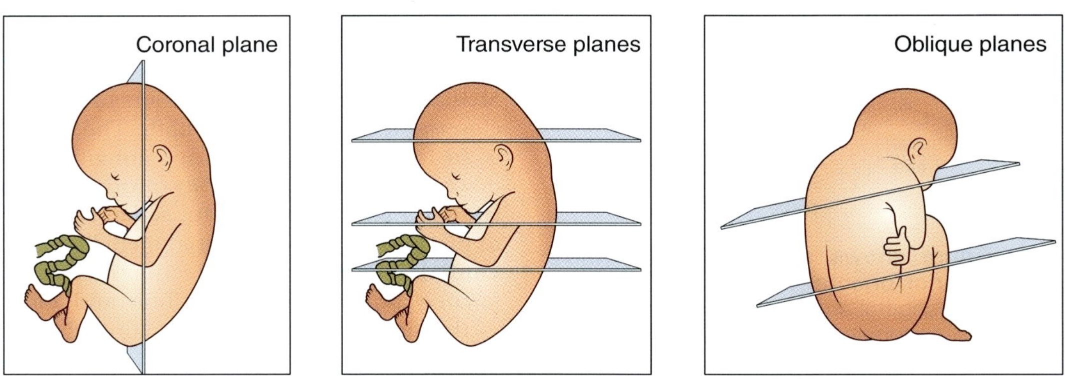

Fig. 1.4 Figure shows coronal, transverse and oblique planes of the foetus.

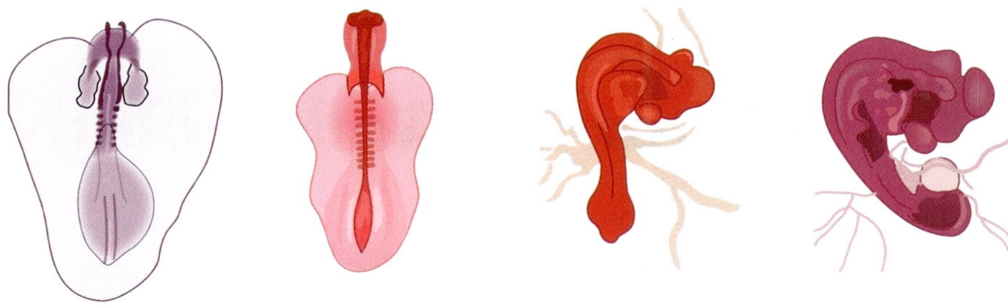

Fig. 1.5 Serial sections of chick embryo whole mount.

plane, which divides the body into front and back halves. These sections are particularly useful for understanding structures that are positioned in a front-to-back direction.

- **Serial sections**: Serial sections are a series of consecutive tissue sections that provide a continuous view of a structure or region. These are especially valuable for reconstructing three-dimensional structures (Fig. 1.5).

BRAIN TEASERS

1. In the context of human embryonic development, what do '*human embryonic coordinates*' primarily refer to?
   A. A system for describing foetal development
   B. A method for tracking the age of the embryo
   C. A set of coordinates for navigation during pregnancy
   D. A system for describing the position of organs in the embryo
2. What is the significance of the cranial–caudal axis in embryology?
   A. It describes the dorsal–ventral orientation of the embryo.
   B. It marks the midline of the embryo.
   C. It represents the growth and development direction in embryos.
   D. It determines the proximal–distal relationships in limb development.
3. Which of the following axis descriptions defines the dorsal–ventral axis in an embryo?
   A. From head to tail
   B. From back to front
   C. From left to right
   D. From the centre to the periphery
4. What are '*coronal sections*' typically used for in embryology?
   A. Studying structures in the anterior–posterior direction
   B. Investigating dorsal–ventral relationships in the embryo
   C. Examining the left–right orientation of organs
   D. Providing a continuous view of a structure
5. In embryology, what do 'serial sections' help with?
   A. Cutting the embryo into left and right halves
   B. Providing a three-dimensional (3D) view of a structure or region
   C. Creating slices perpendicular to the long axis
   D. Analysing the development of the heart

Answers

1. (B); 2. (C); 3. (B); 4. (A); 5. (B).

FURTHER READINGS

Bergmann S, Penfold CA, Slatery E, et al. Spatial profiling of early primate gastrulation in utero. *Nature.* 2022;609(7925):136-143. doi:10.1038/s41586-022-04953-1.

Chen K, Zheng Y, Xue X, et al. Branching development of early post-implantation human embryonic-like tissues in 3D stem cell culture. *Biomaterials.* 2021;275:120898. doi:10.1016/j.biomaterials.2021.120898.

2 History of Embryology

AN 76.1 Describe the stages of human life.
AN 76.2 Explain the terms phylogeny and ontogeny.

ANAMNESE

In a fascinating clinical case, a renowned obstetrician encountered a pregnant patient with an uncommon but intriguing dilemma. The patient had previously undergone a groundbreaking medical procedure involving *in vitro fertilization* (IVF) using a donated egg. During her prenatal checkup, an ultrasound revealed an unusual quirk: the developing embryo exhibited a unique genetic marker not present in the mother or the egg donor. It was a rare case of genetic chimerism where two distinct embryos had fused during the earliest stages of development, forming a single entity with two sets of genetic information. The treating doctor's deep knowledge of human embryology history and the concept of chimerism first observed by early embryologists, enabled her to explain this enigmatic occurrence to the patient. This exceptional case not only showcased the intricacies of embryonic development but also highlighted the enduring significance of historical embryological discoveries in addressing contemporary medical puzzles.

It is truly fascinating to learn what scientists in ancient periods believed about the theory of conception. Tracing the understanding of the steps of embryological development of a human foetus from 3000 BC to the present day arouses an interest in delving deeper into the subject.

- In ancient *Egypt* (3000 BC), it was believed that the soul entered the child through the *placenta*.
- The *first* recorded embryological studies were conducted in *Greece* by Hippocrates.
- *Aristotle* is recognized as the *founder of embryology*.
- *Galen* wrote a book on the formation of the foetus.

EMBRYOLOGY IN MIDDLE AGES

Constantinus Africanus (AD 1020–1087)

Constantinus Africanus made significant contributions to the field of embryology through his work '*De humana natura*'. In this notable text, he explored the development of the foetus within the context of celestial bodies, particularly the planets. What set his work apart was the intriguing correlation he drew between the stages of foetal development and the months of pregnancy.

RENAISSANCE

- **Leonardo da Vinci** (1452–1519) is celebrated as a pioneering figure in the history of science and art. His contributions to embryology were particularly remarkable, as he was the first person to create precise anatomical drawings of dissected pregnant uteri containing foetuses (Fig. 2.1).
- **William Harvey** suggested that the embryo is secreted by the uterus.
- **Fabricius of Acquapendente** studied embryos from various species.

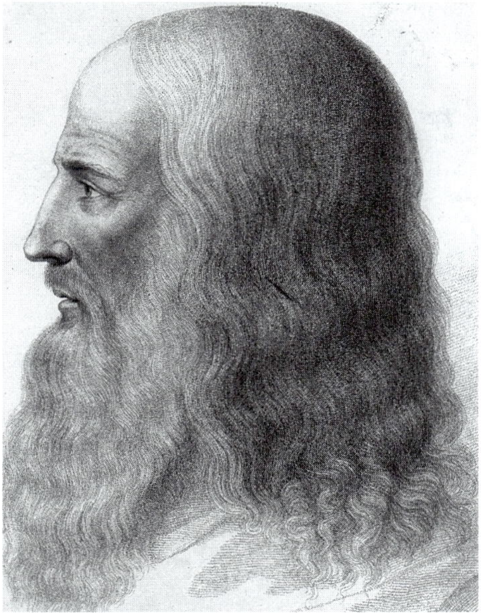

Fig. 2.1 Leonardo da Vinci. (Source: *Introduction to Fluid Mechanics*, Second Edition, 2018.)

- **Girolamo Fabricius**, in his work '*De formato foetu*', described the formed foetus and its stages of development.
- **Regnier de Graaf** once believed that the embryo was secreted from the ovaries.
- **Marcello Malpighi** posited that the egg contained a miniature chick.
- **Johan Ham van Arnheim and Anton van Leeuwenhoek** were the first scientists to observe spermatozoa.
- **Caspar Friedrich Wolff** proposed the following theories:
  - Refuted preformation theory.
  - Proposed layer concept and the basis of theory of *epigenesis*.
  - Discovered the '*Wolffian bodies*' and '*Wolffian ducts*'.
  - Described these in his dissertation '*Theoria Generationis*' after observing them in his studies on chick embryos (Fig. 2.2).
- **Lazzaro Spallanzani** found out that both ovum and sperm are needed for fertilization.
- **Christian Heinrich Pander** studied the chick embryo and discovered the germ layers.
- **Étienne Saint-Hilaire** and his son **Isidore** put forth the science of teratology.
- **Karl Ernst von Baer:**
  - Known as the *father of modern embryology*.
  - Discovered the *blastula* stage of development and the *notochord*.
- **Matthias Schleiden and Theodor Schwann** (Fig. 2.3) formulated the cell theory in 1839.
- **Wilhelm His Sr.** (Fig. 2.4):
  - Invented the microtome.
  - Explained the methods of fixation, sectioning, staining and reconstruction of the embryos.
  - Studied the development of the nervous system in a collection of 12 human embryos.
- **Franklin P. Mall:**
  - Collected embryos for scientific study.
  - His collection was later donated to Carnegie Institution for Science.
- **Hans Spemann** (Fig. 2.5):
  Laid the theory of primary induction by organizing centres and was awarded Nobel Prize in 1935.
- **Robert G. Edwards and Patrick Steptoe:**
  - Pioneers in *in vitro fertilization* (IVF).
  - First test-tube baby, Louise Brown, was born in 1978.

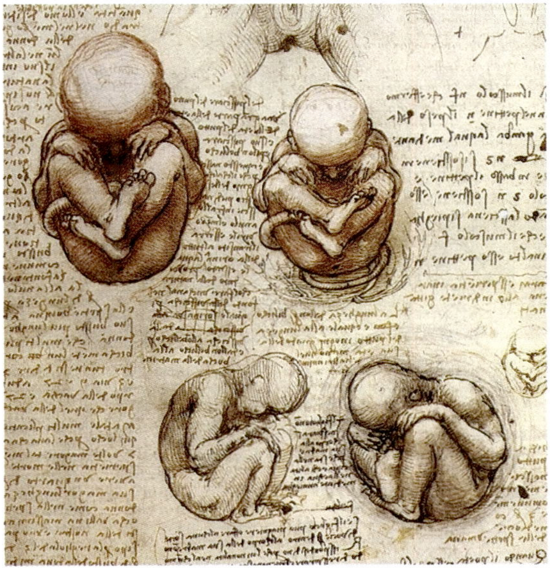

Fig. 2.2 Views of foetus and the womb, Leonardo da Vinci, ca. 1510–1512. (Source: *Reproductive and Developmental Toxicology*, 2011.)

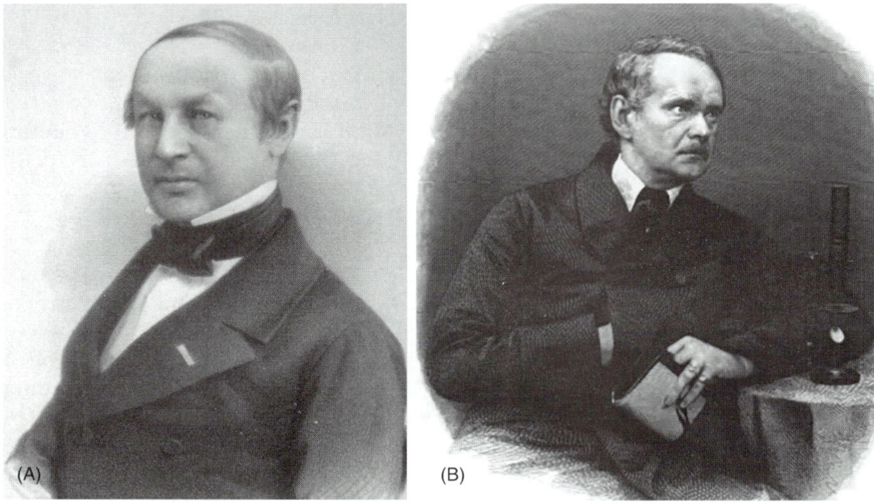

Fig. 2.3 (A) Theodor Schwann (1810–1882). (B) Matthias Schleiden (1804–1881). (Source: Reproduced from Wikipedia.)

RECENT ADVANCES IN EMBRYOLOGY

There have been numerous recent advances in embryology following IVF, often with the contributions of various scientists and researchers. Some notable developments include following:

- **CRISPR-Cas9 gene editing**: The revolutionary CRISPR-Cas9 technology has been applied to edit the genes of embryos to correct genetic mutations. Scientists like **Jennifer Doudna and Emmanuelle Charpentier** played pivotal roles in developing this gene-editing tool.
- **Artificial gametes**: Researchers, like **Karim Nayernia**, have made strides in developing artificial sperm and eggs from stem cells, which holds promise for individuals with fertility issues.
- **Preimplantation genetic testing (PGT)**: PGT has seen significant advancements in recent years and scientists, like **Sir Alec Jeffreys** who developed DNA fingerprinting, have contributed to improving genetic screening methods (Fig. 2.6).
- **Time-lapse imaging**: Time-lapse imaging systems for monitoring embryo development have been refined. Scientists, like **Professor Magdalena Zernicka-Goetz**, have used these technologies to gain insights into early embryo development.
- **Embryo selection algorithms**: Researchers, including **Professor Dagan Wells**, have developed sophisticated algorithms for selecting the most viable embryos for implantation, increasing the success rates of IVF.
- **Artificial uterus**: **Dr. Hung-Ching Liu's** work on developing an artificial womb, or '*Biobag*', is paving the way for potential advancements in neonatal care and assisted reproduction (Fig. 2.7).

STAGES OF HUMAN LIFE (AN 76.1)

As we analyse the development of an individual, we consider *three* important constructs:

- The life stages.
- The family cycle.
- The life course.

THE LIFE STAGES

- According to social scientists, the '*life cycle*' refers to the division of individual lives into a series of sequential stages. The primary stages of human life are as follows:
  - **Infancy**: The infancy stage encompasses the period from birth to approximately 12 months. During this stage, infants rely on caregivers for their basic needs, including

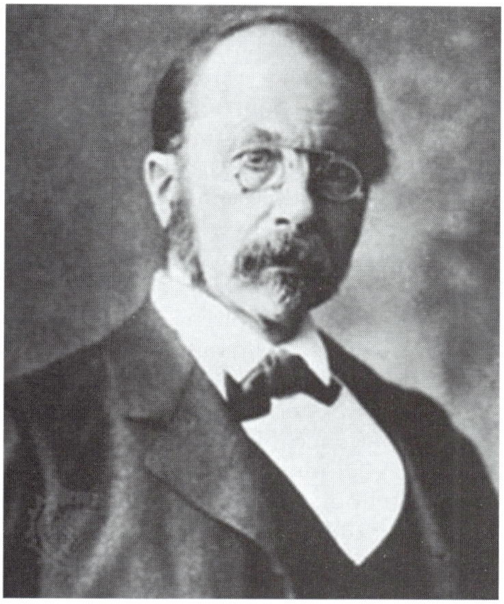

Fig. 2.4 Wilhelm His Sr. (1831–1904). (Source: Reproduced from Wikimedia Commons.)

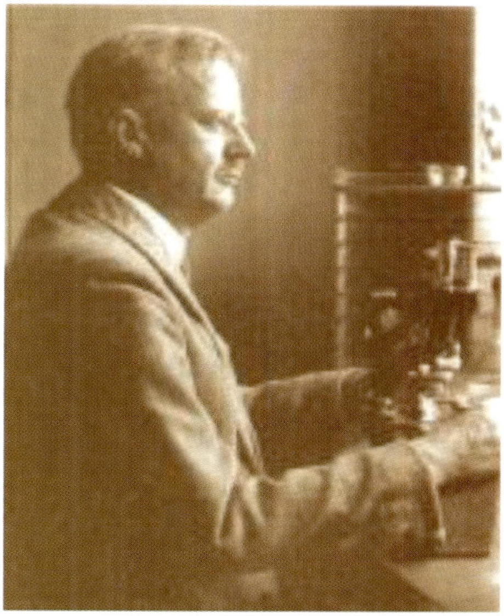

Fig. 2.5 Hans Spemann (1869–1941). (Source: *Biotechnology for Beginners*, Second Edition, 2017.)

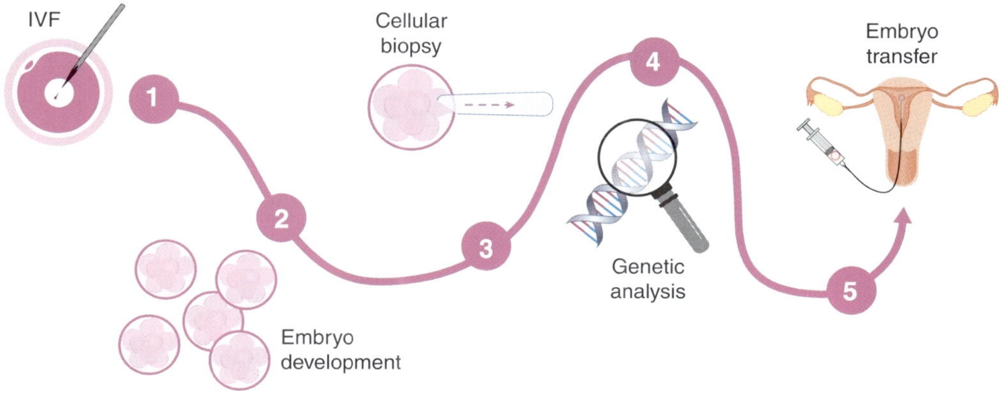

Fig. 2.6 Preimplantation genetic testing (PGT).

nourishment, comfort and security. Major milestones include learning to roll, sit, crawl and walk.

- **Childhood**: Childhood extends up to 12 years. This stage is marked by significant growth and development, as children acquire language, motor skills and cognitive abilities. They begin formal education and develop social skills.
- **Adolescence**: Adolescence spans the teenage years, typically from ages 13 to 19 years. This is a time of rapid physical growth and puberty, as well as emotional and social development. Adolescents explore their identities and gain more independence.
- **Early adulthood**: Early adulthood, from approximately ages 20 to 40 years, is a period of further self-discovery, education, career development, and often, romantic relationships, marriage and starting a family. It is a time of increased responsibility and independence.

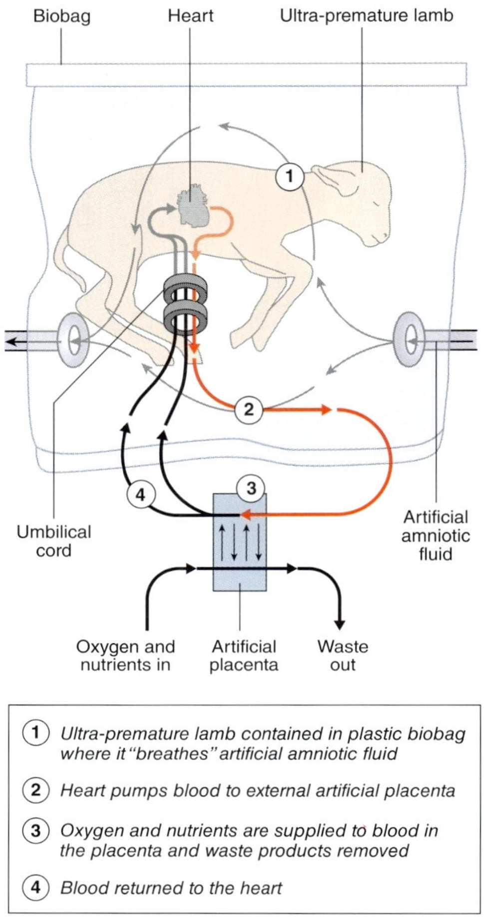

Fig. 2.7 Artificial uterus/Biobag. (Source: *Journal of Reproductive Immunology*: Y. Nami et al., Fig. 6, Page 9, Elsevier B.V., 2023.)

- **Middle age**: Middle age typically spans from early 40s to the late 60s. This stage is characterized by career stability, raising children and potentially caregiving for aging parents. Individuals may reassess their life goals and experience physical changes associated with aging.
- **Late adulthood**: Late adulthood begins in the late 60s and continues throughout one's lifetime. This stage is often marked by retirement, reflecting on life accomplishments, and facing the challenges of aging, including potential health issues. It is also a time of wisdom and reflection.
- **End of life**: The final stage of human life is the end of life, which encompasses the last years and months of a person's existence. During this stage, individuals may require medical care and support as they face the end of their life journey.

- Each stage is defined in terms of three distinct concepts: *biological, psychological and social.*
- For example, in adolescence stage:
  - *Biological* component involves pubertal physical changes, rapid physiological growth and sexual maturation.
  - *Psychological* component involves drastic mood swings, generational conflict and identity crisis.
  - *Social* component involves the shifting social experience, institutional treatment and cultural definition of adolescence.
- Another school of thought is that as we progress through life, we naturally transition from one stage to another. Some individuals might become stuck at a certain stage or even skip a stage without learning its important lessons. The stages are as follows:
  - **Stage 1**: Mimicry (imitation) and education.
  - **Stage 2**: Exploration and self-discovery.
  - **Stage 3**: Dedication and commitment.
  - **Stage 4**: Retirement and passing down your legacy.

THE FAMILY CYCLE

- The stages of the family cycle are described in terms of:
  - Presence or absence of children.
  - Child's age.
  - Employment status of the father.
- According to **Hill,** a **nine-stage model** of the family cycle is as follows:
  - Establishment (newly married, childless).
  - New parents (infant to 3 years).
  - Preschool family (child 3 to 6 years).
  - School-age family (oldest child 6 to 12 years).
  - Family with adolescent (oldest child 13 to 19 years).
  - Family with young adult (oldest child 20 years).
  - Family as launching centre (from departure of first to last child).
  - Postparental family (after children have left home until father retires).
  - Aging family (after retirement of father).

THE LIFE COURSE

It focuses on major life-cycle transitions:

- Marriage.
- Schooling.
- Entry into and exit from the labour force.
- It is based on the changing socioeconomic, cultural and historical conditions.

PHYLOGENY (AN 76.2)

- Phylogeny, a fundamental concept in the field of biology, is intricately tied to ***Charles Darwin's theory of evolution***. According to Darwin's concept, all modern life on Earth is connected through a shared ancestry with a single common ancestor at the root of this vast family tree, often referred to as the ***last universal common ancestor*** **(LUCA)**. This LUCA represents the point from which all living organisms diverged, giving rise to the remarkable diversity of species we observe today.
- The process of evolution is envisioned as a continuous branching or bifurcation in a tree-like structure, which is aptly termed the ***'Tree of Life'***. Each branch of this tree represents a species or a group of related organisms and the points where branches split signify divergence, often due to environmental pressures or genetic mutations.
- Phylogeny itself refers to the sequence of events involved in the evolutionary development of a species or a taxonomic group of organisms. It is a roadmap that maps out the evolutionary history of life on Earth, illustrating the relationships between different species and providing insights into their shared ancestry.
- To construct phylogenetic trees, scientists use various tools and methods, including comparative anatomy, genetics and fossil records. These trees not only help us understand how different species are related but also shed light on the mechanisms of evolution, adaptation and the emergence of biodiversity. In essence, phylogeny is a powerful tool that allows us to trace the path of life's development, uncover the patterns of descent and divergence, and gain a deeper appreciation for the interconnectedness of all living organisms on our planet.

ONTOGENY

- Ontogeny is a crucial concept in biology that refers to the course of development of an individual organism from the moment of fertilization through its various growth stages to reach its mature form.
- It is important to distinguish ontogeny from phylogeny. While phylogeny concerns the evolutionary history of species and the relationships between different species, ontogeny focuses on the developmental history of an individual organism within its lifetime.
- **Ernst Haeckel's** theory of recapitulation, also known as the biogenetic law or embryological parallelism, postulates that '***ontogeny recapitulates phylogeny***'. In other words, this theory suggests that during the course of its development, an individual organism goes through stages that mirror the adult forms of its evolutionary ancestors. Haeckel proposed that the embryonic development of an organism retraces the evolutionary history of its species (Fig. 2.8).

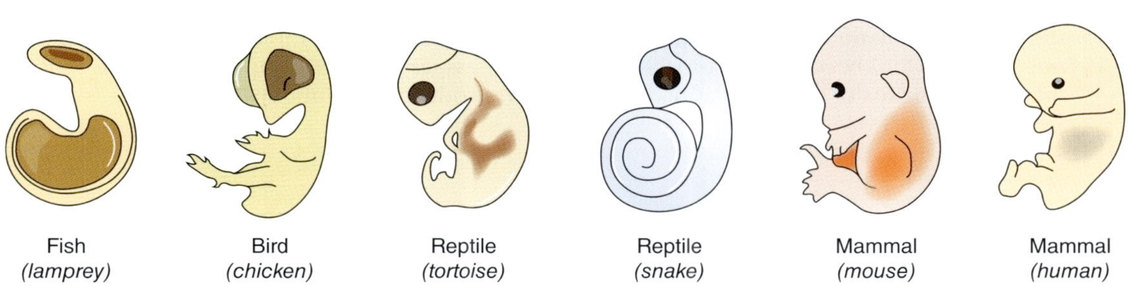

Fig. 2.8 Ontogeny recapitulates phylogeny.

- For instance, according to this theory, early stages of embryonic development in various vertebrate species would display similarities because they would represent common ancestral features from their evolutionary past. This idea was based on the observation that embryos of different species often appear similar during certain stages of development, such as the presence of gill slits in human embryos, which are remnants from our aquatic ancestors.
- It is important to note that Haeckel's theory of recapitulation has been met with criticism and is not universally accepted in its original form. Modern evolutionary biology acknowledges that ontogeny does not strictly recapitulate phylogeny but rather exhibits variations influenced by genetic and environmental factors. Nonetheless, the concept of ontogeny remains vital in understanding how individual organisms develop and grow, and it continues to be a topic of ongoing research and exploration in the field of biology.

HUMAN EMBRYOGENESIS

Human embryogenesis is the process by which a single fertilized egg, known as a zygote, develops into a multicellular embryo and eventually into a foetus. It is a complex and highly regulated series of events that takes place over approximately 9 months. The key stages of human embryogenesis are as follows:

  - **Fertilization**: The process begins with fertilization when a sperm cell penetrates the egg. This forms the zygote, which contains the complete set of 46 chromosomes (23 from each parent).
  - **Cleavage**: In the first few days after fertilization, the zygote undergoes rapid cell division, forming a solid ball of cells called a morula.
  - **Blastocyst formation**: The morula continues to divide and becomes a blastocyst. The blastocyst consists of an outer layer of cells, the trophoblast, which will develop into the placenta, and an inner cell mass, which will give rise to the embryo.
  - **Implantation**: The blastocyst attaches itself to the uterine wall and the trophoblast cells facilitate its implantation. This occurs around 6–10 days after fertilization.
  - **Gastrulation**: Gastrulation is a crucial stage where the three primary germ layers—ectoderm, mesoderm and endoderm—are established. These layers give rise to various tissues and organs in the body.
  - **Neurulation**: Neurulation is the formation of the neural tube, the precursor to the central nervous system, which eventually becomes the brain and spinal cord.
  - **Organogenesis**: During this stage, which spans weeks 4 to 8 of development, the major organ systems and structures begin to form. This includes the heart, lungs, liver and limbs.
  - **Foetal development**: By the end of the eighth week, the embryo is referred to as a foetus. Over the next several months, the foetus undergoes further growth and development, including the maturation of organ systems, the development of external features and the acquisition of reflexes.
  - **Birth**: Human embryogenesis concludes with childbirth, usually occurring around the 38th to 40th week of pregnancy. At birth, the foetus is fully developed and becomes a newborn infant (Fig. 2.9).

- Throughout human embryogenesis, precise genetic and epigenetic signals guide the differentiation and development of cells into specialized tissues and structures. Any disruptions or abnormalities during this process can lead to congenital defects or developmental disorders. A deep understanding of human embryogenesis is vital for both medical science and reproductive technologies, as it allows for the prevention and treatment of developmental issues and the improvement of assisted reproductive techniques like IVF.

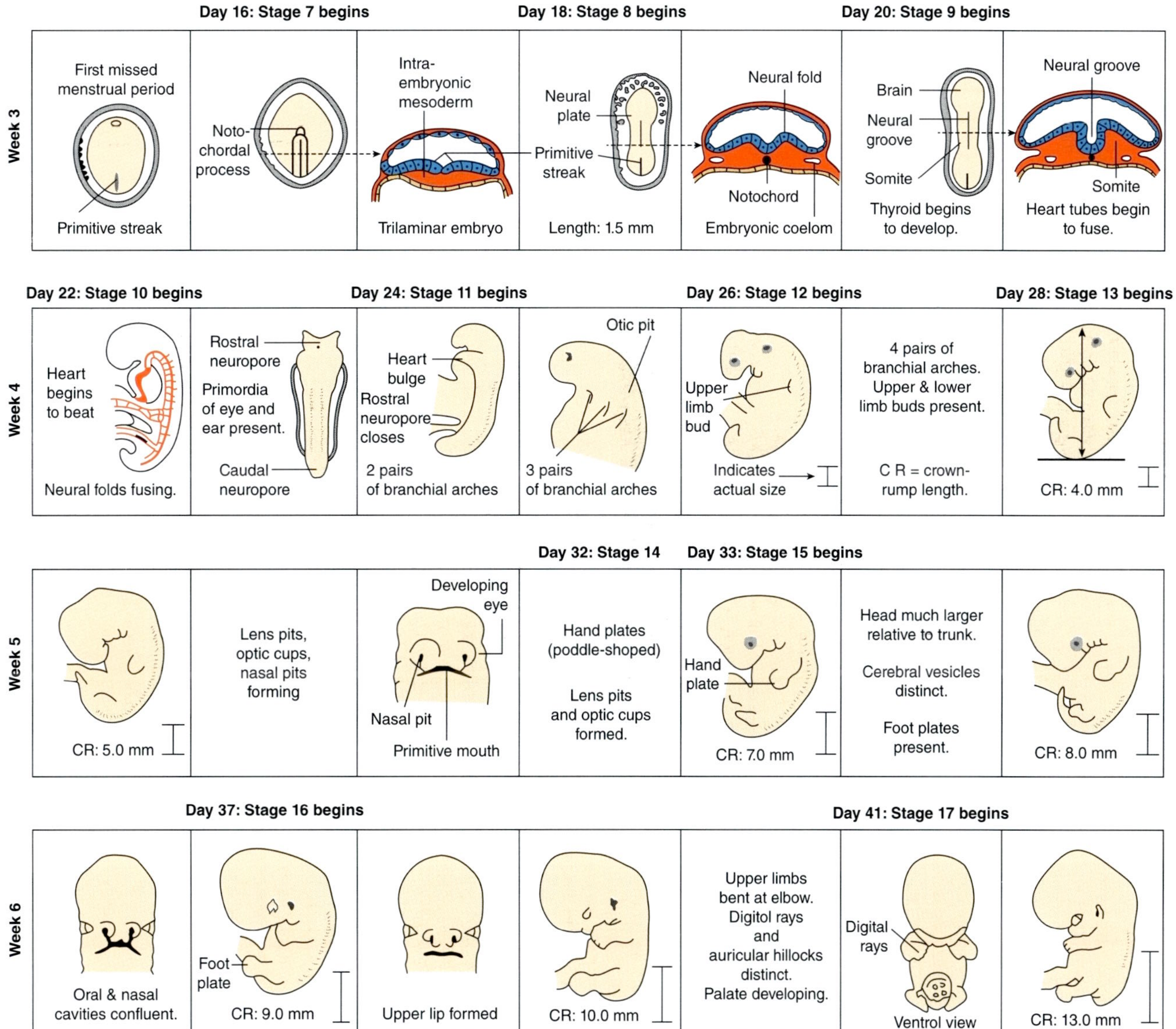

Fig. 2.9 Human embryogenesis.

BRAIN TEASERS

1. Who was the first person to create precise anatomical drawings of dissected pregnant uteri containing foetuses?
   A. William Harvey
   B. Fabricius of Acquapendente
   C. Leonardo da Vinci
   D. Regnier de Graaf
2. What did Lazzaro Spallanzani find out about fertilization?
   A. Both ovum and sperm are needed
   B. Only ovum is needed
   C. Only sperm is needed
   D. Fertilization is not essential
3. Who is known as the '*father of modern embryology*' and discovered the blastula stage of development and the notochord?
   A. Karl Ernst von Baer
   B. Girolamo Fabricius
   C. William Harvey
   D. Franklin P. Mall
4. The biogenetic law, which states that '*ontogeny recapitulates phylogeny*', was proposed by whom?
   A. Ernst Haeckel
   B. Charles Darwin
   C. Karl Ernst von Baer
   D. William Harvey
5. Which scientist made significant contributions to CRISPR-Cas9 gene-editing technology?
   A. Jennifer Doudna
   B. Karl Ernst von Baer
   C. Sir Alec Jeffreys
   D. Franklin P. Mall
6. The process of neurulation is essential for the development of which organ systems?
   A. Digestive system
   B. Nervous system
   C. Respiratory system
   D. Cardiovascular system
7. Who is credited with developing artificial sperm and eggs from stem cells?
   A. Jennifer Doudna
   B. Karim Nayernia
   C. Matthias Schleiden
   D. Leonardo da Vinci
8. What is the primary purpose of preimplantation genetic testing (PGT)?
   A. Embryo selection
   B. Prenatal care
   C. Fertilization
   D. Stem cell research
9. In the family cycle model described by Hill, which stage involves children leaving home and the father's retirement?
   A. Establishment
   B. Early adulthood
   C. Family as launching centre
   D. Aging family
10. What is the main concept of '*ontogeny*' in biology?
   A. Evolutionary history of species
   B. Developmental history of an organism within its lifetime
   C. The Tree of Life
   D. The life cycle

Answers

1. (C); 2. (A); 3. (A); 4. (A); 5. (A); 6. (B); 7. (B); 8. (A); 9. (D); 10. (B).

FURTHER READINGS

Barnes ME. *Ernst Haeckel's Biogenetic Law (1866)*. Embryo Project Encyclopedia; May 3, 2014.

Bayefsky MJ, Berkman BE. Implementing expanded prenatal genetic testing: should parents have access to any and all fetal genetic information? *Am J Bioeth.* 2022;22(2):4-22. doi:10.1080/15265161.2020.1867933.

Brännström M, Racowsky C, Carbonnel M, et al. Uterus transplantation: from research, through human trials and into the future. *Hum Reprod Update.* 2023;29(5):521-544. doi:10.1093/humupd/dmad012.

Gaucher EA, Kratzer JT, Randall RN. Deep phylogeny—how a tree can help characterize early life on Earth. *Cold Spring Harb Perspect Biol.* 2010; 2(1):a002238. doi:10.1101/cshperspect.a002238.

Mintz S. Reflections on age as a category of historical analysis. *J Hist Childhood Youth.* 2008;1(1):91-94.

Gametogenesis 3

AN 77.3 Describe spermatogenesis and oogenesis along with diagrams.

ANAMNESE

In a busy urban hospital, a young couple arrived at the obstetrics and gynaecology department with a history of multiple miscarriages. They had been trying to conceive for years but had experienced the anguish of recurrent pregnancy loss. As the medical team delved into their case, they discovered that the lady had an underlying condition affecting her gametogenesis, leading to chromosomal abnormalities in her ova. This condition played a crucial role in the repeated miscarriages. With the support of reproductive specialists, they explored assisted reproductive techniques to improve their chances of having a healthy pregnancy. This challenging clinical scenario underlines the critical role of gametogenesis in fertility, the significance of early diagnosis and the hope that advances in reproductive medicine can offer couples like them in their quest to build a family.

Retinoic acid (RA), synthesized from the dietary vitamin retinol, is required for male and female gametes to enter meiosis. In the embryonic period, RA acts by inhibiting male germ cells from entering into meiosis until after birth and thereby protecting germ cells. In contrast, deficiency of RA causes the degeneration of germinal epithelium by arresting spermatogenesis. **Stra8** is expressed in embryonic ovaries just before meiotic initiation, whereas its expression in testes is first detected after birth. Signalling by RA is required for *Stra8* expression. Deficiency of RA results in aberrant gametogenesis.

GERM CELL

Primordial germ cells (PGCs) are the precursors of gametes with males developing sperm and females developing oocytes.

PGCs initially emerge within the epiblast, a component of the embryonic disc, during the second week of development. Subsequently, by the third week, they relocate to the wall of the yolk sac, and by the end of the fifth week, they migrate through the dorsal mesentery of the gut to reach their final destination within the developing gonads (Fig. 3.1).

FURTHER DEVELOPMENT OF PRIMORDIAL GERM CELL

Once the PGCs have reached their destination in the developing gonads (testes in males and ovaries in females), they undergo two significant processes:

- **Gametogenesis.**
- **Cytodifferentiation.**

Gametogenesis involves meiosis, a process that leads to a reduction in the number of chromosomes.

Cytodifferentiation is the maturation process that the germ cells undergo to achieve their full development.

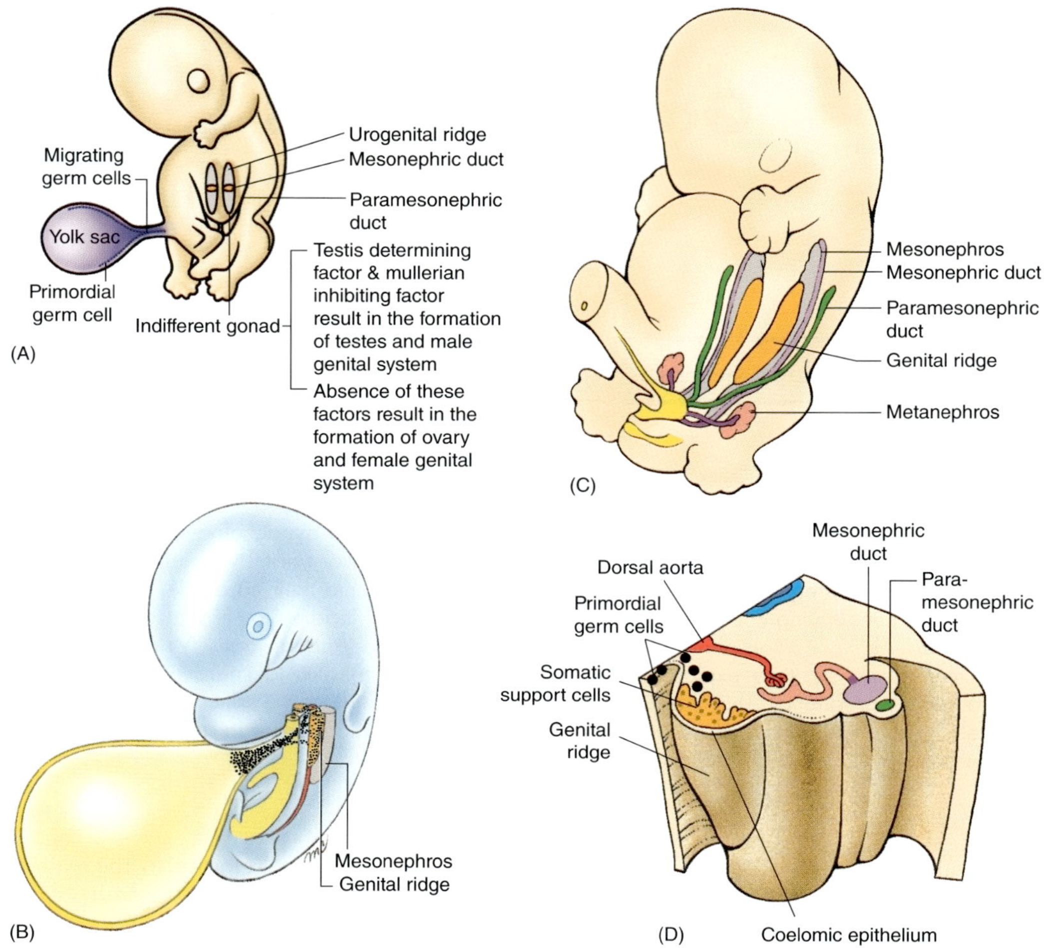

Fig. 3.1 Primordial germ cells migrating from yolk sac to developing gonads. Formation of the genital ridges and paramesonephric ducts. (A, D) During the fifth and sixth weeks, the genital ridges form in the posterior abdominal wall just medial to the developing mesonephroi in response to colonization by primordial germ cells (*black dots*) migrating from the yolk sac. (B) Each paramesonephric duct develops from an invagination and proliferation of coelomic epithelial cells extending caudally (*arrow*) alongside and parallel to the mesonephric duct. (C) The relationship of the mesonephric ducts and paramesonephric ducts to one another and to the developing gonads and kidneys. (D) The primordial germ cells induce the coelomic epithelium lining the peritoneal cavity to proliferate and form the somatic support cells. (Source: Larsen's Human Embryology, Fourth Edition, 2008.)

RESTORATION OF DIPLOID NUMBER

PGCs initially possess a diploid number of chromosomes (44XX or 44XY).

During gametogenesis, they undergo the first meiotic division, resulting in each mature gamete carrying a haploid number of 23 chromosomes (22X or 22Y).

MITOSIS AND MEIOSIS

Before delving into gametogenesis, it is beneficial to review two fundamental cell divisions.

MITOSIS

Mitosis, a critical process in cell division, gives rise to two genetically identical daughter cells through DNA duplication, making it essential for growth, repair and cell replacement. The six distinct phases of mitosis are as follows:

- **Interphase**: This initial stage encompasses the cell cycle, consisting of G1 (gap 1), S (synthesis, where DNA duplication occurs) and G2 (gap 2).
- **Prophase**: During this phase, DNA condenses into chromosomes and mitotic spindles are formed.
- **Prometaphase**: The nuclear membrane vanishes, microtubules attach centrioles to centromeres and chromosome movement commences.
- **Metaphase**: Chromosomes neatly align in the cell's centre.
- **Anaphase**: Chromosome pairs split and each sister chromatid pair moves to opposite cell ends.
- **Telophase**: Sister chromatids reach opposite cell ends and new membranes form around the nuclei of the daughter cells.
- **Cytokinesis**: Finally, the actin ring surrounding the cell's centre contracts, leading to the separation of the two daughter cells (Fig. 3.2).

Clinical Significances

- Errors during mitotic division have the potential to persist in the daughter cells.
- If these errors arise during embryonic development, they can impact a significant number of cells.
- Consequences may include conditions such as trisomy (the presence of an extra chromosome), translocation or inversion.

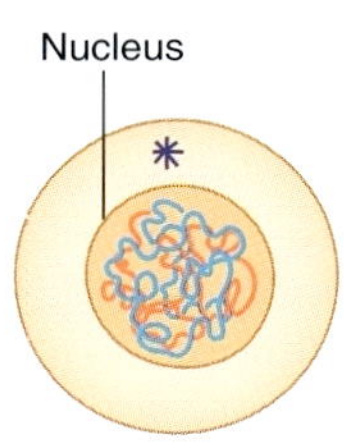

Interphase: The cell prepares for mitosis. At this stage, the chromosomes are not clearly visible.

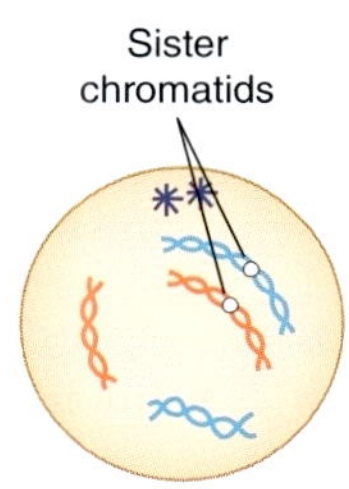

Prophase: The chromosomes, pairs of sister chromatids, condense and become visible. Meanwhile, the nucleolus and nuclear envelope disappear.

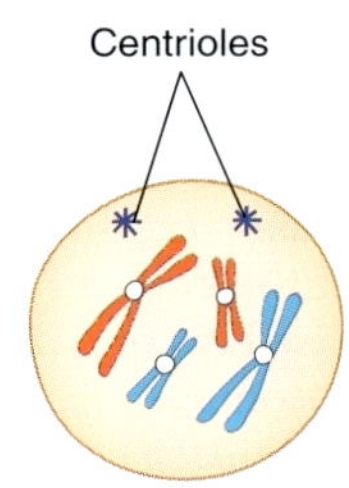

Prometaphase: The centrioles begin moving to opposite ends of the cell and start forming the mitotic spindle.

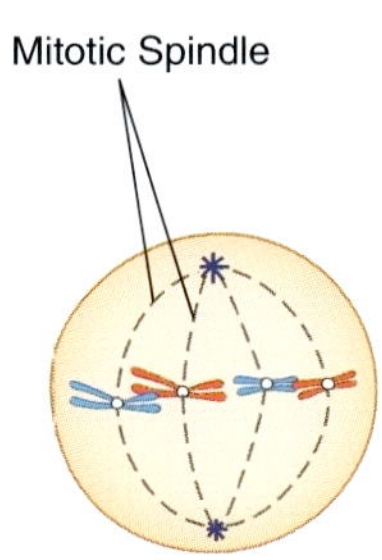

Metaphase: Spindle fibers align chromosomes at the cell's equator, also known as the metaphase plate.

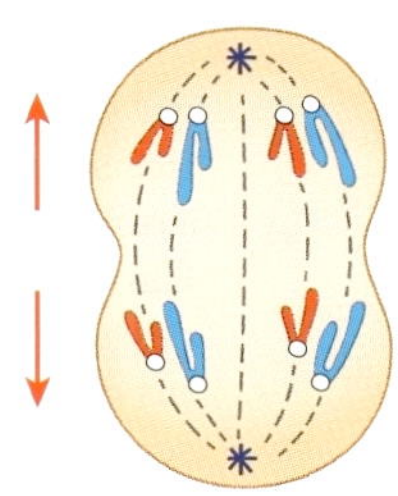

Anaphase: Sister chromatids separate and travel to opposite ends.

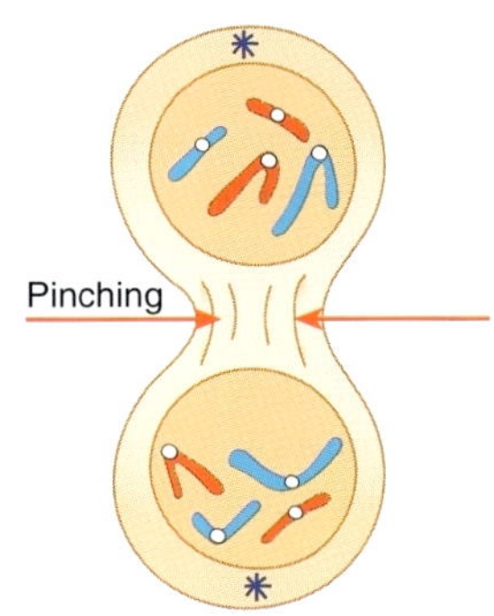

Telophase & Cytokinesis: After new nuclei are formed, the cell membrane pinches the middle of the cell, gradually dividing it into two daughter cells.

Fig. 3.2 Stages of mitosis.

MEIOSIS

- In humans, sexual reproduction involves a distinct form of cell division known as meiosis.
- Meiosis entails two consecutive divisions in a cell known as meiosis I and meiosis II, ultimately yielding four new cells.
- These daughter cells possess only half the usual number of chromosomes, making them haploid.
- The formation of haploid spermatozoa and oocytes through meiosis ensures that upon fertilization, the resulting zygote can reestablish the standard chromosome count.

Meiosis I

Meiosis I involves the following phases:

- **Interphase,** representing the standard diploid phase.
- **Prophase I,** where homologous chromosomes engage in DNA exchange.
- **Prometaphase I,** characterized by the disappearance of the nuclear membrane and the initiation of microtubule-mediated chromosome movement (diploid).
- **Metaphase I,** during which chromosomes align at the cell's midpoint (diploid).
- **Anaphase I,** as one of each pair of homologous chromosomes migrates to opposite ends of the cell (diploid).
- **Telophase I,** culminating in the formation of new membranes around the nuclei of daughter cells (diploid).
- **Cytokinesis,** where an actin ring constricts the cell's centre, resulting in division (haploid).

Following meiosis I, each cell possesses 23 chromosomes, with each chromosome consisting of two chromatids (haploid).

Homologous chromosomes, one inherited from the father and one from the mother, carry genes for the same biological traits, although these genes may exhibit slight variations. For instance, the genes responsible for iris colour represent homologous chromosomes with one encoding blue eyes and the other green eyes (comprising different alleles of the same gene).

Meiosis II

Meiosis II closely resembles mitosis.

- **Prophase II** entails the condensation of chromatids and the formation of microtubules (mitotic spindle) (haploid).
- **Prometaphase II** features the disappearance of the nuclear membrane and the initiation of microtubule-mediated chromosome movement (haploid).
- **Metaphase II** finds chromosomes arranged at the cell's midpoint (haploid).
- **Anaphase II** witnesses the separation of chromosome pairs at centromeres with each pair of sister chromatids moving to opposite ends of the cell (haploid).
- **Telophase II** marks the formation of new membranes around the new nuclei for the daughter cells (haploid).
- **Cytokinesis** involves the splitting of the cell into two (haploid).

In the end, four cells with 23 unpaired chromosomes each are produced (Fig. 3.3).

Clinical Significance

- **Genetic diversity**: During meiosis, homologous chromosomes undergo recombination (crossing over), where genetic material is exchanged between chromatids. This leads to the creation of unique combinations of genes in gametes. This genetic diversity is essential for the adaptation and evolution of species.
- **Inheritance and genetic disorders**: Errors in meiosis, such as nondisjunction, can lead to aneuploidy, where gametes have an incorrect number of chromosomes. For example, in Down syndrome, there is an extra copy of chromosome 21. Understanding meiosis is essential in diagnosing and counselling individuals with genetic disorders and in the development of prenatal genetic testing.
- **Reproductive medicine**: Assisted reproductive technologies like *in vitro* fertilization (IVF) often involve manipulating meiosis. It is crucial for clinicians to understand meiosis to ensure the successful fertilization of eggs and the production of viable embryos.
- **Cancer**: Meiosis, or errors in meiosis-like processes, can be related to cancer. Meiotic-like processes, such as chromosomal crossover and recombination, can contribute to genetic mutations that lead to the development of cancer.
- **Contraception**: Some contraceptive methods, like hormonal birth control pills, work by affecting meiosis. Understanding the mechanisms of meiosis helps in the development of effective contraceptives.

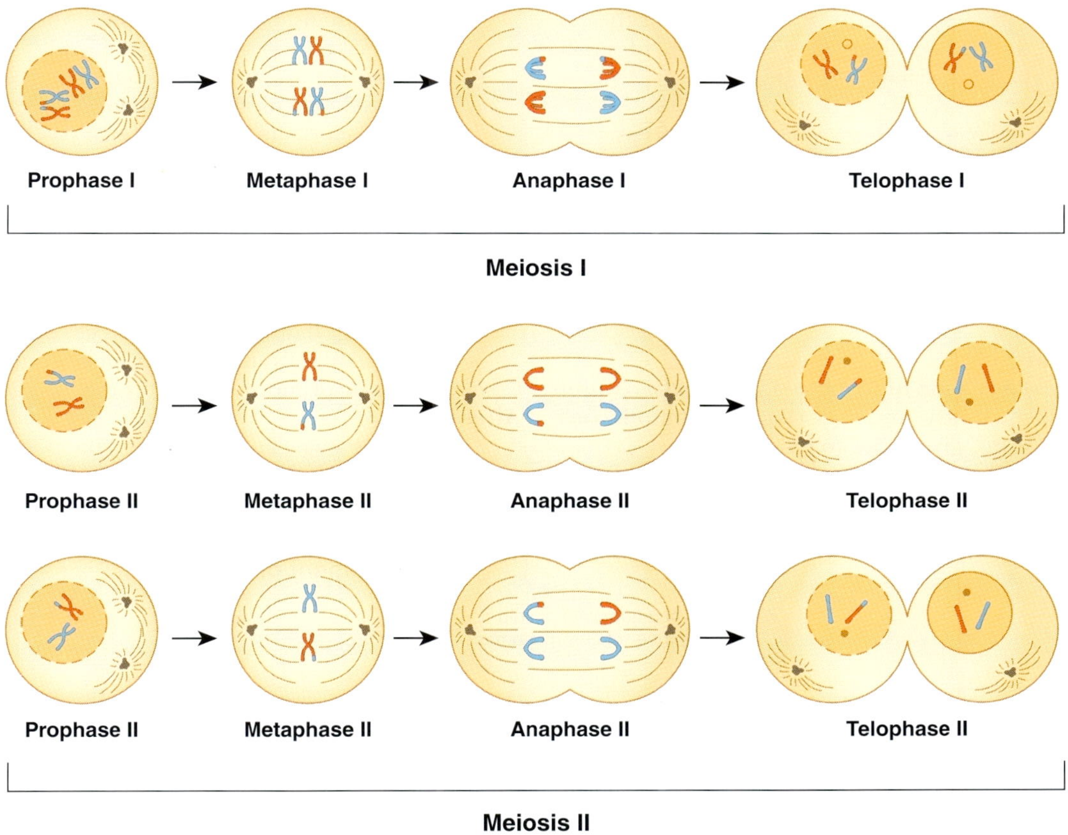

Fig. 3.3 Stages of meiosis.

GAMETOGENESIS (AN 77.3)

Gametogenesis comprises distinct phases that are critical for the development of mature gametes:

- **Formation of germ cells**: The process begins with the extraembryonic origin of germ cells and their subsequent migration into the gonads, where they will ultimately mature into gametes.
- **Proliferation of germ cells**: Germ cells undergo mitotic divisions, leading to an increase in their number. This phase ensures an ample supply of potential gametes for future reproduction.
- **Halving of chromosomes**: The key step involves the reduction of chromosomal material through meiosis, which results in the formation of haploid cells. This halving of chromosomes is crucial for maintaining the diploid number upon fertilization.
- **Maturation**: Finally, the germ cells undergo structural and functional maturation to become fully developed gametes. This phase prepares them for their role in fertilization.

  These processes result in the maturation of PGCs into mature gametes.

Gametogenesis can be categorized into two main types:

- **Oogenesis**: This is the specific process leading to the development of female gametes or ova. It occurs within the ovaries and involves unique features such as the division of cytoplasm and the formation of polar bodies.
- **Spermatogenesis**: In contrast, spermatogenesis pertains to the production of male

gametes or sperm. It takes place in the testes and results in the formation of small, highly specialized sperm cells.

OOGENESIS

Oogenesis is the process through which primordial female germ cells evolve into mature ovum (Fig. 3.4). The distinct phases involved in oogenesis are as follows.

Before birth

- **Formation of oogonia**: Initially, PGCs within the ovary undergo repetitive mitotic divisions, giving rise to oogonia.
- **Differentiation into primary oocytes**: By the end of the third month of development, the oogonia enlarge and differentiate into primary oocytes.
- **Peak oogonia count**: At the fifth month of prenatal development, the maximum number of oogonia, approximately 7 million, is reached.
- **Degeneration and formation of primary oocytes**: By the end of the seventh month, the majority of oogonia undergo degeneration. However, the surviving primary oocytes enter the prophase of the first meiotic division. During this phase, they become enveloped by a layer of flattened epithelial cells, known as follicular cells, to create primary ovarian follicles or primordial follicles (Fig. 3.5).

After birth

- **Diplotene stage**: Following birth, the primary oocytes, which have completed the **Prophase of Meiosis 1**, enter a prolonged resting phase

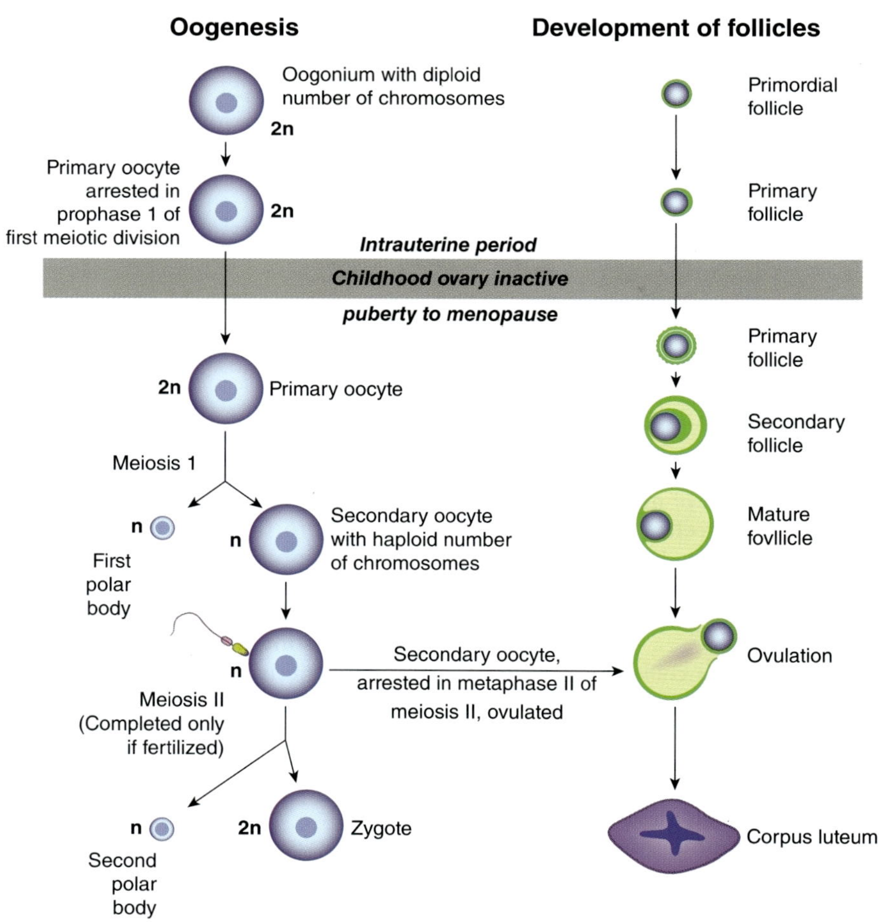

Fig. 3.4 Different stages of oocytes and follicles during oogenesis.

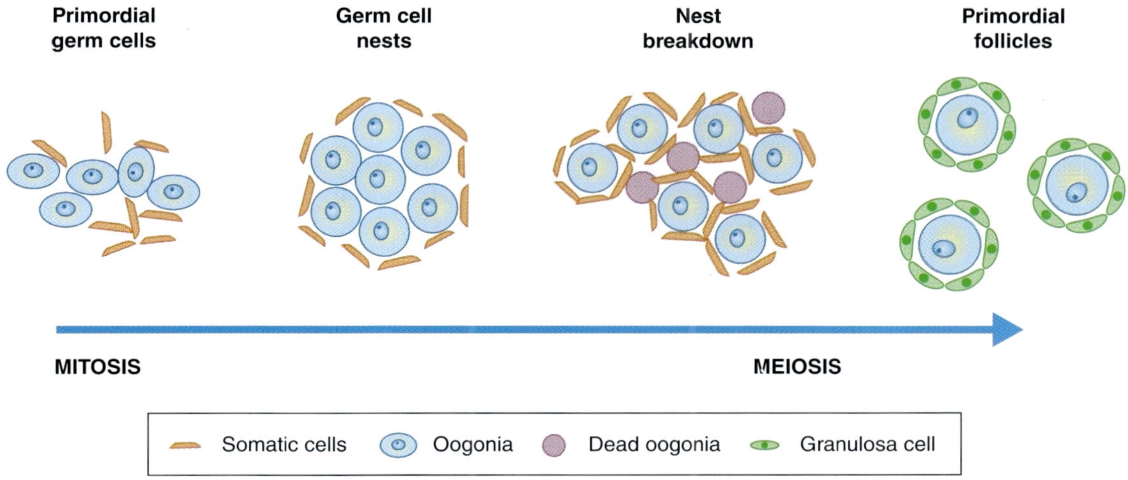

Fig. 3.5 Development of primordial follicles.

known as the dictyotene or diplotene stage, instead of progressing into metaphase.

- **Puberty and oocyte maturation inhibitor (OMI)**: This diplotene stage persists until puberty. It is upheld due to the presence of OMI secreted by the surrounding follicular cells. Throughout this phase, the oocyte accumulates cellular components and cortical granules, making preparations to meet the embryo's requirements.
- **Oocyte count**: Approximately **80,000** primary oocytes remain at birth.

Puberty

- **Ovulation and follicular changes**: At the onset of puberty, the count of oocytes is reduced to approximately **40,000** and only a small fraction, fewer than **500**, will be ovulated during the reproductive years.
- This process involves notable changes in:
  - ➤ **The follicles.**
  - ➤ **The oocyte.**

CHANGES IN THE FOLLICLE

In the course of each reproductive cycle, approximately **15 to 20 follicles** progress through a series of developmental stages: primary, secondary and tertiary follicles (Fig. 3.6).

- **Primary ovarian follicle/primordial follicle**: The primary stage features a central large cell known as the primary oocyte, encircled by a layer of flattened follicular cells.
- **Transition to primary follicle**: During maturation, the follicular cells shift from a flattened shape to a cuboidal form and multiply, creating multiple layers of cells called **Granulosa cells.** This transition marks the progression to the primary follicle.
- **Formation of zona pellucida**: In parallel, the granulosa cells and the oocyte secrete the zona pellucida, a glycoprotein layer that envelops the oocyte. This stage characterizes the **Secondary follicle.**
- **Development of theca folliculi**: Simultaneously, the ovarian tissue that surrounds the granulosa cells evolves into two distinct layers: the outer **theca externa** (a fibrous layer) and the inner **theca interna** (a glandular and vascular layer).
- **Formation of the antrum**: The follicular cells create fluid-filled spaces, which eventually merge to form a larger cavity known as the antrum, housing the follicular fluid.
- **Eccentric position of primary oocyte**: The primary oocyte, once centrally located, shifts to an eccentric position.
- **Maturity as tertiary or vesicular follicle**: This advanced stage is referred to as a vesicular or tertiary follicle.
- **Cumulus oophorus/cumulus ovaricus**: Follicular cells surrounding the oocyte project into the antral cavity, forming a structure called the cumulus oophorus or cumulus ovaricus.
- **Mature Graafian follicle**: A follicle in its mature state, containing a secondary oocyte, is known as a **Graafian follicle.**

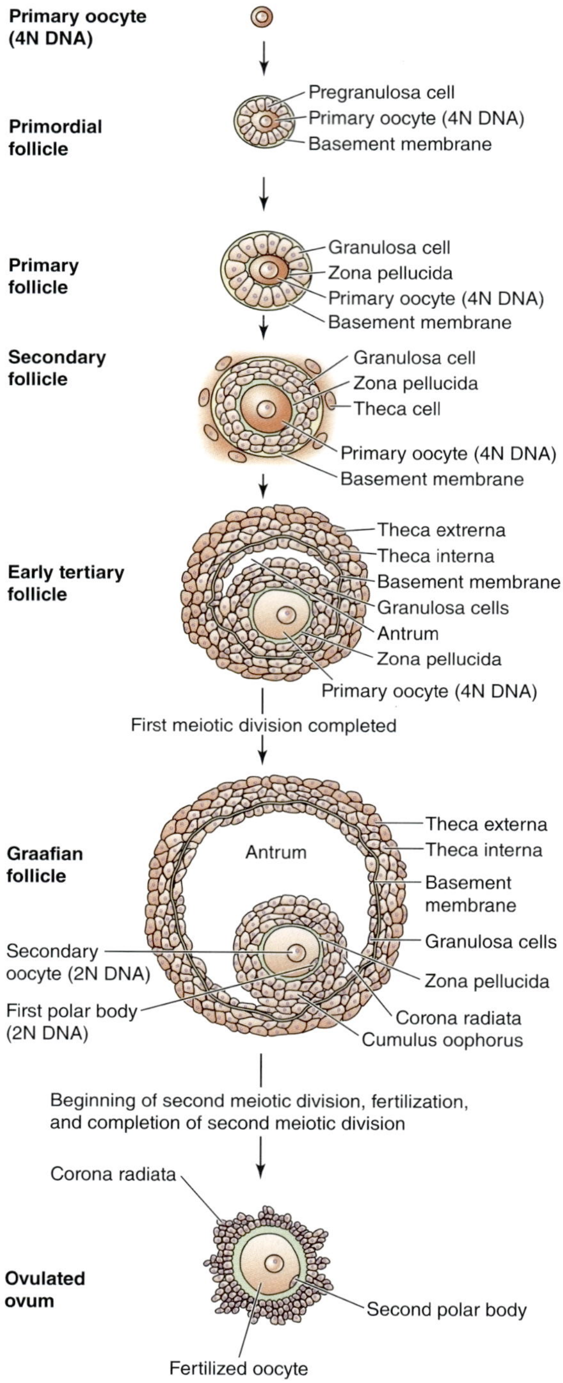

Fig. 3.6 The maturation of the ovarian follicle. (Source: Medical Physiology: A Cellular and Molecular Approach, Updated Second Edition, 2012.)

GRAAFIAN FOLLICLE

The Graafian follicle is the most advanced stage of follicular development, characterized by the following distinctive features:

- **Impressive size**: This follicle attains a considerable size, typically exceeding 25 millimetres in diameter.
- **Presence of secondary oocyte and polar body**: Within the perivitelline space, the Graafian follicle contains the secondary oocyte and the associated polar body.
- **Zona pellucida envelope**: The oocyte is enveloped by the zona pellucida, a glycoprotein layer that plays a crucial role in fertilization.
- **Distinctive cellular components**: The follicle comprises various cell types, including the membrana granulosa, cumulus oophorus, and theca externa and interna. These components collectively contribute to the mature state of the Graafian follicle (Fig. 3.7).

CHANGES IN THE OOCYTE

Primordial germ **cell** (5th week)

↓

Oogonia (44XX)

↓

Primary oocyte (44XX) (3rd month)

↓

Primary oocyte in prophase of first meiotic division

↓

At birth-diplotene/dictyotene stage (arrested prophase of first meiotic division)

↓

Before ovulation first meiotic division completes **Secondary** oocyte + first polar body (22X) (22X)

↓

Second meiotic division (arrested at metaphase of the second meiotic division, which is completed only if fertilization occurs)

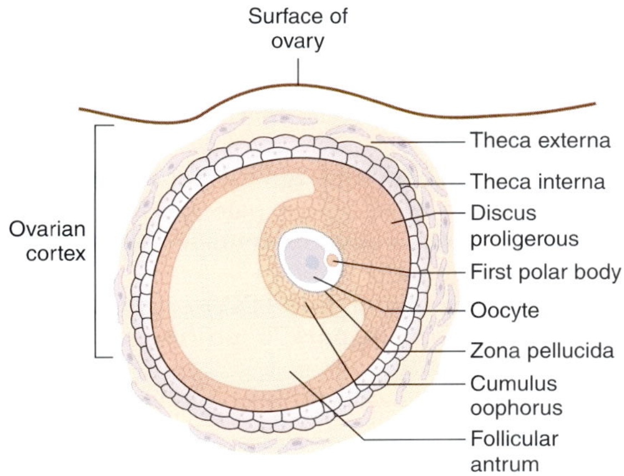

Fig. 3.7 Graafian follicle. (Source: Fundamentals of Oral Anatomy, Physiology and Histology; 2019.)

- During the fifth week of development, PGCs give rise to oogonia, each carrying 44XX chromosomes.
- In the third month of foetal development, some oogonia differentiate into primary oocytes, preserving the 44XX chromosomal composition.
- These primary oocytes advance to the prophase stage of the first meiotic division.
- At birth, many primary oocytes remain arrested in the **diplotene or dictyotene stage of prophase of the first meiotic division**.
- Only before ovulation, selected few primary oocytes restart development and complete the first meiotic division, forming a secondary oocyte and the first polar body, both with 22X chromosomes.
- Subsequently, the secondary oocyte proceeds to the second meiotic division, but it arrests at metaphase and will only complete this division if fertilization occurs.
- At the time of ovulation, the **Oocyte-cumulus complex** is released from the ruptured follicle, including the secondary oocyte arrested at metaphase, surrounded by the zona pellucida, and enveloped by two to three layers of corona radiata.
- In the event of fertilization, the result will be a mature ovum, the first polar body and the second polar body. Additionally, the first polar body may undergo a second meiotic division to produce two polar bodies.
- Notably, the secondary oocyte receives most of the cytoplasm, while the first polar body receives almost none.
- The follicular cells adjacent to the zona pellucida are referred to as **corona radiata** and they play an essential role during fertilization.
- It is important to remember that if fertilization does not occur, the secondary oocyte arrested at metaphase will degenerate over time.

CLINICAL NUGGETS

- In some cases, the **Primary oocyte** can remain arrested in meiosis I for as long as **40–50 years,** particularly if it is not yet its turn in the menstrual cycle. Consequently, **DNA damage** accumulates over time, leading to a higher prevalence of reduced fertility, especially in older women.
- Elevated levels of oestrogens and progesterone can suppress the production of **Gonadotropin-releasing hormone (GnRH)** and subsequently inhibit the release of **Luteinizing hormone (LH)** and **Follicle-stimulating hormone (FSH)**. This principle forms the basis of contraceptive pills.
- Without adequate levels of FSH, follicles will not properly develop. Similarly, the absence of an LH surge can prevent ovulation from occurring.
- Chemotherapy and radiotherapy have the potential to damage primordial ovarian follicles. Thus, it is advisable to consider oocyte **cryopreservation** prior to such treatments, as this allows for the storage of oocytes that can be used for IVF at a later time.
- **Mittelschmerz,** a German word meaning 'middle pain', refers to lower abdominal or pelvic pain that occurs typically midway between two menstrual periods. This pain often coincides with ovulation and is generally felt on one side of the lower abdomen, corresponding to the side from which the egg is released. The pain can vary in intensity and usually lasts a few hours to a couple of days. It is believed to be related to the stretching and irritation of the ovarian follicle or the surface of the ovary as the egg is released.

SPERMATOGENESIS

The process of transformation of spermatogonia into mature spermatozoa involves two major events (Fig. 3.8):

- **Spermatogenesis.**
- **Spermiogenesis.**

SPERMATOGENESIS

- Unlike oogenesis which begins before birth, spermatogenesis initiates at puberty (Table 3.1).
- At birth, germ cells in males are situated in the **sex cords of the testes**.
- All germ cells have an inherent potential to develop as oocytes, regardless of their chromosomal pattern.
- In males, the genital ridge prevents the initiation of prenatal meiosis through a **Male meiosis inhibitor** produced by Sertoli cells.
- Cells derived from the surface epithelium of the testes become **Sustentacular or Sertoli cells**.
- The sex cords later undergo canalization to form seminiferous tubules.
- PGCs undergo mitotic division to produce **Type A spermatogonia (dark type)**, which act as stem cells.
- These stem cells undergo further mitotic divisions to become **Type A pale spermatogonia**, which subsequently differentiate into **Type B spermatogonia**.
- Primary spermatocytes (44XY) originate from type B spermatogonia, a process known as **Spermatocytosis**.
- Primary spermatocytes are the **largest** spermatogenic cells.

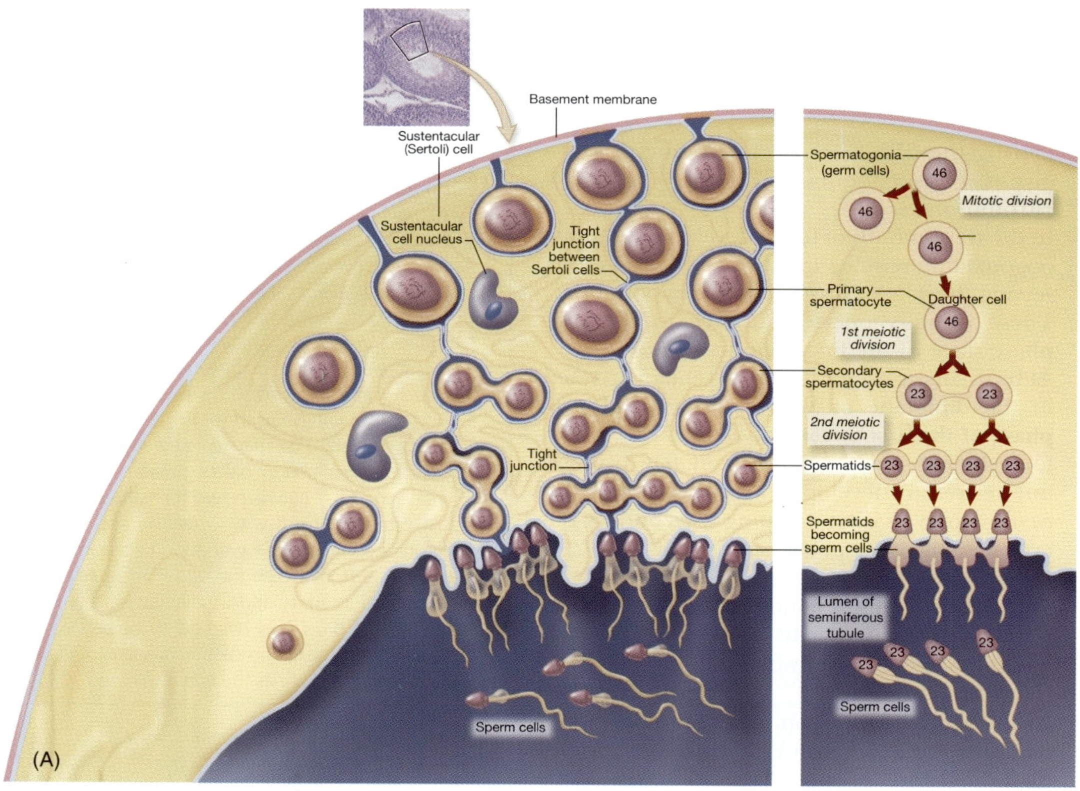

Fig. 3.8 Spermatogenesis. (A) First, spermatogonia in the outer rim of the seminiferous tubule produce daughter cells by mitotic division. These daughter cells, each with 46 chromosomes, become primary spermatocytes. A primary spermatocyte then undergoes meiotic division I to form two secondary spermatocytes, each with a haploid number of chromosomes (23). Each of the two secondary spermatocytes undergoes meiotic division II to form a total of four spermatids. Spermatids then differentiate to form heads and tails, eventually becoming mature spermatozoa, all with 23 chromosomes. Recall the role of the sustentacular cells (Sertoli cells), which support the developing male gametes structurally (by physically supporting them) and functionally (by releasing nutrients to them and by secretion of the hormone

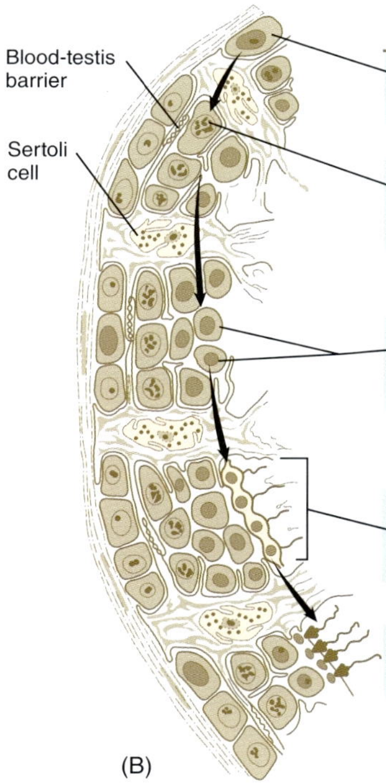

Cell types	Meiotic events	Chromosomal complement	Duration
Spermatogonium (type B)	DNA replication	**2n, 4c**	~16–18 days
Primary spermatocyte	First meiotic division in progress	**2n, 4c**	24–30 days
First meiotic division completed			
Two secondary spermatocytes	Second meiotic division in progress	**1n, 2c**	1 day
Second meiotic division completed			
Four spermatids	Immature haploid gametes	**1n, 1c**	~27 days
Spermiogenesis			
Four spermatozoa	Haploid gametes	**1n, 1c**	~2–3 weeks to attain functional maturity

Fig. 3.8, cont'd inhibin). (B) Summary of the major events in human spermatogenesis. (Source: Part A: Anatomy & Physiology. Adapted International Edition; 2019; Part B: Human Embryology and Developmental Biology. 6th ed.; 2019.)

- Primary spermatocytes then undergo the first meiotic division, producing **Secondary spermatocytes**.
- Since the first meiotic division is a reduction division, secondary spermatocytes can have two chromosomal varieties: **22 + X or 22 + Y**.
- The second meiotic division is then completed to form **haploid spermatids**.
- One primary spermatocyte yields **four spermatids**.
- Throughout this series, cytokinesis remains incomplete, ensuring that successive cell generations are interconnected by cytoplasmic bridges, allowing for synchronous development.

SPERMIOGENESIS

Spermatids are initially large, round cells with dark-stained nuclei.

- Spermiogenesis refers to the metamorphosis of spermatids into spermatozoa without further cell division. It typically involves four main phases (Figs 3.9 and 3.10):
  - **Golgi phase:** During this phase, the Golgi apparatus in the spermatid becomes prominent. The Golgi vesicles fuse to form the acrosome cap, which will later play a role in penetrating the egg during fertilization. The nucleus of the spermatid begins to condense and relocate to a position where it will become the head of the mature spermatozoon.
  - **Cap phase:** The cap, or acrosome, continues to develop over the anterior part of the nucleus. It contains enzymes that are essential for the sperm's ability to penetrate the protective layers of ovum.
  - **Acrosome phase:** In this phase, the acrosome cap is fully formed and covers the nucleus, resembling the head of the sperm. The nucleus continues to condense.

Table 3.1 Comparison of Spermatogenesis and Oogenesis

Characteristics	Spermatogenesis	Oogenesis
Occurs in	Testes of males	Ovaries of females
Timing	Begins at puberty, continues throughout life	Begins before birth, completes during reproductive years
Gamete produced	Sperm (spermatozoa)	Ova (oocyte)
Number of gametes	Many sperm produced continuously	10–15 ova produced cyclically
Chromosome reduction	Four functional sperm from one primary spermatocyte	One functional ovum from one primary oocyte
Meiotic divisions	Two meiotic divisions (meiosis I and II)	Two meiotic divisions (meiosis I and II)
Polar bodies	No polar bodies	Three polar bodies (incomplete meiosis)
Timing of meiosis	Continuous throughout life	Begins before birth and completes in cycles and second meiotic division completed after fertilization
Hormonal regulation	Influenced by testosterone, FSH and LH	Influenced by FSH, LH, oestrogen and progesterone
Gamete size	Small, highly motile sperm	Larger, nonmotile ovum
Timing of gamete maturation	Sperm are mature when produced	Ova require further maturation upon fertilization
Final functional gamete	Spermatozoa	Ovum
Cytoplasmic contents	Limited cytoplasm, mainly for motility	Abundant cytoplasm, nutrients for early embryonic development
Cellular divisions	Equal divisions in both meiotic divisions of spermatogenesis	First meiotic division produces a large secondary oocyte and a small polar body; the second meiotic division occurs only upon fertilization
Cessation of gamete production	Continues throughout a male's life	Usually ceases at menopause with no new ova produced
Chromosome constitution	23X or 23Y	23X

- **Maturation phase:** During the final phase, the sperm's tail and flagellum develop. The centrosome divides into two centrioles with the proximal centriole contributing to the formation of the axial filament in the neck and the distal centriole forming an annulus or ring at the distal end of the middle piece. The axial filament extending from the neck to the annulus is surrounded by mitochondria to form the middle piece. The remaining axial filament extends to become the main piece and endpiece of the tail. Residual bodies are formed, which contain some cytoplasm. Most of this excess cytoplasm is extruded from the spermatid and subsequently phagocytosed by Sertoli cells.

- In humans, the process from spermatogonium maturation into spermatozoa takes approximately 64–74 days, with spermiogenesis requiring about 24 days.
- The spermatozoa within the seminiferous tubules are initially nonmotile and incapable of fertilizing an egg.

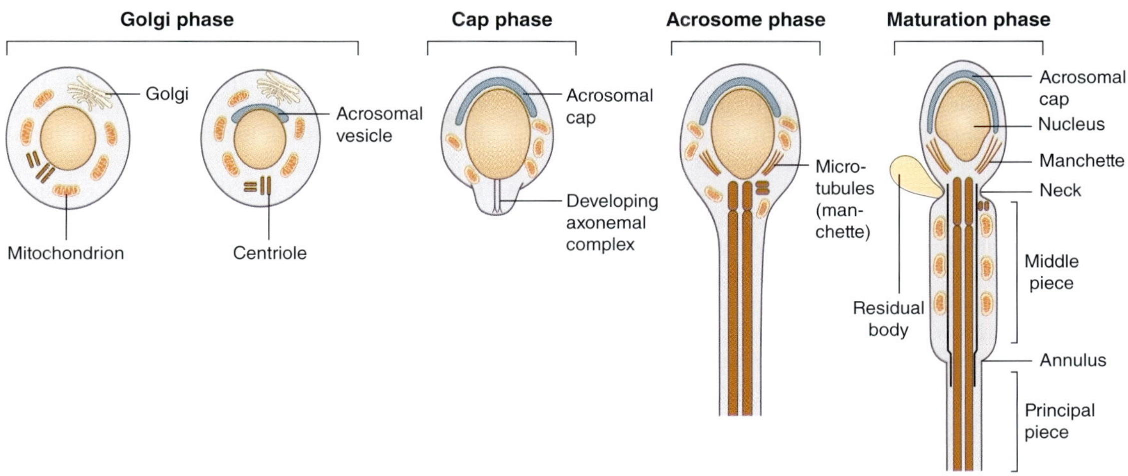

Fig. 3.9 Four phases of spermiogenesis.

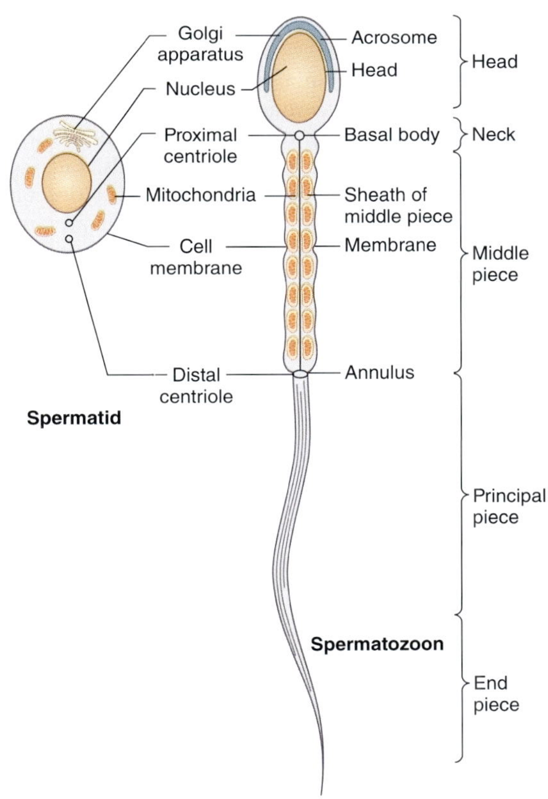

Fig. 3.10 Derivatives of spermatozoon. (Source: Part A: Stevens & Lowe's Human Histology, 4th ed.; Part B: Textbook of Clinical Embryology, 2nd ed., Fig. 3.5, page 28.)

- As spermatozoa pass through the epididymis, they undergo biochemical maturation, including glycoprotein coating and surface modifications.
- The ejaculated spermatozoa are mixed with secretions from the prostate gland and seminal vesicles, creating an environment conducive to independent motion.

CLINICAL NUGGETS

Semen analysis

- The seminal fluid is made up of secretions from the testis, epididymis, prostate and seminal vesicles.
- Seminal fluid volume is markedly reduced in incomplete collection, severe androgen deficiency, obstruction in ejaculatory ducts or bilateral absence of the vas deference.
- Reference limits for fertility: (WHO 2010 manual).
  - **Semen volume:** 1.5 mL (1.4–1.7 mL).
  - **Total sperm number:** 39 million per ejaculate (33–46 million).
  - **Sperm concentration:** 15 million per millilitre (12–16 million).
  - **Vitality:** 58% live (55%–63%).
  - Progressive motility: 32% (31%–34%).
  - Total (progressive and nonprogressive) motility: 40% (38%–42%).
- **Morphologically** normal forms: 4.0% (3.0%–4.0%).
- Spermatozoa can have abnormalities like small or piriform head, double or triple heads, acrosomal defects and double tails.

- Smoking, sexually transmitted diseases, toxins, testicular overheating and radiation affect sperm count and motility.
- **Abnormalities in sperm count**, also known as oligozoospermia or azoospermia, can impact a man's fertility. Some common abnormalities in sperm count are as follows:
  - **Oligozoospermia**: It refers to a lower than normal sperm count in the ejaculate. Typically, a sperm count of less than 15 million sperm per millilitre (mL) of semen is considered low. It can be caused by various factors, including hormonal imbalances, infections, varicoceles (enlarged veins in the testicles) and exposure to environmental toxins.
  - **Azoospermia**: It is the complete absence of sperm in the ejaculate. This can result from obstructive causes, where there is a blockage in the male reproductive tract preventing sperm from reaching the semen or nonobstructive causes, which include problems with sperm production. Nonobstructive azoospermia may be related to genetic factors, testicular injury or hormonal imbalances.
  - **Aspermia**: It is a condition in which a man does not ejaculate any semen and, consequently, there are no sperm in the ejaculate. This can be due to a variety of factors, including retrograde ejaculation (sperm entering the bladder instead of exiting the penis), nerve damage or certain medical conditions.
  - **Hypospermia**: It is characterized by a lower volume of semen during ejaculation, which can result in a lower sperm count due to a more diluted sample. This condition may be associated with dehydration or hormonal imbalances.
  - **Hyperzoospermia**: It is the opposite of oligozoospermia, where there is an abnormally high sperm count in the ejaculate. While having more sperm may sound advantageous for fertility, excessively high sperm counts can sometimes result in reduced sperm motility or other issues.
- **Asthenozoospermia:** It is characterized by reduced sperm motility, meaning that sperm have difficulty swimming effectively. This condition can make it challenging for sperm to reach and fertilize an egg.
- Abnormal spermatozoa, also known as abnormal sperm, refer to sperm cells that deviate from the normal shape, size and structure. Various types of abnormal spermatozoa include (Fig. 3.11).
  - **Teratozoospermia**: It is a condition where a significant percentage of sperm have abnormal morphology or shape. Common abnormalities include misshapen heads, tails or midsections. These morphological defects can hinder sperm's ability to penetrate and fertilize an egg.
  - **Head abnormalities:**
    - Pinhead sperm: Sperm with tiny or pointed heads.

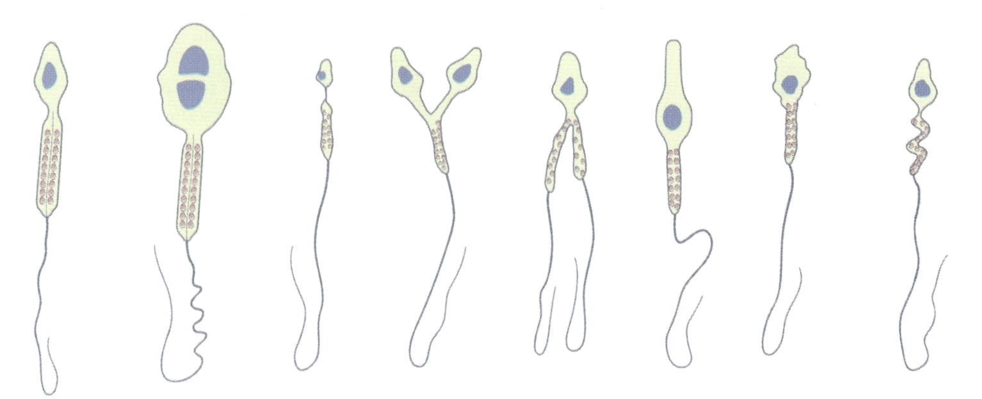

Fig. 3.11 Sperms with abnormal morphology.

- ➢ Large head sperm: Sperm with oversized heads.
- ➢ Amorphous head sperm: Sperm with irregularly shaped heads.
- **Tail abnormalities**:
  - ➢ **Short tail sperm**: Sperm with abnormally short tails, limiting their motility.
  - ➢ **Coiled-tail sperm**: Sperm with twisted or coiled tails, affecting movement.
  - ➢ **Absent Tail Sperm**: Sperm with no tail, rendering them immotile.
- **Midpiece abnormalities:**
  Midpiece defects: Issues with the central part of the sperm that contains mitochondria, affecting energy production and motility.
- **Double-headed sperm**: Sperm with two heads, which typically cannot fertilize an egg effectively.
- **Double-tailed sperm**: Sperm with two tails, reducing motility and fertilization potential.
- **Cytoplasmic droplets**: Excessive amounts of residual cytoplasm on the sperm, which can impair motility and interfere with fertilization.
- **Vacuoles**: Small cavities or irregularities in the sperm head or other regions can negatively impact sperm function.

KLINISCHE PERLEN

ABNORMALITIES IN OVULATION

It refers to irregular or disrupted patterns of ovulation, which can affect a woman's fertility and menstrual cycle. Some common abnormalities in ovulation are as follows:

- **Anovulation:** Anovulation is the absence of ovulation during the menstrual cycle. This condition is a common cause of infertility.
- **Polycystic ovary syndrome (PCOS):** PCOS is a hormonal disorder that often leads to anovulation or oligo-ovulation. Women with PCOS may have multiple small cysts on their ovaries and may experience irregular or absent periods.
- **Luteinized unruptured follicle syndrome (LUFS):** LUFS occurs when a mature egg develops in the ovary, but it does not release during ovulation. This can be challenging for women trying to conceive.
- **Premature/primary ovarian insufficiency (POI):** POI is a condition in which the ovaries stop functioning correctly before the age of 40 years. Women with POI often experience irregular periods and reduced fertility.
- **Hyperprolactinemia:** High levels of the hormone prolactin can suppress ovulation. This condition can be caused by a prolactinoma (a benign pituitary gland tumour) or certain medications.
- **Thyroid disorders:** Both hyperthyroidism and hypothyroidism can impact the menstrual cycle and ovulation.

SPONTANEOUS ABORTIONS

- Fifty percent have major chromosomal abnormalities and gene mutations. Defects in gametogenesis due to various reasons can result in spontaneous abortions:
  - **Chromosomal abnormalities:** During gametogenesis, errors can occur in the distribution of chromosomes either due to nondisjunction of autosomes or sex chromosomes during meiosis (euploid/aneuploid) or nondisjunction during mitosis (translocation, mosaicism), resulting in an abnormal number of chromosomes in the gametes. When a fertilization event involves a gamete with chromosomal abnormalities, it can result in an embryo with too many or too few chromosomes. Most of these embryos are not viable and often lead to spontaneous abortions. Turner syndrome (Fig. 3.12) is one of the most common genetic disorders characterized by short stature, gonadal dysgenesis, cardiac defects, renal defects, webbed neck, low-set ears and skeletal deformities including cubitus valgus, a propensity to ear infections and hearing deficits.
  - **Genetic mutations:** Genetic mutations that affect the genes involved in gametogenesis or early embryo development can lead to miscarriages. These mutations may impact the proper development of the embryo.
  - **Hormonal imbalances:** Hormonal imbalances during gametogenesis can disrupt the normal maturation of gametes. For example, in women, problems with ovulation or hormonal imbalances can result in the release of immature eggs, making successful

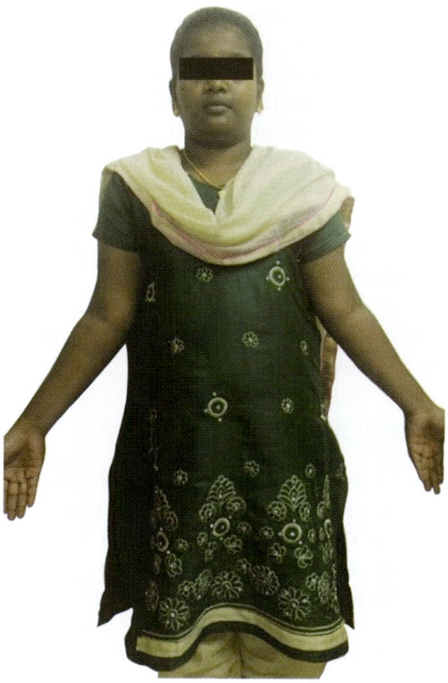

Fig. 3.12 A girl with Turner syndrome having short neck, short stature and cubitus valgus. (Source: Photo courtesy: Dr. Suja.)

fertilization less likely and increasing the risk of miscarriage.

- **Environmental factors:** Exposure to environmental toxins, radiation or certain medications during gametogenesis can damage the DNA of gametes and lead to developmental abnormalities in the embryo, potentially resulting in miscarriage.
- **Structural abnormalities:** In some cases, structural defects in the reproductive organs can affect gametogenesis. These may include abnormalities in the fallopian tubes, uterus or testes, which can hinder fertilization or the implantation of the embryo.

TERATOMAS

- Teratomas are diverse tumours characterized by a mixture of mature and immature cells or tissues originating from one or more of the three PGC layers. They typically arise from **Pluripotent stem cells, PGCs or the Epiblast**, which are capable of differentiating into various tissue types. Hence, they contain bone, teeth, skin, gastrointestinal components, etc.
- These tumours often occur in gonadal regions but can also be found in midline or paraxial locations throughout the body.
- Teratomas are commonly categorized based on their site of origin, distinguishing between intragonadal (occurring within the ovaries or testes) and extragonadal (developing outside these primary sites, such as sacrococcygeal, mediastinal, retroperitoneal or nasopharyngeal teratomas) (Fig. 3.13).
- Teratomas can be histologically classified into three main types:
  - **Mature teratoma:** Comprising well-differentiated, noncancerous tissues resembling normal mature cells and they are commonly seen in gonads, for example, dermoid cyst of ovary.
  - **Immature teratoma:** Comprising poorly differentiated or embryonic-like tissues that may lack the structural organization of mature tissues. They are more likely to be malignant compared to mature teratomas.
  - **Teratoma with a malignant component:** Combining teratomatous elements with a malignant component, such as a germ cell tumour or another aggressive neoplasm.

POINTS TO PONDER

- **PGCs** originating in the yolk sac migrate through the dorsal mesentery to reach the developing gonads.
- **Oogonia** experience mitotic activity during the prenatal period, while **spermatogonia** continue mitosis throughout an individual's life.
- **Oocytes** encounter **two meiotic blocks** during their development, one in diplotene of prophase I and the other in metaphase II.
- **Meiosis** initiates in females during the fifth month of intrauterine life, while in males, it begins at puberty.
- Hormones produced by the pituitary gland, such as **FSH and LH**, stimulate follicular cells to secrete oestrogen and progesterone.
- With hormonal influence, selected follicles grow in size each month, ultimately leading to the ovulation of one dominant follicle in females.
- Spermatogenesis occurs in the **testes,** while functional maturation of spermatozoa takes place in the **epididymis.**
- In males, **Leydig cells** respond to LH stimulation by producing testosterone and **Sertoli cells** support spermatogenesis under the influence of FSH.

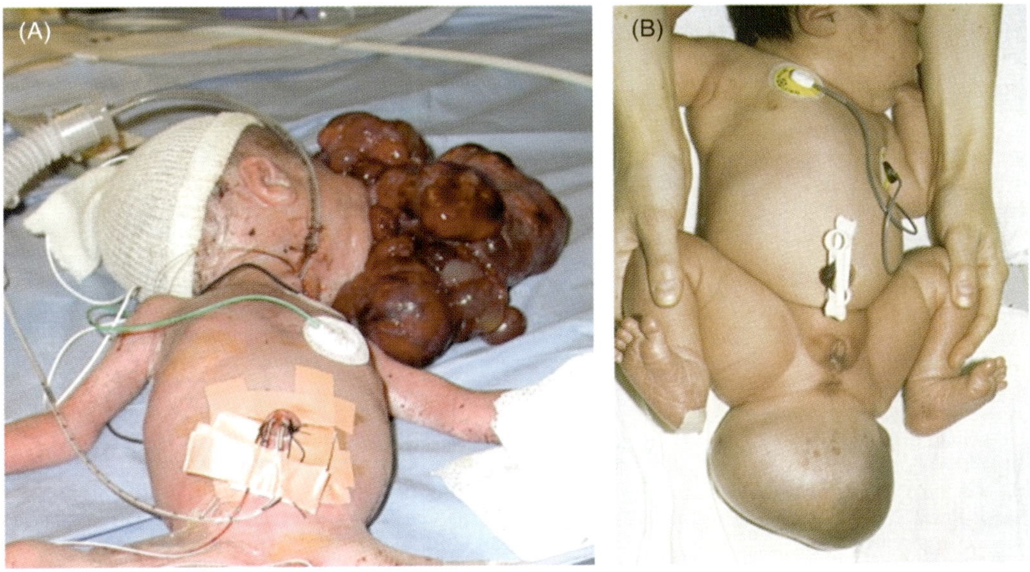

Fig. 3.13 (A) **Oropharyngeal teratoma:** Newborn with a massive oropharyngeal cervical teratoma immediately after ex utero intrapartum treatment (EXIT procedure) was performed to secure the airway. Immediate resection of the teratoma followed in an adjacent operating room. (B) **Sacrococcygeal teratoma:** A female infant with a large sacrococcygeal teratoma that developed from remnants of the primitive streak. (Source: Part A: A Practice of Anesthesia for Infants and Children. 4th ed.; 2009; Part B: Before We Are Born: Essentials of Embryology and Birth Defects. First South Asia Edition; 2016.)

BRAIN TEASERS

1. What is the initial event in gametogenesis that involves the extraembryonic origin of germ cells?
   A. Proliferation of germ cells
   B. Formation of oogonia
   C. Formation of mature gametes
   D. Migration into the gonads
2. What is the specific process leading to the development of female gametes?
   A. Spermatogenesis
   B. Ovulation
   C. Oogenesis
   D. Mitosis
3. At what stage does the majority of oogonia undergo degeneration in Oogenesis?
   A. Before birth
   B. Puberty
   C. After birth
   D. During the diplotene stage
4. What is the role of the acrosome in spermiogenesis?
   A. It forms the neck of the sperm
   B. It contains enzymes for penetrating the egg
   C. It produces cytoplasmic bridges
   D. It covers the tail
5. What is the main function of the zona pellucida in the Graafian follicle?
   A. Protection of oocyte and a role in fertilisation
   B. Formation of the antrum
   C. Synthesis of hormones
   D. Attachment to the follicular cells
6. When does spermatogenesis initiate?
   A. Before birth
   B. At puberty
   C. After puberty
   D. During embryonic development
7. What is the final product of primary spermatocytes after the second meiotic division?
   A. Spermatids
   B. Spermatozoa
   C. Secondary spermatocytes
   D. Sertoli cells
8. What is the approximate duration of spermiogenesis in humans?
   A. 10-20 days
   B. 24 days
   C. 40-50 days
   D. 60-70 days

9. What is the function of residual bodies in spermatogenesis?
   A. Formation of spermatozoa
   B. Extrusion of excess cytoplasm
   C. Maturation of spermatids
   D. Production of hormones
10. Which clinical condition is characterized by the complete absence of sperm in the ejaculate?
   A. Oligozoospermia
   B. Hyperzoospermia
   C. Aspermia
   D. Hypospermia
11. What does teratozoospermia refer to in the context of spermatogenesis abnormalities?
   A. Abnormal sperm morphology
   B. Reduced sperm motility
   C. Increased sperm count
   D. Absence of sperm
12. What is the primary function of the acrosome in spermiogenesis?
   A. Energy production
   B. Motility
   C. Penetration of the egg
   D. Formation of the tail
13. Which event occurs during the Cap Phase of spermiogenesis?
   A. Formation of the acrosome cap
   B. Development of the tail
   C. Maturation of spermatozoa
   D. Division of centrosome
14. What is the role of the epididymis in sperm maturation?
   A. Initial sperm production
   B. Biochemical maturation
   C. Spermatocytosis
   D. Spermiogenesis
15. What happens if fertilization does not occur after the completion of the second meiotic division in oogenesis?
   A. Formation of secondary polar bodies
   B. Degeneration of the secondary oocyte
   C. Ovulation
   D. Activation of Oocyte Maturation Inhibitor (OMI)
16. Which type of cells contribute to the mature state of the Graafian follicle?
   A. Leydig cells
   B. Sertoli cells
   C. Cumulus oophorus
   D. Primordial germ cells

Answers

1. (D); 2. (C); 3. (A); 4. (B); 5. (A); 6. (B); 7. (A); 8. (B); 9. (B); 10. (C); 11. (A); 12. (C); 13. (A); 14. (B); 15. (B); 16 (C).

FURTHER READINGS

Kocaoğlu Ç. Two sisters with Angelman syndrome: a case series report. *J Pediatr Neurosci.* 2017;12(4): 383-385. doi:10.4103/jpn.JPN_55_17.

Kumar V, Abbas AK, Aster JC. *Robbins & Cotran Pathologic Basis of Disease.*

Kurman RJ, et al. *WHO Classification of Tumours of Female Reproductive Organs: World Health Organization Classification of Tumours series.*

Scully RE. *Tumors of the Ovary, Maldeveloped Gonads, Fallopian Tube, and Broad Ligament (Atlas of Tumor Pathology series).*

Song KU, Nam OH, Kim MS, Choi SC, Lee HS. An 18-year-old patient with Prader-Willi syndrome: a case report on dental management under sedation and general anesthesia. *J Dent Anesth Pain Med.* 2015;15(4): 251-255. doi:10.17245/jdapm.2015.15.4.251.

Varma AV, Malpani G, Agrawal P, Malukani K, Dosi S. Clinicopathological spectrum of teratomas: an 8-year retrospective study from a tertiary care institute. *Indian J Cancer.* 2017;54:576-579.

4 Female Reproductive Cycles

AN 77.1 Describe the uterine changes occurring during the menstrual cycle.
AN 77.2 Describe the synchrony between the ovarian and menstrual cycles.

ANAMNESE

A 35-year-old woman was perplexed by her sudden weight gain, irregular menstrual cycles and difficulty conceiving. Concerned about her fertility, she sought medical advice. After a thorough evaluation of her menstrual history, it was discovered that she had been experiencing irregular periods for over a year. Further tests revealed elevated levels of certain hormones. The diagnosis was polycystic ovary syndrome (PCOS), a condition affecting the ovaries and menstrual cycle. Understanding, the connection between her menstrual irregularities and PCOS was pivotal. With treatment and lifestyle adjustments aimed at regulating her cycle, she was not only able to shed the extra weight but also successfully conceived.

Hormonal interaction between the hypothalamus, anterior pituitary and ovaries regulates the female reproductive system. The hypothalamus secretes gonadotropin-releasing hormone (GnRH). GnRH regulates release of luteinizing hormone (LH) and follicle-stimulating hormone (FSH) from specialized cells in the anterior pituitary as short bursts every 1–4 hours. LH and FSH promote ovulation and stimulate secretion of the sex hormones oestrogen and progesterone from the ovaries. They stimulate the target organs of the reproductive system (e.g. breasts, uterus and vagina). The menstrual cycle consists of 28 days (21–35 days). The length of the cycle decreases with advancing age and about 7% of menstrual cycles are shorter than 26 days. In an infertility setting, 5.4% of menstrual cycles are 35 days or longer.

UTERUS

- Uterus is a pear-shaped muscular organ consisting of a body and cervix.
- The walls of the body are made up of 3 layers:
  - **Endometrium**: Thin inner layer.
  - **Myometrium**: Thick layer made of smooth muscle.
  - **Perimetrium**: Thin external layer.
- Endometrium consists of three layers:
  - **Stratum compactum.**
  - **Stratum spongiosum.**
  - **Stratum basale.**
- Stratum compactum and spongiosum are known together as **functional layer** which will be shed during menstruation and after delivery (Fig. 4.1).

UTERINE TUBES

- They are two in number and attached to the horns of the uterus and distal end opens into the peritoneal cavity.
- It has got four parts:
  - **Interstitial/uterine part.**
  - **Isthmus.**

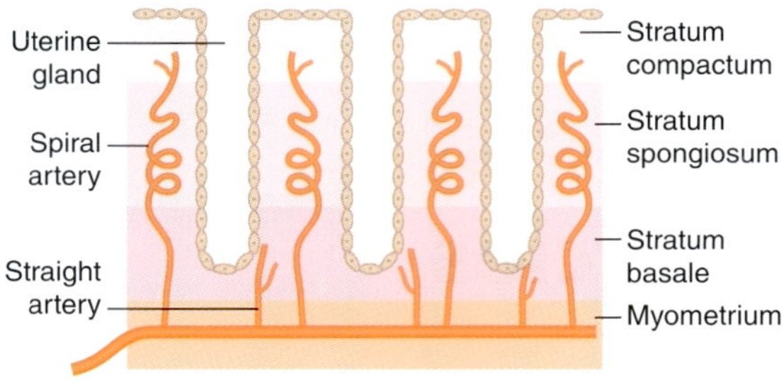

Fig. 4.1 Layers of uterine wall.

   - **Ampulla.**
   - **Infundibulum.**
- Fertilization occurs at the **ampulla** (Fig. 4.2).
- The cleaving zygote is carried to the uterine cavity by the ciliated epithelium lining the uterine tube.

OVARIES

- Ovaries are paired, almond-shaped reproductive glands responsible for producing oocytes.
- They are securely positioned near the pelvic brim, suspended by a specialized peritoneal fold known as the suspensory ligament of the ovary.
- The upper end of each ovary is linked to the ovarian fimbria of the uterine tube, facilitating the capture of released ova during ovulation.
- The lower end is anchored to the cornua of the uterus by the ligament of the ovary, ensuring stability and proper positioning (Fig. 4.2).

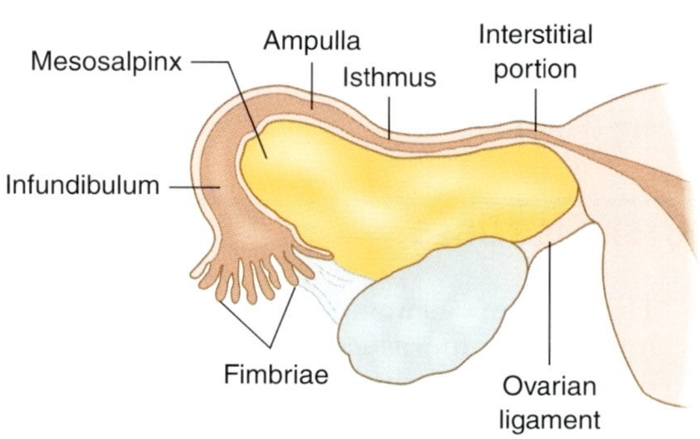

Fig. 4.2 Parts of uterine tube.

- Resting within a peritoneal depression, referred to as the ovarian fossa, situated along the lateral pelvic wall, the ovaries are well protected for their vital reproductive functions.

FEMALE REPRODUCTIVE CYCLES

Females experience monthly reproductive cycles, typically beginning at puberty between the ages of 10–13 years. These cycles are often referred to as reproductive or sexual cycles.

- The initial onset of menstruation is known as menarche, marking the commencement of the reproductive phase in a woman's life.
- Coordinated activities involving the hypothalamus in the brain, the pituitary gland, the ovaries, the uterus, uterine tubes, vagina and mammary glands collectively prepare the female reproductive system for potential pregnancy.
- Within this process, the cyclical changes occurring in the ovaries are referred to as the ovarian cycle, while the changes taking place in the uterus are recognized as the menstrual cycle. These cycles work together to regulate and maintain the female reproductive system.

OVARIAN CYCLE

The ovarian cycle consists of the recurring processes within the ovary, including the development of ovarian follicles, ovulation and the formation of the corpus luteum (Fig. 4.3).

- This cycle typically continues throughout a woman's reproductive years, with the exception of pregnancy, and naturally concludes at menopause.
- FSH and LH play pivotal roles in driving these cyclical changes in the ovary as well as influencing the growth of the endometrium.
- **FSH** is responsible for the growth of ovarian follicles, which, in turn, secrete oestrogen, leading to several significant effects:
   - Development of secondary sexual characteristics.
   - Proliferation of the endometrium prior to ovulation.
   - Feedback inhibition of FSH.
   - Stimulation of **LH** secretion.

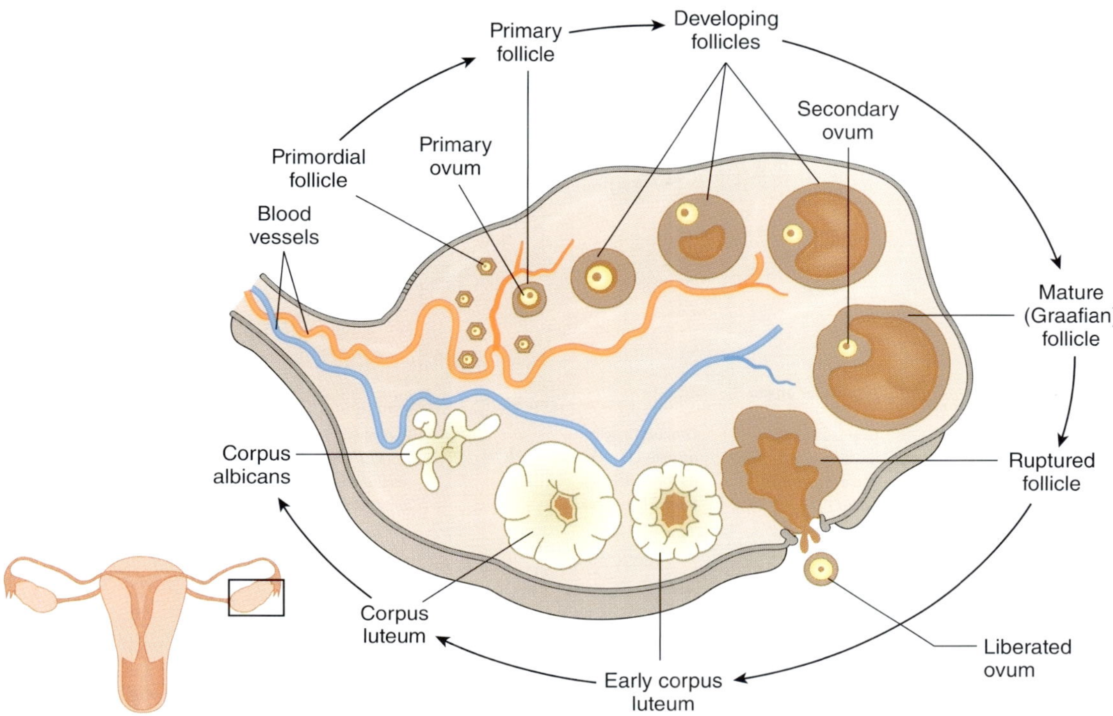

Fig. 4.3 Ovary showing different stages of follicle. Sagittal section of the ovary, showing follicles in different stages of development.

- LH then takes the stage by inducing ovulation and promoting the formation of the corpus luteum, which, in return, secretes progesterone, resulting in effects such as:
  - ➢ Preparing the uterus to receive a fertilized ovum by stimulating the secretory phase.
  - ➢ Preventing the expulsion of the ovum by reducing uterine muscle contractions.
  - ➢ Inhibiting FSH and, consequently, the maturation of follicles during corpus luteum formation.
- This complex hormonal process involves FSH stimulating LH production through oestrogen, while LH counters FSH through the mediation of progesterone.
- The ovarian cycle is divided into two main phases (Fig. 4.4):
  1. **Follicular phase:**
     During the follicular phase, ovarian follicles develop and release a single mature oocyte.
     The developing oocyte secretes oestrogen, which instigates changes in the endometrial lining of the uterus, corresponding to the first half of the menstrual cycle.
  2. **Luteal phase:**
     In the luteal phase, the corpus luteum is formed. The corpus luteum secretes progesterone, which induces changes in the endometrial lining, corresponding to the second half of the menstrual cycle.

Follicular Phase

The process of follicular development includes the following key steps (Fig. 4.3):

i. **Growth and differentiation of primary oocyte:**
Primary oocytes within the follicles undergo growth and differentiation.

ii. **Proliferation of follicular cells:**
Follicular cells surrounding the oocyte proliferate, providing support and nourishment.

iii. **Formation of zona pellucida:**
The protective layer known as the zona pellucida forms around the oocyte.

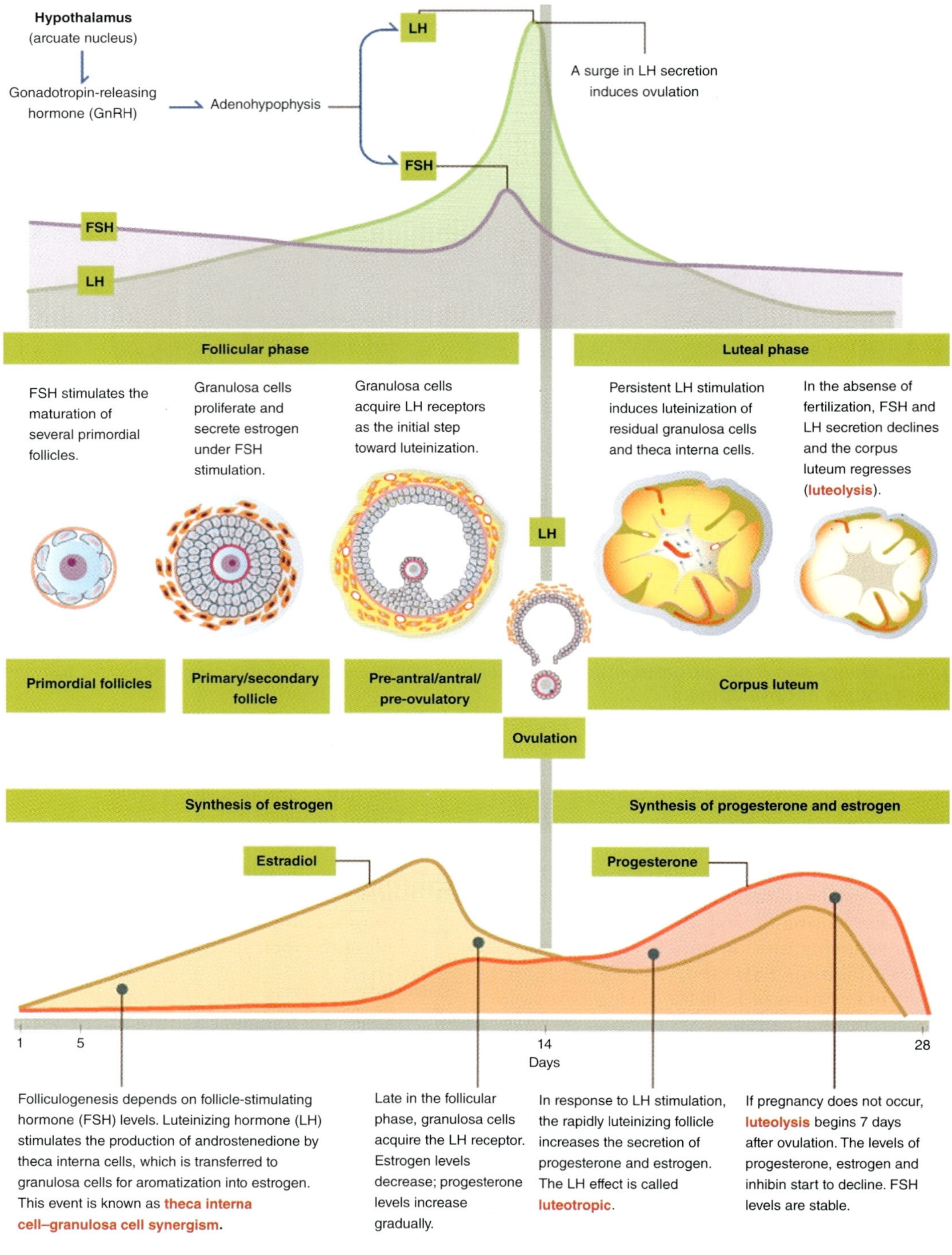

Fig. 4.4 Ovarian cycle and the effects of hormones. (Source: Histology and Cell Biology: An Introduction to Pathology. 5th ed., 2019.)

iv. **Development of theca folliculi:**
The theca folliculi, a vital component of the follicle, undergoes development.

Stimulation of primary follicles:
In each ovarian cycle, approximately 15–20 primary follicles, derived from primordial follicles (containing an oocyte surrounded by a layer of flattened granulosa cells), are stimulated by FSH.

Oocyte discharge and atresia:
Only one oocyte is released from a follicle during ovulation, while the rest of the follicles degenerate and become atretic, forming corpus atreticum.

Antral/vesicular/secondary follicle:
A primary follicle with an antrum and liquor folliculi is referred to as an antral, vesicular or secondary follicle.

Graafian/mature vesicular follicle:
The secondary follicle with its theca layer organized into outer theca externa and inner theca interna is known as the Graafian or mature vesicular follicle.

Theca interna and externa:
The theca interna which is vascular is responsible for producing follicular fluid and some oestrogen, while the theca externa mainly consists of fibroblasts and macrophages.

Meiosis I and formation of secondary oocyte:
Meiosis I is completed within the Graafian follicle, resulting in the formation of a secondary oocyte.

First polar body:
The first polar body is situated between the zona pellucida and the cell membrane of the oocyte in the perivitelline space.

Meiosis II and arrest before ovulation:
Meiosis II is initiated but the oocyte is arrested in metaphase approximately 3 hours before ovulation.

Ovulation:
Ovulation is initiated by an increased level of prostaglandins in response to a surge in LH. This surge triggers local muscular contractions in the ovarian wall, expelling the mature oocyte, which subsequently floats within the peritoneal cavity.

Secondary oocyte release:
The secondary oocyte released during ovulation is enclosed by the zona pellucida and corona radiata with follicular cells arranged radially around it.

Mittelschmerz:
Mittelschmerz, a term of German origin meaning 'middle pain', refers to the discomfort or pain experienced by some women during ovulation. It typically occurs near the middle of the menstrual cycle.

Anovulation:
Anovulation is characterized by the absence of ovulation in the context of the menstrual cycle.

Luteal Phase

During the luteal phase of the ovarian cycle, several important processes occur (Fig. 4.4).

Formation of corpus luteum:
Following ovulation and under the influence of LH, granulosa cells and theca interna cells undergo changes, turning into lutein cells. These lutein cells collectively form the corpus luteum (Fig. 4.3).

Hormone secretion by corpus luteum:
The corpus luteum plays a crucial role by secreting both oestrogen and progesterone. These hormones prepare the uterine endometrium for potential embryo implantation.

Corpus albicans formation:
If fertilization does not occur, the corpus luteum gradually shrinks due to the degeneration of its luteal cells. It transforms into a fibrotic scar tissue known as the corpus albicans (Fig. 4.3).

Progesterone decline and menstrual bleeding:
As the corpus luteum degenerates, the production of progesterone decreases. This hormonal shift triggers menstrual bleeding.

Corpus luteum of pregnancy:
In the case of successful fertilization, the corpus luteum enlarges to become the 'corpus luteum of pregnancy'. It remains active throughout the first 20 weeks of pregnancy, supporting increased progesterone production.

Prevention of corpus luteum degeneration:
Human chorionic gonadotropin (hCG), a hormone secreted by the syncytiotrophoblast of the blastocyst, prevents the degeneration of the corpus luteum during early pregnancy.

Placental hormone production:
Later in pregnancy, the placenta takes over the role of producing oestrogen and progesterone, which are necessary for the maintenance of the pregnancy.

Abortion risk:

If the corpus luteum of pregnancy is prematurely removed before the fourth month of pregnancy, it can result in abortion or miscarriage.

Menopause and climacteric:

Ovarian cycles naturally terminate at menopause, typically occurring between the ages of 48 and 55 years. The climacteric phase refers to the overall changes that occur at the end of the reproductive period and signifies the permanent cessation of menstrual periods (menopause).

MENSTRUAL CYCLE (AN 77.1)

- Uterus (endometrium) receives and maintains the embryo during pregnancy and expels (contraction of myometrium) the foetus at the termination of pregnancy.
- The endometrium changes daily throughout the menstrual cycle.
- **Endometrial structure:**
  The endometrium comprises two distinct layers:
  - ➢ **Functional layer:**
    This layer is regularly shed during each menstrual period or after childbirth.
  - ➢ **Basal layer:**
    The basal layer remains intact and provides the foundation for endometrial regeneration.
- **Endometrial composition:**
  The endometrium is composed of several key elements:
  - ➢ **Columnar epithelium:** Forms the lining of the endometrial surface.
  - ➢ **Uterine glands:** Glands within the endometrium that contribute to the secretion of various substances.
  - ➢ **Specialized connective tissue stroma:** Provides structural support within the endometrium.
  - ➢ **Spiral arteries:** These arteries originate from the basal layer and extend towards the surface of the endometrium.
- **Endometrial/menstrual cycle:** The cyclical changes in the uterine endometrium that occur during the reproductive years are referred to as the endometrial or menstrual cycle.
- **Hormonal control:** The ovarian hormones, oestrogen and progesterone secreted by ovarian follicles and the corpus luteum regulate these cyclical changes.
- **Cycle phases:** The endometrial cycle commences with oocyte maturation, extending until the oocyte enters the uterine tube.
- **Cycle duration:** Typically, each menstrual cycle lasts around 28 days with day 1 designated as the day when menstrual flow begins.

HORMONAL CONTROL OF MENSTRUAL CYCLE

The menstrual cycle is controlled by the hormones secreted by hypothalamus, adenohypophysis and ovary as follows:

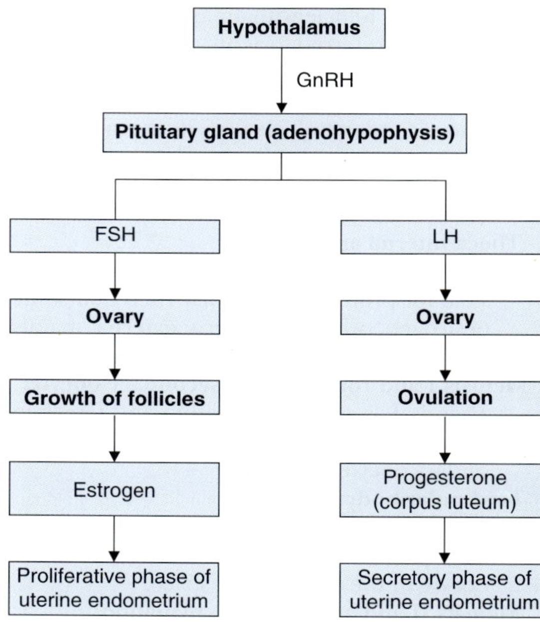

The process of ovarian follicle maturation is regulated by both FSH and LH. LH, in particular, triggers ovulation and also plays a role in promoting the development of the corpus luteum and the proliferation of ovarian follicles.

PHASES OF THE MENSTRUAL CYCLE

The menstrual cycle is divided into four distinct phases based on changes in the endometrium (Fig. 4.5).

1. **Menstrual phase (days 1–4):**
   - ▪ This phase is characterized by the shedding of the functional layer of the uterine endometrium, resulting in menstrual bleeding.

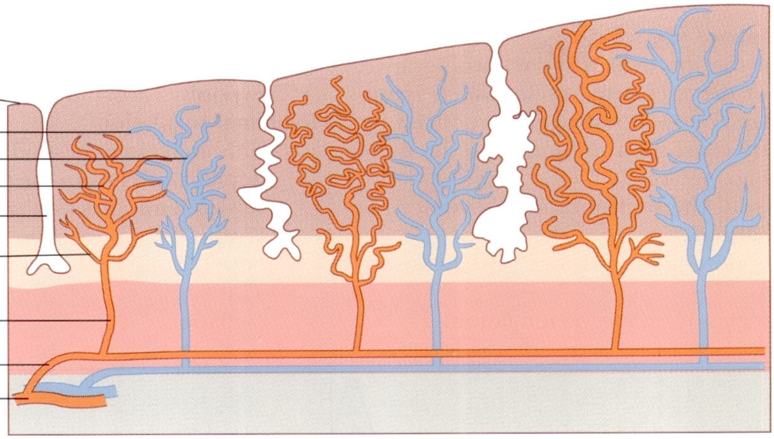

Fig. 4.5 Endometrial changes in menstrual cycle.

- In the absence of fertilization, the corpus luteum degenerates, leading to a decline in progesterone levels.
- The reduced progesterone levels cause spasms in the coiled endometrial arteries, reducing blood supply to the functional layer.
- The functional layer is subsequently sloughed off, while the basal layer remains intact.

2. **Proliferative phase/follicular phase (days 5–14):**
   - During this phase, the functional layer of the endometrium regenerates.
   - The growth of ovarian follicles coincides with this phase and is controlled by the oestrogen secreted by the developing follicles.
   - The endometrial thickness increases two to threefold.
   - Spiral arteries elongate and the number of glands increases.
3. **Secretory phase/luteal phase (days 15–25):**
   - The secretory activity of endometrial glands intensifies, resulting in a thickening and softening of the endometrium.
   - Progesterone is primarily secreted by the corpus luteum during this phase.
   - Spiral arteries, as they penetrate the stratum compactum, become increasingly coiled.
   - The formation of large venous spaces and arteriovenous anastomosis occurs.
4. **Premenstrual phase (days 26–28):**
   Reduced blood supply to the endometrium during this phase leads to ischemia, causing spasmodic pain and spotting of blood.

CLINICAL NUGGETS

Hormonal regulation of reproduction and mammary glands

1. **Anterior pituitary hormones:**
   - In the absence of inhibitory signals, particularly dopamine from the hypothalamus, the anterior pituitary gland produces multiple hormones, including **FSH, LH and prolactin.**
   - Prolactin has a significant role and primarily acts on the mammary glands.
2. **Posterior pituitary hormone:**
   - The posterior pituitary gland releases only one hormone directly involved in reproductive processes: oxytocin.
   - **Oxytocin** plays key roles in childbirth by promoting uterine contractions and in milk ejection (let-down) from the mammary glands during breastfeeding.

SYNCHRONY BETWEEN THE OVARIAN AND MENSTRUAL CYCLE (AN 77.2)

It refers to the coordination between two key processes in the female reproductive system: the ovarian cycle and the menstrual cycle. These cycles are closely interconnected and their timing and hormonal changes are synchronized to facilitate various reproductive events, including ovulation and the preparation of the uterine lining for possible pregnancy (Fig. 4.6).

Proliferative phase (days 5–14):

- During the preovulatory or proliferative phase of the menstrual cycle, which spans from days 5 to 14, oestrogens produced by the ovary exert their influence on the uterine lining.
- As a result, the uterine lining becomes re-epithelialized.
- The endometrial stroma progressively thickens.
- Uterine glands undergo elongation.
- Spiral arteries start to extend towards the surface of the endometrium.
- In the late proliferative phase, elevated levels of oestradiol secreted by the developing ovarian follicle act on the hypothalamo-hypophyseal system.

Hormonal regulation:

- This increase in oestradiol triggers the secretion of GnRH from the hypothalamus, which subsequently acts on the pituitary gland.
- Within 24 hours, a preovulatory surge of both LH and FSH is released into circulation.
- The surge of LH is critical for triggering ovulation.

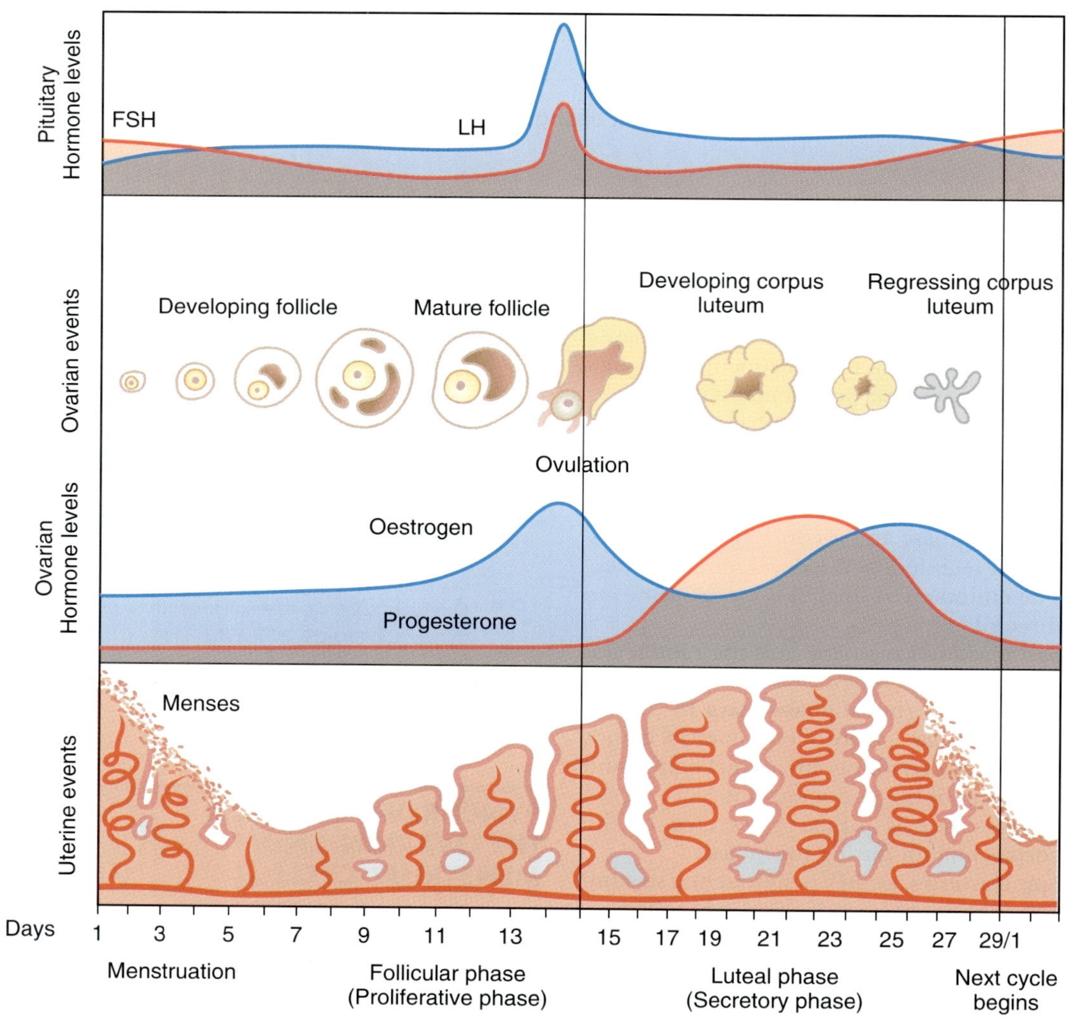

Fig. 4.6 Synchrony between the ovarian and menstrual cycle.

Secretory phase:

- Once ovulation occurs, progesterone takes over and prepares the endometrium for potential embryo implantation.
- During this secretory phase, the straight uterine glands begin to coil and spiral arteries grow closer to the endometrial surface.
- If pregnancy does not occur, the menstrual cycle progresses towards its conclusion.

Feedback mechanisms and menstruation:

- The first feedback mechanism is initiated by inhibin, a hormone produced by granulosa cells.
- Inhibin reaches the anterior pituitary gland and suppresses gonadotropins, particularly FSH (and LH).
- As a result, the corpus luteum regresses and the secretion of progesterone by the ovary decreases.
- The regression of the corpus luteum leads to the breakdown of spiral arteries, resulting in local ischemia and subsequent haemorrhage.
- This cascade of events initiates menstruation.

KLINISCHE PERLEN

MENSTRUAL IRREGULARITIES

Menstrual irregularities refer to deviations from the normal menstrual cycle pattern and can include the following conditions:

1. **Amenorrhoea:**
   - Amenorrhoea is the absence of menstruation.
   - Primary amenorrhoea occurs when a female has not experienced menstruation even after reaching 16 years of age.
   - Secondary amenorrhoea is characterized by the sudden cessation of menstruation that was previously regular (e.g. due to pregnancy).
2. **Hypomenorrhoea:**
   Hypomenorrhoea is a condition where there is very light or scanty blood flow during menstruation.
3. **Oligomenorrhoea:**
   Oligomenorrhoea is defined by menstruation occurring at intervals longer than the typical 28–35 days.
4. **Menorrhagia:**
   Menorrhagia refers to abnormally heavy or prolonged bleeding during menstruation.
5. **Metrorrhagia:**
   Metrorrhagia is characterized by episodes of bleeding that occur between regular menstrual cycles.

CONTRACEPTIVE METHODS

Contraception consists of a variety of methods designed to prevent pregnancy. Some common forms of contraception where the hormones play an important role are as follows.

HORMONAL CONTRACEPTION

- Hormonal contraceptives typically contain oestrogen in combination with progesterone (progestin) or progestin alone.
- These hormones exert their effects by:
  - Inhibiting ovulation, thereby preventing the release of FSH and LH from the pituitary gland.
  - Altering the lining of the uterus.
  - Modifying the consistency of cervical mucus.

MALE CONTRACEPTIVE PILL

- A potential male contraceptive may involve a synthetic androgen, which can inhibit the secretion of FSH and LH.
- These actions aim to either halt sperm production or reduce it to a level of infertility [e.g. synthetic androgen – Dimethandrolone undecanoate (DMAU)].

INTRAUTERINE CONTRACEPTIVE DEVICE

Intrauterine contraceptive devices (IUCDs) come in two main types (Fig. 4.7):

- Copper-based IUCDs, such as Copper T, release copper into the uterus, preventing fertilization, implantation and the entry of sperm.
- Hormonal IUCDs, containing progestin, reduce the activity of sperm, impair the viability of both sperm and ova, and thicken cervical mucus to block sperm entry [e.g. **Mirena IUD (levonorgestrel-releasing intrauterine system)**].

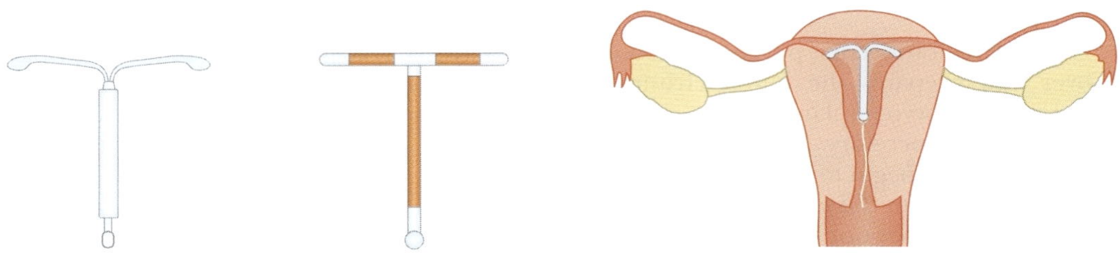

Fig. 4.7 Intrauterine contraceptive devices.

EMERGENCY CONTRACEPTION

- Emergency contraception involves high doses of progestin, sometimes with oestrogen or the use of **RU-486** (Mifepristone).
- These agents should be taken within 120 hours after intercourse.
- Mifepristone can even be used after implantation as an abortifacient.

CONTRACEPTIVE PILLS

- Contraceptive pills, also known as birth control pills, function by suppressing ovulation.
- They act on the hypothalamus and pituitary gland to inhibit the secretion of GnRH, FSH and LH.
- There are three main types of oral contraceptive pills:
  - Combined oestrogen–progesterone pills.
  - Progesterone-only pills.
  - Continuous or extended-use pills.
- Progesterone prevents pregnancy, while the oestrogen component helps regulate menstrual bleeding.

POINTS TO PONDER

Hormonal Control of the Female Reproductive System

The female reproductive system undergoes cyclic, hormonally induced changes in preparation for potential pregnancy. This hormonal control operates in a hierarchical manner:

1. **Hypothalamus-pituitary interaction:** The process begins with the hypothalamus, which signals the adenohypophysis (anterior pituitary gland) to release specific hormones, including FSH and LH.
2. **Pituitary hormones:** FSH and LH, produced by the anterior pituitary, play pivotal roles in regulating the female reproductive cycle. They stimulate ovarian follicles to produce key hormones—oestrogens and progesterone.
3. **Hormone action:**
   - Oestrogens and progesterone, produced by the ovarian follicles, exert profound effects on various female reproductive tissues.
   - Oestrogens stimulate the growth and preparation of the uterine endometrium for possible embryo implantation.
   - In pregnancy, the corpus luteum continues to produce progesterone to maintain the pregnancy.
4. **Menstruation and corpus luteum regression:**
   - In the absence of fertilization, hormonal support is withdrawn, leading to the shedding of the endometrial lining (menstruation).
   - This regression of the corpus luteum results in the end of the current menstrual cycle and the initiation of a new one.

Hormonal control in males:
- In males, LH plays a crucial role in stimulating Leydig cells to produce testosterone, a primary male sex hormone.
- FSH acts on Sertoli cells, supporting the process of spermatogenesis (sperm production).

Feedback mechanisms: Both in males and females, a feedback inhibition mechanism is in place. This mechanism helps to regulate the production of pituitary hormones, ensuring the cyclic nature of the reproductive system.

BRAIN TEASERS

1. During the luteal phase, what triggers the formation of the corpus luteum?
   A. Follicle-stimulating hormone (FSH)
   B. Luteinizing hormone (LH)
   C. Oestrogen
   D. Progesterone

2. Which hormone plays a key role in preparing the uterine endometrium for potential embryo implantation during the luteal phase?
   A. FSH
   B. LH
   C. Oestrogen
   D. Human chorionic gonadotropin (hCG)
3. What happens to the corpus luteum if fertilization does not occur?
   A. It enlarges to support a future pregnancy
   B. It transforms into a fibrotic scar tissue
   C. It continues to produce oestrogen and progesterone
   D. It remains unchanged throughout the menstrual cycle
4. How does the menstrual cycle get initiated during the premenstrual phase?
   A. An increase in progesterone levels
   B. A rise in oestrogen levels
   C. Spasmodic contractions of the myometrium
   D. A reduction in blood supply to the endometrium
5. What hormonal changes stimulate ovulation and regulate the menstrual cycle in females?
   A. Thyroid hormones
   B. Gonadotropin-releasing hormone (GnRH)
   C. Insulin
   D. Human growth hormone (HGH)
6. What is the main function of inhibin in the feedback mechanisms of the menstrual cycle?
   A. Stimulating FSH secretion
   B. Suppressing LH secretion
   C. Supporting progesterone production
   D. Enhancing oestrogen levels
7. Which type of contraceptive involves high doses of progestin and is taken within 120 hours after intercourse?
   A. Hormonal contraception
   B. Emergency contraception
   C. Male contraceptive pill
   D. Intrauterine contraceptive device (IUCD)
8. What is the function of the synthetic androgen in male contraception?
   A. Enhancing sperm viability
   B. Reducing cervical mucus thickness
   C. Stimulating the release of FSH
   D. Halting sperm production
9. Among the types of oral contraceptive pills, which one combines oestrogen and progesterone and helps regulate menstrual bleeding?
   A. Combined oestrogen–progesterone pills
   B. Progesterone-only pills
   C. Continuous or extended-use pills
   D. Synthetic androgen pills
10. What does 'synchrony between the ovarian and menstrual cycle' refer to?
   A. The simultaneous occurrence of ovulation and menstruation
   B. Coordination between the timing and hormonal changes in the ovarian and menstrual cycles
   C. The direct interconnection of the hypothalamus and the pituitary gland
   D. The initiation of the menstrual cycle by hormonal feedback mechanisms

Answers

1. (B); 2. (C); 3. (B); 4. (D); 5. (B); 6. (B); 7. (B); 8. (D); 9. (A); 10. (B).

FURTHER READINGS

Devesa-Peiro A, Sebastian-Leon P, Pellicer A, Diaz-Gimeno P. Guidelines for biomarker discovery in endometrium: correcting for menstrual cycle bias reveals new genes associated with uterine disorders. *Mol Hum Reprod.* 2021;27(4):gaab011. doi:10.1093/molehr/gaab011.

Kiesner J, Eisenlohr-Moul T, Mendle J. Evolution, the menstrual cycle, and theoretical overreach. *Perspect Psychol Sci.* 2020;15(4):1113-1130. doi:10.1177/1745691620906440.

Kim C, Nguyen AT, Berry-Bibee E, Ermias Y, Gaffield ME, Kapp N. Systemic hormonal contraception initiation after abortion: a systematic review and meta-analysis. *Contraception.* 2021;103(5):291-304. doi:10.1016/j.contraception.2021.01.017.

Vidafar P, Spitschan M. Light on Shedding: a review of sex and menstrual cycle differences in the physiological effects of light in humans. *J Biol Rhythms.* 2023;38(1):15-33. doi:10.1177/07487304221126785.

5 Fertilization

> **AN 77.4** Describe the stages and consequences of fertilization.
> **AN 77.5** Enumerate and describe the anatomical principles underlying contraception.
> **AN 77.6** Describe fertility and sterility, surrogate motherhood and social significance of 'sex-ratio'.

ANAMNESE

In a metropolitan fertility clinic, the couple, having struggled for years to conceive, sought the expertise of reproductive specialists. A battery of tests revealed that wife's eggs and husband's sperm were both healthy, but an unusual interaction hindered fertilization. Wife's eggs possessed a thicker-than-normal zona pellucida, making it difficult for the sperm to penetrate. The medical team employed intracytoplasmic sperm injection (ICSI) to manually introduce a single sperm into each of wife's eggs. Fertilization took place and she became pregnant. This case highlighted the critical role of fertilization in human reproduction, demonstrating how scientific innovation and an understanding of the male and female gametes' can overcome nature's obstacles.

Fertilization is a complicated multistage event which involves maturation and development of the spermatozoa and ova, sperm migration into the uterine tube, sperm–ovum interaction and then fusion. The classical models of fertilization focus on sperm-zona binding and the zona-induced acrosome reaction. Fusion can occur either within the female body (*in vivo*) or outside the body (*in vitro*) under specified condition resulting in the formation of a zygote. Recent gene knockout approaches in mice have revealed that what has been observed in In vitro fertilization (IVF) differs significantly from what occurs during 'physiological' fertilization.

FERTILIZATION (*IN VIVO*) (AN 77.4)

- The most prevalent site for fertilization within the female body is the ampulla of the uterine tube (Fig. 5.1).
- Fertilization occurs through a series of three distinct stages:
  - **A. Gamete transport into the uterine tube:** Sperm released during ejaculation must travel from the vaginal canal to the ampulla of the uterine tube to facilitate fertilization.
  - **B. Fusion of gametes:** The critical moment in fertilization takes place when a single spermatozoon successfully penetrates the zona pellucida encapsulating the secondary oocyte.
  - **C. Results of fertilization.**

A. Gamete Transport into the Uterine Tube

- As part of the process of fertilization, sperms travel from the vagina to reach the ampulla, the preferred site for fertilization.
- This journey spans approximately 2 to 7 hours, by the propulsion of sperms which

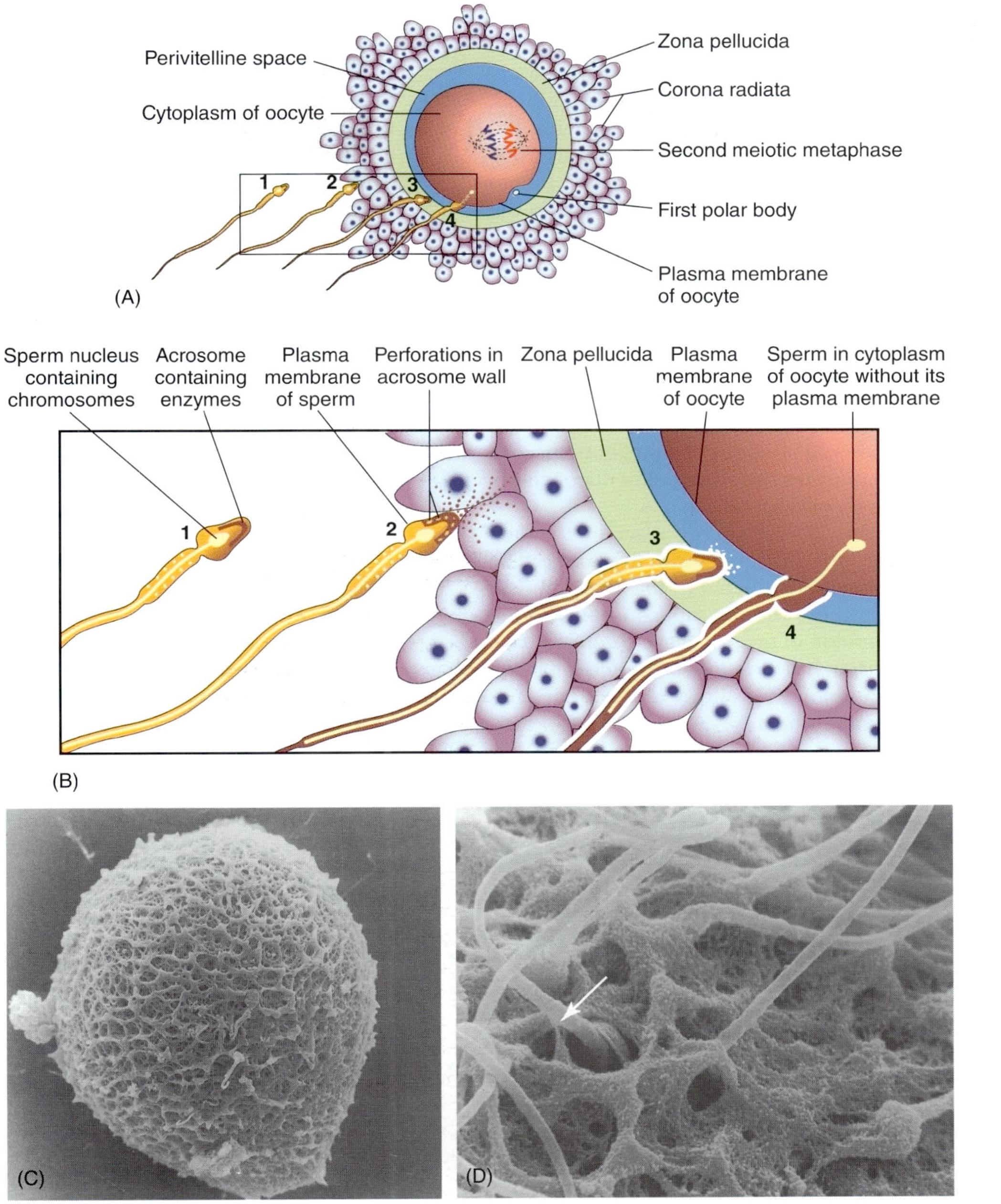

Fig. 5.1 Penetration of Sperm. (A) Acrosome reaction and sperm penetrating an oocyte. **(B)** (*1*) Sperm during capacitation, a period of conditioning that occurs in the female reproductive tract. (*2*) Sperm undergoing the acrosome reaction, during which perforations form in the acrosome. (*3*) Sperm digesting a path through the zona pellucida by the action of enzymes released from the acrosome. (*4*) Sperm after entering the cytoplasm of the oocyte. Note that the plasma membranes of the sperm and oocyte have fused and that the head and tail of the sperm enter the oocyte, leaving the sperm's plasma membrane attached to the oocyte's plasma membrane. **(C)** Scanning electron microscopy of an unfertilized human oocyte showing relatively few sperms attached to the zona pellucida. **(D)** Scanning electron microscopy of a human oocyte showing penetration of the sperm (*arrow*) into the zona pellucida. (Source: *The Developing Human: Clinically Oriented Embryology*. 11th ed., 2020. Courtesy P. Schwartz and H.M. Michelmann, University of Göttingen, Göttingen, Germany.)

occurs by the combined action of seminal **prostaglandins** (contraction of uterine muscles) and **oxytocin** from the neurohypophysis.

- A large number of sperms sets in for the journey but only a fraction (typically 300–400) ultimately reach the destination due to the barriers presented by the cervix and the ostium of the uterine tube.
- Concurrently, oocytes are propelled towards the uterine tube through a combination of contractions within the tube and the coordinated ciliary action of its epithelium.

B. Fusion of Gametes

- The critical moment in fertilization takes place when a single spermatozoon successfully penetrates the zona pellucida enveloping the secondary oocyte.
- Out of the 300–400 sperms reaching the uterine tube, only one unites with the oocyte. The remaining sperms, aided by the hyaluronidase found in the acrosome cap, contribute to the disintegration of the protective corona radiata.
- The three hurdles for the sperm before penetration are as follows (Fig. 5.2):
  - ➢ **Corona radiata.**
  - ➢ **Zona pellucida.**
  - ➢ **Vitelline membrane of secondary oocyte.**
- **Prefertilization sperm changes:**
  Before the spermatozoa can engage in fertilization, they undergo two significant alterations within the female genital tract.
  - **Capacitation:**
    - This transformation occurs primarily within the female genital tract, particularly in the uterine tube, and typically extends over approximately **7 hours**.
    - During this process, the glycoprotein coat covering the acrosomal region of the spermatozoa is removed (Fig. 5.3). This crucial step renders the spermatozoa 'capacitated', ensuring that only these primed spermatozoa are capable of undergoing the acrosome reaction.
  - **Acrosome reaction:**
    - The acrosomal cap of the sperm contains essential enzymes, such as **hyaluronidase** and **acid phosphatase**.
    - Once capacitated, the sperm makes multiple contacts with the oocyte,

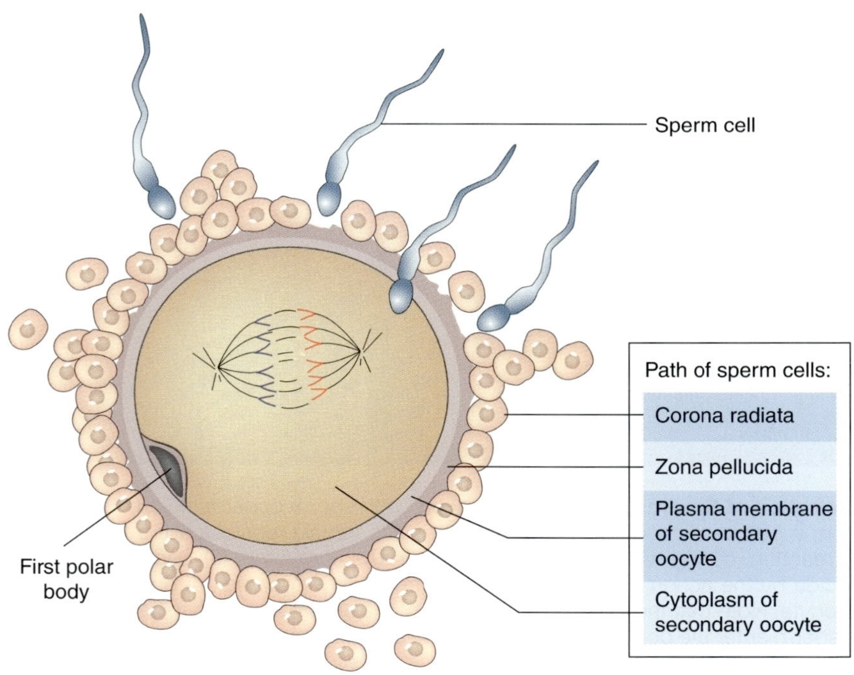

Fig. 5.2 Hurdles for the sperm entry.

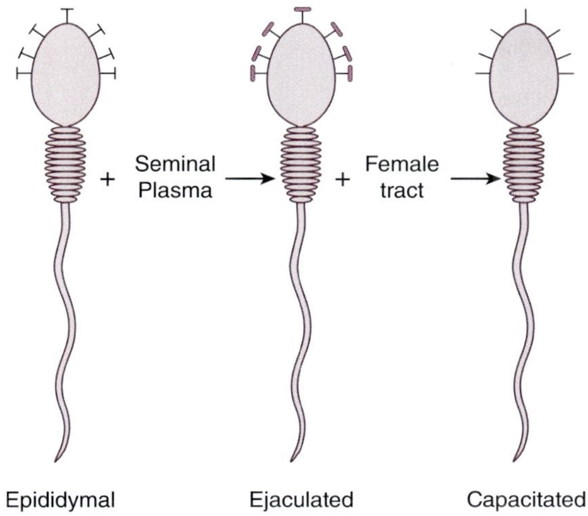

Fig. 5.3 Capacitation of sperm.

releasing these enzymes to overcome the various barriers (corona radiata, zona pellucida and vitelline membrane) in the acrosome reaction (Fig. 5.4).

- **Chemical mediators for barrier dissolution:** Several chemicals play a crucial role in disintegrating the protective barriers:
  - **Corona radiata**: Hyaluronidase.
  - **Zona pellucida**: Acrosin.
  - **Vitelline membrane**: Integrin peptides.
- **Cortical reaction**
  It occurs immediately after the sperm penetrates the oocyte. The primary purpose of the cortical reaction is to prevent multiple sperm from fertilizing the same egg, ensuring that only one sperm successfully fertilizes the egg. The steps involved are as follows (Fig. 5.5):
  1. **Sperm penetration**: When a sperm penetrates the zona pellucida, it triggers a series of biochemical changes within the egg.
  2. **Cortical granule release**: The egg contains cortical granules, which are small membrane-bound vesicles located just beneath the egg's surface. Upon fertilization, the sperm's entry into the egg leads to an increase in **intracellular calcium levels**. This rise in calcium levels triggers the release of the contents of the cortical granules into the perivitelline space (the space between the egg cell membrane and the zona pellucida).
  3. **Formation of fertilization envelope**: The released contents from the cortical granules include enzymes that modify the zona pellucida, making it impermeable to other sperm. This is known as the fertilization envelope or the slow block to polyspermy. The fertilization envelope hardens and lifts away from the egg's surface, creating a physical barrier that prevents additional sperm from binding to or penetrating the egg (Fig. 5.5).
  4. **Completion of fertilization**: Once the cortical reaction is initiated and the fertilization envelope is formed, no other sperm can enter the egg. This ensures that the genetic material of only one sperm successfully combines with the genetic material of the egg, resulting in a viable zygote.

C. Results of Fertilization

a. **Postfusion effects:**
After the fusion of gametes, the female gamete completes its second meiotic division, yielding the formation of a mature ovum. In the perivitelline space, one may occasionally observe the division of the first polar body into two polar bodies, resulting in a total of three polar bodies in some cases.

b. **Formation of female pronucleus:**
The vesicular nucleus of the mature ovum is recognized as the female pronucleus. This female pronucleus carries a haploid set of chromosomes, consisting of 22 autosomes and one X chromosome.

c. **Formation of male pronucleus:**
The head of the spermatozoon undergoes a distinct transformation, swelling to form the male pronucleus, which also contains a haploid set of chromosomes consisting of 22 autosomes and one X or one Y chromosome.

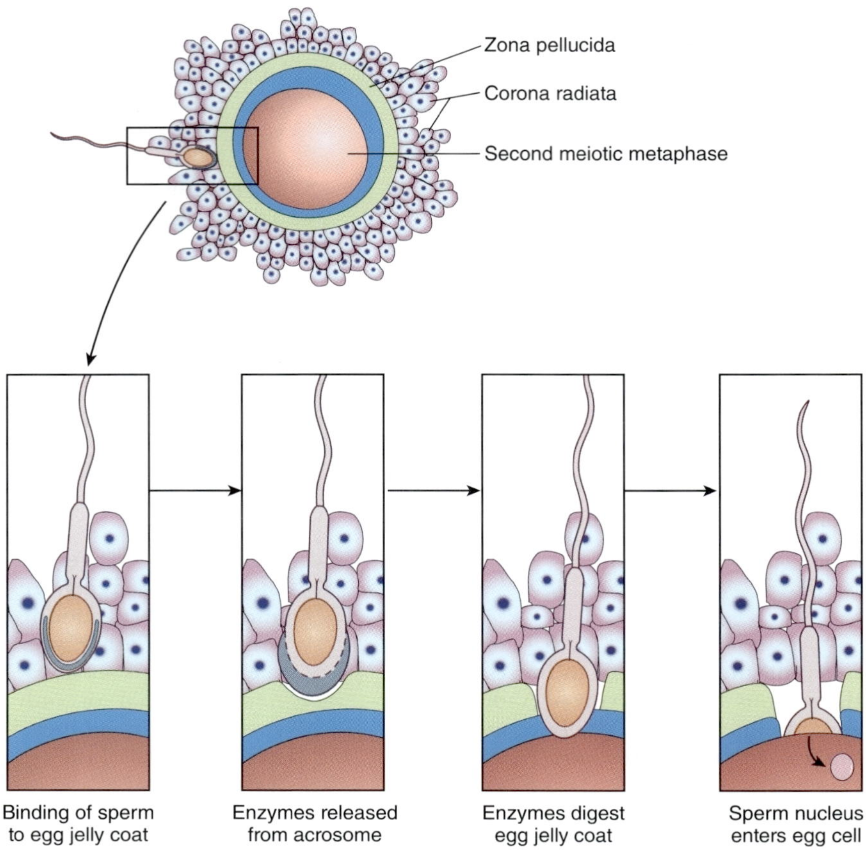

Fig. 5.4 Acrosome reaction.

d. **Restoration of diploid chromosome number in zygote:**
   The male and female pronuclei come together and the nuclear membranes surrounding them dissolve. This union results in the formation of a zygote with a diploid complement of chromosomes. While chromosomes are contributed in equal measure from both parents, the zygote's cytoplasm is exclusively inherited from the mother—a vital factor for early development.
e. **Determination of offspring's chromosomal sex by the father:**
   The chromosomal sex of the offspring is ultimately dictated by the father's contribution:
   - When an X-bearing spermatozoon unites with a mature ovum (containing an X-chromosome), it gives rise to a female child.
   - Conversely, when a Y-bearing spermatozoon fuses with the ovum, a male child is conceived.
f. **Onset of cleavage:**
   - The initial cleavage division occurs as chromosomes align in the equatorial region and subsequently migrate to opposite poles. This process is accompanied by an equitable division of cytoplasm, resulting in the formation of two daughter cells known as **blastomeres**.
   - In determining the age of the embryo, two distinct systems are employed:
     - **Fertilization age**: This is calculated from the moment of fertilization.
     - **Menstrual age**: It is computed from the commencement of the mother's last

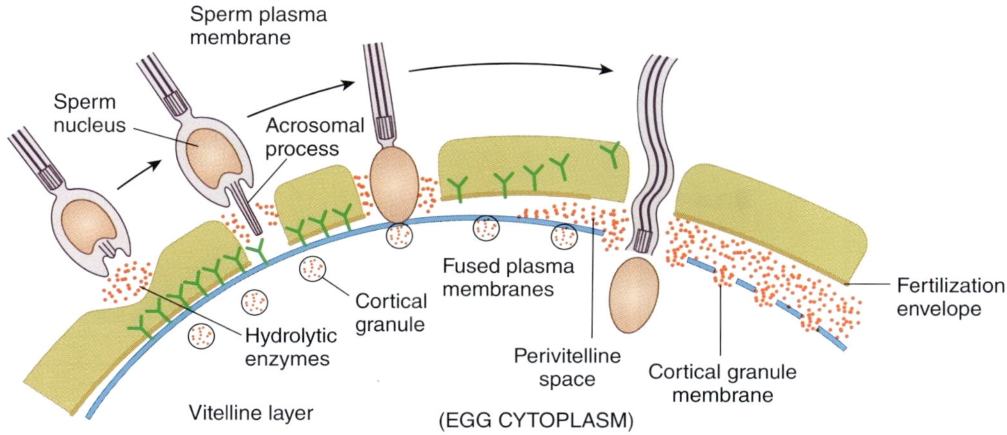

Fig. 5.5 Cortical reaction.

menstrual period and is typically two weeks greater than the fertilization age.

ASSISTED REPRODUCTIVE TECHNOLOGY

- Approximately one in six couples encounter challenges when attempting to conceive naturally. 90% of these couples experiencing infertility can conceive with the assistance of various medical options.
- Assisted reproductive technology (ART) consists of a diverse range of medical techniques aimed at overcoming infertility issues.
- **Artificial insemination (AI):** This method involves the deliberate introduction of sperm into the female reproductive tract to facilitate fertilization.
- **Hormonal therapies:** Hormonal interventions are frequently employed in cases of hormonal imbalances or irregularities that might hinder successful conception.
- ***In vitro* techniques:** In cases where natural conception fails, *in vitro* techniques play an important role in those who seek infertility treatment (Fig. 5.6):
  - **IVF and embryo transfer:** IVF is a widely recognized and successful procedure where an egg and sperm are fertilized outside the body, with the resulting embryos subsequently transferred into the woman's uterus.
  - **Intracytoplasmic sperm injection (ICSI):** ICSI is a specialized technique where a single sperm is injected directly into an egg, proving invaluable in cases of male infertility or where conventional fertilization methods have not succeeded.
  - **Gamete intrafallopian transfer (GIFT):** GIFT involves the collection of eggs and sperm, followed by their immediate placement into the woman's fallopian tube. This method allows for natural fertilization to take place within the body in conditions like hostile cervical mucus.
  - **Zygote intrafallopian transfer (ZIFT):** ZIFT combines elements of both IVF and GIFT, with fertilized eggs (zygotes) being transferred into the fallopian tube, where they have the opportunity to develop before descending into the uterus.

FERTILIZATION (*IN VITRO*)

Infertility due to anomalies in the uterine tube and inadequate number of sperms/decreased motility can be treated by fertilizing the ovum *in vitro* and transferring it into the uterine cavity of the biological/surrogate mother.

IVF is a complex ART and the process involves several distinct steps (Fig. 5.7):

I. **Ovarian stimulation**: The woman is administered hormonal medications to stimulate the ovaries to produce multiple mature eggs.

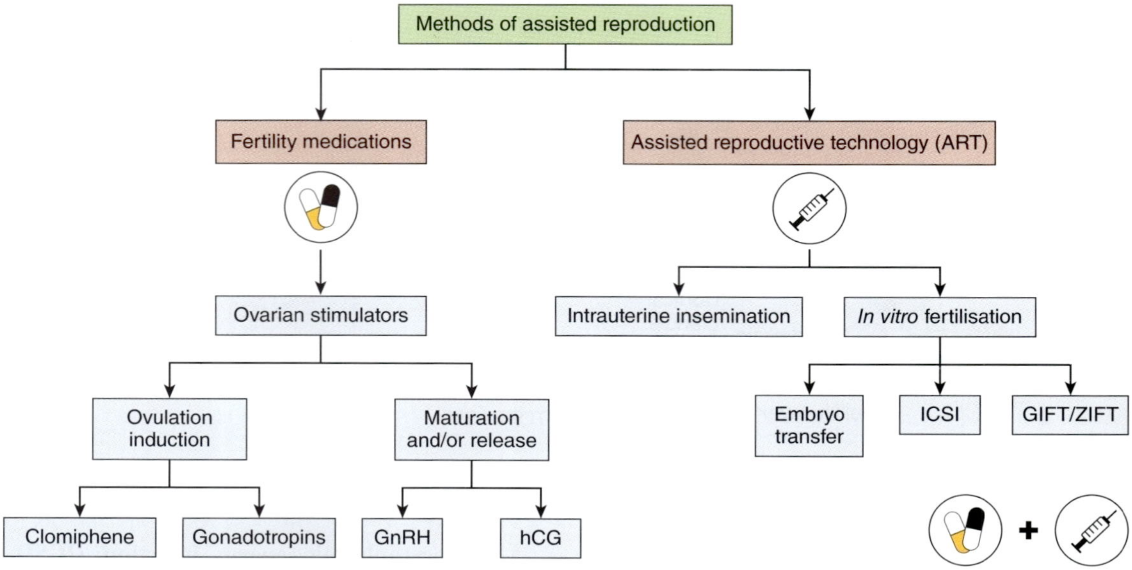

Fig. 5.6 Assisted reproductive technology.

Monitoring via ultrasound and hormone tests ensures the eggs are developing correctly.

II. **Egg retrieval**: When the eggs are mature, a minor surgical procedure is performed to remove the eggs from the ovaries.

III. **Sperm collection**: On the same day as the egg retrieval, a sperm sample is collected from the male partner or a sperm donor.

IV. **Fertilization**: The eggs and sperm are combined in a laboratory dish for fertilization. There are two primary methods:
   - **Conventional IVF**: In this method, eggs and sperm are placed together in a dish and left to fertilize naturally.
   - **ICSI**: In ICSI, a single sperm is injected directly into an egg. This is used when there are male fertility issues or if previous IVF attempts were unsuccessful.

V. **Embryo culture**: The fertilized eggs (embryos) are cultured in a special incubator for a few days to allow them to develop and grow.

VI. **Embryo selection**: Embryos are typically assessed for quality and the best ones are selected [**Preimplantation Genetic Diagnosis (PGD)**] for transfer into the uterus. Extra embryos can be cryopreserved for future use.

VII. **Embryo transfer**: One or more selected embryos are carefully placed into the woman's uterus. This is done through the cervix using a thin catheter. The number of embryos transferred depends on various factors, including the woman's age and the quality of the embryos.

VIII. **Luteal phase support**: Hormonal medications may be given to support the uterine lining and encourage embryo implantation.

IX. **Pregnancy test**: Approximately 10–14 days after the embryo transfer, a blood test is performed to determine if the IVF cycle was successful and if the woman is pregnant.

SINGLE EMBRYO TRANSFER

Rather than implanting multiple embryos, a more advanced approach involves the transfer of a single embryo that has been allowed to develop for a few additional days. This extended cultivation period enhances the chances of successful implantation and minimizes the risk of preterm labour, offering a more controlled and potentially safer option for those undergoing assisted reproduction.

SURROGACY (AN 77.6)

- In certain cases, a woman may possess viable eggs but is unable to conceive and carry a pregnancy to term. An example includes a woman who has undergone a hysterectomy,

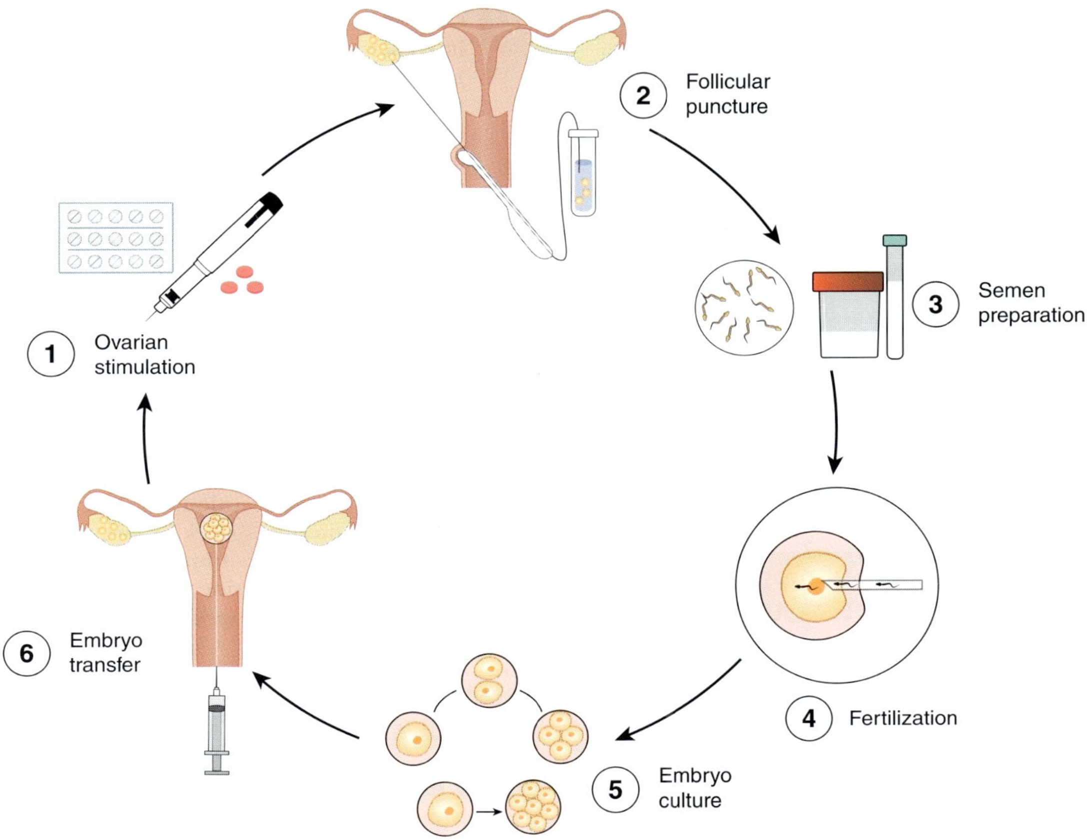

Fig. 5.7 ***In vitro* fertilization.**

thus lacking a functioning uterus. In such instances, IVF offers a promising solution by extracting the eggs from the woman with functional ovaries and transferring the resulting embryos into the uterus of another woman, commonly referred to as the surrogate mother. Surrogacy, however, is a multifaceted concept consisting of not only medical procedures but also raising psychological and religious considerations.

- The surrogacy process involves several key steps, including:
  - Stimulating gamete production using medications like clomiphene citrate.
  - Laparoscopic retrieval of eggs.
  - Isolation of the most viable and active sperm for fertilization.
  - Fertilization of both eggs and sperm under optimal laboratory conditions.
  - Culturing of the developing embryos.
  - Typically, up to three embryos are implanted into the surrogate's uterine cavity.
  - Any remaining embryos are preserved through cryopreservation for potential future use.

CLINICAL NUGGETS

Polyspermy

- It is the fertilization of an egg by more than one spermatozoon.
- **Prevention mechanisms:** To prevent polyspermy, two primary mechanisms come into play:
  - **Fast electrical block:** Upon the sperm's initial contact with the egg, a swift electrical block occurs on the egg's plasma membrane, preventing additional sperm from entering.
  - **Zona reaction:** Products released from the cortical granules, situated just beneath the

egg's plasma membrane, trigger the zona reaction/cortical reaction. This response leads to the inactivation of sperm receptors on the zona pellucida, further safeguarding against multiple sperm penetration.

- In some advanced reproductive technology centres, spermatozoa can be carefully introduced under the zona pellucida or directly into the oocyte. This approach is employed when there are concerns about compatibility between the sperm and the egg, issues with sperm motility or deficiencies in the sperm's ability to interact with the zona pellucida. By introducing sperm directly into or near the egg, potential barriers in the reproductive process can be bypassed, increasing the chances of successful fertilization.
- It is important to distinguish between fertility, which is the capacity to conceive, and sterility, which represents the inability to achieve conception.

ANATOMICAL PRINCIPLES UNDERLYING CONTRACEPTION (AN 77.5)

Anatomical principles underlying contraception involve understanding the reproductive anatomy and how different contraceptive methods work to prevent pregnancy. Here are some key anatomical principles related to contraception:

I. **Female reproductive anatomy**: Understanding the female reproductive system is essential for effective contraception. This includes knowledge of the ovaries, fallopian tubes, uterus, cervix and vagina.

II. **Ovulation and fertilization**: Contraception aims to prevent fertilization by blocking or interfering with the release of an egg (ovulation) and the subsequent fertilization of the egg by sperm in the fallopian tube.

III. **Cervical mucus**: The cervix produces mucus that changes in consistency throughout the menstrual cycle. Effective contraception methods may target this mucus to inhibit sperm from passing through the cervix and reaching the egg.

IV. **Endometrial changes**: Some contraceptive methods work by altering the endometrial lining of the uterus, making it less receptive to a fertilized egg for implantation.

V. **Barrier methods**: Barrier contraceptives, like condoms, diaphragms and cervical caps, physically block the passage of sperm into the female reproductive tract.

VI. **Hormonal methods**: Hormonal contraceptives, such as birth control pills, patches and injections, work by altering hormonal signals to the ovaries, preventing ovulation and affecting the cervical mucus to inhibit sperm penetration.

VII. **Intrauterine devices (IUDs)**: IUDs are inserted into the uterus and can work by releasing hormones or copper, which affects sperm motility and fertilization.

VIII. **Sterilization**: Sterilization procedures involve the permanent blocking or sealing of the fallopian tubes in women or the vas deferens in men, preventing eggs and sperm from meeting.

IX. **Emergency contraception**: Emergency contraception methods work by preventing or delaying ovulation, inhibiting fertilization or altering the uterine lining to prevent implantation after unprotected intercourse.

SOCIAL SIGNIFICANCE OF SEX RATIO (AN 77.6)

- **Sex ratio at birth**: The 'sex ratio at birth' is the ratio of male live births for every 100 female births. In the absence of manipulation, this ratio remains relatively consistent across human populations, typically ranging from 105 to 107 male births for every 100 female births.
- **Factors affecting sex ratio at birth**: Several factors can influence the sex ratio at birth, including family size, parental age and occupation, birth order, hormonal treatments, exposure to environmental toxins and stress.
- **Population sex ratio**: The 'population sex ratio' refers to the total number of males for every 100 females in the entire population. It depends on three primary factors:
  - The sex ratio at birth.
  - Differential mortality rates between the sexes at various ages.
  - Gains and losses due to migration.
- **Impact of son preference**: Deviations from these norms often result from the deeply rooted tradition of son preference. This preference is manifest in multiple ways:
  - Prenatally, through practices like sex determination and sex-selective abortion.

  - Postnatally, through the neglect and abandonment of female children, which can lead to higher female mortality rates.
  - Sex selection can also be influenced by the gender of the preceding child, affecting family dynamics.
- **Consequences of a high sex ratio**: A skewed sex ratio can have far-reaching consequences, including:
  - Increased levels of violence, which pose a threat to the stability and security of society.
  - A significant number of men remaining single and unable to form families.
  - The potential for a large expansion of the sex industry and human trafficking.
  - The implementation of laws forbidding practices like infanticide, abandonment and neglect of female children can help mitigate this situation, promoting gender equity and social well-being.

KLINISCHE PERLEN

INNOVATIVE FERTILITY PRESERVATION TECHNIQUES

- **Ovarian tissue freezing technique:**
  - Ovarian tissue freezing involves the process of removing, freezing and subsequently reimplanting ovarian tissue (Fig. 5.8). This technique is particularly vital for women facing radiation or chemotherapy, as it offers a means of preserving fertility. By safeguarding their ovarian tissue, women can hope to regain their reproductive capabilities after medical treatment.
- **Uterine transplant:**
  - Uterine transplants are a groundbreaking solution for women who desire to conceive but lack a uterus while still possessing functioning ovaries. In 2013, a case unfolded at Sahlgrenska University Hospital in Gothenburg, Sweden. A 35-year-old woman, diagnosed with congenital absence of the uterus (Mayer-Rokitansky-Küster-Hauser syndrome), received a uterus transplant from a living 61-year-old donor (P2). Before the transplantation, the recipient and her partner underwent IVF treatment, resulting in the cryopreservation of 11 embryos. A year post-transplantation, the recipient underwent her first single embryo transfer, resulting in a successful pregnancy. Immunosuppressive agents were administered and continued throughout the pregnancy, ultimately leading to the birth of a healthy male baby with a normal birth weight for gestational age (1775 g). This remarkable procedure offers new hope for women with uterine-related infertility, highlighting the potential for achieving motherhood through innovative medical interventions.

PREGESTATIONAL GENETIC DIAGNOSIS (PGD)

It is a process of genetic testing and screening that is performed before conception or early in pregnancy to assess the risk of passing on specific genetic conditions or chromosomal abnormalities to a child. This type of genetic testing is typically carried out when individuals or couples have concerns about their genetic heritage or have a family history of genetic disorders. Pregestational genetic diagnosis involves several key components:

1. **Genetic counselling**: Before undergoing genetic testing, individuals or couples often receive genetic counselling. This process helps them understand the implications of their genetic risk factors and the available testing options.
2. **Genetic testing**: Various genetic tests may be conducted to assess the risk of passing on genetic conditions. These tests can include carrier screening, which identifies whether individuals carry specific genetic mutations, and preconception testing to identify potential genetic risks.
3. **PGD**: For couples undergoing IVF, PGD can be performed. This involves testing embryos created through IVF for specific genetic conditions before they are implanted in the uterus.
4. **IVF**: In cases where PGD is necessary, couples may undergo IVF to create embryos that can be tested for genetic abnormalities.
5. **Prenatal testing**: If pregnancy has already occurred, prenatal testing can be conducted. This includes procedures such as chorionic villus sampling (CVS) or amniocentesis, which can diagnose genetic conditions in the developing foetus.

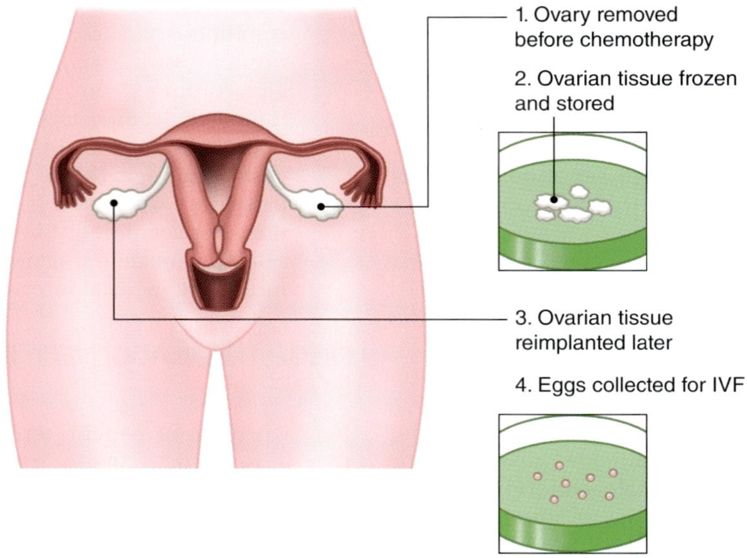

Fig. 5.8 Ovarian tissue freezing technique.

POINTS TO PONDER

The process of fertilization unfolds through a series of sequential events, each with its own vital role:

- **Penetration of the corona radiata**: Sperm must first navigate through the protective layer known as the corona radiata, which surrounds the egg.
- **Attachment to the zona pellucida**: Following penetration, the sperm attaches itself to the zona pellucida, a specialized glycoprotein matrix surrounding the egg.
- **Acrosomal reaction and zona pellucida penetration**: To proceed, the sperm undergoes the acrosomal reaction, releasing enzymes that enable it to penetrate the zona pellucida, a crucial step in reaching the egg.
- **Binding and fusion of sperm and egg**: The union occurs as the sperm binds to and fuses with the egg, resulting in the formation of a zygote.
- **Prevention of polyspermy**: Complex mechanisms come into play to prevent polyspermy, ensuring that only one sperm successfully fertilizes the egg.
- **Metabolic activation of the egg**: Fertilization activates the egg metabolically, setting the stage for subsequent developmental processes.
- **Decondensation of the sperm nucleus**: The sperm nucleus undergoes decondensation, preparing it for integration with the egg's genetic material.
- **Completion of meiosis in the egg**: The egg completes its second meiotic division, resulting in the formation of the female pronucleus.
- **Fusion of male and female pronuclei**: The male pronucleus, derived from the sperm, fuses with the female pronucleus, combining the genetic material of both parents.
- **Overcoming three hurdles for sperm entry**: Sperm must overcome three hurdles on their path to fertilization: the corona radiata, the zona pellucida and the vitelline membrane.

The outcomes of this process are:

- **Completion of female gamete's second meiotic division**: Fertilization triggers the completion of the second meiotic division in the female gamete, resulting in a mature ovum.
- **Formation of female pronucleus**: A vesicular nucleus forms in the mature ovum, known as the female pronucleus, containing a haploid set of chromosomes (22 + X).
- **Formation of male pronucleus**: The head of the spermatozoon swells to form the male pronucleus, also carrying a haploid set of chromosomes.
- **Restoration of diploid chromosome number**: The fusion of male and female pronuclei restores the diploid number of chromosomes in the zygote.
- **Chromosomal sex determination by the father**: The father's contribution of either an X or a Y-bearing

spermatozoon during fertilization determines the chromosomal sex of the offspring.

- **Commencement of cleavage**: Fertilization marks the beginning of cleavage, where the zygote divides into two daughter cells, called blastomeres, initiating the early stages of embryonic development.

BRAIN TEASERS

1. What is the main role of hyaluronidase found in the acrosome cap of sperm during fertilization?
   A. To digest the zona pellucida
   B. To promote capacitation of sperm
   C. To break down the corona radiata
   D. To facilitate the acrosome reaction
2. What triggers the release of the contents of cortical granules during the cortical reaction in fertilization?
   A. Fertilization of the egg
   B. Sperm penetration of the zona pellucida
   C. Increase in intracellular calcium levels in the egg
   D. Formation of the fertilization envelope
3. What purpose does the fertilization envelope serve in fertilization?
   A. It prevents the zona pellucida from hardening.
   B. It facilitates the binding of additional sperm to the egg.
   C. It acts as a physical barrier to prevent other sperm from entering the egg.
   D. It enhances the movement of the zygote within the female reproductive tract.
4. What is the primary purpose of the cortical reaction in fertilization?
   A. To trigger the release of acrosomal enzymes from sperm
   B. To promote capacitation of spermatozoa
   C. To prevent multiple sperm from fertilizing the same egg
   D. To facilitate the formation of male and female pronuclei
5. How many autosomes are typically present in the male pronucleus formed during fertilization?
   A. 23
   B. 22
   C. 24
   D. 20
6. In which part of the female genital tract does capacitation primarily occur?
   A. Uterus
   B. Vagina
   C. Uterine tube
   D. Cervix
7. What is the main function of the enzyme found in the acrosome cap of sperm?
   A. To trigger the release of cortical granules
   B. To break down the zona pellucida
   C. To facilitate the formation of the fertilization envelope
   D. To promote the acrosome reaction
8. How is the chromosomal sex of the offspring determined in fertilization?
   A. By the number of X chromosomes in the egg
   B. By the number of X chromosomes in the sperm
   C. By the presence of maternal chromosomes
   D. By the father's contribution of an X or Y chromosome
9. What is the main goal of artificial insemination (AI) in assisted reproductive technology (ART)?
   A. To perform in *vitro* fertilization (IVF)
   B. To introduce sperm directly into the female reproductive tract
   C. To promote the acrosome reaction in spermatozoa
   D. To assist with hormonal therapy
10. Which ART technique combines elements of both IVF and GIFT and involves transferring fertilized eggs into the fallopian tube for development?
    A. Artificial insemination (AI)
    B. Intracytoplasmic sperm injection (ICSI)
    C. Gamete intrafallopian transfer (GIFT)
    D. Zygote intrafallopian transfer (ZIFT)

Answers

1. (C); 2. (C); 3. (C); 4. (C); 5. (B); 6. (C); 7. (B); 8. (D); 9. (B); 10. (D).

FURTHER READINGS

Brannstrom M, Johannesson L, Bokstrom H, Kvarnstrom N. Livebirth after uterus transplantation. *Lancet.* 2015;385(9968):607-616.

Hesketh T, Xing ZW. Abnormal sex ratios in human populations: causes and consequences. *Proc Natl Acad Sci.* 2006;103(36):13271–13275. doi:10.1073/pnas.0602203103.

Sugishita Y, Taylan E, Kawahara T, Shahmurzada B, Suzuki N, Oktay K. Comparison of open and a novel closed vitrification system with slow freezing for human ovarian tissue cryopreservation. *J Assist Reprod Genet.* 2021;38(10):2723-2733. doi:10.1007/s10815-021-02297-9.

Zhu Y, Zhang F, Chen H, Sun X, Jiang F. The use of frozen embryos and frozen sperm have complementary IVF outcomes: a retrospective analysis in couples experiencing IVF/Donor and IVF/Husband. *BMC Pregnancy Childbirth.* 2022;22(1):776. doi:10.1186/s12884-022-05088-x.

SECTION 2

EARLY EMBRYONIC DEVELOPMENT

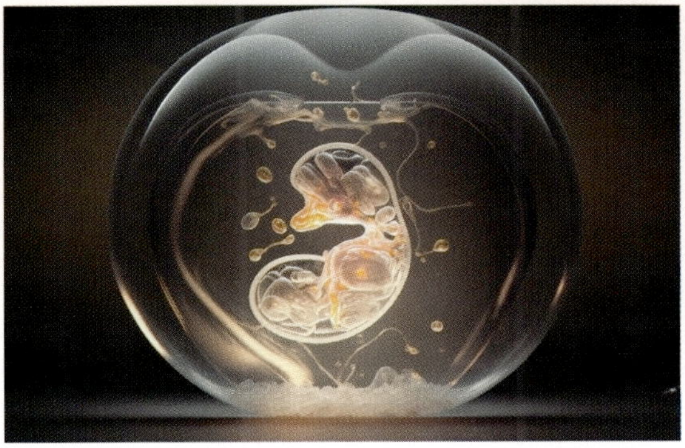

6 First Week of Development

AN 78.1 Describe cleavage and formation of blastocyst.
AN 78.2 Describe the development of trophoblast.
AN 78.3 Describe the process of implantation.
AN 78.3 Describe the common abnormal sites of implantation.

ANAMNESE

A 35-year-old woman presented with unusual abdominal discomfort and intermittent bleeding during her fourth pregnancy. Initial ultrasound examination revealed a rare case of abdominal pregnancy, where the embryo had implanted outside the uterus, specifically within the peritoneal cavity. Despite the challenges associated with abdominal pregnancies, such as the risk of massive haemorrhage and maternal complications, a surgical team successfully removed the ectopic pregnancy. This case showed the need for early and accurate diagnosis of abnormal implantation, which allowed for timely intervention and ultimately a healthy outcome for the patient.

A fertilized egg must successfully attach itself to uterine tissue in order to survive. Failure in implantation and placental development are the two important contributors to infertility and recurrent miscarriage. The process of implantation has two main components, a healthy embryo and a receptive endometrium that should enable implantation. The interference between the embryo and the endometrium leads to apposition and invasion of embryos. This is mandatory for successful implantation and normal placentation. These processes seem to involve many mediators originating in the embryo, as well as in the endometrium, and also involve the maternal immunologic system.

GESTATION PERIOD

- The typical gestation period for human pregnancy spans 40 weeks or 280 days, starting from the last menstrual period (LMP).
- This duration is calculated as LMP (first day of the last menstrual period) plus 9 months with a margin of about 7 days (9 months ± 7 days), which amounts to 266 days or roughly 38 weeks after fertilization.
- The gestation period can be divided into two distinct stages:
  - **The embryonic period**, spanning from fertilization to 8 weeks.
  - **The foetal period**, extending from the ninth week (third month) until the completion of the pregnancy.
- The embryonic period is further subdivided into two critical phases:
  - **The germinal period**—the time from fertilization to 3 weeks.
  - **The embryonic period proper**—the development from 4 to 8 weeks.

CHANGES IN THE FIRST WEEK (AN 78.1)

- It includes the journey of zygote from the time of fertilization to the point of implantation (Fig. 6.1).

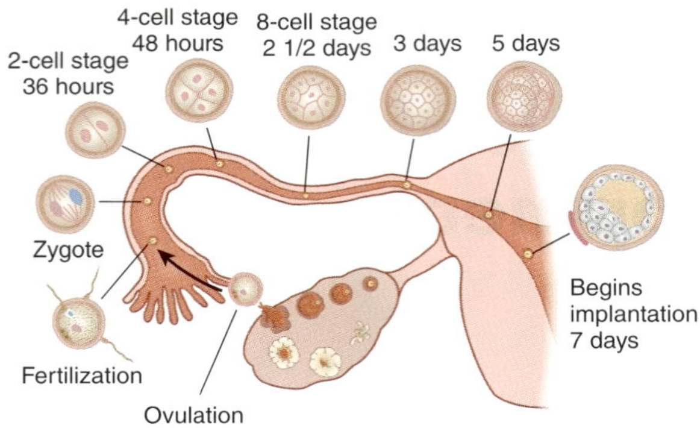

Fig. 6.1 Different stages of the fertilized ovum. Fertilization, implantation, and growth of the embryo. A mature ovum is released in ovulation. The ovum is fertilized by a sperm, and the product of fertilization, the zygote, undergoes rapid cell division, finally implanting in the endometrium on approximately day 7. (Source: *Quick & Easy Medical Terminology*, 9th ed. 2020.)

- The chief events are:
  - **Cleavage division.**
  - **Formation of morula.**
  - **Formation of blastocyst.**
  - **Implantation.**

CLEAVAGE DIVISION

This represents a process in which the zygote undergoes repeated mitotic division.

- The zygote is enveloped by the **zona pellucida** throughout this division.
- The resulting smaller cells are termed **blastomeres**.
- Cleavage division serves to restore the cells to their normal size.
- The cleavage pattern can be categorized into four distinct stages:
  - ➢ 2-cell stage.
  - ➢ 4-cell stage.
  - ➢ 12-cell stage.
  - ➢ 16-cell stage.
- These stages unfold between 30 and 96 hours following fertilization.
- During the 2-cell stage, the cells exhibit size **asymmetry (unequal size)**.
- By the 12–16 cell stage, the cells have achieved nearly uniform size **(equal size)**.

FORMATION OF MORULA

- The 12–16 cell stage is referred to as the morula.
- At this point, the zygote reaches the uterine cavity, typically occurring about 3 days after fertilization.
- **Factors** facilitating the transport of zygote are:
  - **Ciliary beats** of the tubal lining.
  - **Contraction** of the uterine tube.
- During this stage, the spherical blastomeres undergo a process known as **compaction**, where the cells flatten against each other.
- This compaction increases intercellular contact through the formation of tight junctions.
- The cells in the morula are categorized into **two groups**:
  - **The outer cell mass** consists of cells at the periphery, which possess tight junctions and eventually form protective and nutritive coverings for the embryo, namely trophoblasts and chorion.
  - **The inner cell mass** comprises cells in the centre, characterized by gap junctions, and these cells give rise to the embryo proper (Table 6.1).
- Importantly, the morula remains enveloped by the **zona pellucida**.

Table 6.1 Changes in Outer and Inner Cell Mass

Stage of Development	Outer Cell Mass (Trophoblast)	Inner Cell Mass
Morula (12–16 cells)	Cells at the periphery, forming tight junctions.	Cells in the centre, characterized by gap junctions.
Blastocyst (32–64 cells)	Outer cell mass, consisting of flattened cells.	Attached to the trophoblast, forming the embryoblast.

FORMATION OF BLASTOCYST (AN 78.2)

- Mitotic activity persists within the morula.
- Uterine fluid, referred to as '**uterine milk**', permeates the morula via diffusion through the zona pellucida and the outer cell mass. This fluid accumulates in the spaces between the inner cell mass. Subsequently, a singular fluid-filled cavity, known as the **blastocele,** is formed.
- The **blastocyst**, a stage comprising 32–64 cells, is essentially a morula with a blastocele. This transition takes place between the fourth and fifth day following fertilization, with the blastocyst still enclosed by the zona pellucida (as shown in Fig. 6.2).

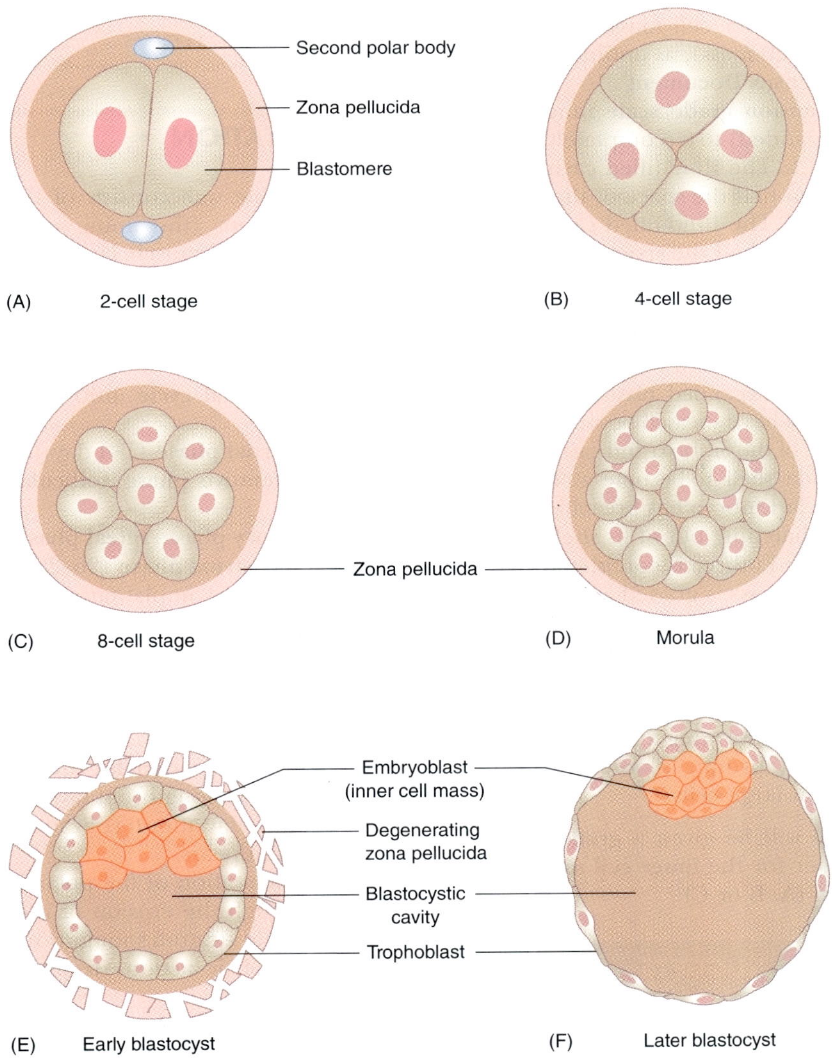

Fig. 6.2 Blastocyst. The process of cleaving the zygote and forming the blastocyst is illustrated in various stages. The zona pellucida disappears by the late blastocyst stage, and although cleavage increases the number of blastomeres, there is no increase in the embryo's size until the zona pellucida degenerates, allowing the blastocyst to enlarge significantly.

- The outer cell mass, consisting of flattened cells, is now referred to as the **trophoblast**. The inner cell mass, which remains attached to the trophoblast, is termed the **embryoblast**.
- The nomenclature of the trophoblast depends on its attachment to the embryoblast:
  - **Polar trophoblast** (covering the embryonic pole).
  - **Mural trophoblast** (covering the rest of the wall and the abembryonic pole).
- **Blastocysts** are classified based on criteria such as expansion, inner cell mass and trophectoderm (outer cell mass), as outlined in '**The Istanbul Consensus Document**'.
  - The **expansion grade scale** ranges from 1 (least expanded) to 6 (completely hatched):
    - **Grade 1:** The fluid-filled cavity takes up less than half the space of the embryo.
    - **Grade 2:** The fluid-filled cavity takes up more than half the space of the embryo.
    - **Grade 3:** The blastocyst cavity has expanded into the entire volume of the embryo, pressing the trophectoderm cells up tightly against the inside of the zona.
    - **Grade 4:** Expanded blastocyst, where the blastocyst has increased beyond the original volume of the embryo and caused the zona pellucida 'shell' to become super thin.
    - **Grade 5:** Embryo has breached the zona and is hatching out of its shell.
    - **Grade 6:** Embryo is completely hatched.
- The **inner cell mass** is graded as follows:
  - **A:** Many cells, tightly packed.
  - **B:** Several cells, loosely packed.
  - **C:** Very few cells.
- The **trophectoderm** grading is as follows:
  - **A:** Many cells, forming a cohesive layer.
  - **B:** Few cells, forming a loose layer.
  - **C:** Very few large cells.

The **embryo** will be given a **grade (1–6),** followed by a letter for the **inner cell mass** and the **trophectoderm (A, B or C)**.

CLINICAL NUGGETS

Functions of zona pellucida

- It acts as a **selective barrier**, permitting only sperm of the same species to access the egg.
- It initiates the **acrosomal reaction** in sperm, facilitating their penetration into the egg.
- After fertilization, it acts as a safeguard, preventing additional sperm from reaching the zygote.
- It facilitates the transmission of substances secreted by the uterine tube to the developing embryo during cleavage.
- It serves as an **immunological barrier** due to the absence of histocompatibility antigens, thus safeguarding the interface between the mother and the embryo.
- It holds the blastomeres together, promoting **cohesion** during early development.
- It plays a role in the **differentiation** of trophoblastic cells.
- It **prevents premature implantation** of the cleaving embryo into the uterine tube's wall, regulating the implantation process.

IMPLANTATION (AN 78.3)

- The uterine wall consists of three layers: the endometrium (the lining mucosa), myometrium (smooth muscle layer) and perimetrium (outer peritoneal covering).
- The cyclical changes occurring in the endometrium have been extensively discussed in previous chapters.
- The **menstrual cycle** unfolds in four distinct phases:
  - **Menstrual phase** (1–4 days).
  - **Proliferative phase/follicular phase** (5–14 days).
  - **Secretory phase/luteal phase** (15–25 days).
  - **Premenstrual phase** (26–28 days).
- At the time of implantation, the uterus is in the secretory phase.
- During this phase, the endometrium exhibits three distinct layers: **the stratum compactum, stratum spongiosum and stratum basale** (Fig. 6.3). The functional layer, referred to as the **stratum functionale**, consists of the compactum and spongiosum layers.
- By the fifth day after fertilization, the zona pellucida disappears.
- The implantation of the polar trophoblast occurs through the erosion of the stratum compactum and stratum spongiosum, facilitated by the proteolytic action (**trypsin-like enzymes**) of the trophoblast.
- The apical **glycocalyx** coating the uterine epithelium diminishes in quantity, and apical microvilli retract to establish a flattened surface in many areas of the epithelium.
- **Embedding or implantation** takes place on the sixth or seventh day following fertilization.

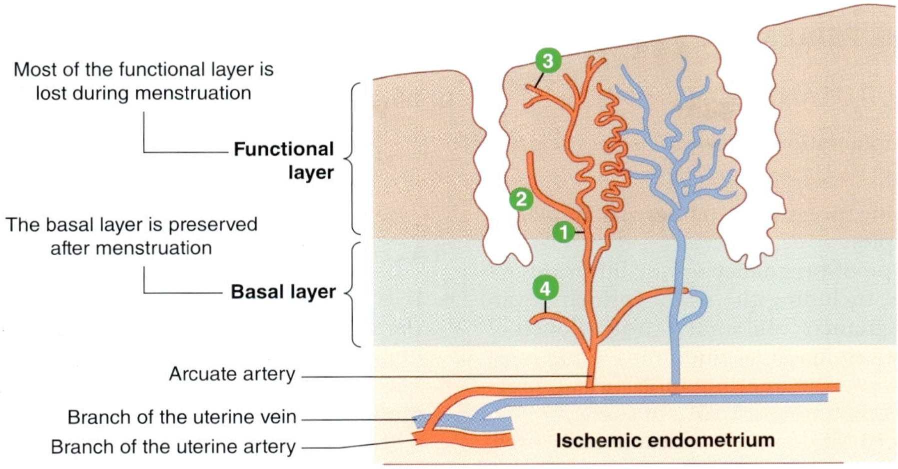

Pre-menstrual or ischemic stage

1. Periodic contractions of the spiral artery, triggered by a reduction in progesterone, deprive the supply of oxygen (hypoxia) to the functional layer.
2. A breakdown of the spiral artery floods the lamina propria with blood.
3. The functional layer, consisting of glands and decidual-like cells, detaches and sheds into the uterine cavity (**menses**).
4. The basal layer is not affected because basal straight arteries provide independent blood supply to this layer.

Fig. 6.3 Endometrium showing different layers. Premenstrual or ischaemic stage of the endometrium. (Source: *Histology and Cell Biology: An Introduction to Pathology*, 5th ed. 2020.)

- The implantation site can be found at the junction of the fundus and posterior wall of the uterine body or anywhere in the upper part of the uterine cavity.

CLINICAL NUGGETS

- **Blastocyst abnormalities** are frequent and typically incompatible with sustaining life.
- These abnormalities often result in either failed implantation within the uterus or the absence of pregnancy signs.
- Failed implantation, caused by a variety of factors at any stage of the process, is a prevalent reason for miscarriages among couples undergoing IVF treatment.
- During implantation, **immunosuppressant cytokines** are produced to prevent an immune response between the embryo and the mother. In certain autoimmune diseases like **Systemic lupus erythematosus (SLE) and Antiphospholipid antibody syndrome,** and antiphospholipid antibody syndrome, the mother's body can attack the embryo at the implantation stage.

- The **fertile window** refers to the specific period during a woman's menstrual cycle when she is most likely to conceive if she has unprotected sexual intercourse. Ovulation is when the ovary releases an egg into the fallopian tube, making it available for fertilization by sperm. The fertile window may vary from woman to woman but is generally considered to be the days around the middle of the menstrual cycle, usually **between days 10 and 17 in a 28-day cycle**. The fertile window can be influenced by factors such as the length of the menstrual cycle, irregular periods and individual variations. Couples trying to conceive often track ovulation and monitor their fertile window to increase the chances of pregnancy (Fig. 6.4).
- **Parental imprinting**, a phenomenon in which the expression of specific genes from the egg differs from the expression of the same genes from the spermatozoon, leads to diverse manifestations. Parental imprinting takes place during gametogenesis and is not passed on to subsequent generations. Examples of conditions related to parental imprinting include **Hydatidiform mole, Beckwith-Wiedemann syndrome, Prader-Willi syndrome and Angelman syndrome.**

KLINISCHE PERLEN (AN 78.3)

ABNORMAL IMPLANTATION

Abnormal implantation is a critical aspect of pregnancy (see Fig. 6.4).

A) **Extrauterine pregnancy (abnormal implantation/ectopic):**
   - This type of pregnancy occurs in various locations, including the ovary (primary ovarian pregnancy), abdominal cavity (Pouch of Douglas or greater omentum) and, most commonly, the uterine tube (tubal pregnancy, accounting for 95% of cases).
   - **Advanced abdominal (extrauterine) pregnancy (AAP)** is defined as a situation where a foetus either currently lives or shows signs of previous development within the mother's abdominal cavity after 20 weeks of gestation.
   - AAP can be categorized as primary or secondary:
     - ➢ **Primary AAP** involves the direct implantation of the fertilized ovum into the peritoneal cavity, although it is less common.
     - ➢ **Secondary AAP** occurs when the fertilized ovum initially implants in the fallopian tube or uterus, and due to fimbrial abortion or rupture, the foetus subsequently resides and develops in the mother's abdominal cavity. In rare cases, an embryo that has fully developed within the abdominal cavity may not be delivered, leading to calcification and the formation of a **Lithopaedion**.

B) **Intrauterine abnormal implantation:**
   - In this scenario, the blastocyst attaches to the lower part of the uterine cavity, a condition known as placenta praevia.

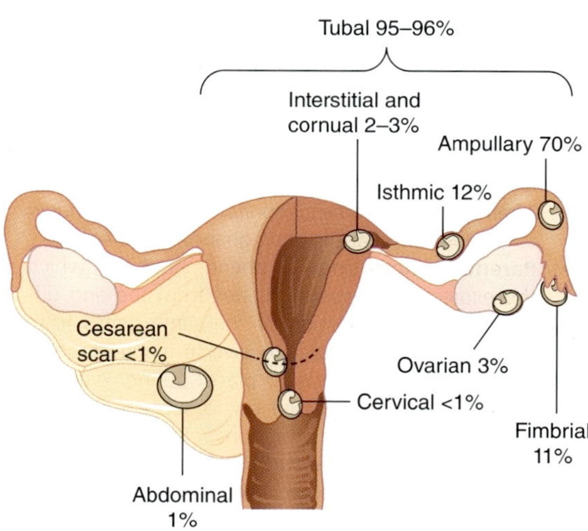

Fig. 6.4 Different sites of abnormal implantation.

PLACENTA PRAEVIA

- It is characterized by severe bleeding during the second trimester of pregnancy and during delivery.
- Placenta praevia is classified into distinct grades (Fig. 6.5).
  - **Grade I**: The placenta is located in the lower segment.

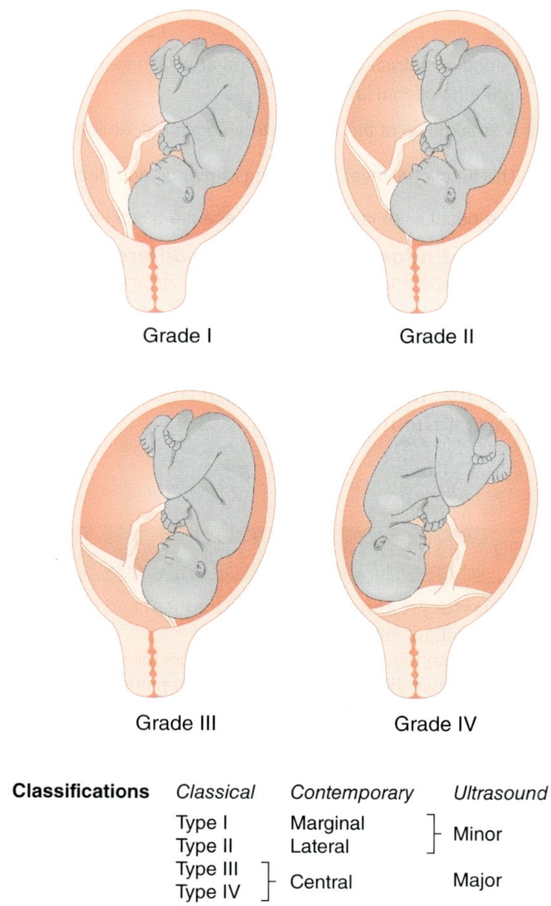

Fig. 6.5 Different grades of placenta previa. (Source: *Essentials of Obstetrics and Gynaecology*, 2nd ed., 2012)

- **Grade II**: The placenta is positioned near the internal os.
- **Grade III**: The placenta covers the internal os but does not obstruct the lumen upon os dilatation.
- **Grade IV**: The placenta entirely covers the internal os.

STEM CELLS

There are two primary types of stem cells (Table 6.2):

1. **Embryonic stem cells:**
   - These stem cells are derived from the **inner cell mass**.
   - They are pluripotent, meaning they have the capacity to develop into various tissue types.
   - Embryonic stem cells are typically obtained from embryos following in vitro fertilization (IVF).
   - There are two key methods of obtaining them:
     - ➢ **Therapeutic cloning**: This involves creating blastocysts from enucleated oocytes fused with the nuclei of adult cells.
     - ➢ **Reproductive cloning**: These cells can be obtained from embryos resulting from IVF.
   - Embryonic stem cells have potential applications in treating conditions such as diabetes, Parkinson's disease, anaemia and spinal cord injuries, among others.
2. **Adult stem cells:**
   - These cells are multipotent, meaning they have the capacity to give rise to a range of cell types within the same lineage, rather than being pluripotent and capable of differentiating into various cell types.
   - Adult stem cells can be sourced from various locations, including bone marrow, adipose tissue (fat), peripheral blood, human umbilical cords and placental tissue.
   - Their primary clinical applications involve the treatment of haematological malignancies and cartilage defects.

Table 6.2 Differences Between Embryonic and Adult Stem Cells

Characteristic	Embryonic Stem Cells	Adult Stem Cells
Source	Derived from early-stage embryos (typically within the first few days after fertilization).	Found in various tissues and organs in mature organisms.
Pluripotency	Pluripotent: Can differentiate into cells of all three germ layers (ectoderm, mesoderm and endoderm) and give rise to various cell types.	Multipotent: Can differentiate into a limited range of cell types within a specific tissue or organ.
Differentiation potential	High differentiation potential and versatility.	Limited differentiation potential within their tissue.
Tissue compatibility	Less tissue-compatible; may lead to immune rejection.	More tissue-compatible; lower risk of immune rejection when used within the same individual.
Research and therapeutic applications	Valuable for studying early embryonic development, disease modelling and drug testing.	Valuable for tissue repair, regeneration and treatment of degenerative diseases.
Ethical considerations	Ethical concerns due to the destruction of embryos.	Ethical considerations may be reduced since they are derived from adult tissues.

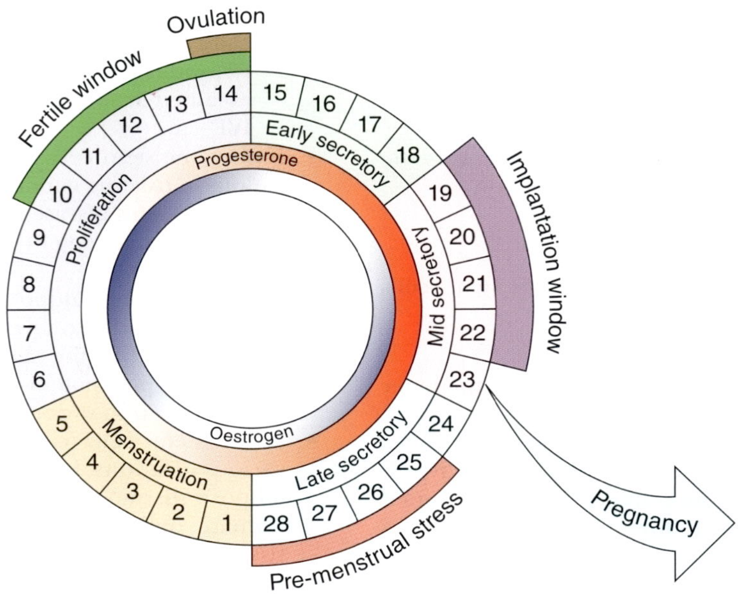

Fig. 6.6 The menstrual cycle. typically depicted as a 28-day period, varies in length among women and across different stages of reproductive life (Bull et al., 2019). It involves fluctuations in oestradiol and progesterone levels, as shown in the inner circles. The fertile window represents the days leading up to ovulation, presenting the highest likelihood of pregnancy through intercourse. The implantation window aligns with the mid-secretory phase of the cycle.

POINTS TO PONDER

- In the first week of development, several key events occur:
  - The zygote undergoes **cleavage division**, with stages from 2-cell to 16-cell.
  - Formation of the **morula**, which enters the uterine cavity.
  - The morula undergoes compaction, with outer cells forming protective coverings (**trophoblasts**) and inner cells giving rise to the **embryo.**
  - The blastocyst forms as the morula develops a fluid-filled cavity (**blastocele**).
  - Implantation occurs during the secretory phase of the menstrual cycle, with the **zona pellucida** disappearing and the trophoblast eroding the endometrium (Fig. 6.6).
- Under light microscope, the **zona pellucida** appears as a translucent membrane surrounding the following structures till it is shed off before implantation:
  - **Primary oocyte.**
  - **Zygote.**
  - **Morula.**
  - **Very early blastocyst.**

BRAIN TEASERS

1. What is the typical human gestation period, starting from the last menstrual period (LMP)?
   A. 38 weeks
   B. 40 weeks
   C. 42 weeks
   D. 36 weeks
2. During which stage of pregnancy does the embryonic period occur?
   A. First trimester
   B. Second trimester
   C. Third trimester
   D. Fourth trimester
3. The embryonic period includes two distinct phases, one of which is the germinal period. How long does the germinal period last?
   A. 3 weeks
   B. 4 weeks
   C. 8 weeks
   D. 12 weeks
4. What is the name of the stage that follows the morula during early embryonic development?
   A. Blastocyst
   B. Zygote

C. Trophoblast
D. Foetus

5. What is the primary function of the zona pellucida during early embryonic development?
   A. To provide nutrition to the embryo.
   B. To act as a barrier for sperm entry.
   C. To initiate the acrosomal reaction in sperm.
   D. To regulate implantation.
6. Which process increases intercellular contact during the morula stage of embryonic development?
   A. Compaction
   B. Cleavage division
   C. Formation of trophoblast
   D. Implantation
7. The nomenclature of the trophoblast depends on its attachment to the embryoblast. What is the term for the trophoblast covering the embryonic pole?
   A. Polar trophoblast
   B. Mural trophoblast
   C. Inner cell mass
   D. Trophoblastic cavity
8. During which phase of the menstrual cycle does implantation typically occur?
   A. Menstrual phase
   B. Proliferative phase
   C. Secretory phase
   D. Premenstrual phase
9. What term is used for pregnancy that occurs outside the uterus, such as in the fallopian tube?
   A. Extrauterine pregnancy
   B. Intrauterine pregnancy
   C. Placenta praevia
   D. Stem cell implantation
10. During which week of pregnancy does the embryonic period extend up to?
   A. 6th week
   B. 8th week
   C. 10th week
   D. 12th week

Answers

1. (B); 2. (A); 3. (A); 4. (A); 5. (B); 6. (A); 7. (A); 8. (C); 9. (A); 10. (B).

FURTHER READINGS

Alpha Scientists in Reproductive Medicine and ESHRE Special Interest Group of Embryology. The Istanbul consensus workshop on embryo assessment: proceedings of an expert meeting. *Hum Reprod.* 2011;26:1270-1283.

Deng W, Wang H. Efficient cell chatting between embryo and uterus ensures embryo implantation†. *Biol Reprod.* 2022;107(1):339-348. doi:10.1093/biolre/ioac135.

Muter J, Lynch VJ, McCoy RC, Brosens JJ. Human embryo implantation. *Development.* 2023;150(10): dev201507. doi:10.1242/dev.201507.

Ray, P., De, A., Yaghoubi, S., & Khanna, A. (2015). Application of Adult Stem Cells in Medicine. *Stem cells international, 2015,* 258313. https://doi.org/10.1155/2015/258313

7 Second Week of Development

AN 78.4 Describe the formation of extraembryonic mesoderm and coelom, bilaminar disc.
AN 78.5 Describe in brief abortion, decidual reaction and pregnancy test.
AN 80.1 Describe formation, functions and fate of chorion, amnion, yolk sac and decidua.

ANAMNESE

A 29-year-old woman presented for her first prenatal visit during the second week of her pregnancy with mild nausea and abdominal discomfort. Routine ultrasound revealed an unexpected finding—a vesicular mole in her uterus, characterized by the presence of grape-like clusters of fluid-filled vesicles. Beta-hCG levels were notably elevated. This unexpected diagnosis raised concerns about the viability of her pregnancy. The patient was counselled about the nature of the vesicular mole and its potential risks, including the risk of developing into a gestational trophoblastic neoplasm. An immediate suction dilation and curettage (D&C) procedure was performed to remove the abnormal tissue. Subsequent histopathological examination confirmed the presence of a complete hydatidiform mole.

Yolk sac is the first recognizable structure inside the gestational sac. Its size in relation to the gestational age can be indicative of outcomes, with a smaller yolk sac often associated with less favourable results and an unusually large yolk sac raising concerns. It is important to ensure that the number of yolk sacs aligns with the number of embryos present.

During the **second week of development**:

- The blastocyst's **implantation** concludes around the 12th day.
- The penetration site in the endometrium is sealed by a **fibrin plug**.
- Morphological changes in the embryoblast lead to the formation of a **bilaminar germ disc**, composed of the epiblast and hypoblast.
- This bilaminar germ disc gives rise to all the embryonic tissues and organs.
- The second week also witnesses the development of **extraembryonic structures**, including the amniotic cavity, yolk sac (umbilical vesicle), chorionic sac, amnion, chorion, primary villus and connecting stalk.

CHANGES IN THE GERM DISC (AN 78.4; AN 80.1)

- Cells of the inner cell mass or embryoblast differentiate into **two layers** (eighth day) (Fig. 7.1):
  1. **Epiblast/primary ectoderm.**
     The thicker layer consisting of high columnar cells related to the amniotic cavity.
  2. **Hypoblast/primary endoderm.**
     Consisting of flattened or cuboidal cells adjacent to the exocoelomic cavity.
- **Two cavities** develop in relation with epiblast and hypoblast.
- The space created within the epiblast due to its separation from the cytotrophoblast is termed

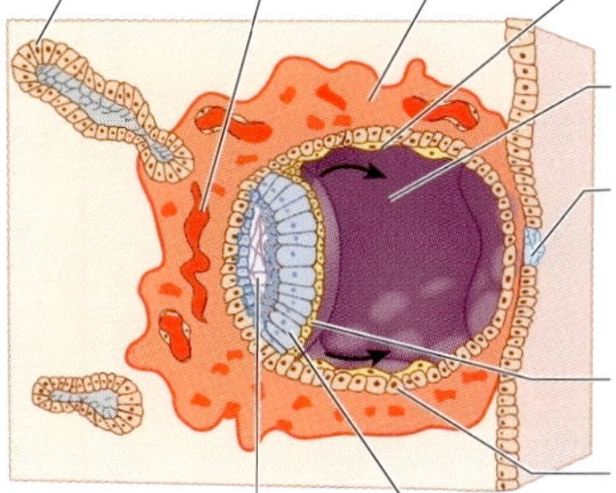

Fig. 7.1 An implanted blastocyst showing bilaminar germ disc.

the **amniotic cavity**. This amniotic cavity is filled with amniotic fluid, known as 'liquor amnii' in Latin.

- Epiblast cells adjacent to the cytotrophoblast are referred to as amnioblasts. Along with the rest of the epiblast, they form the lining of the amniotic cavity.
- Flattened cells originating from the hypoblast, often referred to as **Heuser's membrane**, extend to line the inner surface of the blastocystic cavity.
- This membrane, in conjunction with the hypoblast, collectively comprises the lining of the exocoelomic cavity, also known as the **Primitive Yolk sac**. (It is worth noting that some authors suggest that the cells lining the primitive yolk sac may have their origins in the cytotrophoblast).
- Simultaneously, the cells of the trophoblast (occasionally originating from the yolk sac) give rise to a cluster of cells termed the **extraembryonic mesoderm or primary mesoderm**. This layer is situated between the trophoblast and the flattened endodermal cells that line the yolk sac.
- The extraembryonic mesoderm serves to separate the wall of the amniotic cavity from the trophoblast, but it does not contribute to the development of any embryonic tissues.
- Over time, small cavities emerge within the extraembryonic mesoderm, which eventually merge to form a larger cavity known as the extraembryonic or **chorionic cavity** (refer to Fig. 7.2).
- The chorionic cavity encircles both the primitive yolk sac and the amniotic cavity, except at the point where the germ disc remains connected to the trophoblast through the **connecting stalk**.
- As blood vessels develop, the connecting stalk transforms into the **umbilical cord**.
- The sole location where the extraembryonic mesoderm traverses the chorionic cavity is within the connecting stalk.
- As the chorionic cavity forms, the extraembryonic mesoderm undergoes a division into two distinct layers:
  - The mesoderm that lines the inner aspect of the trophoblast and the outer aspect of the amniotic cavity is termed the **Parietal or Somatopleuric Extraembryonic mesoderm**.
  - The mesoderm that lines the outer aspect of the primitive yolk sac is referred to as the **Visceral or Splanchnopleuric Extraembryonic mesoderm**.
- Concurrently, the hypoblast generates additional cells that migrate along the inner surface of Heuser's membrane.
- These cells subsequently undergo proliferation, gradually giving rise to a novel cavity within the exocoelomic cavity, now recognized as the **Secondary Yolk sac or Definitive Yolk sac** (as depicted in Fig. 7.3).
- It is important to note that the secondary yolk sac is notably smaller in size when compared to the primitive yolk sac.
- During its development, a significant portion of the primitive yolk sac undergoes pinching-off, leading to the formation of **two distinct yolk sacs** by the end of the 13th day:
  - The primitive yolk sac, which eventually degenerates.
  - The secondary yolk sac.
- The somatopleuric layer of extraembryonic mesoderm in conjunction with the trophoblast is referred to as the **chorion**.
- Separating the embryo, along with its amnion and yolk sac, from the outer wall of the blastocyst (now termed the chorion) is the **extraembryonic coelom**.
- The amnion, yolk sac and chorion all adopt a **two-layered structure** as a consequence of the division of the extraembryonic mesoderm into two distinct layers.
- Consequently, the amnion and chorion comprise extraembryonic ectoderm and mesoderm, while the yolk sac is composed of extraembryonic endoderm and mesoderm.

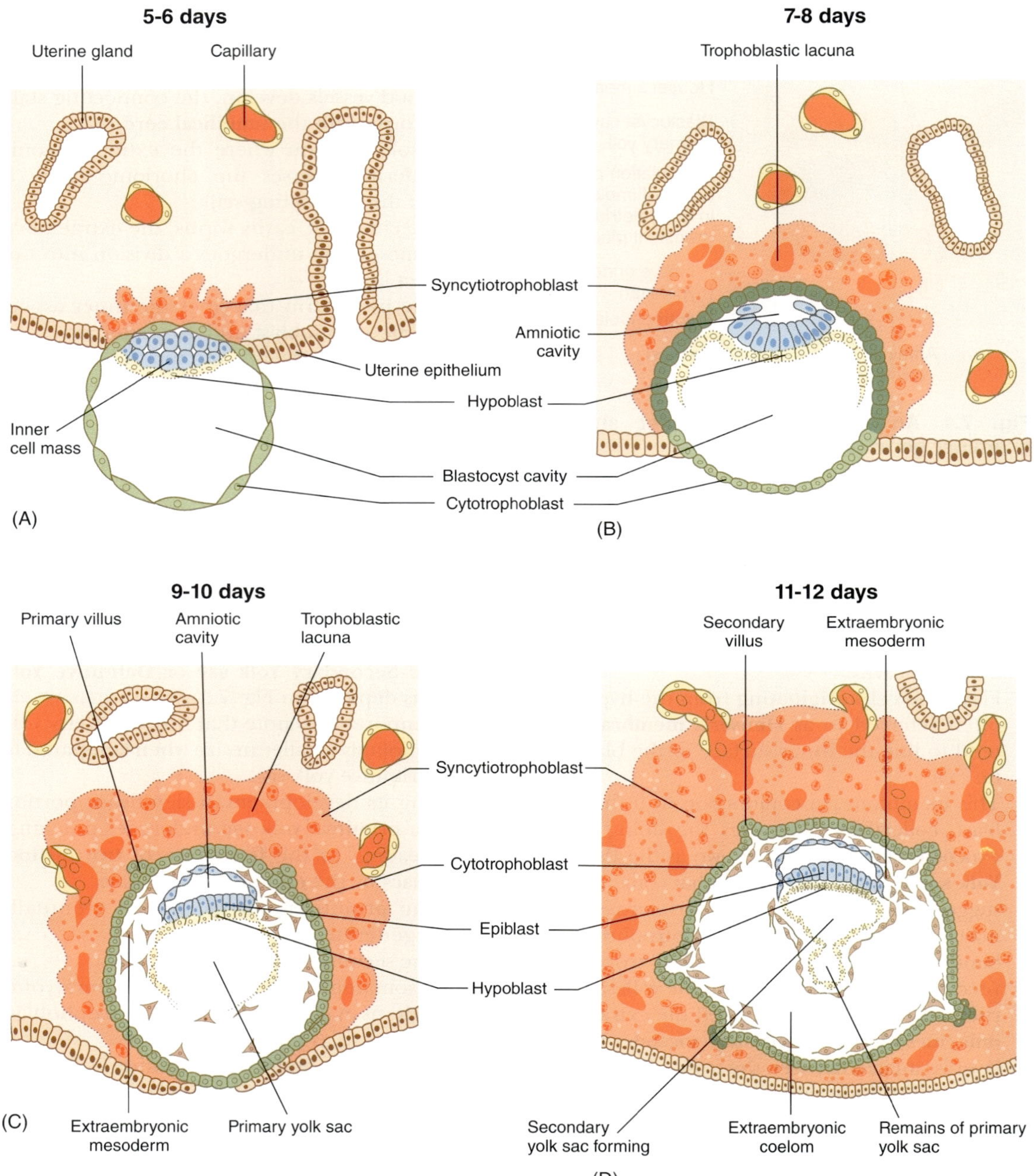

Fig. 7.2 Human blastocyst showing formation of secondary yolk sac. Major stages in implantation of a human embryo. (A) The syncytiotrophoblast is just beginning to invade the endometrial stroma. (B) Most of the embryo is embedded in the endometrium; there is early formation of the trophoblastic lacunae. The amniotic cavity and yolk sac are beginning to form. (C) Implantation is almost complete, primary villi are forming, and the extraembryonic mesoderm is appearing. (D) Implantation is complete; secondary villi are forming. (Source: *Human Embryology and Developmental Biology.* 4th ed. 2009.)

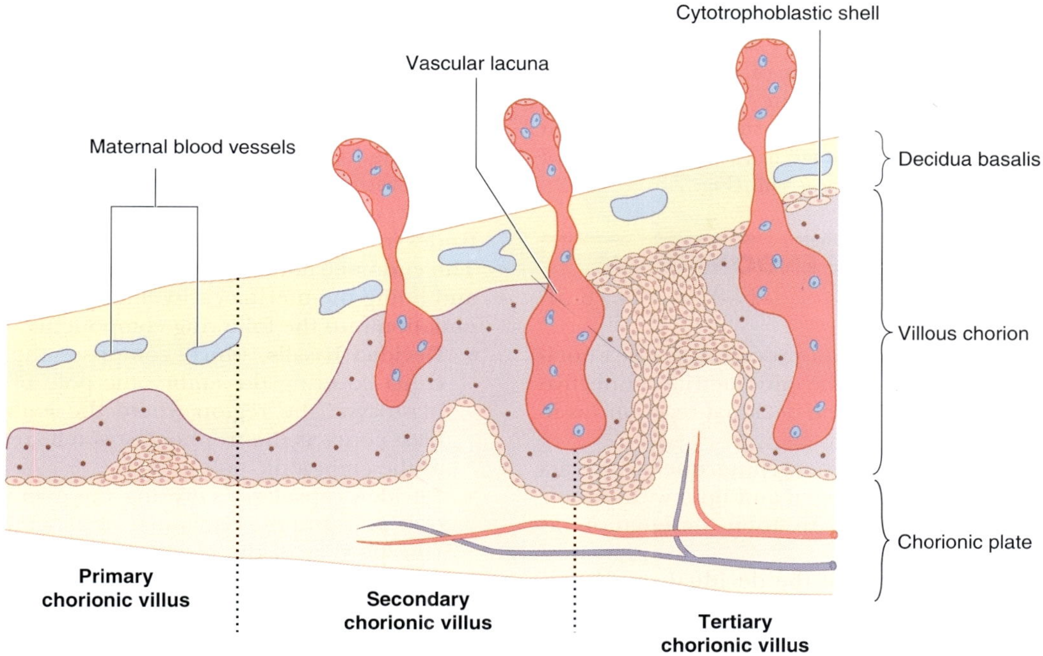

Fig. 7.3 Formation of chorionic villi.

CHANGES IN THE TROPHOBLAST

- By the eighth day of development, the blastocyst becomes partially embedded within the endometrial stroma (see Fig. 7.2).
- Over the embryoblast region, the trophoblast undergoes differentiation into two distinct layers:
  - **The cytotrophoblast**, a layer of actively dividing cells that generate new cells. These cells migrate into the growing syncytiotrophoblast mass, where they merge, losing their individual cell membranes.
  - **The syncytiotrophoblast**, a rapidly expanding, multinucleated structure with no distinct cell boundaries.
- The erosive syncytiotrophoblast infiltrates the endometrial connective tissue, gradually facilitating the embedding of the blastocyst into the endometrium.
- Syncytiotrophoblastic cells displace endometrial cells at the implantation site.
- Endometrial cells undergo **apoptosis**, or programmed cell death, further aiding in the invasion process.
- Within the syncytiotrophoblast, **lacunar spaces** begin to appear and are separated by **trabeculae** (syncytiotrophoblast).
- This stage of trophoblast development is known as the **lacunar stage**.
- Soon, these lacunae become filled with a mixture of maternal blood from ruptured endometrial capillaries.
- The fluid within the lacunar spaces, known as **embryotroph** (with 'trophe' denoting nourishment in Greek), diffuses into the embryonic disc and provides essential nutrients to the developing embryo.
- The connection between eroded endometrial capillaries and the lacunae establishes the **primordial uteroplacental circulation** (as depicted in Fig. 7.2).
- Oxygenated blood enters the lacunae from the spiral **endometrial arteries**, while poorly oxygenated blood is removed from them through the **endometrial veins**.
- As the trophoblast continues to erode an increasing number of sinusoids, maternal blood begins to flow through the trophoblastic system, thus establishing the **uteroplacental circulation**.

- The conclusion of the second week is marked by the emergence of **primary chorionic villi**, which involve the proliferation of cytotrophoblast as cellular extensions within the syncytiotrophoblast. This formation of primary chorionic villi represents the **first stage** in the development of the placenta's chorionic villi (Fig. 7.3).

CHANGES IN THE ENDOMETRIUM (AN 80.1; AN 78.5)

During the implantation process, there is a notable transformation in the endometrial connective tissue cells, known as the decidual reaction (as illustrated in Fig. 7.4).

- These cells undergo swelling due to the accumulation of glycogen and lipid within their cytoplasm, leading to their designation as **decidual cells**.
- The primary role of the decidual reaction is to provide essential **nourishment for the early embryo** and to create an immunologically privileged site for the developing conceptus.
- The endometrium consists of three distinct layers:
  - **Stratum compactum.**
  - **Stratum spongiosum.**
  - **Stratum basale.**
- Following implantation, the blastocyst initially lodges within the **stratum compactum**.
- As the embryo grows, it subsequently protrudes into the uterine cavity.
- The endometrium surrounding the conceptus and lining the uterine cavity undergoes differentiation into the following components:
  - **Decidua basalis**, which comprises the decidua covering the embryonic pole of the blastocyst (the region where the embryoblast contacts the trophoblast is referred to as the embryonic pole).
  - **Decidua capsularis**, covering the abembryonic pole and the remainder of the embryo (the portion of the blastocyst opposite the embryonic pole where the embryoblast is attached is known as the abembryonic pole).
  - **Decidua parietalis**, which represents the remainder of the decidua lining the uterine cavity.

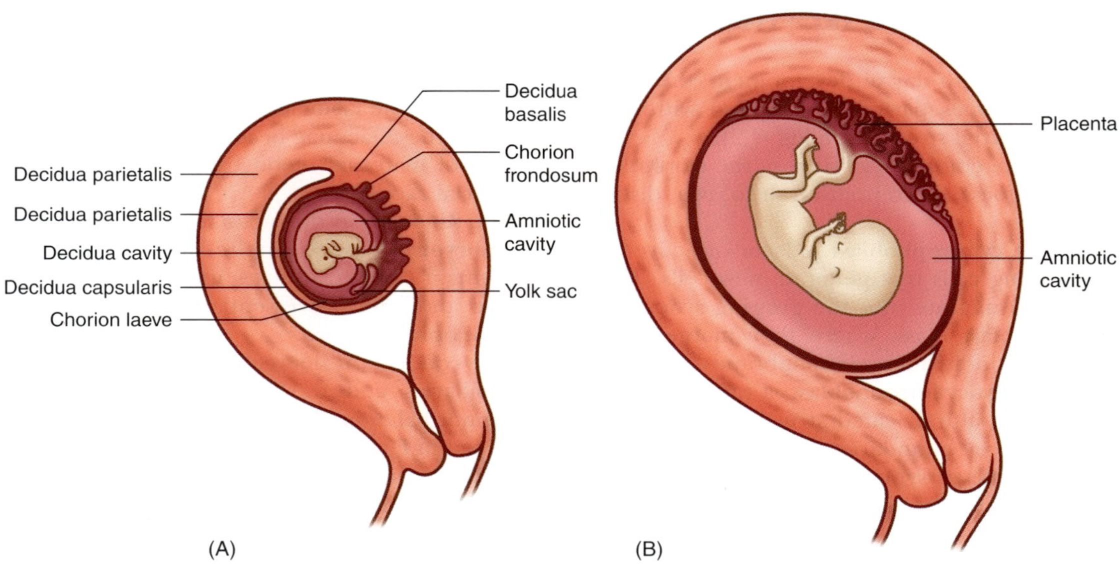

Fig. 7.4 The uterine cavity with the foetus showing deciduas. (A) The inner ring of decidua capsularis and the outer ring of decidua parietalis with the intervening uterine cavity (not labelled) known as 'double decidual sign' allows discrimination of deciduas in USG (at eight weeks of gestation). (B) The amnion is fused with chorion obliterating chorionic cavity and yolk sac. Further growth of the foetus results in the fusion of decidua capsularis with decidua parietalis, thus eliminating double decidual sign.

CLINICAL NUGGETS (AN 78.5)

Pregnancy tests

- **Early pregnancy factor** (a member of the heat-shock protein family) becomes detectable in maternal blood within **36–48 hours after fertilization**.
- This factor is commonly referred to as the **pregnancy-specific protein** and serves to offer immunological protection to the developing embryo.
- While it is produced by the embryo, its presence in the **maternal serum** is attributed to its synthesis and secretion by the ovary.
- The diagnosis of early pregnancy can be established with an accuracy of 88.6% by detecting **early pregnancy factor (EPF)** activity in maternal serum within 2 days after ovulation.
- This breakthrough provides a valuable foundation for pregnancy diagnosis, particularly for women seeking safe termination or those who experience unexpected conception.
- The syncytiotrophoblast of the placenta actively generates **human chorionic gonadotropin (hCG)** during the initial two months of pregnancy.
- This hormone is produced by foetal tissues and is excreted in the mother's urine, serving as the foundation for **urine pregnancy tests (UPT)**.

Abortion

Miscarriages and induced abortions:

- Approximately 50% of fertilized eggs that do not reach maturity undergo spontaneous abortion.
- These spontaneous abortions, also known as miscarriages, often transpire during the **first three weeks** of pregnancy.
- Due to the small size of the embryo during this early stage, they frequently go unnoticed by the mother and are mistaken for a heavy menstrual period.
- A significant portion of the embryos that are aborted in this manner exhibit **chromosomal abnormalities**, serving as a natural mechanism to mitigate the occurrence of severely malformed infants.
- Folic acid antagonists, such as **Aminopterin**, have been employed in clinical trials as abortifacients.
- Embryos that manage to survive the abortion process after the administration of this drug often exhibit severe **malformations**, including conditions like anencephaly and cleft lip and palate.
- This underscores the critical importance of ensuring an adequate intake of **folic acid** in one's diet to support normal development.
- Abortion, whether spontaneous or induced, can be brought about through chemical, surgical or other means prior to **20 weeks of gestation**, a point often considered nonviable.
- The act of abortion may be conducted legally or illegally. When performed legally, it is referred to as **Medical Termination of Pregnancy (MTP)**.

KLINISCHE PERLEN

HYDATIDIFORM MOLE (MOLAR PREGNANCY) AND GESTATIONAL TROPHOBLASTIC DISEASE

- A hydatidiform mole, also known as a **molar pregnancy**, is a form of gestational trophoblastic disease.
- It occurs when a **nonviable fertilized egg** implants in the uterus.
- In these instances, trophoblastic tissue is present in the **absence of female pronuclei**, suggesting that the development of the trophoblast is primarily regulated by **paternal genes**.
- There are two main types of molar pregnancy, as illustrated in Fig. 7.5:
  - **Partial mole:**
    - A haploid egg is fertilized either by two sperm or by one sperm.
    - It contains some foetal tissue but **lacks a viable foetus.**
    - Sperm undergoes mitosis, resulting in genotypes of **69,XXY (triploid) or 92, XXXY (tetraploid).**
  - **Complete mole:**
    - Represents a pregnancy **without an embryo.**
    - Occurs when a single (monospermic) or two sperms (dispermic) combine with **an egg that has lost its DNA.**
    - In the case of a single sperm, the male pronucleus reduplicates, forming a 'complete' 46-chromosome set.
    - The genotype is **46,XX (diploid)** due to the mitosis of the fertilizing sperm, but it can also be **46,XY (diploid).**

      Note: Complete hydatidiform moles may progress into **choriocarcinoma** or evolve into **invasive moles.**

GENOMIC IMPRINTING

- Genomic imprinting involves the differential expression of homologous chromosome regions based on whether the **genetic material is inherited from the mother or the father.**
- Distinct clinical symptoms seen in **Angelman syndrome** (maternal) and **Prader-Willi syndrome** (paternal) result from microdeletions occurring on the same **chromosome 15.**

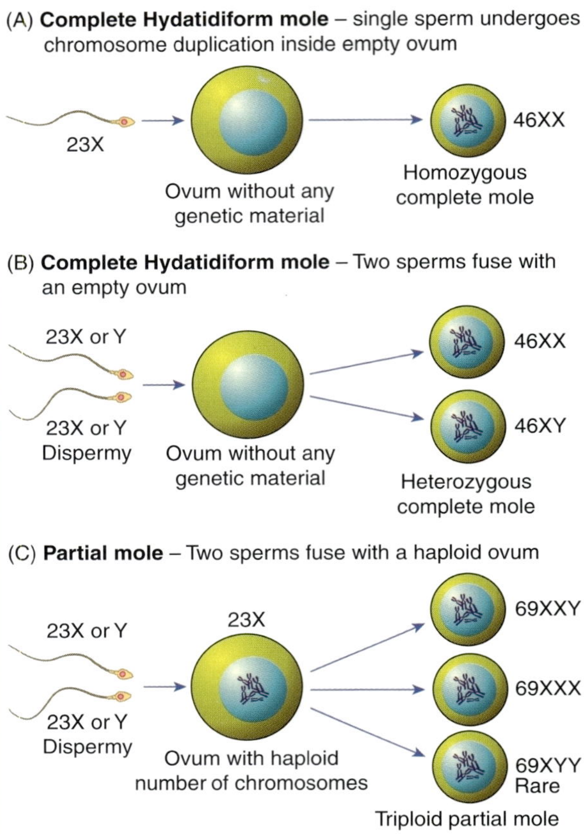

Fig. 7.5 Different types of hydatidiform mole.

Angelman Syndrome

- Angelman syndrome arises from deletions or mutations within the **maternal chromosome 15q11-q13 region.**
- This condition is associated with the acronym **SAPI,** characterized by:
  - **S**eizures.
  - **A**phasia.
  - **P**aroxysms of laughter.
  - **I**ntellectual disability.

Prader-Willi Syndrome

- Prader-Willi syndrome is caused by the absence of expression of imprinted genes in the **paternally derived region (i.e. 15q11.2-q13) of chromosome 15**, resulting from several genetic mechanisms, including paternal deletion, maternal uniparental disomy 15 and, rarely, an imprinting defect.
- This syndrome is marked by the acronym **HHOS**, presenting with:
  - **H**ypotonia.
  - **H**ypogonadism.
  - **O**besity.
  - **S**evere intellectual disability.

X CHROMOSOME INACTIVATION

- X chromosome inactivation is a crucial process in female development.
- To compensate for the single X chromosome in males, one of the two active X chromosomes in a female blastocyst is randomly inactivated.
- The **inactivated X chromosome** undergoes condensation to form a structure known as the **Barr body** (Fig. 7.6).
- Importantly, during the early stages of embryonic development, both X chromosomes in female embryos remain active.
- X-chromosome inactivation involves the transcriptional silencing of one X chromosome.
- Both X chromosomes have an equal probability of being silenced.
- Once the silencing is established, it remains stable across all subsequent cell generations, with the same X chromosome continuing to be inactivated.

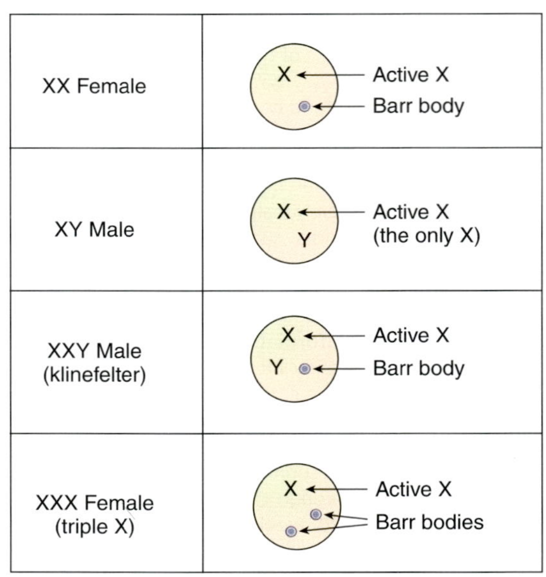

Fig. 7.6 Barr body and X inactivation.

POINTS TO PONDER

Second Week of Development

- In the second week, the embryoblast undergoes differentiation into **two distinct layers**, the epiblast and the hypoblast, forming a **bilaminar embryonic germ disc.**
- Within the embryonic pole of the blastocyst, the **amniotic cavity** begins to develop, positioned between the epiblast and the trophoblast.
- The **amnion**, one of the four extraembryonic membranes, lines the amniotic cavity.
- Cells from the embryonic disc give rise to both the embryo itself and the various extraembryonic membranes.
- This includes the formation of the **primary yolk sac**, which is lined by the exocoelomic membrane or Heuser's membrane, as well as the **secondary yolk sac**, also known as the definitive yolk sac.
- Another important development is the emergence of a new cavity, the **extraembryonic coelom, or chorionic cavity**, which forms as the extraembryonic mesoderm splits into two layers.
- With the splitting of the extraembryonic mesoderm, both the amnion and yolk sac become double-layered structures:
  - The **amnion** now consists of an inner ectoderm and an outer mesoderm layer.
  - The **yolk sac** is composed of an inner endoderm and an outer mesoderm layer.
- The outer wall of the blastocyst is referred to as the **chorion**, which also contains a layer of mesoderm.
- The trophoblast undergoes differentiation into **cytotrophoblast and syncytiotrophoblast**, both of which contribute to the formation of the extraembryonic membranes.

Event	Description
Rule of twos	Memory aid for second-week developmental events
Embryoblast split	Division of the embryoblast into epiblast and hypoblast
Trophoblast differentiation	Trophoblast giving rise to cytotrophoblast and syncytiotrophoblast
Yolk sac formation	Formation of two yolk sacs—primary and secondary
New cavity development	Emergence of two new cavities: amniotic cavity and chorionic cavity
Extraembryonic mesoderm split	Splitting of the extraembryonic mesoderm into two layers
Membrane development	Development of two-layered membranes: amnion, yolk sac and chorion

BRAIN TEASERS

1. What is the function of the extraembryonic mesoderm in the early development of the embryo?
   A. It contributes to the formation of embryonic tissues.
   B. It helps create the amniotic cavity.
   C. It produces the yolk sac.
   D. It separates the wall of the amniotic cavity from the trophoblast.
2. What is the role of the secondary yolk sac in embryonic development?
   A. It primarily functions as a nutrient reservoir.
   B. It is the first structure to develop in the embryo.
   C. It is larger in size compared to the primary yolk sac.
   D. It is much smaller than the primitive yolk sac.
3. What does the term 'chorion' refer to in the context of embryonic development?
   A. The outer wall of the blastocyst.
   B. The lining of the amniotic cavity.
   C. The primary yolk sac.
   D. The extraembryonic ectoderm.
4. What is the term for the stage of trophoblast development characterized by the appearance of lacunar spaces filled with maternal blood within the syncytiotrophoblast?
   A. Syncytial stage
   B. Erosive stage
   C. Lacunar stage
   D. Apoptotic stage
5. What is the role of the embryotroph within the lacunar spaces in the syncytiotrophoblast during the second week of development?
   A. It facilitates the formation of primary chorionic villi.
   B. It provides nourishment to the developing embryo.
   C. It aids in the differentiation of cytotrophoblast.
   D. It contributes to the establishment of uteroplacental circulation.
6. What is the primary function of the decidual reaction in the endometrium during implantation?
   A. It aids in the attachment of the embryo to the uterine wall.
   B. It promotes the proliferation of decidual cells.
   C. It provides nourishment for the early embryo and creates an immunologically privileged site.
   D. It facilitates the development of the embryonic pole.
7. Which part of the endometrium is referred to as decidua basalis?
   A. The region surrounding the embryonic pole of the blastocyst.
   B. The region where the embryo initially lodges within the endometrium.
   C. The portion opposite the embryonic pole.
   D. The part that lines the uterine cavity.
8. What is the primary characteristic that distinguishes a complete mole from a partial mole in gestational trophoblastic disease?
   A. The presence of foetal tissue.

B. The occurrence of two sperm fertilizing a haploid egg.
C. The diploid genotype.
D. The potential for progression into choriocarcinoma.

9. In the context of molar pregnancies, what is the role of paternal genes in the development of trophoblastic tissue?
A. They do not play a role in trophoblast development.
B. They regulate the development of the female pronuclei.
C. They control the development of the male pronucleus.
D. They primarily regulate the development of the trophoblast.

10. What is the term for the condensed, inactivated X chromosome in a female cell?
A. Barr chromosome
B. Silent X
C. Inactive X
D. Barr body

Answers

1. (D); 2. (D); 3. (A); 4. (C); 5. (B); 6. (C); 7. (A); 8. (C); 9. (D); 10. (D).

FURTHER READINGS

Lin M, Chen J, Liao B, He Z, Lin S, Luo Y. When a vesicular placenta meets a live fetus: case report of twin pregnancy with a partial hydatidiform mole. *BMC Pregnancy Childbirth.* 2021;21(1):694. doi:10.1186/s12884-021-04160-2.

Mengel-From J, Lindahl-Jacobsen R, Nygaard M, et al. Skewness of X-chromosome inactivation increases with age and varies across birth cohorts in elderly Danish women. *Sci Rep.* 2021;11(1):4326. doi:10.1038/s41598-021-83702-2.

Tang Y, Zhu C, Zhu C, et al. The impact of pre-evacuation ultrasound examination in histologically confirmed hydatidiform mole in missed abortion. *BMC Womens Health.* 2020;20(1):196. doi:10.1186/s12905-020-01064-9.

Wang TS, Tsai WH, Tsai LP, Wong SB. Clinical characteristics and epilepsy in genomic imprinting disorders: Angelman syndrome and Prader-Willi syndrome. *Ci Ji Yi Xue Za Zhi.* 2019;32(2):137-144. doi:10.4103/tcmj.tcmj_103_19.

8 Third Week of Development

AN 78.4 Describe the formation of prochordal plate.
AN 79.1 Describe the formation and fate of the primitive streak.
AN 79.2 Describe formation and fate of notochord.
AN 79.5 Explain embryological basis of sacrococcygeal teratomas.
AN 79.5 Explain embryological basis of nucleus pulposus.
AN 80.1 Describe formation of allantois.

ANAMNESE

A pregnant woman presented with recurrent miscarriages, prompting a thorough investigation. Genetic testing revealed a mutation affecting the formation of the primitive streak in the developing embryo. The primitive streak plays a fundamental role in establishing the body's overall structure, and its impairment resulted in failed embryonic development. This case emphasized the importance of the primitive streak in early embryogenesis the underlying cause of the recurrent miscarriages and future management and counselling for the patient.

Gastrulation is a remarkable developmental process that takes the undifferentiated mass of cells from the blastula stage and transforms it into a gastrula, characterized by the emergence of three distinct germ layers: the **endoderm, mesoderm** and **ectoderm**. This process involves the specialization of pluripotent embryonic cells into specific cell types like muscles and neurons, resulting in a shift from a two-dimensional blastula to a complex three-dimensional model.

- A pivotal event in the third week of embryonic development, gastrulation defines the formation of the **trilaminar germ disc**, as intraembryonic mesoderm inserts itself between the two primary germ layers (Fig. 8.1).
- The third week of development is a critical period during which the embryo is particularly vulnerable to the detrimental effects of **teratogenic factors** (teratogenic insult).

CHANGES IN THE GERM DISC

GASTRULATION

- The circular bilaminar germ disc, initially formed during the second week of development, undergoes a transformation, becoming more oval in shape.
- This alteration results in the formation of a pear-shaped disc characterized by a broader cephalic (head) region and a narrower caudal (tail) end.
- The bilaminar embryonic disc evolves into a **trilaminar germ disc** through the invagination of pluripotent cells originating from the epiblast layer, which migrate into the space between the two primary layers.
- The three primary germ layers are now distinctly established: ectoderm, mesoderm and endoderm.

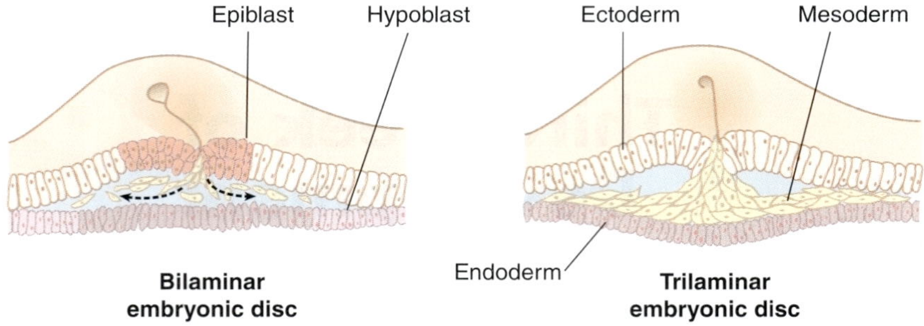

Fig. 8.1 Formation of trilaminar germ disc.

- This crucial process is important in defining the embryo's axial orientation and signifies the initiation of morphogenesis.
- Within the epiblast layer, further differentiation leads to the development of several structures:
  - **Surface ectoderm**, responsible for forming the epidermis of the skin.
  - **Neuroectodermal cells**, which play a role in shaping the neural plate, a crucial structure for central nervous system development.
  - **The primitive streak**, located in the caudal portion of the epiblast, forms a distinct elevation that protrudes into the amniotic cavity.

PRIMITIVE STREAK (AN 79.1)

- Gastrulation initiates with the emergence of the primitive streak on the surface of the epiblast, as illustrated in Fig. 8.2.

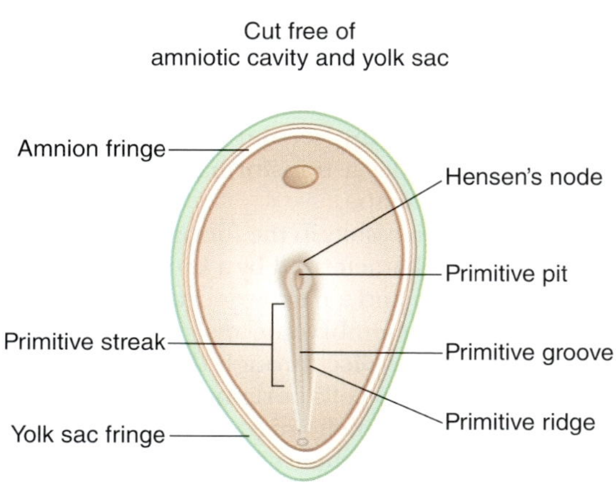

Fig. 8.2 Formation of primitive streak on the surface of epiblast.

- By the **15th day** of development, the craniocaudal axis is firmly established, setting the stage for further embryonic differentiation.
- The primitive streak serves as the **primary organizer**, inducing the differentiation of critical structures such as the notochord and intraembryonic mesoderm.
- At the cephalic end, a distinctive knob-like thickening known as the **primitive node (or Hensen's node)** becomes apparent.
- A depression forms at the centre of the Hensen's node, referred to as the **primitive pit**.
- A narrow groove, known as the **primitive groove**, appears within the primitive streak and maintains continuity with the primitive pit.
- Pluripotent ectodermal cells rapidly proliferate, filling the space between the epiblast and hypoblast during the process of gastrulation, leading to the development of **intraembryonic mesoderm** (depicted in Fig. 8.3).
- Epiblast cells displace the hypoblast layer to establish the **definitive endoderm**.
- Subsequently, the epiblast is redesignated as the **definitive ectoderm.**
- Ultimately, the three primary germ layers—ectoderm, mesoderm and endoderm—all originate from these pluripotent epiblast cells.

FUNCTIONS OF PRIMITIVE STREAK

The primitive streak plays a significant role in embryonic development and gives rise to various essential structures and functions:

1. **Intraembryonic Mesoderm:** The primitive streak is responsible for the formation of intraembryonic mesoderm, a fundamental tissue that contributes to the development of various

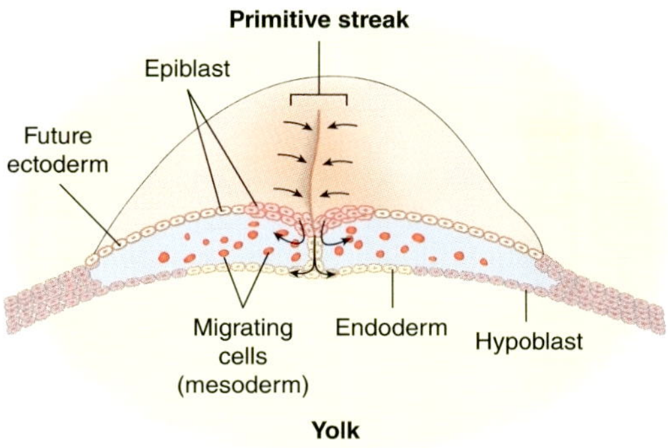

Fig. 8.3 Formation of intraembryonic mesoderm.

organ systems, including the skeletal, muscular and circulatory systems.

2. **Notochord:** It serves as the origin of the notochord, a critical structure that plays a central role in the formation of the axial skeleton and the development of the nervous system.
3. **Septum Transversum:** The primitive streak also contributes to the septum transversum, which is essential for the formation of the diaphragm, separating the thoracic and abdominal cavities.
4. **Determining the Future Craniocaudal Axis:** Through the formation of the primitive streak, the embryo's future craniocaudal (head-to-tail) axis is established, laying the foundation for the body's overall orientation and development.
5. **Embryo Bilateral Demarcation:** Additionally, the primitive streak demarcates the embryo into distinct left and right halves, facilitating the development of bilateral symmetry and the differentiation of structures on both sides of the body.

FATE OF PRIMITIVE STREAK (AN 79.5)

As embryonic development progresses, the primitive streak undergoes several significant changes:

- **Gradual Diminishment:** After the fourth week of development, the primitive streak gradually decreases in size and becomes less prominent.
- **Sacrococcygeal Tumours (Teratomas):** Remnants of the primitive streak can sometimes persist and give rise to sacrococcygeal tumours, also known as teratomas. These tumours, found in the sacral region, are the **most common neonatal tumours**, with an incidence of approximately 1 in 35,000–40,000 live births.
- **Females** are more frequently affected by sacrococcygeal teratomas (with a 4:1 female-to-male ratio).
- **Congenital Anomalies:** Around 18% of infants with sacrococcygeal teratomas may have additional congenital anomalies.
- **Benign and Malignant Tumours:** Sacrococcygeal teratomas can be categorized as benign (mature) or malignant (immature), depending on their composition of embryonic elements.
- **Trilaminar Tissue Composition:** One distinctive characteristic of these tumours is that they contain tissues derived from **all three germ layers** (endoderm, mesoderm and ectoderm).
- **Altman Classification:** Researchers, including Altman et al., have classified sacrococcygeal teratomas into four groups (Fig. 8.4):
  - **Type I:** Type I tumours are mainly exterior, with minimal pelvic components.
  - **Type II:** Type II tumours exhibit a significant pelvic component, often resembling an hourglass shape.
  - **Type III:** Type III tumours have a larger proportion of intraabdominal and intrapelvic components compared to the external component.
  - **Type IV:** Type IV tumours are exclusively located in the presacral region, with no external component.
- **Teratogenic Effects:** Teratogens, which are agents that can cause congenital malformations, typically affect the germ disc between the 15th and 18th day of development. Consequently, both the primitive streak and notochord can be affected by these teratogenic influences.

FORMATION OF NOTOCHORD (AN 79.2)

The notochord is a midline structure that develops in the region between the cranial end of the primitive streak and the caudal end of the prechordal plate. This process can be described in the following stages:

- **Initiation of Notochord Formation:** The process begins as cells in the region of the primitive node proliferate and migrate cranially through the primitive pit, giving rise to a median solid

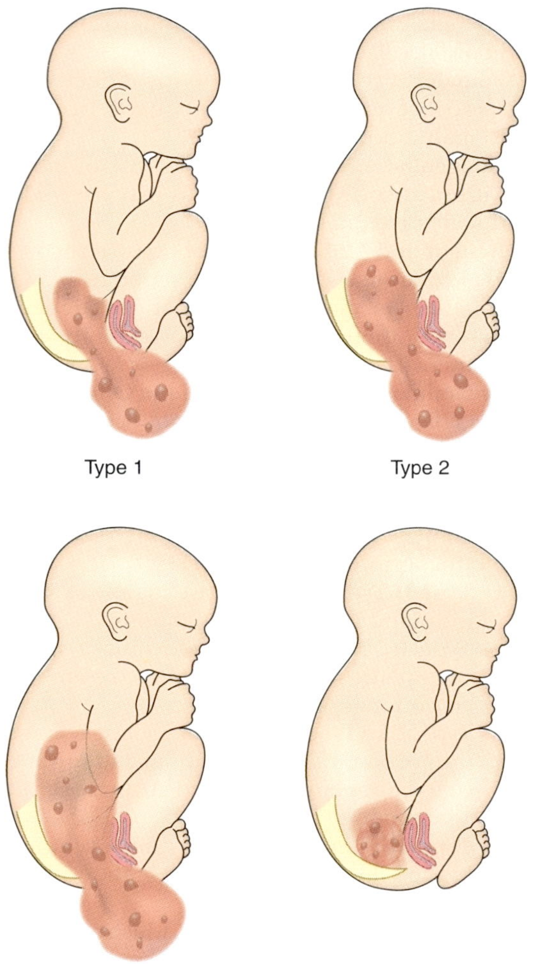

Fig. 8.4 Different types of sacrococcygeal teratomas.

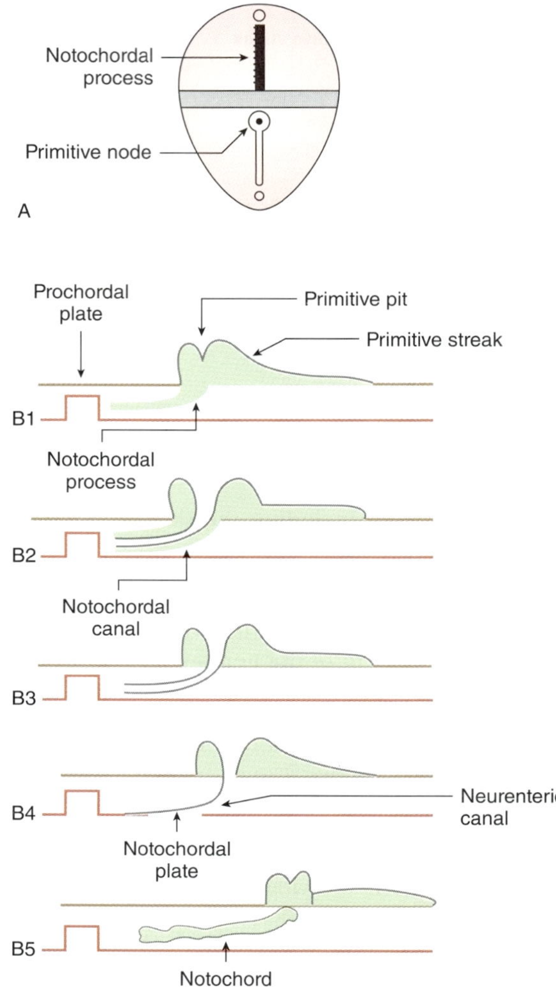

Fig. 8.5 Formation of notochord.

cellular cord called the **notochordal process or head process.**

- **Development of the Notochordal Canal:** The primitive pit extends into the notochord, leading to the formation of the **notochordal canal.**
- **Fusion With the Endoderm:** The floor of the notochordal canal fuses with the adjacent endoderm.
- **Breakdown of Fused Layer:** Subsequently, the fused layer starts to break down, creating openings in the floor of the notochordal canal (refer to Fig. 8.5).
- **Formation of the Neurenteric Canal:** This breakdown establishes a communication channel between the **amniotic cavity and the yolk sac**, which is known as the **neurenteric canal**. The neurenteric canal serves as a means for nutritional exchange through diffusion to the ectodermal surface since the embryo's circulatory system has not yet been established.
- **Remodelling of Canal Walls:** Over time, the walls of the neurenteric canal undergo reformation and become flattened.
- **Conversion into Notochordal Plate:** This transformation process results in the notochordal canal evolving into the notochordal plate (as shown in Fig. 8.5).

- **Formation of Definitive Notochord:** The notochordal plate subsequently undergoes a curved configuration, and cell proliferation within it converts it into a solid rod of cells, referred to as the definitive notochord (see Fig. 8.5).
- **Detachment and Ascension:** The definitive notochord detaches from its previous position and rises from the roof of the yolk sac. As a result, the endodermal layer becomes continuous.

FUNCTIONS OF NOTOCHORD

- **Establishment of Embryonic Disc's Central Axis:** The notochord plays a fundamental role in establishing the central axis of the embryonic disc, providing structural support and guidance for the developing embryo.
- **Induction of Neural Tube Formation:** It acts as a critical inducer for the formation of the neural tube from the ectoderm located above it. This process is essential for the development of the **nervous system.**
- **Scaffolding for Vertebral and Intervertebral Disc Formation:** The notochord serves as a central column around which the vertebral bodies and intervertebral discs develop, contributing to the structural framework of the vertebral column.

FATE OF NOTOCHORD (AN 79.5)

- **Replacement by Vertebral Column:** As development progresses, the notochord undergoes a transformation in which it is eventually replaced by the formation of the vertebral column.
- **Formation of Nucleus Pulposus:** Following the establishment of the vertebral column, the part of the notochord located between the vertebral bodies evolves into the nucleus pulposus, located at the central core of the vertebral discs (Fig. 8.6). The nucleus pulposus is a gel-like material composed of water and loosely bound collagen fibres. It is encircled by the **annulus fibrosus**, which originates from the sclerotomal cells. The presence of the nucleus pulposus within each intervertebral disc enables these structures to withstand the forces of compression and torsion, contributing to the spine's flexibility and shock-absorbing properties.
- **Remnants of Notochord:** Notable remnants of the original notochord persist in the adult body, primarily represented by the **nucleus pulposus** of each intervertebral disc and the **apical ligament of the dens** (Fig. 8.7). These structures, derived from the embryonic notochord, serve essential roles in the maintenance of the vertebral column's functionality and stability.

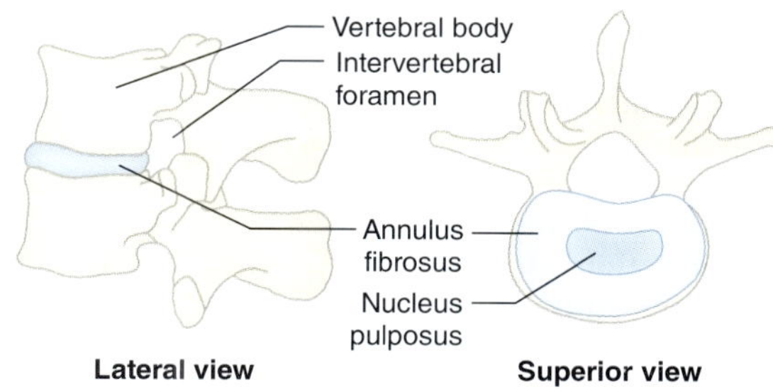

Fig. 8.6 Nucleus pulposus.

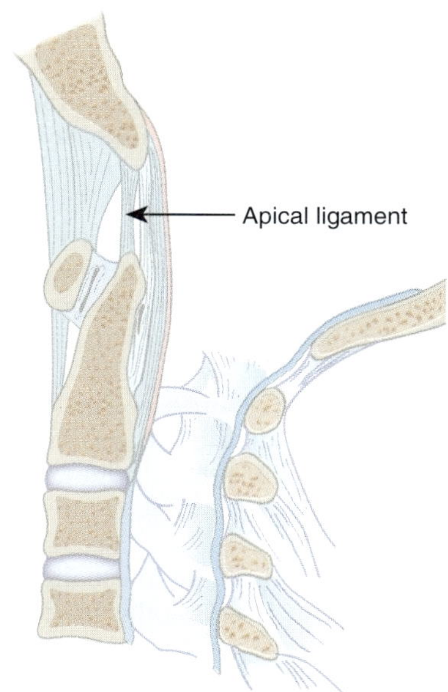

Fig. 8.7 Apical ligament of the dens (from the tip of the dens to the anterior margin of foramen magnum).

ALLANTOIC DIVERTICULUM (AN 80.1)

- The allantoic diverticulum is a small endodermal outgrowth that emerges from the caudal end of the **umbilical vesicle (yolk sac)** and extends towards the connecting stalk. This development typically occurs around the 16th day of embryonic development.

- **Vascularization of Chorion:** One of its vital functions is to facilitate the vascularization of the chorion and villi by establishing connections with the allantoic or umbilical blood vessels.
- **Formation of Umbilical Arteries:** The blood vessels within the allantoic stalk eventually transform into what will become the umbilical arteries, playing a crucial role in the circulatory system of the developing foetus.
- **Persistence as Urachus:** The proximal part of the allantoic diverticulum persists as the urachus, which is a tubular structure located between the bladder and the umbilicus throughout the developmental process (Fig. 8.8).
- **Adult Remnant:** In adults, the urachus is represented by the **median umbilical ligament**, serving as a remnant of this embryonic structure (Fig. 8.9).
- **Clinical Significance:** Defects or abnormalities in the development of the allantoic diverticulum are associated with various bladder-related issues and can impact overall urinary system development.
- **Absorption Into Hindgut:** As development progresses, the allantoic diverticulum undergoes absorption into the hindgut, marking the completion of its role in the embryonic development process.
- **Urachus anomalies:** The anomalies can result in a connection between the bladder and the umbilicus.
  1) **Patent Urachus/urachal fistula:** This occurs when the urachus fails to close completely after birth, leading to a persistent communication between the bladder and the umbilicus. This can result in urine leakage from the umbilicus.
  2) **Urachal Cyst:** In this case, the urachus partially closes, forming a cyst that may be filled with mucus. The cyst can become infected, causing pain and discomfort.
  3) **Urachal Sinus:** A urachal sinus is a blind-ending tract that extends from the bladder to the umbilicus. It may intermittently drain fluid or become infected.

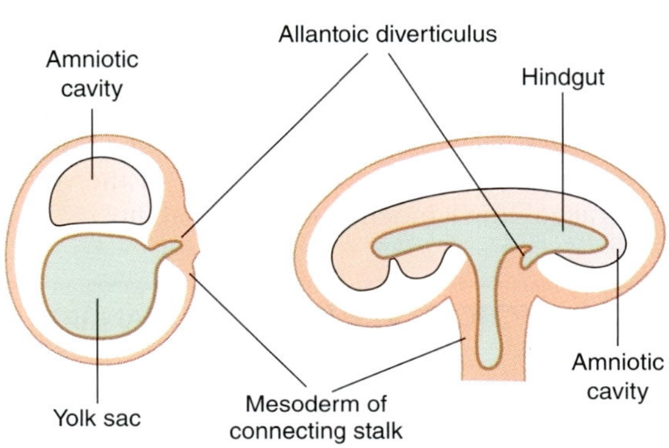

Fig. 8.8 Allantoic diverticulum.

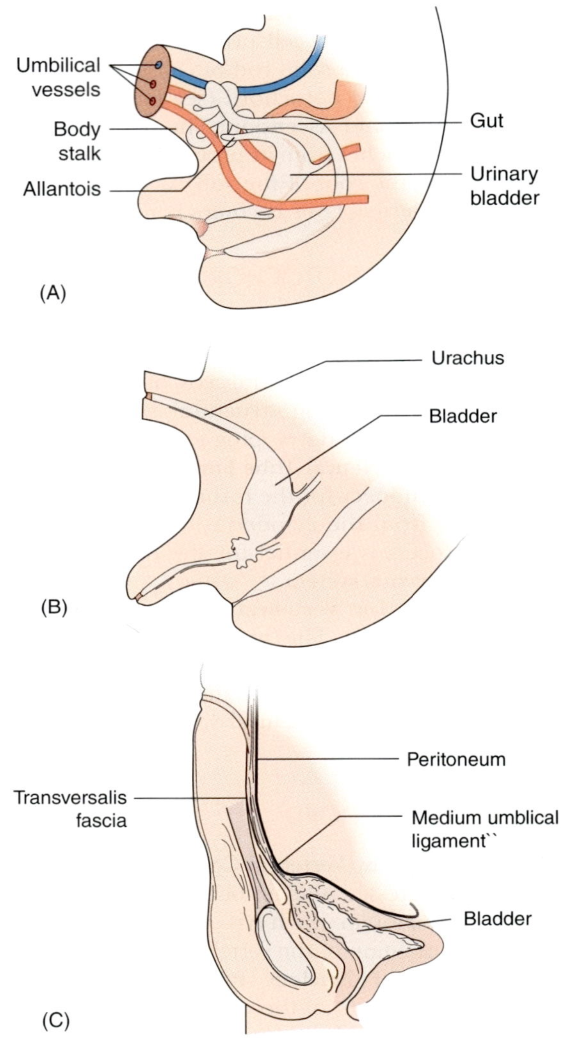

Fig. 8.9 Urachus and median umbilical ligament.

DIFFERENTIATED REGIONS IN THE EMBRYONIC DISC (AN 78.4)

- **Prechordal Plate (Prochordal Plate)** (Fig. 8.10):
  - The prechordal plate forms from the first cells that travel towards the cephalic end from the primitive streak, situated beneath the buccopharyngeal (or oropharyngeal) membrane.
  - It arises from the cranial end of the primitive streak and intercalates into the endodermal layer, resulting in a thickened structure. The columnar cells in the oval area of prechordal plate are tightly adherent to the ectodermal layer.This is the first sign of differntiation of the germ disc. Cephalo-caudal axis and bilateral symmetry of the embryo is thus established.
  - Some portions of the prechordal plate undergo an epithelial-to-mesenchymal transformation, giving rise to head mesenchyme cells beneath the forebrain located just cranial to the notochord.
  - The prechordal plate is considered by some as a mesendodermal structure because it contributes to head mesenchyme (mesodermal) and is part of the oropharyngeal membrane, which ruptures to form the mouth opening (endodermal).
- **Cloacal Membrane:**
  - Situated in the area caudal to the primitive streak, between the primitive streak and the connecting stalk.
  - The cloacal membrane eventually divides into the **anal and urogenital membranes.**

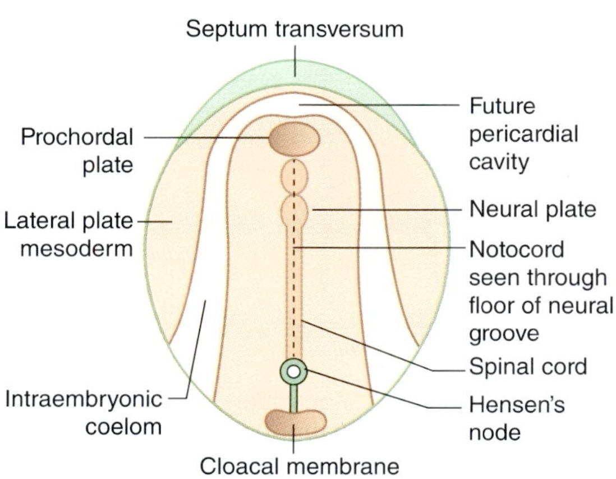

Fig. 8.10 Differentiated regions of embryonic disc.

- **Notochord:**
  - Positioned in the midline, caudal to the prechordal plate and cranial to the primitive streak.
- **Oropharyngeal Membrane:**
  - A two-layered membrane found at the cranial end of the embryonic disc, consisting of ectoderm and endoderm.
  - It ruptures to form the mouth opening.
- **Pericardial Bar:**
  A horse-shoe-shaped intraembryonic mesoderm structure located cranial to the buccopharyngeal membrane.
- Regarding the distribution of intraembryonic mesoderm, it spreads throughout the embryonic disc, except in three specific regions:
  - **Oropharyngeal membrane.**
  - **Cloacal membrane.**
  - **Notochord.**

CLINICAL NUGGETS

- During the formation of the neural plate, **Sonic hedgehog (Shh)** secreted by the underlying prechordal plate plays a critical role in the division of the initially single eye field into two distinct optic primordia.
- Without proper Shh signalling, the eye field remains undivided, leading to the development of conditions such as **holoprosencephaly and cyclopia**, characterized by the presence of a single, midline eye (Fig. 8.11).

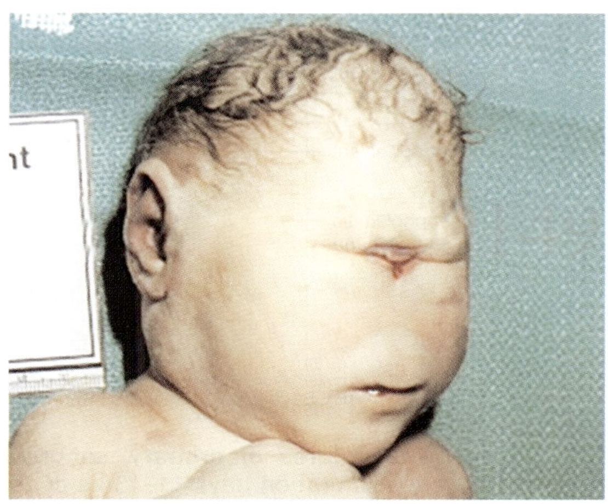

Fig. 8.11 Foetus with cyclopia. (Courtesy: Dr. A.E. Chudley, Department of Pediatrics and Child Health, University of Manitoba, Children's Hospital.)

CHANGES IN TROPHOBLAST

During the early stages of the third week of development, the trophoblast undergoes significant transformations, which are essential for the progression of embryonic development:

- **Formation of Primary Villi:** Initially, the trophoblast is characterized by primary villi, which are composed of a central core of cytotrophoblast cells covered by a layer of syncytiotrophoblast.
- **Development of Secondary Villi:** As development proceeds, mesodermal cells penetrate the primary villi, giving rise to secondary villi.
- **Penetration of Chorionic Blood Vessels:** Subsequently, chorionic blood vessels extend into the core of secondary villi, resulting in the formation of tertiary villi (Fig. 8.12).
- **Composition of Tertiary Villi:** Each tertiary villus is organized from centre to periphery as follows:
  - Endothelial cells of the chorionic capillaries.
  - Primary mesodermal cells.
  - Cytotrophoblast.
  - Syncytiotrophoblast.
- **Intervillous Space:** The intervillous space is filled with maternal blood, facilitating the exchange of gases and nutrients between the maternal and foetal circulatory systems.

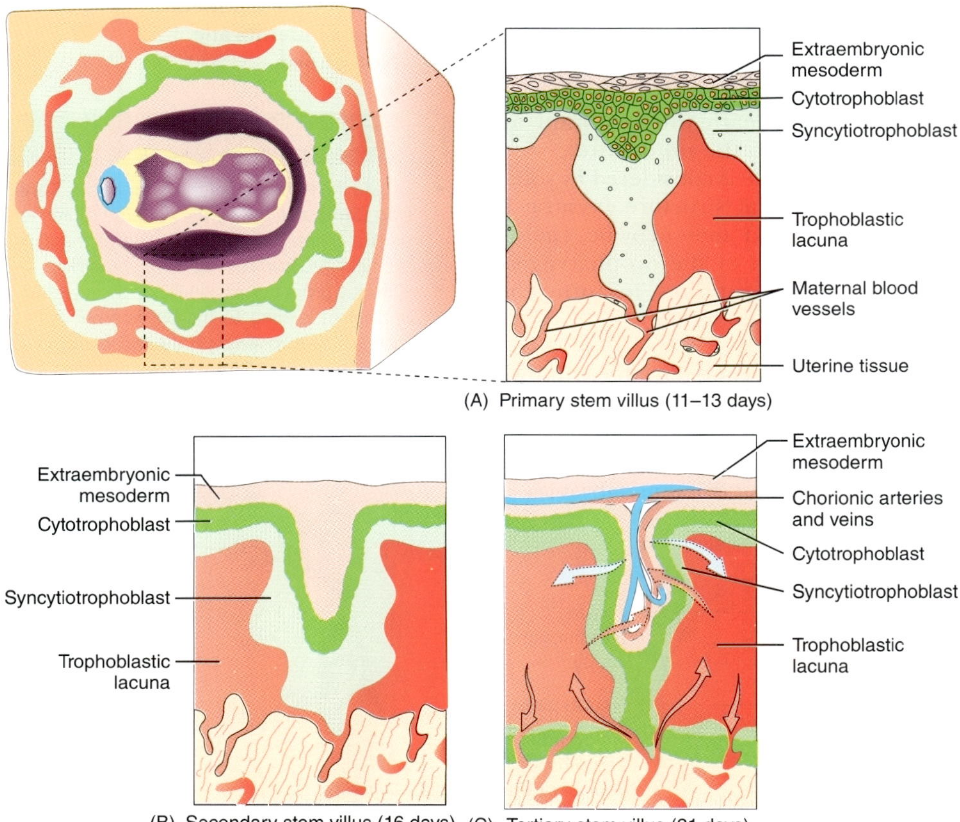

Fig. 8.12 The structures of primary, secondary and tertiary villus. Formation of chorionic villi. (A) Primary stem villi form on days 11–13 as cytotrophoblastic proliferations that bud into the overlying syncytiotrophoblast. (B) By day 16, the extraembryonic mesoderm begins to proliferate and invade the centre of each primary stem villus, transforming each into a secondary stem villus. (C) By day 21, the mesodermal core differentiates into connective tissue and blood vessels, forming the tertiary stem villi. (Source: *Larsen's Human Embryology*, 4th ed. 2008.)

- **Branching Villi:** Tertiary villi give rise to numerous branching villi that project into the intervillous space, increasing the surface area for efficient exchange between maternal and foetal blood.
- **Formation of Cytotrophoblastic Shell:** The cytotrophoblastic cells within the chorionic villi undergo proliferation and extend through the syncytiotrophoblast to create an outer cytotrophoblastic shell. This structure surrounds the chorionic sac and plays a crucial role in attaching the developing embryo to the maternal endometrium.
- **Isolation of Mesodermal Cells and Chorionic Blood Vessels:** It is important to note that the mesodermal cells and the chorionic blood vessels do not reach the cytotrophoblastic shell of the blastocyst. This separation is essential for the establishment of the **placental barrier**, which maintains the necessary separation between maternal and foetal circulatory systems while allowing for essential exchanges.
- These changes in the trophoblast are important in creating the placental structures required for the nourishment, oxygenation and waste removal that support the developing embryo throughout the course of pregnancy.

KLINISCHE PERLEN

CAUDAL DYSGENESIS (SIRENOMELIA)

- Often referred to as '**Mermaid syndrome**' due to the fusion of the lower limbs, resembling a mermaid tail (see Fig. 8.13A and B).
- Results from **improper mesoderm formation** in the caudal region of the embryo during gastrulation.
- Affects the development of lower limbs, the urogenital system and vertebrae in the lumbosacral region.
- Caudal dysplasia is associated with **gestational diabetes** and elevated insulin levels.

SITUS INVERSUS

- Involves the transposition of viscera in both the thorax and abdomen (refer to Fig. 8.14). In individuals with **situs inversus totalis**, the most common form, all of the internal organs are reversed. This includes the heart, liver, stomach, spleen, and other organs in the chest and abdomen.
- **Kartagener's Syndrome (Immotile Cilia Syndrome):**
  - Presents with **complete situs inversus**, a condition where the major organs are mirrored from their normal positions.
  - Associated with **bronchiectasis and chronic sinusitis.**

LATERALITY SEQUENCE

- Laterality sequence can be predominantly bilaterally left-sided or right-sided.
- In some cases, organs may exhibit symmetrical positioning, referred to as '**heterotaxy**'.
- '**Isomerism**' represents the most extreme form of heterotaxy, characterized by the development of two right sides or two left sides.

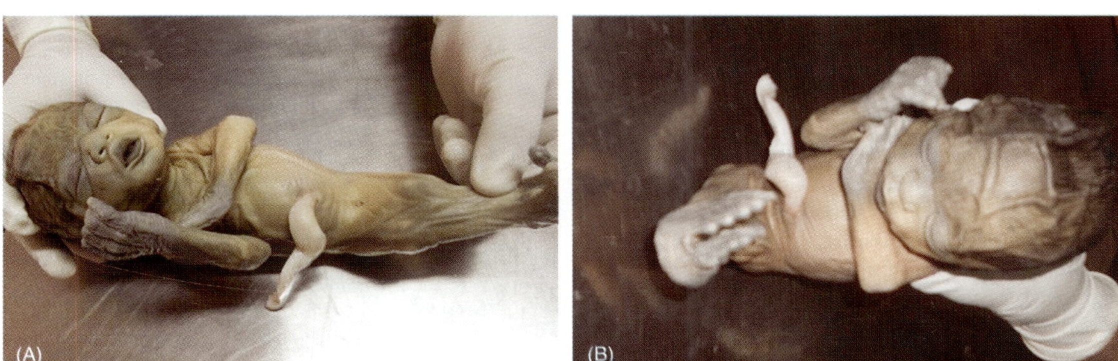

Fig. 8.13 (A) A foetus with sirenomelia. (B) The lower limbs fused resembling a mermaid's tail. (Photo courtesy: Dr Ramakrishnan.)

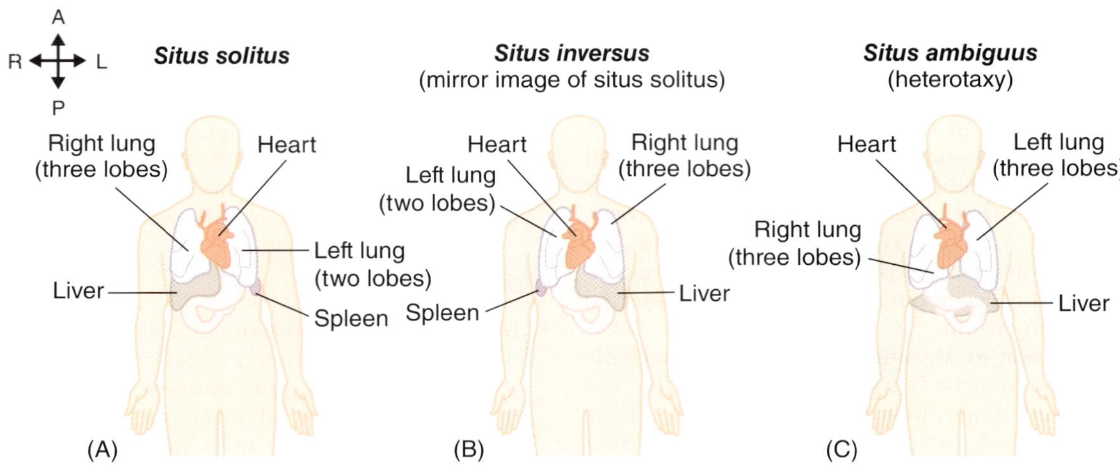

Fig. 8.14 Abnormalities of left/right (L/R) asymmetry in humans. (A) The normal L/R positions of organs arranged along midline (situs solitus). The apex of the heart points towards the left. The right lung is trilobed and the left lung is bilobed. In the abdominal cavity, the spleen and stomach are positioned on the left side and the liver is on the right. The small bowel is looped in a counterclockwise direction. (B) A complete mirror image of organ arrangement along the midline is called situs inversus. Persons with situs inversus might have no symptoms. (C) Randomization of the arrangement of the heart, lungs, liver, spleen and stomach along the midline (situs ambiguus or heterotaxy). Situs ambiguus is often associated with congenital heart defects. (Source: *Medical Genetics*, 4th ed. 2010.)

- The presence or absence of a **spleen** is a crucial factor in determining laterality.
  - **Left-sided** laterality is often associated with **polysplenia**.
  - **Right-sided** laterality may result in **asplenia or a hypoplastic spleen**.
- **Role of Serotonin (5HT) in Establishing Laterality:**
  - The signal molecule serotonin (5HT) plays a crucial role in establishing the proper laterality during embryonic development.
  - Children born to mothers using **SSRIs (selective serotonin reuptake inhibitors)**, which are commonly used as antidepressants, may be at risk for laterality-related developmental issues.

These developmental conditions and syndromes highlight the processes involved in embryonic development and the significance of proper mesodermal formation and molecular signalling in determining organ positioning and function.

POINTS TO PONDER

- **Gastrulation, the Onset of the Third Week**
  - The third week of embryonic development is marked by a significant event known as gastrulation.
  - Gastrulation initiates with the formation of the **primitive streak**, which emerges in the epiblast, typically near the caudal end of the bilaminar embryonic disc.
  - Subsequent to the primitive streak's formation, other critical structures develop, including the **primitive node, primitive pit and primitive groove.**
- **Germ Layer Formation**
  - During gastrulation, cells from these structures displace the original hypoblast cells, leading to the formation of the **definitive endoderm.**
  - Simultaneously, other cells migrate bilaterally between the endoderm and epiblast to give rise to the **intraembryonic mesoderm.**
- **Three Primary Germ Layers**
  - Upon the completion of gastrulation, the epiblast undergoes a transition and becomes known as the **ectoderm.**

- Gastrulation is process responsible for the formation of the three primary germ layers: **the ectoderm, mesoderm and endoderm.**
- **Establishment of Major Body Axes**
  - The formation of the primitive streak plays a central role in defining all major body axes, contributing to the development of:
    - The **cranio-caudal axis**, which governs head-to-tail orientation
    - The **dorso-ventral axis**, determining the back-to-belly orientation
    - The **medio-lateral axis**, responsible for the midline-to-side orientation
    - The **left-right axis**, critical in distinguishing left from right sides
- Gastrulation is an important step in development that forms the basic germ layers and sets the foundation for body structure in embryonic development.

BRAIN TEASERS

1. Which of the following structures is primarily responsible for the formation of the axial skeleton and the development of the nervous system?
   A. Primitive node
   B. Primitive groove
   C. Intraembryonic mesoderm
   D. Definitive endoderm
2. What is the function of the septum transversum, which is influenced by the primitive streak?
   A. Formation of the nervous system.
   B. Separation of the thoracic and abdominal cavities.
   C. Development of the circulatory system.
   D. Establishment of the embryo's left-right axis.
3. Which germ layer(s) originate from pluripotent epiblast cells during gastrulation?
   A. Ectoderm
   B. Mesoderm
   C. Endoderm
   D. All of the above
4. What is the function of the notochord in embryonic development?
   A. Formation of the axial skeleton.
   B. Establishment of the embryo's dorso-ventral axis.
   C. Induction of gut tube.
   D. Development of the circulatory system.
5. Which structure is responsible for the establishment of the embryo's left-right axis?
   A. Primitive node
   B. Primitive groove
   C. Notochord
   D. Urachus
6. What is the clinical significance of defects in the development of the allantoic diverticulum?
   A. Impaired blood circulation in the embryo.
   B. Urinary system abnormalities.
   C. Abnormal development of the nervous system.
   D. Circulatory system malformations.
7. Which structure provides structural support and guidance for the developing embryo?
   A. Primitive node
   B. Primitive groove
   C. Notochord
   D. Urachus
8. The remnant of the allantoic diverticulum in adults is represented by which structure?
   A. Median umbilical ligament
   B. Primitive node
   C. Nucleus pulposus
   D. Cloacal membrane
9. The notochord contributes to the development of which organ system?
   A. Skeletal system
   B. Respiratory system
   C. Digestive system
   D. Nervous system
10. What is the fate of the notochord in the course of embryonic development?
   A. It persists as alar ligament.
   B. It transforms into the nucleus pulposus.
   C. It forms the central nervous system.
   D. It differentiates into the endodermal layer.

Answers

1. (C); 2. (B); 3. (D); 4. (A); 5. (C); 6. (B); 7. (C); 8. (A); 9. (A); 10. (B).

FURTHER READINGS

Chen CY, Yu IS, Pai CH, et al. Embryonic Cul4b is important for epiblast growth and location of primitive streak layer cells. *PLoS One.* 2019;14(7):e0219221. doi:10.1371/journal.pone.0219221.

Eitler K, Bibok A, Telkes G. Situs inversus totalis: a clinical review. *Int J Gen Med.* 2022;15:2437-2449. doi:10.2147/IJGM.S295444.

Ivanovitch K, Soro-Barrio P, Chakravarty P, et al. Ventricular, atrial, and outflow tract heart progenitors arise from spatially and molecularly distinct regions of the primitive streak. *PLoS Biol.* 2021;19(5):e3001200. doi:10.1371/journal.pbio.3001200.

Liu S, Chen W, Zhan Y, et al. DNAH11 variants and its association with congenital heart disease and heterotaxy syndrome. *Sci Rep.* 2019;9(1):6683. doi:10.1038/s41598-019-43109-6.

9 Fourth Week to Eighth Week of Development

AN 79.3 Describe the process of neurulation.
AN 79.4 Describe the development of somites and intraembryonic coelom.
AN 79.5 Explain embryological basis of neural tube defects.

ANAMNESE

A 26-year-old first-time expectant mother at 18 weeks of pregnancy, presented with concerns after a routine ultrasound revealed her foetus had anencephaly, a severe neural tube defect. This diagnosis points to the critical role of early embryonic development, specifically between weeks 4 and 8 of gestation, in forming essential structures like the brain and spinal cord. Her past medical history was uneventful, and she had been diligent in her prenatal care and nutrition. This case serves as a reminder of the importance of early prenatal care, proper nutrition and patient-centred counselling in managing complex foetal anomalies.

Designing the human body plan to meet its specific requirements is a complex architectural challenge. A defining characteristic that sets vertebrates apart is the mesodermal segmentation within the somite. This process, known as **somitogenesis**, requires a precise coordination of various factors, including somite definition, the timing of formation and segmentation. The communication between neighbouring structures and the paraxial mesoderm plays a crucial role in shaping the neural tube and its derivatives, and vice versa. The **Sonic hedgehog (Shh) gene**, produced by the notochord and the **Zone of Polarizing Activity** (ZPA) in the limb bud, influences the determination of sclerotome and myotome lineages within the somites.

- The main events of fourth week:
  - Differentiation of **three germ layers**.
  - Formation of **somites**.
  - Formation of **folds** of the embryo.
- Development of face and limb buds-second month (Fig. 9.1).

DIFFERENTIATION OF INTRAEMBRYONIC MESODERM

- The intraembryonic mesoderm undergoes differentiation into three distinct regions, demarcated by a longitudinal groove (as illustrated in Fig. 9.2):
  - **Paraxial mesoderm**, positioned on either side of the notochord and beneath the neural plate.
  - **Intermediate mesoderm**, extending along the base of the longitudinal groove.
  - **Lateral plate mesoderm**, which extends towards the periphery of the germ disc and ultimately merges with the extraembryonic primary mesoderm.

PARAXIAL MESODERM (AN 79.4)

- The paraxial mesoderm, located on both sides of the notochord, extends from the primitive streak to the prechordal plate, positioned

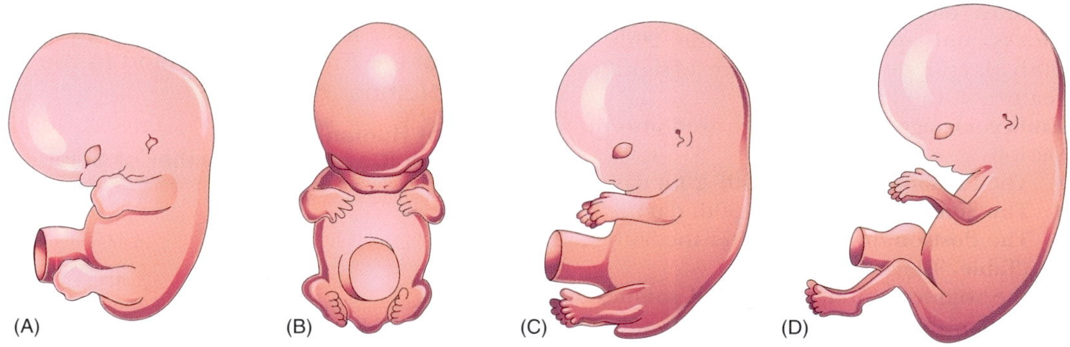

Fig. 9.1 Changes in the developing embryo from 4 to 8 weeks. Illustrations of positional changes of the developing limbs of embryos. (A) At approximately 48 days, the limbs extend ventrally, and the hand plates and foot plates face each other. (B) At approximately 51 days, the upper limbs are bent at the elbow, and the hands are curved over the thorax. (C) At approximately 54 days, the soles of the feet face medially. (D) At approximately 56 days (end of embryonic stage), the elbows point caudally and the knees cranially. (Source: *The Developing Human: Clinically Oriented Embryology*, 11th ed.)

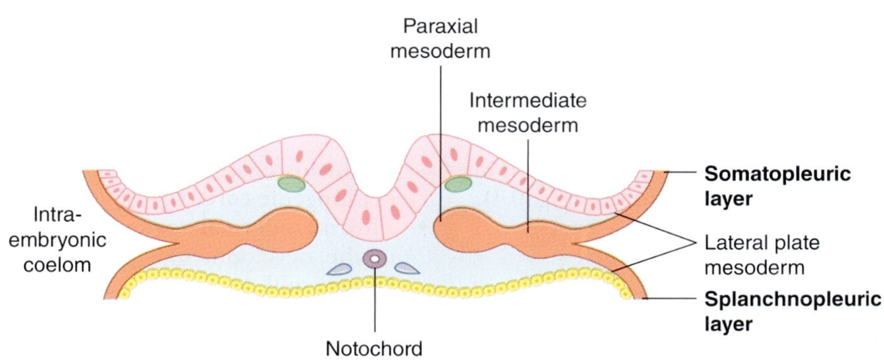

Fig. 9.2 Differentiation of intraembryonic mesoderm.

beneath the neural tube and caudal to the otic vesicle.

- The process of somite formation initiates with the organization of paraxial mesoderm cells into clusters known as **somitomeres**. These somitomeres undergo a gradual compaction and become enveloped by an epithelial layer. Eventually, they detach from the presomitic paraxial mesoderm, evolving into discrete and individual somites.
- Rostrally, unsegmented mesenchymal cells (1–7 somitomeres) give rise to the base of the skull and all the striated muscles of the head. **Preotic somites** specifically contribute to the formation of extrinsic eye muscles.
- Caudal to the otic vesicle, mesenchymal cells become segmented, forming **postotic somites** (Fig. 9.3).

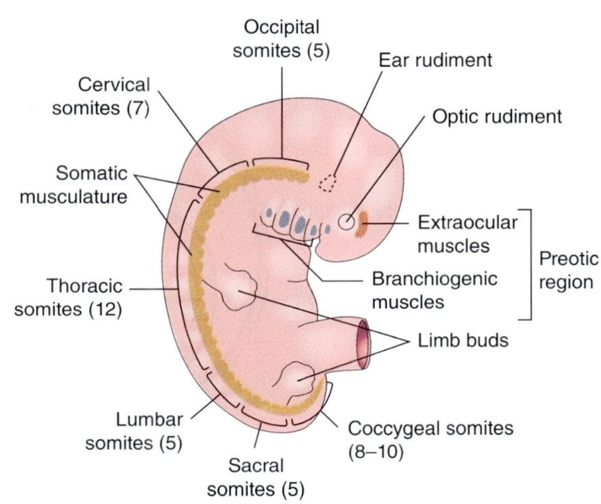

Fig. 9.3 Distribution of somites.

- **Somites/metameres,** which resemble cubical blocks and appear between the 20th and 30th day of development, are a significant feature of the fourth week.
- **Embryonic age** is often categorized into three periods:
  - **The Presomite Period** (15th–20th day).
  - **The Somite Period** (20th–30th day).
  - **The Postsomite Period** (after the 30th day) (Table. 9.1).
- In the somite period, **44 pairs** of somites are formed by the end of the first month, with four to five pairs of **occipital somites** located beside the hindbrain contributing to skull formation.
- Each somite consists of two components:
  - **Dorsolateral,** responsible for generating the **dermomyotome**.
    - ➢ The dermomyotome consists of the lateral dermal plate, contributing to the formation of dermis and subcutaneous tissue, and the medial muscle plate, involved in the development of skeletal muscles, the tongue and the diaphragm.
  - **Ventromedial**, which gives rise to the **sclerotome**.
    - ➢ The sclerotome is responsible for forming the vertebral column and ribs (Fig. 9.4).

Table 9.1 Approximate Age of the Embryo According to the Number of Somites

Age of Human Embryo (Days)	Number of Somites
20	1–4
21	4–7
22	7–10
23	10–13
24	13–17
25	17–20
26	20–23
27	23–26
28	26–29
29	29–34
30	34–35

INTERMEDIATE MESODERM

- Intermediate mesoderm is a slender, elongated band of mesodermal tissue that bridges the gap between the paraxial and lateral plate mesoderms.
- In its upper segment, the intermediate mesoderm is segmented, while in the lower portion, it remains unsegmented, ultimately forming a **nephrogenic cord**.
- This mesodermal region plays a crucial role in the developmental processes of both the kidneys and gonads.

LATERAL PLATE MESODERM

- The lateral plate mesoderm is positioned laterally within the embryonic structure.

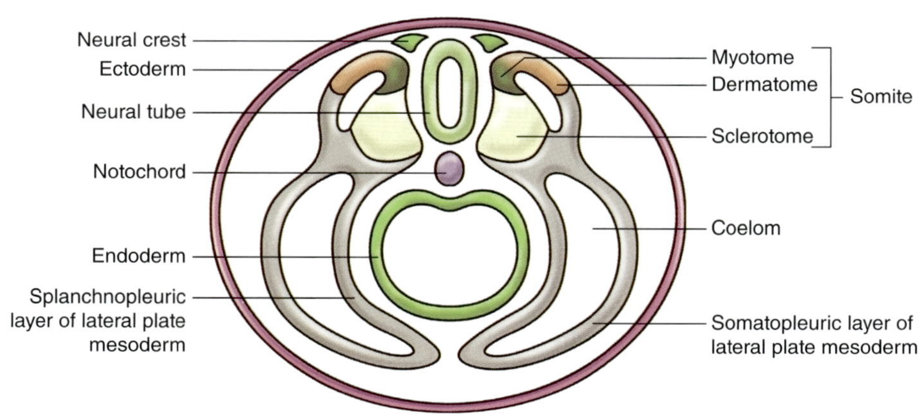

Fig. 9.4 Somites differentiating into sclerotome, myotome and dermatome.

- Derived from the primitive streak, this mesoderm is unsegmented and extends towards the peripheral margin of the embryonic region.
- It maintains continuity with the pericardial bar situated cranially to the buccopharyngeal membrane (Fig. 9.2).
- After the formation of intraembryonic coelom, the lateral plate mesoderm differentiates as **somatopleuric and splanchnopleuric parts** as discussed below.

INTRAEMBRYONIC COELOM (AN 79.4)

- Intraembryonic coelom formation commences with the emergence of small clefts in the lateral plate mesoderm. These clefts later coalesce to create a large, inverted 'U' -shaped cavity, referred to as the **intraembryonic coelom** (as depicted in Fig. 9.5).
- Subsequently, the intraembryonic coelom establishes communication with the extraembryonic coelom, which serves as a vital source of nutrition for the embryonic area until the establishment of the circulatory system.
- The **Pericardial, Pleural and Peritoneal Cavities** are derived from the intraembryonic coelom.
- The intraembryonic coelom plays a role in dividing the lateral plate mesoderm into two distinct parts:
  - **Somatopleuric (Parietal Part)**: This portion of the lateral plate mesoderm, in contact with the ectoderm, gives rise to the **parietal layers** of the peritoneal, pleural and pericardial sacs, as well as contributing to the development of dermal tissues and skeletal elements within the pectoral and pelvic girdles.
  - **Splanchnopleuric (Visceral Part)**: This segment is closely associated with the endoderm and is responsible for forming the **visceral layers** of serous sacs, as well as musculature and connective tissues within the gut, respiratory tubes and heart.
- Cranially, anterior to the prechordal plate, the two halves of the intraembryonic coelom are in continuity with one another. The **pericardium** originates from this part of the intraembryonic coelom.
- The splanchnopleuric layer that forms the floor of this coelomic region is recognized as the **cardiogenic area, cardiogenic plate or heart-forming plate**.
- Positioned cranially to the cardiogenic area, the somatopleuric and splanchnopleuric mesoderm fuse to create the **Septum transversum**, depicted in Fig. 9.6. The septum transversum contributes significantly to the future development of the diaphragm.

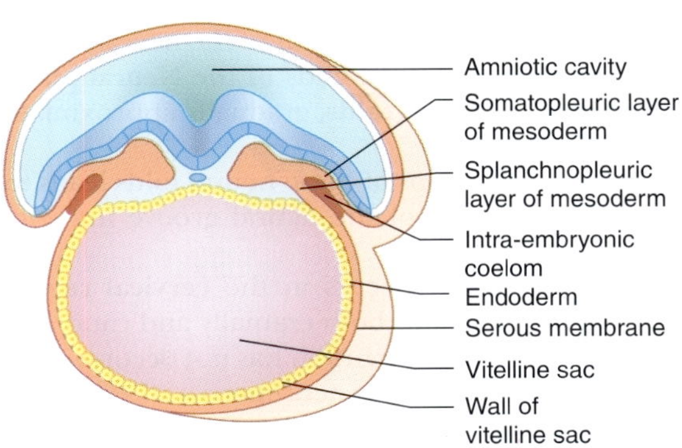

Fig. 9.5 Formation of intraembryonic coelom.

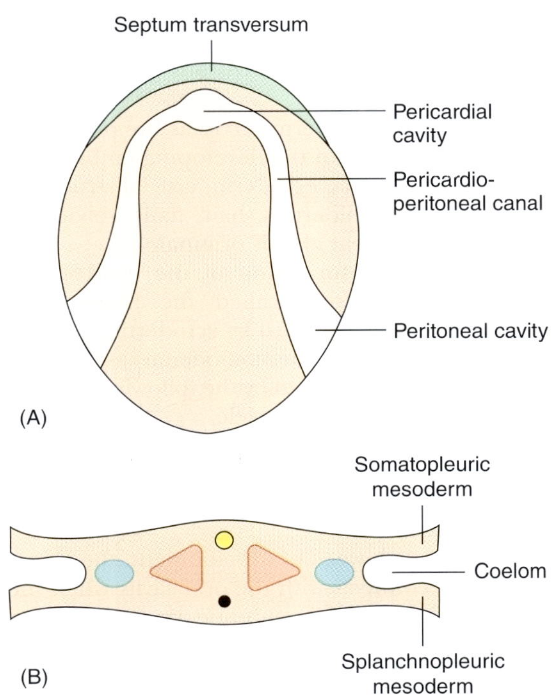

Fig. 9.6 Formation of septum transversum.

DERIVATIVES OF MESODERM

Mesoderm gives rise to various important derivatives, including:

- Mesothelial lining found within body cavities such as the pericardial, pleural and peritoneal cavities.
- Nearly all muscles throughout the body, with the exception of the muscles in the iris and arrector pili.
- The formation of all connective tissues.
- Development of key systems, including the cardiovascular, lymphatic and urogenital systems, which consists of the kidneys, gonads and the suprarenal cortex.
- Mesoderm also plays a role in the development of teeth, except for the enamel.

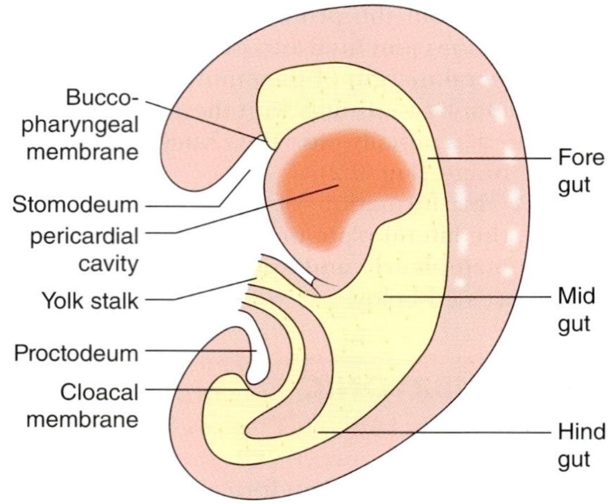

Fig. 9.7 Stomodeum and proctodeum.

DIFFERENTIATION OF ECTODERM

The ectoderm situated above the notochord undergoes differentiation into neurectoderm, which is responsible for the formation of the neural tube. The rest of the ectoderm is subsequently redesignated as surface ectoderm.

SURFACE ECTODERM

- The surface ectoderm serves as the outer protective covering of the developing embryo.
- From the surface ectoderm, crucial structures such as the epidermis, hair, nails, sebaceous glands and sweat glands originate.
- Following the formation of the head-fold, a surface depression called the **Stomodeum** emerges, which is lined by ectoderm.
- The boundaries of the stomodeum (as depicted in Fig. 9.7) are defined by the following regions:
  - **Above**: Forebrain vesicle.
  - **Below**: Pericardial swelling.
  - **Floor**: Buccopharyngeal membrane.
- The stomodeum ultimately shapes the **Primitive oral cavity**.
- By the fourth week of development, the primitive gut connects with the oral cavity when the buccopharyngeal membrane ruptures, allowing amniotic fluid to access the gut.
- With the formation of the tail-fold, a depression forms at the caudal end, known as the **Ectodermal cloaca or Proctodeum**.
- The floor of the proctodeum is established by the **Cloacal membrane** (Fig. 9.7).
- The cloacal membrane further divides into the anal and urogenital membranes, which eventually rupture to form the anal and urogenital orifices.

NEURECTODERM (AN 79.3)

- The neural plate originates as a thickened region of ectoderm located over the notochord.
- The cells within the neural plate are referred to as neurectoderm.
- **Neurulation** (illustrated in Fig. 9.8) is the process through which the neural tube and its derivatives are formed from the neural plate, and the **Notochord** plays an important role in inducing neurulation.
- A midline **Neural groove** develops due to the elevation of both lateral ends of the neural plate.
- The elevated lateral ends of the **Neural plate**, known as **Neural folds**, gradually approximate each other.
- Fusion of the tips of these neural folds leads to the conversion of the neural groove into the **Neural tube**.
- Fusion initially occurs in the **cervical region** and then extends both cranially and caudally.
- The regions where fusion has not occurred are termed the **Anterior neuropore** and **Posterior neuropore**.
- Neuropores allow communication between the neural tube and the amniotic cavity, and

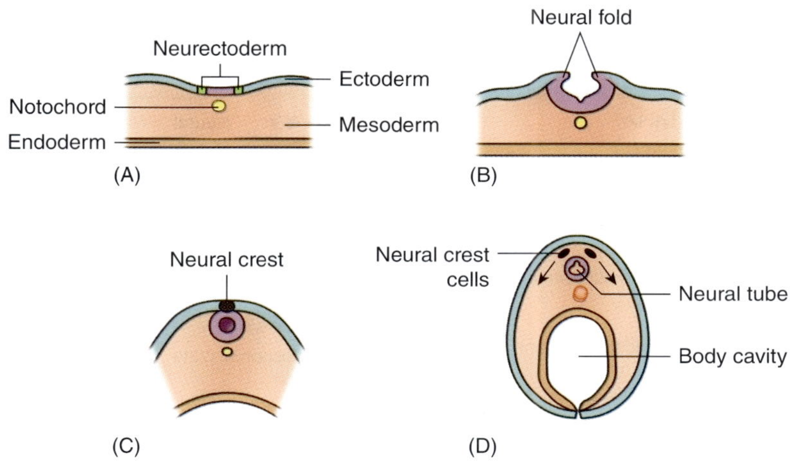

Fig. 9.8 Formation of neural tube from neurectoderm (see the text for description).

amniotic fluid provides nutrition until the establishment of the circulatory system.

- Eventually, both the anterior and posterior neuropores close, resulting in the formation of a completely sealed neural tube.
- The anterior neuropore closes around the **25th day** of development, during the **20 somite** stage, marking the middle of the fourth week. In contrast, the posterior neuropore closes by the **28th day** of development, at the **25 somite** stage, which signifies the end of the fourth week. The neural tube can be regarded as the embryonic foundation of the central nervous system (CNS).
- The cranial end of the neural tube enlarges and develops into the brain, while the caudal tubular end forms the spinal cord.
- The sealed neural tube detaches from the surface ectoderm, with the space between the neural tube and surface ectoderm being occupied by neural crest cells.

NEURAL CREST CELLS

- During neurulation (as depicted in Fig. 9.9), the specialized cells originating from the neurectoderm become dissociated from the neural plate.
- Initially, they are positioned dorsolateral to the neural tube.
- Subsequently, they undergo separation from each other and embark on migrations to various regions within the developing embryo.
- Neural crest cells give rise to a wide range of structures as follows:
  - Schwann cells.
  - Cells of adrenal medulla.
  - Neurons of autonomic ganglia.
  - Cells of dorsal root ganglia.
  - **Sensory ganglia** of cranial nerves (fifth, seventh, eighth, ninth, and tenth).
  - Chromaffin tissue.
  - Pigment cells of skin.
  - Meningeal layers (forebrain).
  - **C cells** of thyroid gland.
  - Odontoblasts.

CLINICAL NUGGETS

- **Neural crest cells** exhibit a highly coordinated migration pattern, essential for the proper development of various body structures.
- Disrupted migration can lead to a shortage of neural crest cells required to form mesenchymal tissues. In cases where this occurs during facial development, it can result in conditions such as **cleft lip and cleft palate**.
- Erroneous migration of neural crest cells into the pharyngeal arches can give rise to malformations in the parathyroid glands, thymus, facial skeleton, heart, aorta and pulmonary trunk. This condition is known as **DiGeorge syndrome**, often referred to as **CATCH 22 syndrome** (Fig. 9.10).

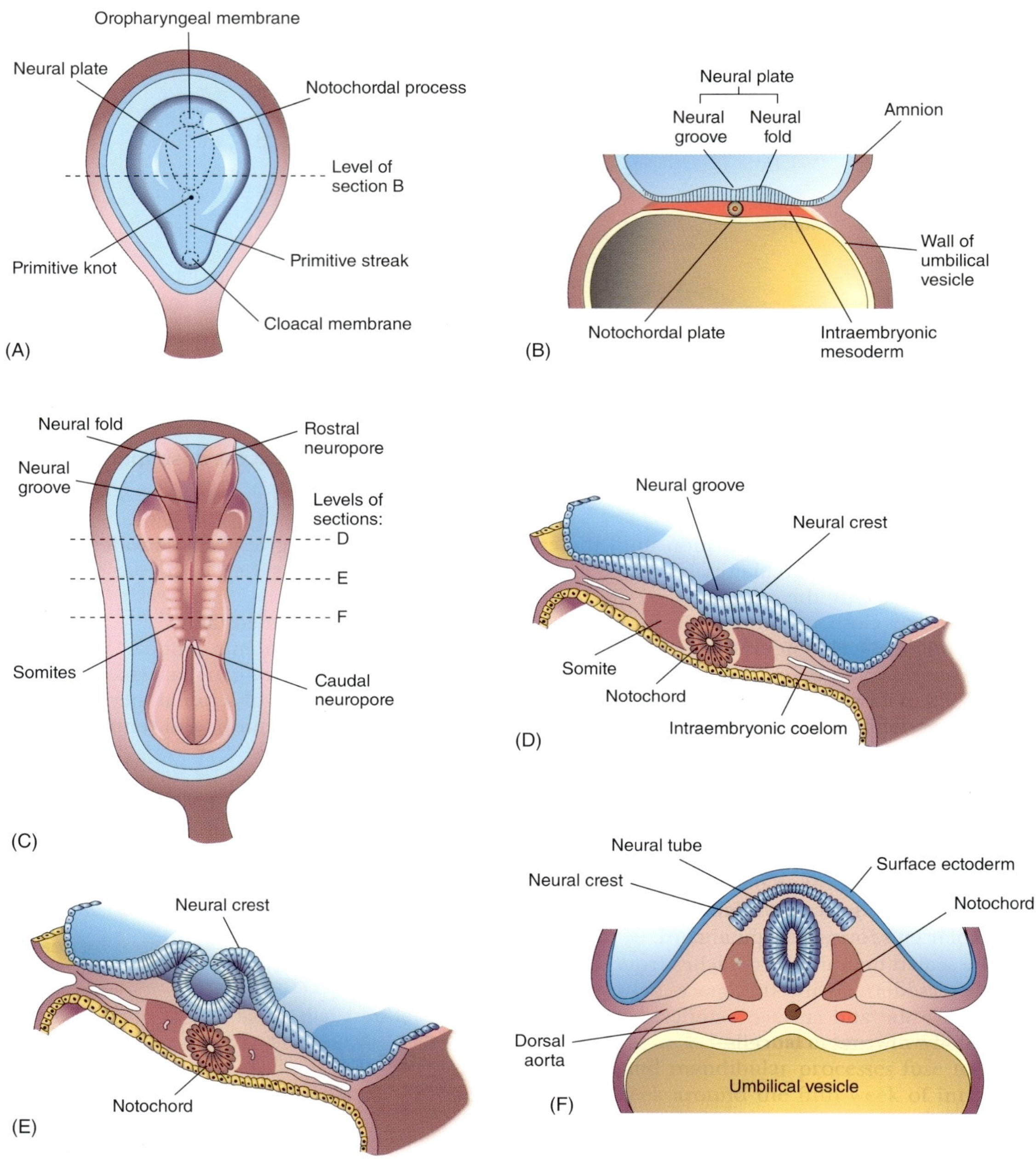

Fig. 9.9 Formation of neural crest cells from neural folds. Illustrations of the neural plate and folding of it to form the neural tube. (A) Dorsal view of an embryo of approximately 17 days, exposed by removing the amnion. (B) Transverse section of the embryo showing the neural plate and early development of the neural groove and neural folds. (C) Dorsal view of an embryo of approximately 22 days. The neural folds have fused opposite the fourth to sixth somites but are open at both ends. (D–F) Transverse sections of this embryo at the levels shown in (C) illustrating formation of the neural tube and its detachment from the surface ectoderm. Note that some neuroectodermal cells are not included in the neural tube but remain between it and the surface ectoderm as the neural crest. (Source: *Before We Are Born: Essentials of Embryology and Birth Defects*, First South Asia ed. 2016.)

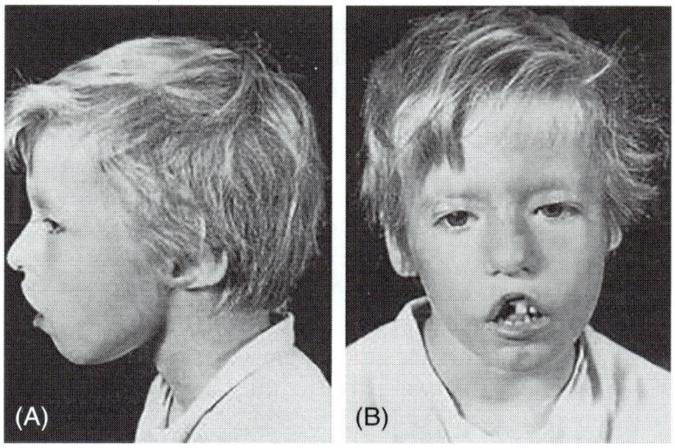

Fig. 9.10 DiGeorge syndrome. (Source: From Male, D., Brostoff, J., Roth, D., et al. [2013]. Immunology [8th ed.]. Mosby.)

FOLDING OF EMBRYO

The embryonic disc undergoes continuous growth, leading to its folding at both the head and tail ends, forming the head and tail folds (cephalo-caudal folding).

- **Cephalo-caudal** folding results from the longitudinal growth of the CNS (Fig. 9.11).
- Simultaneously, **lateral folds** develop on each side of the embryo, driven by the rapid expansion of somites (Fig. 9.12).
- All these folds converge on the ventral surface of the embryo.
- The amniotic membrane envelops the connecting stalk and transforms it into the

DERIVATIVES OF ECTODERM

The ectoderm primarily gives rise to:

- Central nervous system.
- Peripheral nervous system.
- Ganglia.
- Sensory epithelium of ear, nose and eye.
- Epidermis of skin.
- Hair and nails.
- Glands-subcutaneous glands, mammary glands, pituitary gland, sebaceous and sweat glands.
- Muscles of the iris and arrector pili (rest are mesodermal in origin).

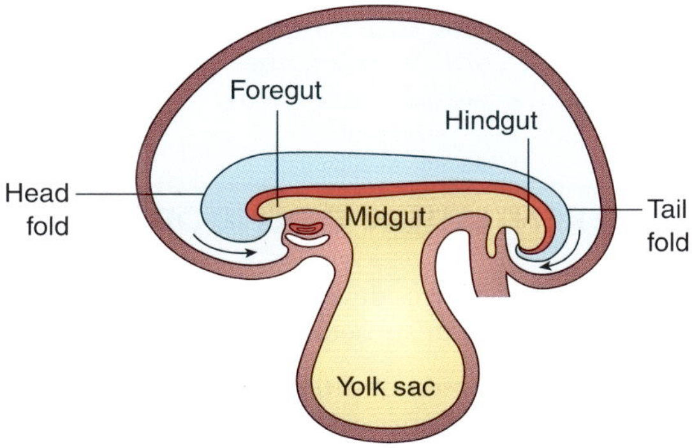

Fig. 9.11 Cephalo-caudal folding of embryo.

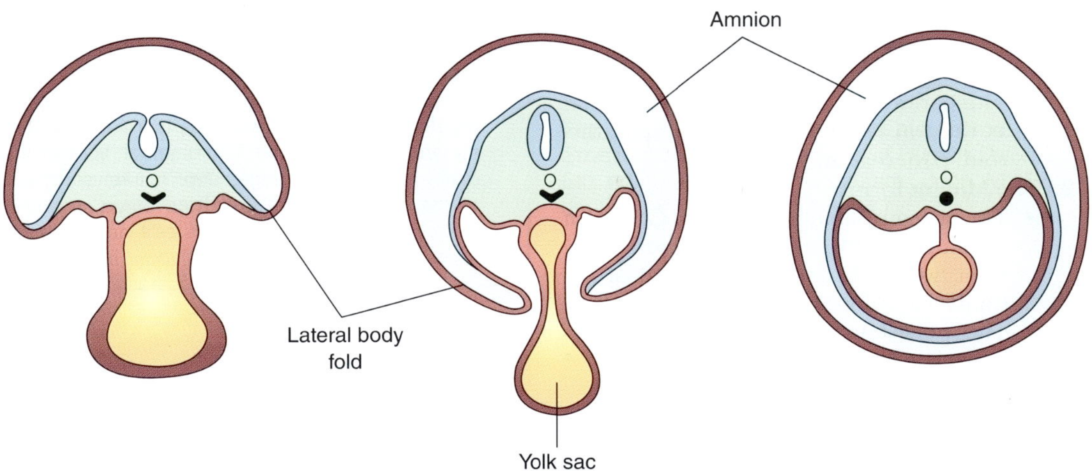

Fig. 9.12 Lateral folding of the embryo.

Umbilical cord. This process causes a reduction in the yolk sac cavity, giving it an hourglass-like shape.

- The yolk sac is divided into two portions: the part enclosed within the embryo forms the **Primitive gut,** while the remaining extraembryonic region becomes the **Umbilical vesicle or Definitive yolk sac**.
- A significant portion of the gastrointestinal tract originates from the primitive gut.
- Initially, the gut maintains a wide connection with the umbilical vesicle.
- The portion of the gut cranial to this connection is referred to as the **Foregut**, while the part caudal to it is known as the **Hindgut**.
- The section of the gut situated between the foregut and hindgut is termed the **Midgut**.
- Over time, the channel facilitating communication between the gut tube and yolk sac narrows. This connecting structure, passing through the umbilical cord, is called the **Vitello-intestinal duct** and eventually disappears.

DIFFERENTIATION OF ENDODERM

The comprehensive development of gut tubes will be discussed in subsequent sections.

The gut is composed of three primary segments:

1. **The Foregut** gives rise to:
   - ➢ The epithelial lining of the gastrointestinal tract (GIT) from the tongue to the ampulla of Vater in the duodenum.
   - ➢ The epithelial lining of the respiratory system, which includes the auditory tube and tympanic cavity.
   - ➢ The parenchyma of various glands, such as the tonsils, thymus, thyroid, parathyroid, pancreas and liver.
2. **The Midgut** forms:
   - ➢ The mucous membrane of the GIT from the ampulla of Vater to the junction of the right two-thirds and left one-third of the transverse colon.
   - ➢ The persistent vitello-intestinal duct is known as **Meckel's diverticulum**.
3. **The Hindgut** forms:
   - ➢ The mucous membrane extending from the left one-third of the transverse colon to the pectinate line of the anal canal.
   - ➢ The mucous membrane of the urinary bladder, urethra and its associated glands.
   - ➢ The epithelial lining of the vagina.

Detailed information on the derivatives is provided in Fig. 9.13.

CLINICAL NUGGETS

Secondary neurulation

- The remnants of the primitive streak undergo enlargement, giving rise to the tail bud or caudal eminence, primarily composed of mesoderm. This region later contributes to the formation of many caudal structures within the body.
- The process of **Gastrulation** concludes with the establishment of the tail bud.
- Secondary neurulation refers to the formation of the neural tube from the tail bud, distinguishing it from primary neurulation, which involves neural tube formation from the neural plate.
- During secondary neurulation, the central cells within the tail bud aggregate to form a solid mass known as the **medullary cord**.
- Subsequently, a lumen develops within the medullary cord, eventually merging with the neural canal of the neural tube (Fig. 9.14).
- Neural crest cells, originating from the neural tube, migrate to establish the **Caudal spinal ganglia**.
- The lateral cells of the tail bud contribute to the formation of the **Caudal somites**.
- Disordered secondary neurulation at each phase of development may cause corresponding lesions, such as failed junction with the primary neural tube (junctional neural tube defect and segmental spinal dysgenesis), dysgenesis or duplication of the caudal cell mass (**caudal agenesis and caudal duplication syndrome**), failed ingression of the primitive streak to the caudal cell mass (**myelomeningocele**), focal limited dorsal neuro-cutaneous nondisjunction (limited dorsal **myeloschisis** and congenital dermal sinus), neuro-mesenchymal adhesion (lumbosacral lipomatous malformation) and regression failure spectrum of the medullary cord (low-lying conus, retained medullary cord, terminal myelocele and terminal **myelocystocele**).

KLINISCHE PERLEN

NEURAL TUBE DEFECTS (NTD) (AN 79.5)

Failure of proper neural tube closure during the fourth week of development leads to neural

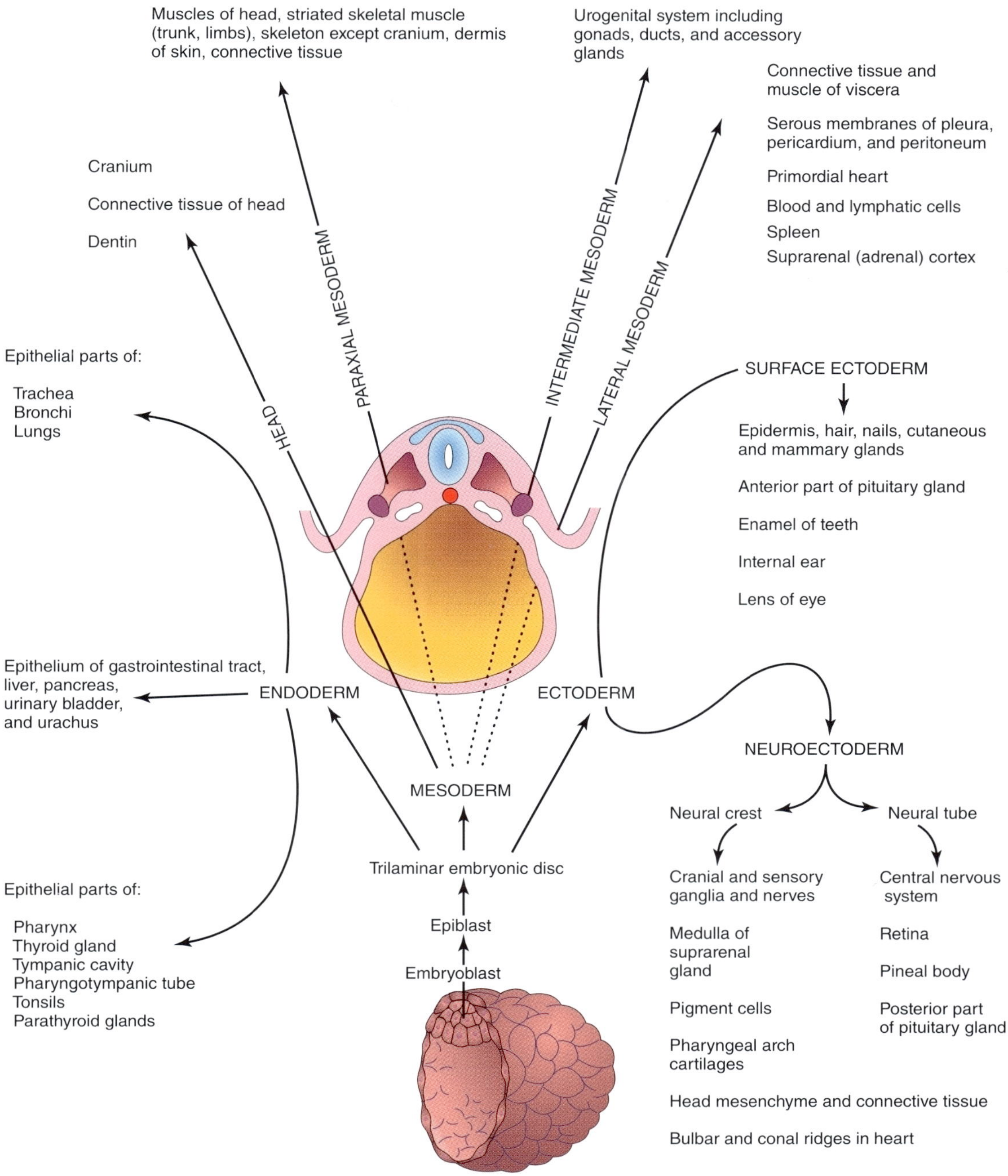

Fig. 9.13 The derivatives of germ layers. Schematic drawing of derivatives of the three germ layers: ectoderm, endoderm and mesoderm. Cells from these layers contribute to the formation of different tissues and organs, for example the endoderm forms the epithelial lining of the gastrointestinal tract and the mesoderm gives rise to connective tissues and muscles. (Source: *The Developing Human: Clinically Oriented Embryology*, 8th ed. 2008.)

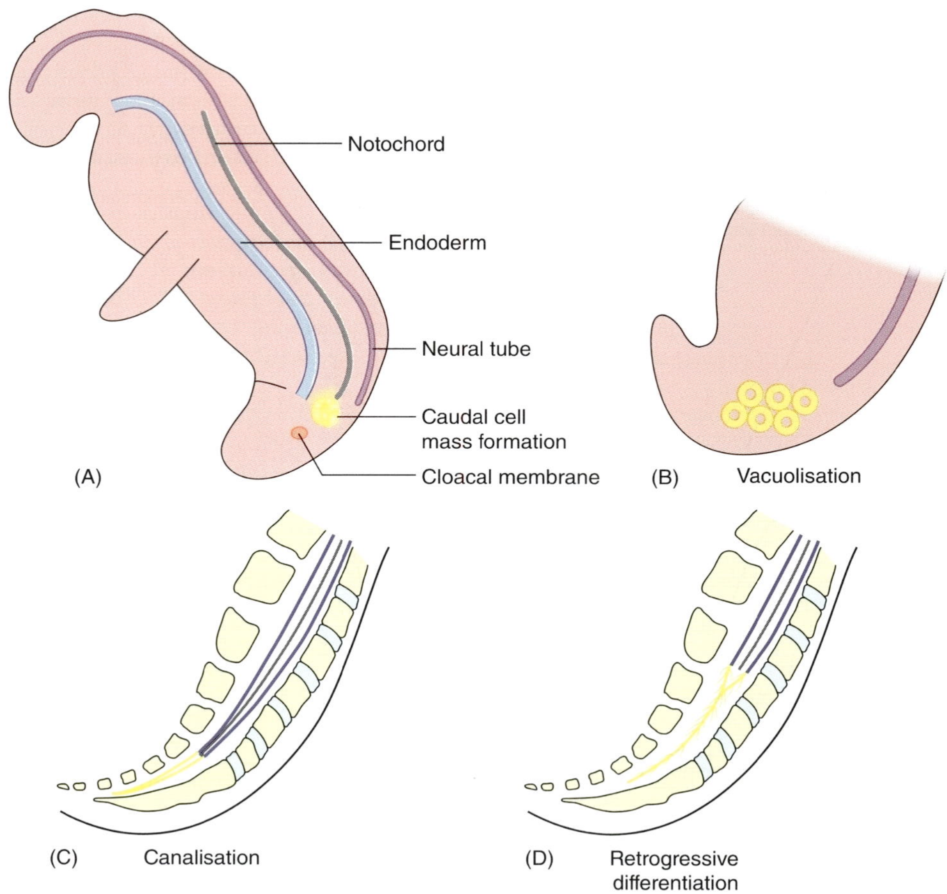

Fig. 9.14 Secondary neurulation.

tube defects. These defects impact the tissues covering the neural tube, including the cranial vault, vertebral arches, meninges, muscles and skin. The specific presentation of the defect varies depending on which components are affected.

Anencephaly (Fig. 9.15)

Resulting from the failure of neural tube closure in the cranial region.

- Characterized by the lack of brain development.
- Prenatal diagnosis often leads to pregnancy termination.
- Daily intake of **400 μg of Folic acid** for three months before conception and throughout pregnancy may help prevent NTDs.

Spina bifida

- Occurs due to the failure of neural tube closure anywhere from the cervical to caudal regions, with the lumbosacral region being the most common site.
- Three main types include:
  1. **Spina Bifida Occulta (Hidden):**
     - The vertebra is not completely closed, but the spinal cord does not protrude.
     - Typically presents as a skin dimple with a tuft of hair, and it is not associated with increased **Alpha-feto protein (AFP)**.
  2. **Meningocele:**
     - In this form, meninges herniate between vertebrae.
     - The nervous system remains intact.
     - Meningocele is the least common type.

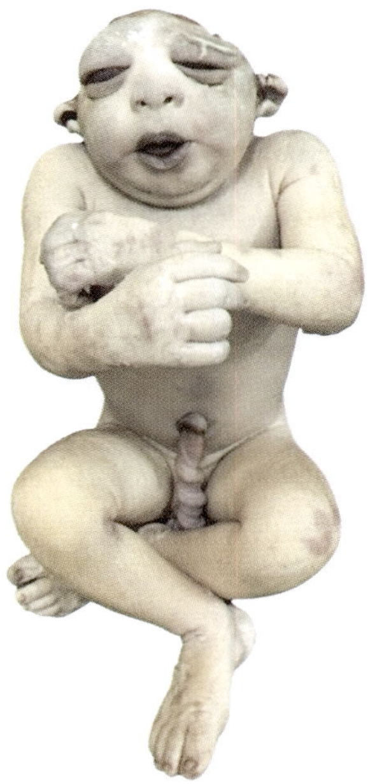

Fig. 9.15 Foetus with anencephaly. (Photo courtesy: Dr Nandagopalan.)

3. **Myelomeningocele:**
   - This is the most severe form with the spinal cord protruding through the defect in the spinal column.
   - **Myeloschisis** is the most severe type of myelomeningocele where the nervous tissue is exposed without an overlying membrane.
- **Neurocutaneous signatures** (hairy tuft, pigmented nevus, angioma, lipoma or dimple) in the lumbosacral region suggest an underlying NTD.

POINTS TO PONDER

During neurulation, the neural plate transforms into a neural tube, which is covered by the ectoderm.

- **The Neural tube** differentiates to give rise to the brain and spinal cord.
- The forebrain, midbrain and hindbrain start taking shape, and the differentiation of neurons and glial cells commences within the neuroepithelium of the neural tube before the start of the fifth week.
- **Somites** form from the paraxial mesoderm in a cranial-to-caudal progression, extending until day 30 of development.
- The somites give rise to three distinct mesodermal components: myotomes, dermatomes and sclerotomes.
  - **Myotomes** contribute to the muscles of the back, ventrolateral body wall and limb musculature.
  - **Dermatomes** are responsible for forming the dermis of the neck and trunk.
  - **Sclerotomes** play a crucial role in the development of vertebral bodies, vertebral arches and the base of the skull.

BRAIN TEASERS

1. What is the primary role of paraxial mesoderm?
   A. Formation of the neural tube.
   B. Development of the gastrointestinal tract.
   C. Differentiation of muscles in the head.
   D. Formation of the kidneys.
2. What does the ventromedial part of a somite give rise to?
   A. Dermis and subcutaneous tissue.
   B. Skeletal muscles and diaphragm.
   C. Vertebral column and ribs.
   D. Base of the skull.
3. What is the primary function of the intermediate mesoderm?
   A. Formation of the head muscles.
   B. Development of the heart.
   C. Differentiation of kidneys and gonads.
   D. Generation of the neural tube.
4. Where is the lateral plate mesoderm derived from?
   A. Primitive streak.
   B. Prechordal plate.
   C. Otic vesicle.
   D. Buccopharyngeal membrane.
5. What does the intraembryonic coelom communicate with to provide nutrition to the developing embryo?
   A. Paraxial mesoderm.
   B. Extraembryonic coelom.
   C. Notochord.
   D. Amniotic fluid.
6. Which part of the lateral plate mesoderm gives rise to the parietal layers of peritoneal, pleural and pericardial sacs?
   A. Somatopleuric.
   B. Splanchnopleuric.
   C. Pericardial bar.
   D. Cardiogenic area.
7. What does the splanchnopleuric layer of the lateral plate mesoderm contribute to?
   A. Formation of skeletal elements in the pectoral girdle.
   B. Development of the gut and respiratory tubes.
   C. The dermis of the neck and trunk.
   D. Musculature and connective tissue in the head.

8. What is the purpose of the septum transversum?
   A. Formation of the neural tube.
   B. Contribution to the development of the diaphragm.
   C. Development of the heart.
   D. Differentiation of the limbs.
9. Which mesodermal layer gives rise to the musculature of the back, ventrolateral body wall and limb musculature?
   A. Dermatomes
   B. Sclerotomes
   C. Myotomes
   D. Somatopleuric layer
10. What is the origin of the neural plate during embryonic development?
   A. Mesoderm
   B. Endoderm
   C. Ectoderm
   D. Notochord
11. What is the process through which the neural tube and its derivatives are formed from the neural plate called?
   A. Neoplasia
   B. Neurulation
   C. Neurogenesis
   D. Neurapraxia
12. What is the role of the notochord in neurulation?
   A. Formation of neural crest cells.
   B. Inducing the formation of the neural tube.
   C. Development of the brain.
   D. Closure of neuropores.
13. Where does fusion of the neural folds initially occur during neurulation?
   A. Caudal region
   B. Lumbar region
   C. Cervical region
   D. Sacral region
14. What are the regions where fusion has not occurred termed during neurulation?
   A. Neuropores
   B. Somites
   C. Neurectoderm
   D. Neural crest cells
15. How does the neural tube obtain nutrition before the establishment of the circulatory system?
   A. From the placenta.
   B. Through diffusion with surrounding tissues.
   C. From the amniotic fluid.
   D. By direct contact with the yolk sac.

Answers

1. (C); 2. (C); 3. (C); 4. (A); 5. (B); 6. (A); 7. (B); 8. (B); 9. (C); 10. (C); 11. (B); 12. (B); 13. (C); 14. (A); 15. (C).

FURTHER READINGS

Maschner A, Krück S, Draga M, Pröls F, Scaal M. Developmental dynamics of occipital and cervical somites. *J Anat.* 2016;229(5):601-609. doi:10.1111/joa.12516.

Vijayraghavan DS, Davidson LA. Mechanics of neurulation: from classical to current perspectives on the physical mechanics that shape, fold, and form the neural tube. *Birth Defects Res.* 2017;109(2):153-168. doi:10.1002/bdra.23557.

Yang J, Lee JY, Kim KH, Wang KC. Disorders of secondary neurulation: mainly focused on patho-embryogenesis. *J Korean Neurosurg Soc.* 2021;64(3):386-405. doi:10.3340/jkns.2021.0023.

10 Third Month to Birth

AN 76.2 Explain the terms—trimester and viability.
AN 80.6 Explain embryological basis of estimation of foetal age.
AN 81.1 Describe various methods of prenatal diagnosis.
AN 81.2 Describe indications, process and disadvantages of amniocentesis.
AN 81.3 Describe indications, process and disadvantages of chorionic villus biopsy.

ANAMNESE

In a high-risk pregnancy scenario, a 35-year-old expectant mother was referred for an amniocentesis procedure. At 16 weeks of gestation, her obstetrician recommended the test due to her advanced maternal age, which posed an increased risk for chromosomal abnormalities in the foetus. The amniocentesis was conducted to collect a small sample of amniotic fluid surrounding the developing baby, allowing for genetic analysis. She had received thorough counselling about the procedure, its risks and benefits, and she decided to proceed with the test in order to understand her baby's health and to assist her in making informed decisions about the pregnancy. She was anxious but hopeful that the results of the amniocentesis would provide the reassurance she needed and guide her prenatal care journey.

The second trimester of pregnancy is often referred to as the **'golden period'** due to the alleviation of many early pregnancy discomforts. Inadequate maternal weight gain during pregnancy has been suggested as a potential contributor to **Intrauterine growth retardation** (IUGR). In the third trimester, the foetus experiences a fourfold increase in fat mass, highlighting the significance of sufficient foetal nutrition during this phase. The maternal weight gain during the third trimester may account for as much as half of the total weight gain.

- Clinically, pregnancy is divided into three trimesters, each lasting approximately 3 months.
  - By the end of the **first trimester**, all major organ systems are typically developed.
  - The **second trimester** witnesses the enlargement of the uterus, foetal growth and increased visibility of anatomical details through ultrasonography. Morning sickness tends to subside, and most major foetal anomalies become detectable during this period.
  - The **third trimester**, often referred to as the foetal period, is characterized by tissue and organ maturation, along with rapid foetal body growth. While head growth decelerates relative to the body, the foetal head descends into the pelvic cavity (Engagement) in preparation for birth.
- In the event of premature birth during the third trimester, newborns may survive with the assistance of intensive care measures.

ESTIMATION OF FOETAL AGE (AN 80.6)

- Foetal length is commonly expressed through two key measurements:
  - **Crown-rump length (CRL):** Measured from the top of the head (crown) to the bottom of the buttocks (rump), it is the preferred method for first-trimester assessment (as depicted in Figs 10.1 and 10.2).
  - **Crown-heel length (CHL):** This measurement extends from the crown of the head to the heel in embryos/foetuses (as illustrated in Fig. 10.1) and is equivalent to the standing height in adults.
- Ultrasound measurements of CRL are instrumental in determining the foetus's size, probable age and the expected delivery date (as seen in AN 80.6).
- Pregnancy duration is typically calculated as:
  - **280 days or 40 weeks** from the onset of the last menstrual period (LMP) (equivalent to 10 lunar months).
  - **266 days or 38 weeks** from fertilization (equivalent to 9 and 1/2 lunar months).
- Pregnancy is traditionally divided into **three trimesters**, each coinciding with different phases of foetal development:
  - The **first trimester** marks the initiation of basic cell differentiation.

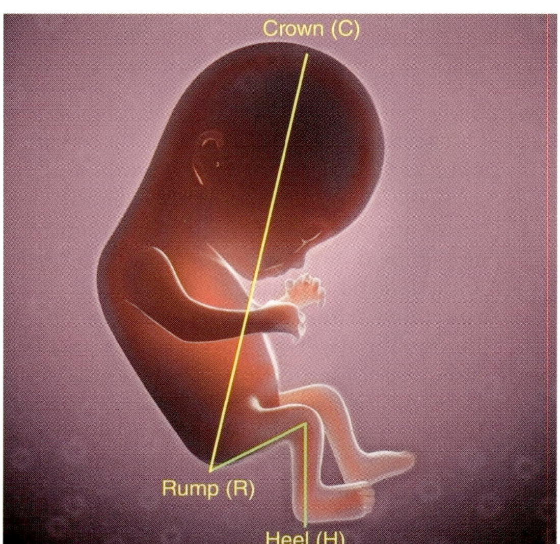

Fig. 10.1 Foetus showing CRL (Crown Rump Length)—CR and CHL (Crown Heel Length)—CRH.

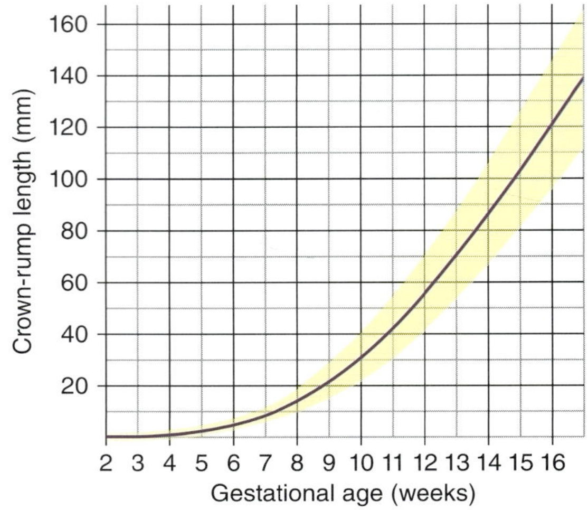

Fig. 10.2 Graph correlating the values of CRL and gestational age.

  - The **second trimester** is characterized by rapid foetal growth and the maturation of various body systems.
  - The **third trimester** represents the final stage of foetal growth, where the development of systems is completed, concluding with childbirth.
- Key measurements during foetal assessment include:
  - Biparietal diameter (the diameter of the head between two parietal eminences).
  - Head circumference.
  - Abdominal circumference.
  - Femur length.
  - Foot length (which exhibits a strong correlation with CRL).
  - Foetal weight, which can vary.

THE CHANGES IN FOETUS

The foetal period consists of the time from 9 weeks until birth and is divided into several stages, each lasting approximately 4–5 weeks.

- **Nine to twelve weeks:**
  - During this phase, the foetal head accounts for half of the CHL.
  - The body experiences rapid lengthening.
  - Facial features become distinct (at 9 weeks).
  - Primary ossification centres appear (at 12 weeks).

  - The upper limbs reach their final relative length while the lower limbs are still comparatively shorter (at 12 weeks).
  - By the 12th week, the external genitalia of both sexes are clearly differentiated.
  - The physiological umbilical hernia typically resolves by the 11th week.
  - Erythropoiesis gradually transitions from the liver (at 9 weeks) to the spleen (at 12 weeks).
  - Urine production commences during this period and is released into the amniotic fluid.
- **Thirteen to sixteen weeks:**
  - The foetus exhibits rapid growth.
  - Limb length and movement increase (although quickening, foetal movements may not be felt by the mother yet).
  - Bones become visible through ultrasound imaging.
  - Primordial ovarian follicles form.
  - The patterning of scalp hair begins.
  - By the 12–14 week period, the sex of the foetus can be determined.
  - The eyes and ears are positioned.
- **Seventeen to twenty weeks:**
  - Growth slows down compared to previous weeks.
  - Mothers typically start feeling **quickening**, the baby's movements.
  - A protective substance called **vernix caseosa** covers the skin, secreted by the foetal sebaceous glands, shielding the delicate skin from the effects of amniotic fluid.
  - Fine hair known as **lanugo** aids in retaining vernix caseosa.
  - Brown fat begins to accumulate.
- **Twenty-one to twenty-five weeks:**
  - There is a rapid gain in foetal weight.
  - The skin takes on a pink to red hue.
  - Rapid eye movements commence (at 21 weeks).
  - **Type 2 pneumocytes** start secreting surfactants (at 24 weeks).
- **Twenty-six to twenty-nine weeks:**
  - The foetus reaches a stage of **viability,** indicating the potential to survive if born prematurely.
  - The central nervous system now controls breathing and regulates body temperature.
  - **Erythropoiesis** primarily occurs in the bone marrow (at 28 weeks).
  - Eyelids open by the 26th week, and toenails become visible.
- **Thirty to thirty-four weeks:**
  - The pupillary light reflex is observable.
  - Premature infants born after the 32nd week have a good chance of survival.
- **Thirty-five to thirty-eight weeks:**
  - The foetus displays a firm grasp and reacts to light.
  - The head and abdominal circumferences initially equalize, but later on, the abdominal circumference surpasses the head circumference.
- **At full term:**
  - The CRL is approximately 360 mm.
  - The average weight is around 3400 g.
  - Male foetuses tend to be longer and heavier than female foetuses.
  - The testes descend into the scrotum.

VIABILITY OF FOETUS (AN 76.2)

- Foetal viability pertains to the foetus's ability to survive outside the uterus.
- Currently, a foetus born after 24 weeks has a considerably higher chance of survival compared to those born before 24 weeks.
- Viability is primarily influenced by gestational age and the baby's weight, with infants weighing less than 500 g facing exceptionally challenging survival odds.
- The maturity of the baby's lungs is a critical factor. Foetal lung development is essential for the baby to breathe independently after birth.
- **Surfactants**, which help keep the lung's air sacs open, are typically produced in adequate amounts after 24–28 weeks of gestation.
- The following factors enhance foetal viability:
  - Good perinatal care.
  - Intensive foetal therapy.
  - Early detection of foetal distress.
- The viability of a foetus is typically assessed by a combination of clinical and diagnostic criteria.
  - **Gestational Age Assessment:** This is typically based on the woman's LMP and confirmed by early ultrasound scans. Gestational age is measured in weeks and days.
  - **Foetal Heartbeat:** The presence of a foetal heartbeat is a significant indicator of foetal viability. Typically, a foetal heartbeat can be detected by ultrasound as early as 6–7 weeks of gestation. By 12 weeks, it should be easily detectable with a Doppler device during prenatal checkups.

- **Foetal Movement:** Foetal movement, or **'quickening'**, is another sign of foetal well-being. Usually, pregnant individuals start feeling foetal movements between 18 and 25 weeks of gestation, depending on various factors.
- **Ultrasound Imaging:** Ultrasonography is an essential tool for assessing foetal viability. Ultrasound scans can help determine gestational age, evaluate foetal anatomy, check amniotic fluid levels and assess blood flow in the umbilical cord and foetal vessels. The presence of foetal movements, a strong heartbeat and appropriate foetal growth are positive indicators.
- **Nonstress Test (NST):** NST is a common prenatal test used to assess foetal well-being during the third trimester. It measures the **baby's heart rate** in response to its movements. A healthy foetus will have an increased heart rate with movements.
- **Biophysical Profile (BPP):** A BPP is a more comprehensive assessment of foetal well-being, combining the NST with ultrasound imaging to evaluate foetal movements, amniotic fluid levels, muscle tone and breathing movements. A higher **BPP score** indicates better foetal health.
- **Amniocentesis:** In some cases, amniocentesis may be performed to assess foetal lung maturity. The level of **surfactant**, a substance crucial for lung function, in the amniotic fluid can provide information about foetal lung development and potential viability.
- **Maternal Health and Conditions:** The health and underlying medical conditions of the pregnant individual also play a significant role in assessing foetal viability.

PRENATAL DIAGNOSIS (AN 81.1)

Various methods are employed to evaluate the growth and development of the foetus in utero, which include:

- **Ultrasonography:** A noninvasive imaging technique using high-frequency sound waves to visualize the foetus, assess its growth and monitor its well-being. It provides valuable information about foetal anatomy, size and position.
- **Maternal Serum Screening:** A blood test performed on the mother to screen for markers that can indicate the risk of certain foetal abnormalities or genetic conditions, such as **Down syndrome**. It helps in assessing the likelihood of foetal health issues.
- **Chorionic Villus Sampling (CVS):** A prenatal diagnostic procedure involving the sampling of chorionic villi from the placenta. CVS is used to detect **chromosomal abnormalities** and genetic conditions in the foetus.
- **Amniocentesis:** A diagnostic test that involves the withdrawal of a small amount of amniotic fluid from the amniotic sac surrounding the foetus. Amniocentesis provides genetic and chromosomal information and can help assess lung maturity.
- **Foetal Blood Sampling (PUBS—Percutaneous Umbilical Cord Blood Sampling):** A procedure that involves the direct sampling of foetal blood from the **umbilical cord** to assess the foetus's blood composition and oxygen levels, particularly in cases of foetal distress.
- **Preimplantation Genetic Diagnosis:** A genetic testing method performed during **In vitro fertilization (IVF)** to screen embryos for genetic disorders before implantation in the uterus.
- **Cardiotocography (CTG):** A monitoring technique that records the foetal heart rate and uterine contractions during pregnancy and labour. It is used to assess the well-being of the foetus and detect signs of foetal distress.

ULTRASONOGRAPHY (USG)

A noninvasive imaging technique utilizing high-frequency sound waves.

- Can be performed **transabdominally or transvaginally** for various purposes.
- **Key parameters** assessed include:
  - Foetal age and growth.
  - Determination of single or multiple gestations.
  - Identification of foetal presentation.
  - Detection of congenital anomalies.
  - Evaluation of uterine anomalies.
  - Assessment of amniotic fluid levels.
  - Localization of the placenta's position.
  - Examination of blood flow through the umbilical cord.
  - Estimation of the expected date of confinement (EDC).
  - Pelvic assessment.
- **Foetal age** is calculated using various measurements such as:
  - Crown-rump length.

- Biparietal diameter of the foetal skull.
- Femur length.
- Abdominal circumference.

• **Congenital anomalies** that can be detected include:
  - Neural tube defects (e.g. anencephaly and spina bifida).
  - Cardiovascular malformations consisting of valve defects, septal defects and major vessel malformations.
  - Facial defects like cleft lip and cleft palate.
  - Abdominal wall defects such as omphalocele and gastroschisis.
  - Genetic conditions like Down syndrome, assessed partly through nuchal translucency measurements.

The main types of ultrasound scans during pregnancy:

- **Transabdominal Ultrasound:** This is the most common type of prenatal ultrasound. A transducer, which emits and receives sound waves, is moved across the mother's abdomen to create images of the developing foetus. It is often used in the first trimester for dating the pregnancy and checking the baby's heartbeat. Later in pregnancy, it is used to monitor foetal growth, amniotic fluid levels and the position of the placenta.
- **Transvaginal Ultrasound:** In the early stages of pregnancy, particularly during the first trimester, a transvaginal ultrasound may be performed. A small, wand-like transducer is inserted into the vagina to provide a closer and clearer view of the uterus and developing foetus. This type of ultrasound is especially useful for dating pregnancies, detecting ectopic pregnancies and assessing the viability of the embryo.
- **Doppler Ultrasound:** Doppler ultrasound is used to assess **blood flow** in the umbilical cord, placenta and foetal heart. It can help identify any potential circulation problems or foetal distress. This type of ultrasound is particularly valuable in high-risk pregnancies and when monitoring the well-being of the foetus (Fig. 10.3).
- **3D and 4D Ultrasound:** These advanced ultrasound techniques provide three-dimensional or real-time **'live' images** of the foetus. While 3D ultrasounds offer static, detailed images, 4D ultrasounds provide moving, real-time views of the baby in utero. These scans are primarily used for the enjoyment and bonding experience of parents and are not typically considered diagnostic tools.

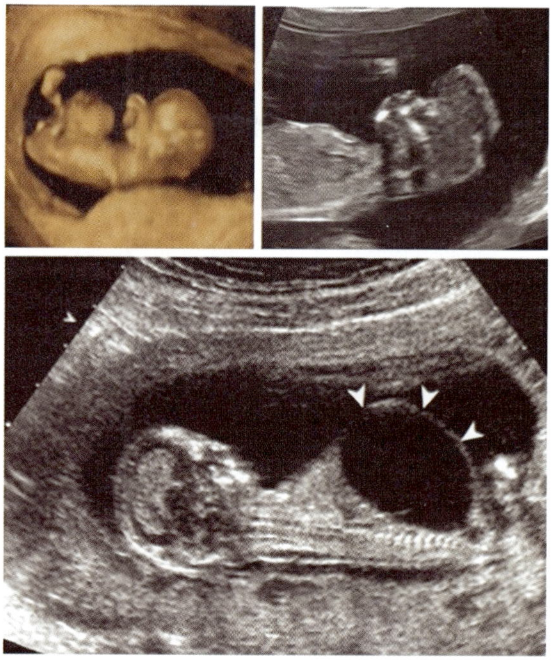

Fig. 10.3 Foetus seen on three-dimensional ultrasound. (Source: Diagnostic Ultrasound, 6th ed.: Deborah Levine, Carol M. Rumack, Fig. 32.6, Elsevier Inc., 2024.)

- **Level II or Targeted Ultrasound:** This is a comprehensive, detailed ultrasound typically performed in the second trimester, around 18–22 weeks. It assesses the foetus's anatomy, looking for any structural abnormalities or birth defects. It is also used to evaluate the placenta, amniotic fluid levels and foetal growth.
- **Biophysical Profile:** A BPP combines ultrasound imaging with a **NST** to assess the foetal well-being, particularly in cases where there may be concerns about the baby's health. It evaluates various factors, including foetal movements, foetal breathing, amniotic fluid levels and the reactivity of the baby's heart rate.
- **Growth Ultrasound:** This type of ultrasound is used to monitor foetal growth throughout the pregnancy. It tracks the baby's size, estimated weight and measurements of specific body parts. Growth ultrasounds can

help identify potential **growth restrictions or macrosomia** (excessive foetal growth).

- **Foetal Echocardiography:** When there are concerns about the baby's heart, a foetal echocardiography, or **foetal cardiac ultrasound**, is performed. This specialized scan focuses on assessing the structure and function of the foetal heart and identifying any congenital heart defects.

MATERNAL SERUM SCREENING

SERUM ALPHA-FETOPROTEIN (AFP)

- Originating from the foetal liver around the 14th week of gestation, AFP enters the maternal circulation via the placenta.
- **Elevated AFP** levels in maternal serum and amniotic fluid are associated with conditions such as:
  - **Neural tube defects.**
  - **Sacrococcygeal teratoma.**
  - **Abdominal wall defects (omphalocele, gastroschisis, bladder exstrophy).**
  - **Amniotic band syndrome.**
  - **Intestinal atresia.**
- Conversely, **decreased AFP levels** are observed in cases of:
  - **Down syndrome.**
  - **Trisomy 18.**
  - **Triploidy.**
  - **Sex chromosomal anomalies.**

Triple Test (Kettering/Bart's Test):

- Conducted during the second trimester of pregnancy (15–18 weeks), this screening test is used to assess the risk of chromosomal abnormalities and neural tube defects.
- It involves measuring the serum levels of AFP, unconjugated estriol (UE3) and beta-hCG.
- In **Trisomy 18 (Edwards syndrome),** all values are low.
- In **Down syndrome,** hCG levels are high, while AFP and UE3 levels are low.

Quadruple Test/Quad Test

The quadruple test includes the triple test components along with **inhibin A.**

- Inhibin A is:
  - High in **Down** syndrome.
  - Low in **Edwards** syndrome.

CHORIONIC VILLUS SAMPLING (AN 81.3)

- A needle is carefully inserted into the placenta either transvaginally or transabdominally, with the assistance of ultrasound guidance (Fig. 10.4).
- Approximately 5–30 mg of **placental tissue** is aspirated and subsequently cultured for genetic analysis.
- This procedure is typically performed around the **10–11 weeks** of gestation.
- **Genetic analysis** of the cultured DNA helps identify and rule out chromosomal abnormalities.
- The tissue obtained during CVS can also be employed for various molecular-genetic analyses.
- In some instances, CVS results may be inconclusive due to chromosomal mosaicism, which can stem from a mosaic foetus or confined placental mosaicism. Such cases require confirmation through amniocentesis.
- Complications associated with CVS include an increased frequency of **limb malformations** when performed early in pregnancy. Additionally, a tear in the amnion during the CVS procedure can lead to the development of an **amniotic band** that may encircle and compromise the blood supply to foetal digits, resulting in degeneration and eventual loss of the affected digits.

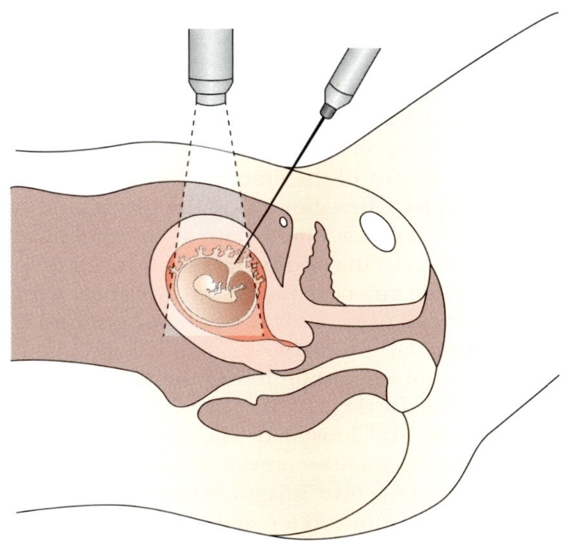

Fig. 10.4 Chorionic villi sampling.

AMNIOCENTESIS (AN 81.2)

- A needle is carefully inserted transabdominally into the amniotic cavity, guided by USG. (Fig. 10.5)
- Approximately 20–30 mL of **Amniotic fluid** is withdrawn for analysis.
- Amniocentesis is not typically performed before 14 weeks of gestation due to the lower volume of amniotic fluid at earlier stages, which increases the risk of foetal injury.
- The extracted amniotic fluid is analysed for:
  - Assessing the levels of **AFP** and **acetylcholinesterase**.
  - Additionally, the fluid contains sloughed-off foetal cells, which can be used for **karyotyping**.
  - PCR **(polymerase chain reaction)** and genotyping to identify and rule out genetic abnormalities.
- This procedure is usually conducted between **14 and 16 weeks** of gestation.
- Amniotic fluid contains metabolic byproducts of the foetus, as well as cells sloughed from the foetus, possibly from the lungs and amniotic membrane.
- Elevated levels of **AFP** may indicate the presence of an open neural tube defect (such as anencephaly) or other open defects like gastroschisis.
- Amniocentesis has limitations in early gestation due to the challenge of performing it when amniotic fluid volume is small, and a small sample may not provide enough cells for analysis.
- In later stages of pregnancy, amniocentesis is utilized to assess foetal lung maturity, Rh sensitization and foetal infections.

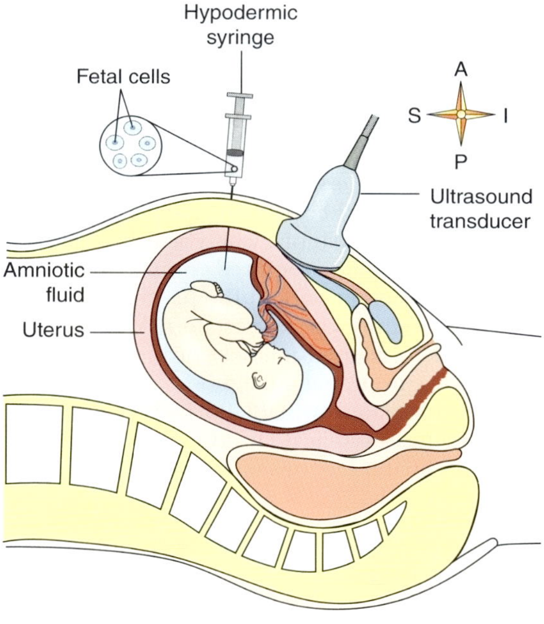

Fig. 10.5 Amniocentesis.

FOETAL BLOOD SAMPLING

- Foetal blood sampling, also known as Percutaneous **Umbilical Cord Blood Sampling (PUBS),** is a medical procedure performed during pregnancy (Fig. 10.6).
- It involves the insertion of a thin needle directly into the umbilical cord under the guidance of USG.
- PUBS allows for the direct collection of a small sample of foetal blood from the umbilical cord.
- The collected foetal blood can be used for various diagnostic and genetic tests to assess foetus.

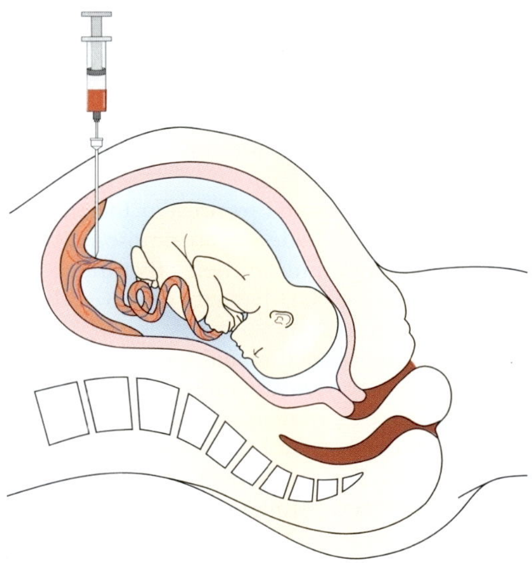

Fig. 10.6 Foetal blood sampling.

- This procedure is typically carried out during the second or third trimester (**24–34 weeks**) of pregnancy.
- PUBS provides valuable information about the foetus, including blood type, oxygen levels,

haemoglobin concentration and the presence of any genetic disorders or infections.

- It is a diagnostic tool used to evaluate the foetal condition when other prenatal tests, such as amniocentesis and CVS, may not provide sufficient information.
- PUBS is considered a more invasive procedure compared to other prenatal tests and is usually reserved for situations where specific diagnostic information is required to make informed medical decisions about the pregnancy.
- The procedure carries certain risks and is performed by trained medical professionals with expertise in prenatal diagnosis.
- Risks associated with PUBS include injury to the foetus, umbilical cord or placenta, as well as potential infections or bleeding.

PREIMPLANTATION GENETIC DIAGNOSIS

- **Preimplantation genetic diagnosis (PGD)** is a specialized genetic testing technique used in conjunction with IVF during assisted reproductive procedures.
- PGD is performed before the embryo is implanted into the woman's uterus (Fig. 10.7).
- It involves the **genetic analysis of embryos** created through IVF to identify specific genetic abnormalities or traits.
- PGD is primarily used to prevent the transmission of genetic disorders or chromosomal abnormalities from parents to their offspring.
- The process of PGD typically involves the following steps:
  1. **Ovulation Induction and Egg Retrieval:** The woman's ovaries are stimulated to produce multiple eggs, which are then collected during an egg retrieval procedure.
  2. **In Vitro Fertilization:** The retrieved eggs are fertilized with sperm in a laboratory to create embryos.
  3. **Embryo Culture:** The embryos are allowed to develop in the laboratory for several days.
  4. **Biopsy:** Typically on the third day or at the blastocyst stage (around five days), one or more cells are removed from the embryo.
  5. **Genetic Testing:** The biopsied cells are genetically analysed for specific genetic mutations, chromosomal abnormalities or desired genetic traits.

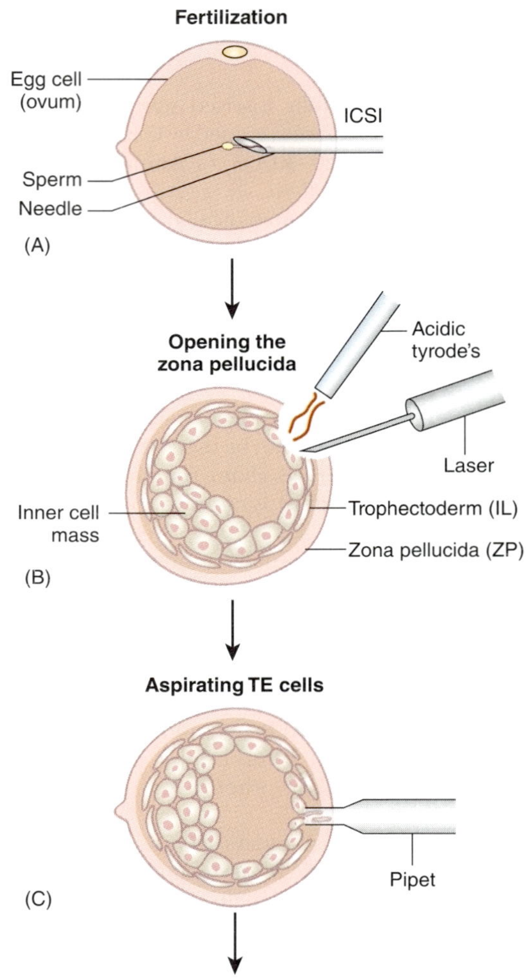

Preimplantation Genetic Testing–Aneuploidy
Next generation sequencing
or
Single nucleotide polymorphism array

Preimplantation Genetic Testing–Monosomic disorder
Single nucleotide polymorphism array

(D)

Fig. 10.7 Preimplantation genetic diagnosis.

  6. **Embryo Selection:** Based on the genetic test results, only embryos without the identified genetic issues are selected for implantation.
  7. **Embryo Transfer:** The selected embryo(s) are transferred into the woman's uterus.

- PGD can be used for a variety of genetic purposes, including identifying single gene disorders, chromosomal abnormalities, gender selection and screening for specific genetic traits.
- PGD can provide prospective parents with information about the genetic health of embryos before pregnancy is established, which can help reduce the risk of having a child with a genetic condition.
- PGD is often considered in cases where one or both parents carry a known **genetic mutation** or have a history of genetic diseases in the family.
- It offers the potential to increase the chances of a successful pregnancy while minimizing the risk of passing on genetic disorders to the next generation.

CARDIOTOCOGRAPHY

- It is a technical means of recording the **foetal heartbeat** and the **uterine contractions** during pregnancy.
- Done in **third trimester** to monitor foetal well-being (Fig. 10.8).
- Cardiotocography, often abbreviated as CTG, is a medical monitoring technique used during pregnancy and labour to assess the well-being of the foetus and to monitor

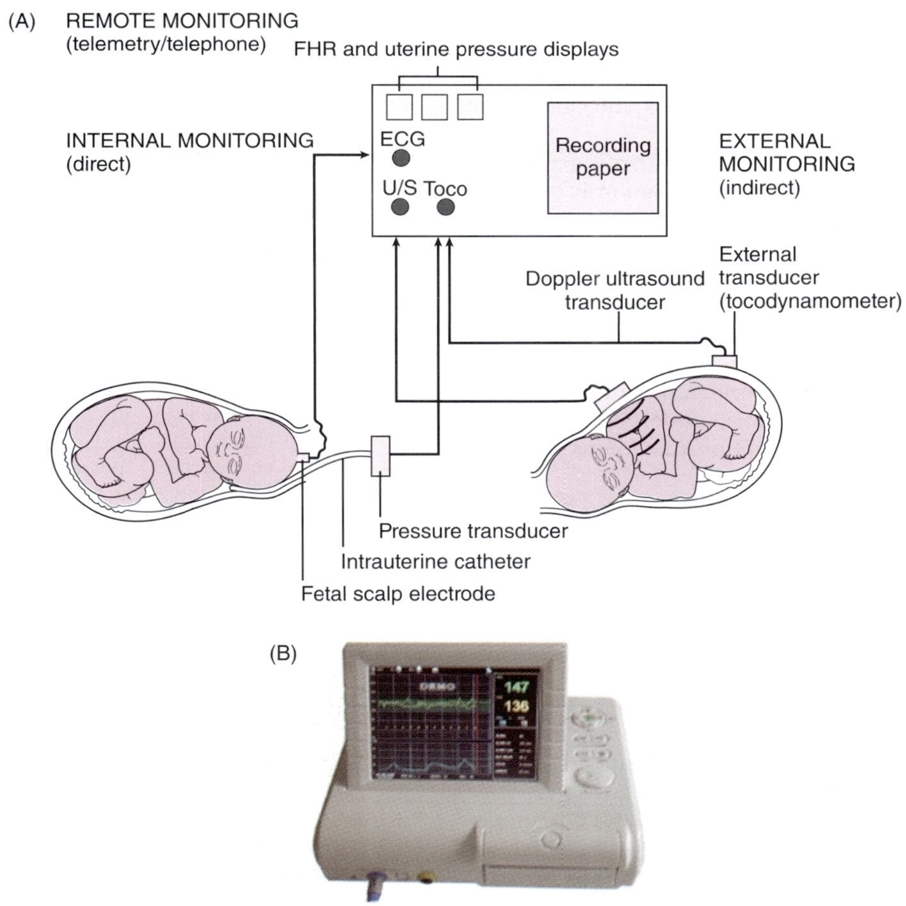

Fig. 10.8 Cardiotocograph to record foetal heart rate and uterine contractions. (A) Cardiotocography monitor. (B) Cardiotocographe. (Source (Fig. 10.8 A): *Skills for Midwifery Practice*, 4th ed. 2017.) (Source (Fig. 10.8 B): *Obstétrique: pour le praticien*, 6th ed. 2013.)

the uterine contractions of the pregnant woman.

- CTG involves the simultaneous recording of two essential parameters:
  - **Foetal Heart Rate (FHR):** This is the recording of the baby's heart rate, which is a vital indicator of foetal well-being. It helps identify signs of distress or abnormal heart rhythms.
  - **Uterine Contractions:** The uterine contractions experienced by the mother are recorded. The frequency, duration and strength of these contractions are essential in evaluating the progress of labour and identifying any potential issues.
- CTG is typically used in the following situations:
  - **Antenatal Monitoring:** In this context, CTG is used to monitor the foetal heart rate during routine check-ups, especially in high-risk pregnancies. This helps in early detection of any potential issues and allows for timely intervention.
  - **Intrapartum Monitoring:** During labour, CTG is widely used to continuously monitor both the foetal heart rate and uterine contractions. It helps ensure the safety and well-being of the baby during the birthing process.
  - **High-Risk Pregnancies:** Women with high-risk pregnancies, such as those with gestational diabetes, preeclampsia or other medical conditions, may undergo CTG more frequently to monitor the foetus's condition.
- CTG is typically conducted using two transducers placed on the mother's abdomen:
  - One transducer records the **foetal heart rate**, often using Doppler ultrasound or direct foetal electrocardiography (FECG).
  - The second transducer measures **uterine contractions**. It is often done by measuring changes in pressure within a belt placed around the abdomen.
- The CTG machine records the data on a paper strip or digitally in real-time.
- The patterns observed during CTG can be classified into different categories, such as **reassuring, nonreassuring or ominous**. A reassuring pattern indicates a healthy and well-oxygenated foetus, while nonreassuring or ominous patterns may signify potential issues that require further evaluation or intervention.

CLINICAL NUGGETS

Treating foetus in utero

The medical management of a foetus in utero aims to lessen the impact of prenatally diagnosed birth defects. There are two primary approaches to foetal intervention:

1. **Surgical Intervention:**
   - Surgical procedures may be employed to address specific congenital anomalies that have been identified before birth. Some conditions that may require surgical intervention include **congenital diaphragmatic hernia, spina bifida** and **hydrocephalus.**
   - In cases of **sacrococcygeal teratomas**, particularly when they are large and require a substantial blood supply, surgical removal is often necessary to prevent heart failure.
   - It is important to note that while foetal surgery is occasionally considered, the survival benefit compared to postnatal surgery is limited in many cases. Consequently, postnatal repair remains the primary treatment approach for most conditions.
2. **Drug Intervention:**
   - Drug therapies during pregnancy can help manage certain foetal conditions. These interventions are typically medical treatments aimed at minimizing potential complications.
   - For example, prenatal supplementation with **folic acid** is recommended to reduce the risk of neural tube defects in the developing foetus.
   - In cases of foetal congenital adrenal hyperplasia (CAH), expectant mothers may be treated with medications like **dexamethasone** during pregnancy to manage the condition and its potential effects on the developing baby.

The choice of treatment approach depends on the specific foetal diagnosis, the gestational age, the severity of the condition and the potential benefits and risks associated with intervention.

KLINISCHE PERLEN

LOW-BIRTH WEIGHT (LBW)

- A newborn's size is typically within the range of 2500–4000 g, with an average length of approximately 51 cm. When an infant's weight falls below 2500 g, it is categorized as having a LBW. LBW can result from various factors, including:
  - **Intrauterine Growth Restriction (IUGR) in Full-Term Infants:** In some cases, full-term infants may experience restricted growth in the womb, leading to a LBW. This could be due to

placental insufficiency, maternal health issues or other factors that limit foetal growth.
   - **Shortened Gestation in Preterm Infants:** Preterm infants, born before completing the full term of pregnancy (usually 37 weeks or earlier), often have LBW due to their shorter time in the womb.
- The key growth-promoting factor before and after birth is **Insulin-like Growth Factor 1 (IGF-1)**. Genetic mutations involving IGF-1 can lead to IUGR and growth retardation after birth.
- Following birth, IGF-1 synthesis is regulated by the influence of growth hormone (GH). Mutations in the growth hormone receptor (GHR) can result in conditions such as **Laron's dwarfism,** characterized by short stature and blue sclera. Interestingly, individuals with Laron's dwarfism do not typically exhibit IUGR since prenatal IGF-1 production is not governed by GH.
- In addition to these factors, maternal health conditions can contribute to LBW:
   - **Preeclampsia:** Preeclampsia is a condition characterized by maternal hypertension and proteinuria, typically occurring anytime between 20 weeks of pregnancy and term. If left untreated, preeclampsia can progress to eclampsia, which is marked by seizures. This condition not only poses risks to the mother's health but can also lead to foetal growth retardation, foetal death or even maternal death in severe cases.
   - **Postterm Syndrome:** When a pregnancy extends for three or more weeks beyond the expected due date, it is referred to as postterm syndrome. Prolonged gestation increases the risk of various complications, including higher foetal and neonatal mortality rates.

POINTS TO PONDER

Foetal Development and Pregnancy Stages

The foetal period is characterized by remarkable growth in both length and mass of the embryo. During the early stages, the developing foetus is relatively thin, but as pregnancy progresses, subcutaneous fat is deposited, contributing to a more rounded appearance.

- Key developmental milestones and changes during this period include:
   - **Cardiac development:** The foetal heart exhibits significant changes. At around 5 weeks, the heart rate is approximately 100 beats per minute, which increases to about 160 beats per minute by 8 weeks. Subsequently, the heart rate undergoes a slight decrease during the remainder of the intrauterine period.
   - **Ductus arteriosus patency:** The ductus arteriosus, a foetal blood vessel that connects the pulmonary artery to the descending aorta, is kept open by prostaglandin E2 during foetal development.
   - **Pulmonary surfactant production:** Pulmonary surfactant, a vital substance for proper lung function, is secreted by the foetal lungs at approximately 24 weeks of gestation. Large quantities of surfactant are synthesized in the weeks leading up to birth, contributing to lung maturation.
   - **Foetal movements:** Foetal movements commence around the seventh week of gestation. The matured foetal movements observed later in pregnancy are a result of functional maturation of the central nervous system.
   - **Gastrointestinal development:** Meconium, the earliest stool of a newborn, begins to fill the lower gastrointestinal tract by midpregnancy, reflecting the maturation of the digestive system.
- **Ultrasonography:** Ultrasonography has become the predominant imaging technique in obstetrics, providing details of foetal development and overall pregnancy progress.
- **Sampling techniques:** Procedures such as amniocentesis and chorionic villus sampling are employed to analyse fluids or cells from the embryo and foetus. These diagnostic tests offer essential information for monitoring foetal health and development.
- **Parturition (Childbirth):** The process of childbirth unfolds in several stages, ensuring a safe and healthy delivery for both the mother and baby. These stages include:
   - **Stage I:** Dilatation of the cervix.
   - **Stage II:** Expulsion of the foetus.
   - **Stage III:** Expulsion of the placenta.
   - **Stage IV:** Reestablishment of uterine tone.

BRAIN TEASERS

1. At what gestational age does the central nervous system control breathing and body temperature in the foetus?
   A. 21 weeks
   B. 26 weeks
   C. 30 weeks
   D. 35 weeks
2. When does erythropoiesis primarily occur in the bone marrow of the foetus?
   A. 21 weeks
   B. 24 weeks
   C. 28 weeks
   D. 32 weeks

11 Development of Gut Tubes

AN 52.4 Describe the development of anterior abdominal wall.
AN 52.5 Describe the development and congenital anomalies of diaphragm.
AN 52.6 Describe the development and congenital anomalies of foregut, midgut and hindgut.

ANAMNESE

A 32-year-old female presented with recurrent abdominal pain and discomfort over the past several months. The patient reported episodes of nausea and occasional vomiting associated with the pain. Imaging studies revealed a gut rotation anomaly, specifically a malrotation of the intestines. Further investigations, including a contrast-enhanced Computed Tomography (CT) scan, confirmed the diagnosis. The anomaly was characterized by abnormal positioning of the intestines during foetal development, leading to a potential risk of **volvulus**. The patient underwent surgery to correct the malrotation and prevent complications. The case highlights the importance of recognizing and promptly addressing gut rotation anomalies to prevent complications and ensure optimal patient outcomes (Fig. 11.1).

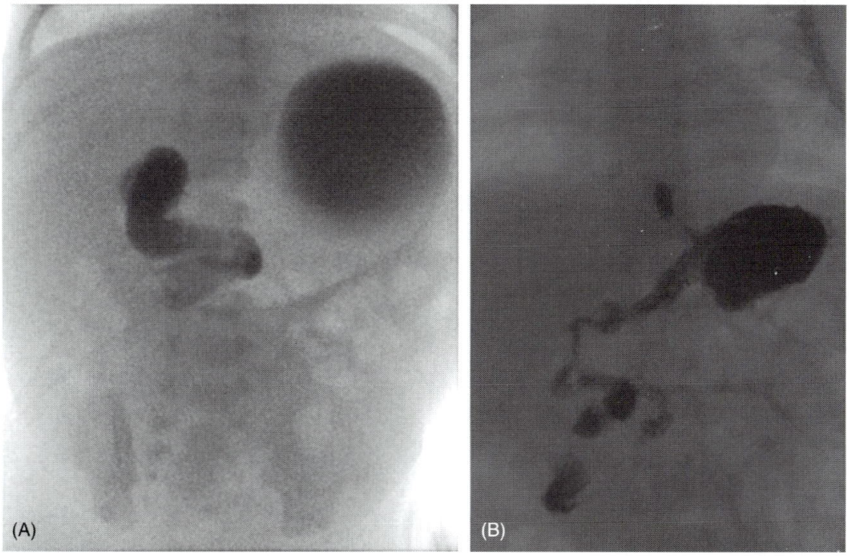

Fig. 11.1 Upper gastrointestinal series showing malrotation with and without obstruction/volvulus. (Source: Avery's Diseases of the Newborn, Eleventh Edition: Taylor Sawyer, Christine A. Gleason, Fig. 6.12, Elsevier Inc., 2024.)

The function of an organ is dependent on its cellular components as well as how they are assembled into a single unit. The developing gut faces unique challenges as it is one of the longest and largest organs in the body, and hence its positioning in the abdomen and the structures derived from it also undergo a complicated mode of development. The aligning of the gut along its longitudinal, dorsoventral, left-right and radial axes is one of the fascinating events in the development of gastrointestinal system.

CONSEQUENCES OF LATERAL FOLDING AND FORMATION OF ANTERIOR ABDOMINAL WALL (AN 52.4)

- **Lateral Folding in Embryonic Development:**
  - Simultaneous with longitudinal folding, the embryo undergoes lateral folding.
  - The left and right flanks of the embryonic disc roll anteriorly, compressing the yolk sac.
  - Germ layers on each side meet and fuse, ensuring continuity in the external surface formation for the embryo, specifically shaping the anterior thoracic and abdominal wall.
- **Ectoderm Fusion:**
  - Ectoderm on the left side merges with the ectoderm on the right side, establishing a continuous external surface for the embryo.
- **Mesodermal and Endodermal Fusion:**
  - Mesodermal and endodermal layers also undergo simultaneous fusion.
  - The endoderm forms a tube that extends between the buccopharyngeal and cloacal membranes while maintaining a connection with the yolk sac. This **endodermal tube** serves as the precursor to the **gastrointestinal tract lining**.
- **Tube Within a Tube Body Plan:**
  - As a consequence of this folding, the embryo adopts a 'tube within a tube' body plan.
  - The outer tube is composed of ectoderm. The inner tube is formed by endoderm. Mesoderm and the early body cavity (coelom) are situated in between these two tubes.

FORMATION OF PRIMITIVE GUT TUBE (AN 52.6)

- **Transformation of the Endodermal Tube:**
  - The endodermal tube undergoes transformation to become the **Primitive gut**. This primitive gut tube serves as the precursor to both the **respiratory** and **digestive systems**.
  - The epithelial lining of both the respiratory and digestive systems originate from the endoderm, except for the regions around the mouth and anal canal, which have an ectodermal origin.
- **Division into Foregut, Midgut and Hindgut:**
  - The primitive gut has a part in free communication with the yolk sac which forms the midgut.
  - The cephalic region forms the foregut, a blind-ended tube cranial to the communication with the yolk sac.
  - In the caudal region, the hindgut is a blind-ended tube caudal to the free communication with the yolk sac (Fig. 11.2).
- **Cloaca Division and Urorectal Septum:**
  - In the ventral aspect of the hindgut, an out-pouching called the **Allantoic diverticulum** arises.
  - The hindgut caudal to this out-pouching is termed the **Cloaca**.
  - The cloaca divides into a broad-ventral **Primitive urogenital sinus** (urogenital system) and a narrow-dorsal **Primitive rectum** (rectum and anal canal).
  - Separation is facilitated by the **urorectal septum**, which fuses with the cloacal membrane, dividing it into a ventral **urogenital membrane** and a dorsal **anal membrane**.

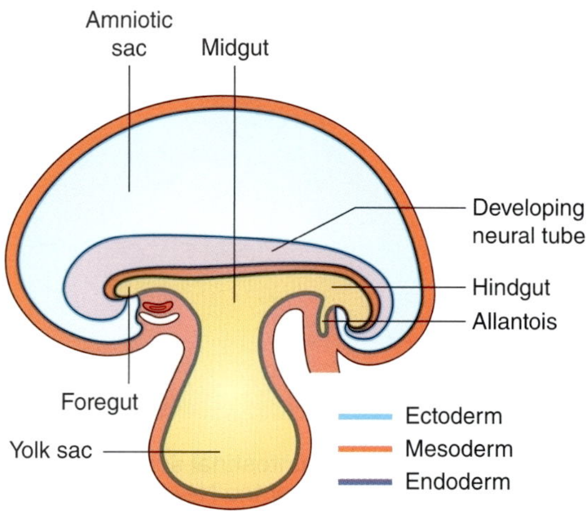

Fig. 11.2 Primitive gut tube showing foregut, midgut and hindgut.

- **Formation of Midgut**
  - The middle part of the primitive gut, in free communication with the yolk sac, is termed the midgut.
  - This communication gradually narrows to form the **vitello-intestinal duct, vitelline duct, yolk stalk or omphalomesenteric duct.** Meckel's diverticulum is the persistent proximal part of vitello-intestinal duct.
  - The midgut undergoes tubularization and forms a loop. Depending on the position of the **Superior mesenteric artery**, the midgut is distinguished into proximal and distal segments.
  - The **Caecal bud** arises from the distal segment of the midgut.
- **Umbilical Opening and Membrane Separation:**
  - After the lateral folding of the embryo, the ectoderm exhibits a defect at the region where the vitello-intestinal duct passes, known as the umbilical opening.
  - The cranial end of the foregut is separated from the stomodeum by the **buccopharyngeal membrane**, while the caudal end of the hindgut is separated from the proctodeum by the **cloacal membrane**.

DERIVATIVES OF GUT TUBE

DERIVATIVES OF FOREGUT

- **Epithelial Lining:**
  - Pharynx, oesophagus, stomach, duodenum (up to ampulla of Vater), respiratory system, auditory tube, tympanic cavity. (The epithelial lining of these structures contributes to the formation of essential passages in the upper gastrointestinal and respiratory systems.)
  - Mucous membrane of tongue.
- **Parenchyma:**
  - Liver and pancreas.
  - Thyroid and parathyroid.
  - Thymus and tonsil.

DERIVATIVES OF MIDGUT

Mucous Membrane of:

- Duodenum. (Second part distal to the major papilla, third part and fourth part.)
- Jejunum.
- Ileum.
- Caecum and appendix.
- Ascending colon.
- Right two-thirds of transverse colon.

DERIVATIVES OF HINDGUT

- **Epithelial Lining and Mucous Membrane of:**
  - Vagina.
  - Alimentary tract. (From the left third of the transverse colon to the pectinate line of the anal canal.)
  - Urinary bladder and urethra.
- **Parenchyma of:**
  - Prostate.
  - Bulbourethral/greater vestibular glands.

ARTERIAL SUPPLY

FOREGUT

- The abdominal derivatives of the foregut receive their arterial supply from branches of the **Coeliac artery** (Fig. 11.3).
- This vascular network covers the region extending from the lower part of the oesophagus to the middle of the second part of the duodenum.

MIDGUT

- Derivatives of the midgut are nourished by branches originating from the **Superior mesenteric artery**.
- This arterial supply extends from the middle of the second part of the duodenum to the junction of the right two-thirds and left one-third of the transverse colon.

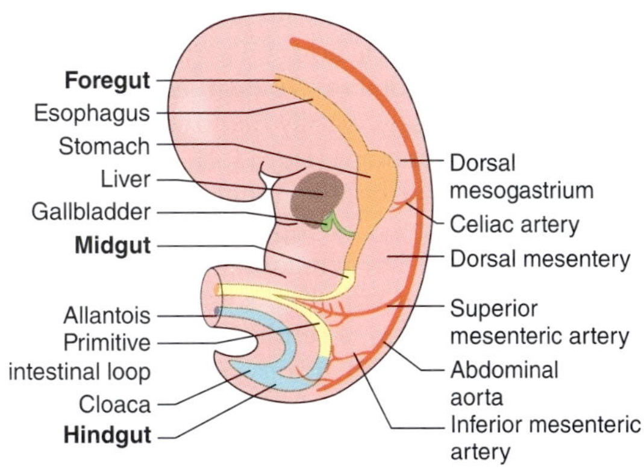

Fig. 11.3 Arterial supply of gut tube.

- The superior mesenteric artery courses up to the apex of the midgut loop through its mesentery, creating a proximal or **Prearterial segment** and a distal or **Postarterial segment** within the midgut.

HINDGUT

- The derivatives of the hindgut are supplied by the **Inferior mesenteric artery**.
- This arterial domain extends from the junction of the right two-thirds and left one-third of the transverse colon to the urogenital sinus.

ROTATION OF GUT

- The midgut loop undergoes elongation, forming a ventral **U-shaped loop** of gut that extends into the proximal umbilical cord, a part of the extraembryonic coelom. This protrusion occurs due to the growing organs' size, resulting in a **Physiological umbilical hernia.**
- The midgut loop, divided into prearterial and postarterial segments based on the position of the superior mesenteric artery, experiences a **90-degree** anticlockwise rotation around the **axis of Superior mesenteric artery** within the umbilical cord when viewed from the front, aligning itself in a horizontal plane.
- During this rotation, the prearterial segment shifts to the right, while the postarterial segment moves to the left.
- The prearterial segment elongates to give rise to:
  a) **Distal duodenum.**
  b) **Coils of jejunum** and **ileum**, initially located outside the abdominal cavity.
- Subsequently, these coils undergo an additional **180-degree** anticlockwise rotation, returning to the abdominal cavity by passing behind the superior mesenteric artery. The complete rotation involves a total of **270 degrees (90 + 180)**, and this process is usually finalized by the **10th week** of development (Fig. 11.4).
- From the postarterial segment, a **Caecal diverticulum** emerges, developing into the caecum and appendix. The remaining part of the postarterial segment contributes to the formation of the lower ileum, ascending colon and proximal two-thirds of the transverse colon.
- The herniated loops ultimately return to the abdominal cavity by the **10th week**, and as the postarterial segment re-enters, it undergoes an anticlockwise rotation. This results in the transverse colon positioning anteriorly to the superior mesenteric artery, with the caecum on its right side.

FIXATION OF GUT

- Initially, all gut derivatives are suspended by a common mesentery during early development.
- Upon completion of rotation, certain parts become retroperitoneal due to the fusion of their mesenteries. These include:
  - **Duodenum** (excluding the proximal few centimetres derived from the foregut).
  - **Ascending colon.**
  - **Descending colon.**
  - **Rectum.**
- Conversely, certain segments retain their original mesentery, contributing to their continued suspension and mobility within the abdominal cavity. These segments include:
  - **Small intestine** (mesentery of the jejunum and ileum).
  - **Transverse colon** (transverse mesocolon).
  - **Sigmoid colon** (sigmoid mesocolon).
- The fixation of gut tubes is a process that ensures the proper organization of gastrointestinal structures as the embryo develops, setting the foundation for their functional roles in digestion and absorption.

DEVELOPMENT OF MESENTERIES

- Mesentery refers to the double layer of peritoneum that encloses an organ and connects it to the body wall, providing structural support.
- Mesenteries suspend the gut tube from both the ventral and dorsal body walls, creating pathways for vessels, nerves and lymphatics to and from abdominal organs.
- Organs enclosed by peritoneum are termed **intraperitoneal**, (covered by peritoneum but not inside the peritoneal cavity) while those against the posterior abdominal wall are termed **retroperitoneal**.
- Initially, the foregut, midgut and hindgut have extensive contact with the posterior abdominal wall.

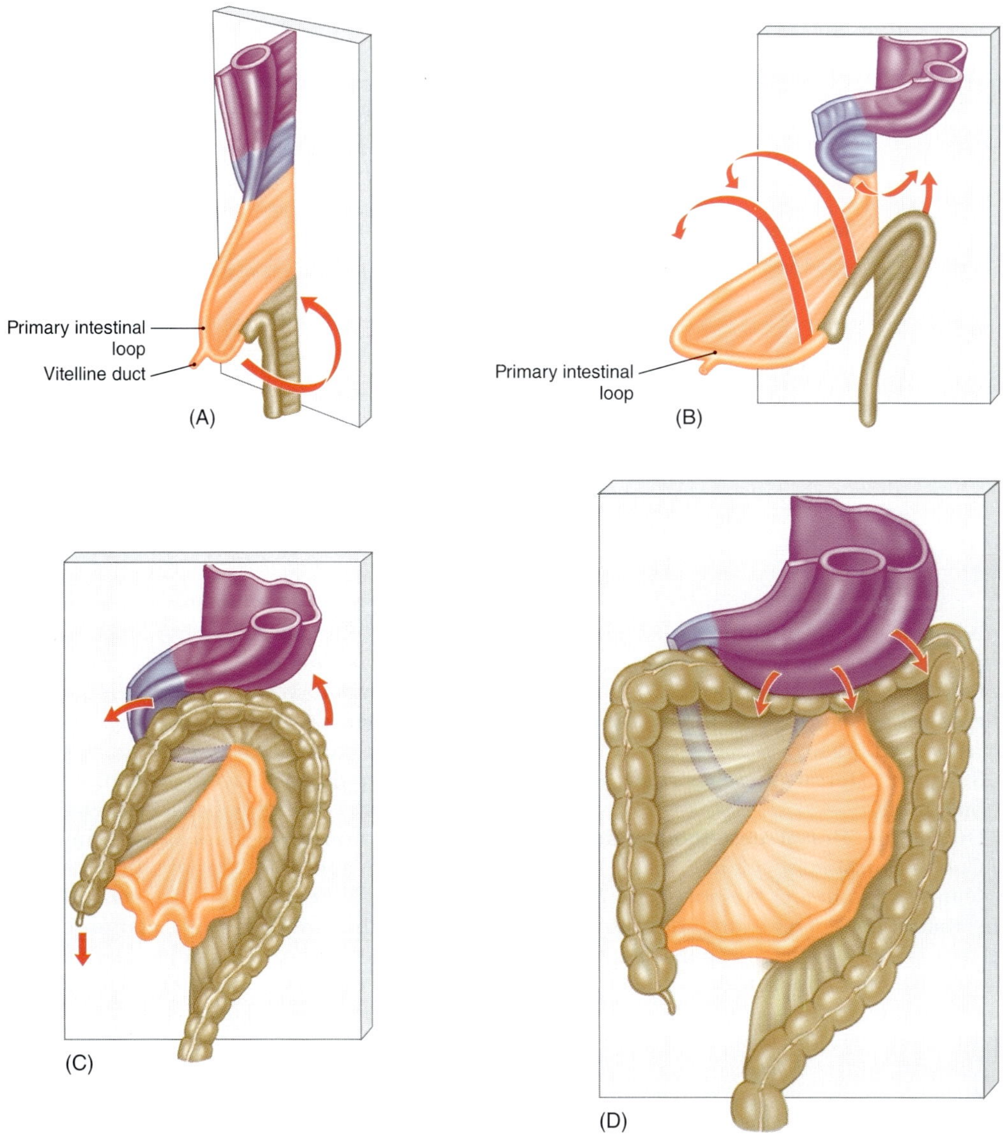

Fig. 11.4 The midgut loop formation and rotation of gut. Schematic illustrations of the intestinal rotation. Intestinal segments and their mesenteries are highlighted in different colours: gaster and mesogastrium (*purple*), duodenum and mesoduodenum (*blue*), jejunum and ileum with associated mesenteries (*orange*), colon and mesocolon (*ochre*). (according to [A]) (A) Caused by the longitudinal growth of the primordial gut, a ventrally oriented loop forms (primary intestinal loop). The proximal (upper) limb of this loop develops into the major part of the small intestine, the distal (lower) limb develops into the colon including the colon transversum. The distal large intestine develops from the hindgut and, thus, differs in its neurovascular supply. (B) Due to a lack of space, the primary intestinal loop is temporarily located outside of the embryo in the umbilical cord (physiological umbilical hernia) and remains connected to the yolk sac via the ductus vitellinus. If the intestines fail to relocate entirely into the embryo, a congenital umbilical hernia (omphalocele) remains which contains portions of the intestinal segments and their mesenteries. Because this congenital hernia traverses through the later umbilical ring, it is covered by amnion only but not by muscles of the abdominal wall. (C) Remnants of the ductus vitellinus may remain as Meckel's diverticulum located at the small intestine. (D) The elongation of the intestines initiates a 270 degree counter-clockwise rotation, resulting in the colon to surround the small intestine like a frame. (Source: *Sobotta Atlas of Human Anatomy: Internal Organs.* 15th ed. 2011.)

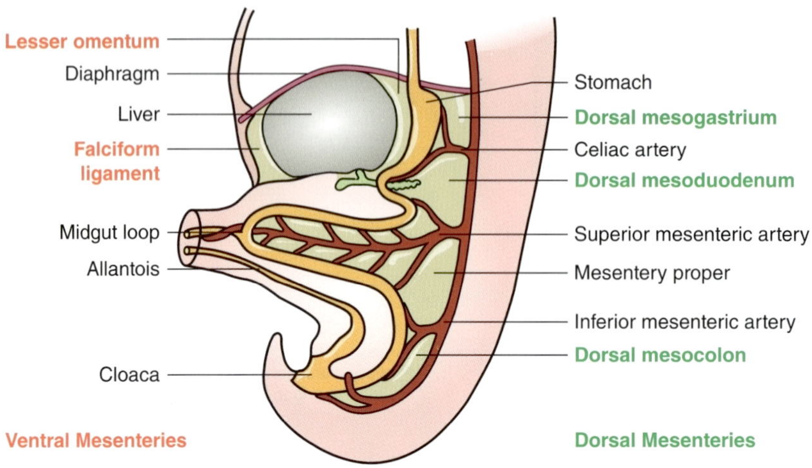

Fig. 11.5 Formation of dorsal and ventral mesenteries.

- The region from the lower end of the oesophagus to the cloacal region of the hindgut is suspended from the posterior abdominal wall by the **Dorsal mesentery** (Fig. 11.5).
- The dorsal mesentery is further named based on associated organs:
  - Stomach: **Dorsal mesogastrium** (greater omentum).
  - Duodenum: **Dorsal mesoduodenum**.
  - Colon: **Dorsal mesocolon**.
  - Jejunum and ileum: **Mesentery proper**.
- The **Ventral mesentery** is present in the terminal part of the oesophagus, stomach and upper part of the duodenum. It originates from the septum transversum.
- As the liver develops, the ventral mesentery gets divided into:
  - **Lesser omentum** (extending from the oesophagus, stomach and upper duodenum to the liver).
  - **Falciform ligament** (extending from the liver to the ventral body wall).

DEVELOPMENT OF BODY CAVITIES

- By the end of the third week, the three germ layers—ectoderm, intraembryonic mesoderm and endoderm—are established.
- The paraxial mesoderm, situated on either side of the notochord, is distinct from the lateral plate mesoderm, with both connected by intermediate mesoderm.
- Cavities appear within the lateral plate mesoderm, eventually coalescing to form the **Intraembryonic coelom**.
- The intraembryonic coelom divides the lateral plate mesoderm into an outer **Parietal or somatopleuric layer** and an inner **Visceral or splanchnopleuric layer**, with the primitive body cavity emerging between them.
- Initially horseshoe-shaped, the primitive body cavity consists of a narrow midline portion and two lateral parts, positioned near the cranial end of the embryonic disc and on either side of the notochord. This single space transforms into three major body cavities: **pericardial, pleural** and **peritoneal** (Fig. 11.6).

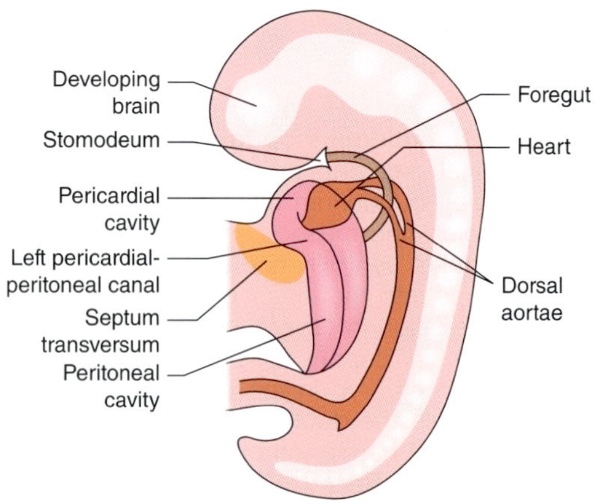

Fig. 11.6 Formation of body cavities.

- As the lateral body wall folds, the body cavity moves ventrally and fuses at the midline, except in the region of the connecting stalk where the gut tube is connected to the yolk sac.
- The midline part evolves into the pericardial cavity, while the two lateral limbs give rise to the peritoneal cavity. Initially, pericardial and peritoneal cavities are connected by narrow **Pericardio-peritoneal canals**, later developing into the pleural cavity (Fig. 11.7).
- The **Parietal layer** of lateral plate mesoderm forms the outer layer of serous membranes lining the peritoneal, pleural and pericardial cavities, while the **Visceral layer** covers the lungs, heart and abdominal organs.

PERICARDIAL CAVITY

- The cranial portion of the intraembryonic coelom forms the pericardial cavity.
- During craniocaudal folding, the pericardial cavity moves to the ventral aspect and is subsequently invaginated by the heart tube.
- Derivatives include the **Parietal layer** of serous and fibrous pericardium (from the somatopleuric mesoderm) and the **Visceral layer** (from the splanchnopleuric mesoderm).

PLEURAL CAVITY

- During the ventral movement of the midline part of the intraembryonic coelom, the pericardio-peritoneal canals extend backward on either side of the foregut.
- These canals fuse on the ventral and dorsal aspects, with lung buds emerging from the foregut and invaginating the pericardio-peritoneal canals, eventually expanding into the **pleural cavities.**
- Initially communicating with the pericardial and peritoneal cavities through canals, they later give rise to the **Pericardio-pleural** (forming the fibrous pericardium) and **Pleuro-peritoneal membranes** (fusing with the septum transversum to form the diaphragm).
- The **Phrenic nerve** runs through the pericardio-pleural membrane (which forms the fibrous pericardium) and hence it provides the embryological basis of course of phrenic nerve over fibrous pericardium

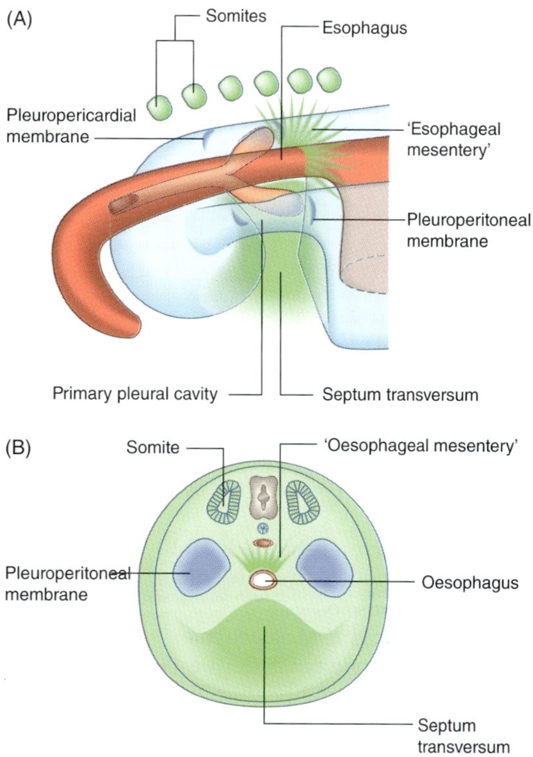

Fig. 11.7 Formation of pericardio-peritoneal canal and diaphragm. (A) Dorsolateral view of the foregut between the pericardio-peritoneal canals. The respiratory diverticulum arises from the ventral side of the pharynx and grows caudally. Bilateral lung buds extend dorsally into the pericardio-peritoneal canals dorsolaterally. Later changes in position of the common cardinal veins contribute to the formation of the pericardio-pleural membranes cranial to the developing lungs, whereas folds of coelomic epithelium, pleuroperitoneal membranes, separate the pleural cavities from the peritoneal cavity. (B) Components of the diaphragm. (Source: *Gray's Anatomy: The Anatomical Basis of Clinical Practice*. 40th ed. 2009.)

DEVELOPMENT OF DIAPHRAGM (AN 52.5)

- The diaphragm originates from four distinct embryonic structures, (Figs 11.7 and 11.8).
  1. **Septum Transversum:**
     Gives rise to the **central tendon** of the diaphragm.
  2. **Pleuroperitoneal Membranes:**
     Contribute to the formation of the diaphragm.

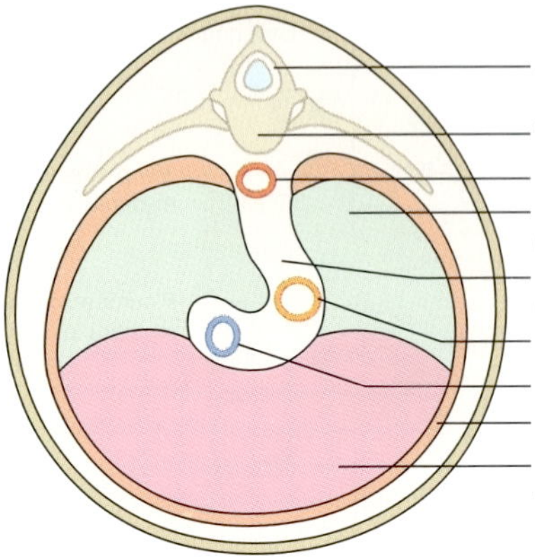

Fig. 11.8 Development of diaphragm.

3. **Mesoderm of the Body Wall:**
   Contributes to the outer rim of the diaphragmatic muscle.
4. **Oesophageal Mesenchyme:**
   The mesentery of the oesophagus merges into the central tendon, facilitating the passage of the aorta, vena cava and oesophagus.

- As myoblasts (from cervical myotomes 3, 4 and 5) descend to form the diaphragm, they carry branches of the **Phrenic nerve** with them. This unique migration explains why a thoracic/abdominal structure is innervated by nerves originating from the cervical region.
- The central tendon, derived from the septum transversum, serves as a crucial anchor point for the diaphragm. It allows the passage of **Inferior vena cava**.
- The bulk of the diaphragm muscle is predominantly innervated by the **phrenic nerve**. In contrast, the outer rim of the diaphragmatic muscle, originating from somatic mesoderm (body wall), is invaded by myoblasts from adjacent somites. Consequently, this outer rim is innervated by **Thoracic spinal nerves** (T7–T12).
- Further differentiation occurs as mesoderm from vertebral levels L1–L3 condenses to form the right and left crura of the diaphragm:
  - The right crus originates on **L1–L3**.
  - The left crus originates on **L1–L2**.

Evolution of the Diaphragm

- In the fourth week of intrauterine life, the septum transversum initially resides in the cervical region and receives its neural supply from the phrenic nerve, which originates from spinal segments C3, C4 and C5.
- As the neck elongates, the heart descends, and the pleural cavities expand, a coordinated process unfolds, leading to the descent of the diaphragm.
- By approximately the **sixth week**, the diaphragm assumes its definitive position at the thoracoabdominal junction, aligning itself against the T7–T12 spinal segments. This relocation explains the rationale for its innervation by thoracic spinal nerves.

CLINICAL NUGGETS

Real-time B-mode ultrasonography

Real-time B-mode ultrasonography is a widely utilized imaging technique for examining the foetus during pregnancy. This advanced ultrasound modality provides dynamic, real-time images, allowing clinicians to assess various aspects of foetal development. Key applications of B-mode ultrasonography in foetal imaging include:

1. **Anatomic assessment:**
   Detailed visualization of foetal anatomy, including the head, face, spine, limbs and internal organs.
2. **Craniofacial evaluation:**
   Detection of craniofacial defects and abnormalities in the development of the foetal skull and facial structures.
3. **Limb anomalies:**
   Identification of abnormalities or irregularities in the development of foetal limbs.
4. **Diaphragmatic hernias:**
   Diagnosis of diaphragmatic hernias, where abdominal organs protrude into the chest cavity.
5. **Caudal dysgenesis syndromes:**
   Assessment of conditions affecting the lower part of the foetal body.
6. **Teratoma detection:**
   Recognition of teratomas, which are tumours arising from multiple cell types and tissues.
7. **Spina bifida screening:**
   Early detection and evaluation of spina bifida, a neural tube defect affecting the spinal cord.
8. **Renal agenesis assessment:**
   Identification of renal agenesis, a condition characterized by the absence of one or both kidneys.

PERITONEAL CAVITY

- During the process of lateral folding, the horseshoe-shaped intraembryonic coelom fuses ventrally, giving rise to the peritoneal cavity—the **largest** among the three body cavities.

- Initially connected to the extraembryonic coelom at the umbilicus, the peritoneal cavity undergoes significant changes by the 10th week of intrauterine life.
- As the midgut loop re-enters the abdomen, the peritoneal cavity loses its connection with the extraembryonic coelom.
- The mesothelial lining of the peritoneal cavity, known as the **visceral layer** of the peritoneum, originates from the **Splanchnopleuric intraembryonic mesoderm**.
- The **parietal layer**, lining the body wall, derives from the **Somatopleuric mesoderm**.
- The line of reflection from the parietal to visceral layers forms the mesentery that suspends the abdominal organs.
- Initially attached to the posterior abdominal wall in the midline, the mesentery's connection becomes complicated due to the rotational movements of the gut.
- The folds of the mesentery, or peritoneum, subdivide the peritoneal cavity into several compartments.
- The **lesser sac** resides behind the stomach, and the lesser omentum establishing communication with the peritoneal cavity through a small opening—the **Epiploic foramen or the Foramen of Winslow**. The remaining part of the peritoneal cavity forms the **greater sac**.

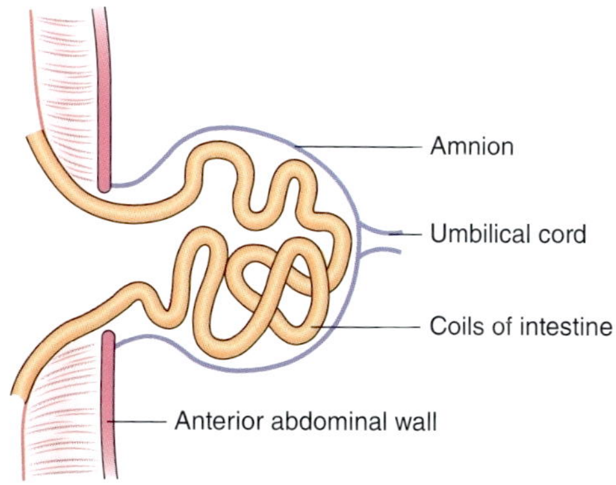

Fig. 11.9 Schematic representation of omphalocele-the loop of intestine covered by amnion.

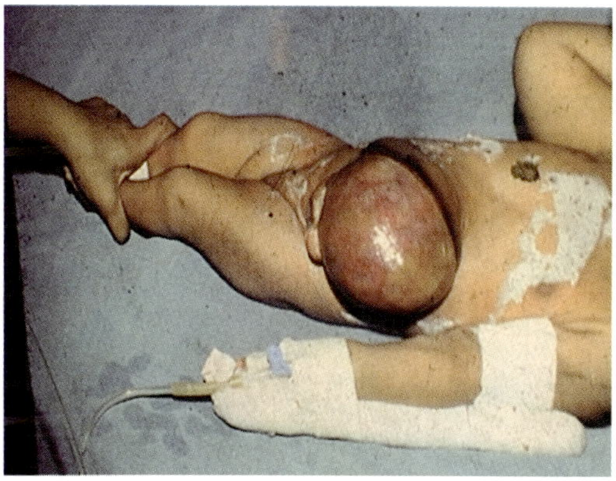

Fig. 11.10 A case of exomphalos (omphalocele) with gut tubes covered by amnion. (Photo courtesy: Dr Aswin.)

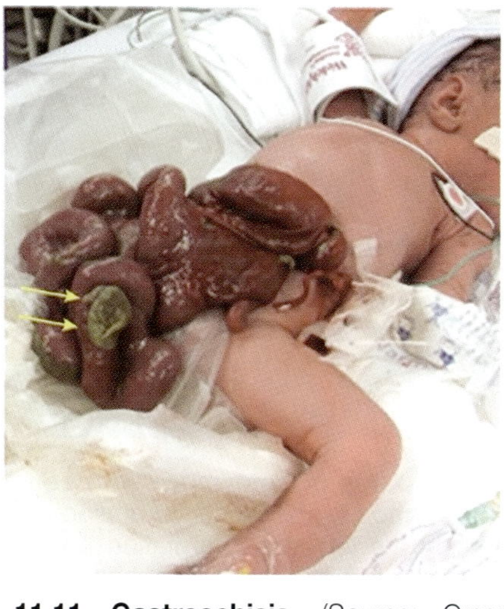

Fig. 11.11 Gastroschisis. (Source: Creasy & Resnik's Maternal-Fetal Medicine: Principles and Practice, 9th ed., Fig. 24.24, Elsevier Inc., 2023.)

KLINISCHE PERLEN

ANTERIOR BODY WALL DEFECTS

Thoracic Defects:

- **Ectopia Cordis:** Unusual positioning of the heart outside the thoracic cavity.

Abdominal Defects:

- **Omphalocele/Exomphalos:** Failure of the gut tube to return to the abdominal cavity after **physiological herniation** (6–10 weeks). Gut tubes covered by the amnion (see Figs 11.9 and 11.10). Associated with **cardiac and neural tube defects**

  Diagnostic Indicators:

  a) Elevated **AFP** (alpha-fetoprotein).

  b) Presence of **Chromosomal abnormalities**.
- **Gastroschisis:** Abdominal viscera protrude outside, typically on the **right side of the umbilicus** (Fig. 11.11).

Urogenital Region Defects:

Bladder or Cloacal Exstrophy (the bladder and a part of the intestine open to the exterior).

Cantrell Pentalogy:

1. **Ectopia cordis.**
2. **Omphalocele or gastroschisis.**
3. Absent **pericardium**.
4. Defects in **sternum**.
5. Defects in the **anterior diaphragm** region.

CONGENITAL DIAPHRAGMATIC HERNIA (AN 52.5)

- Congenital diaphragmatic hernia (CDH) is a developmental anomaly where there is a failure in the fusion of the **pleuroperitoneal membranes** during embryonic development.
- This results in a communication between the pleural and peritoneal cavities, allowing abdominal organs such as stomach,intestines and liver to herniate into the thoracic cavity (Fig. 11.12).
- **Clinical Presentation:**
  - **Pulmonary Hypoplasia:** The herniation of abdominal organs into the chest restricts the normal growth of the lungs, leading to pulmonary hypoplasia.
  - **Respiratory Distress:** Newborns with CDH often present with severe respiratory distress shortly after birth.
  - **Cyanosis:** The inadequate lung development results in poor oxygenation, leading to cyanosis.
  - **Cardiovascular Effects:** CDH can also affect the cardiovascular system, leading to persistent pulmonary hypertension.
- **Types of CDH:**
  1. **Bochdalek Hernia:** Most common type, characterized by a posterior defect in the diaphragm. (Left sided hernia is more common than right sided hernia.)
  2. **Morgagni Hernia:** Anatomical defects in the anterior diaphragm allowing abdominal viscera herniation into the thorax. This type is the rarest, constituting 2%–3% of cases.
- **Diagnosis:**
  - **Prenatal Ultrasound:** CDH can be diagnosed during routine prenatal ultrasound examinations.
  - **Postnatal Imaging:** X-rays and other imaging studies are used to confirm the diagnosis after birth.

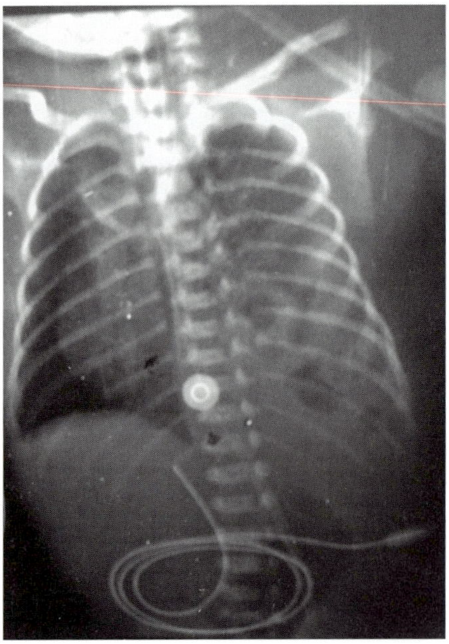

Fig. 11.12 X-ray of a newborn with congenital diaphragmatic hernia. (Absence of diaphragmatic shadow on the left side. Herniating bowel loops seen in the left lung field. Significant mediastinal shift to the right.) (Photo courtesy: Dr Nitya.)

DIAPHRAGMATIC EVENTRATION

- Diaphragmatic eventration is a congenital or acquired condition characterized by the **abnormal elevation** of all or part of the diaphragm.
- Unlike CDH, eventration does not involve a structural defect but rather a weakness or abnormality in the muscular portion of the diaphragm.
- **Causes:**
  1. **Congenital:** The condition may result from a failure of muscular development during foetal life.
  2. **Acquired:** Eventration can also occur later in life due to trauma, neuromuscular diseases or surgical procedures.
- **Clinical Presentation:**
  - **Asymptomatic Cases:** In some individuals, diaphragmatic eventration may be asymptomatic and incidentally discovered during imaging studies.
  - **Respiratory Symptoms:** Symptomatic cases may present with respiratory distress, especially during exertion.
  - **Abdominal Symptoms:** In some cases, there may be associated abdominal symptoms, such as discomfort or a feeling of fullness.

- **Diagnosis:**
  - **Imaging Studies:** X-rays, ultrasound or other imaging studies can reveal the abnormal elevation of the diaphragm.
  - **Pulmonary Function Tests:** Assessing lung function may be done to understand the impact on respiratory capacity.

CENTRAL TENDON DEFECTS

- Central tendon defects refer to abnormalities or openings in the central portion of the diaphragm's central tendon.
- Central tendon defects can be congenital or acquired.
- Congenital defects may result from incomplete fusion or development during foetal life.
- Acquired defects can occur due to trauma, surgical procedures or other pathological processes affecting the diaphragm.
- The clinical presentation of central tendon defects can vary based on the size and nature of the defect. Some individuals may be asymptomatic, while others may experience respiratory or gastrointestinal symptoms.

POINTS TO PONDER

Development of body cavities

- Partitions play a crucial role in subdividing the **Intraembryonic coelom** into distinct cavities, including the pericardial, pleural and peritoneal cavities. The initial partition, known as the **Septum transversum**, is the first to form. It separates the coelom into a thoracic primitive pericardial cavity and an abdominal peritoneal cavity.
- As the embryo undergoes cranial folding and experiences differential body growth, the septum transversum is translocated from the cranial edge of the embryonic disc to its future position as the diaphragm.
- Coronal pleuropericardial folds emerge from the lateral body wall, growing medially and fusing with the ventral surface of the foregut and with each other. This transformative process results in the division of the primitive pericardial cavity into a **definitive pericardial cavity** and **two pleural cavities**.
- A transverse **Pleuroperitoneal membrane** plays a crucial role in closing the pericardioperitoneal canals. This membrane effectively separates the pleural and peritoneal cavities, contributing to the distinct and organized arrangement of the developing body cavities.

BRAIN TEASERS

1. What is the result of the division of the cloaca?
   A. Formation of the hindgut.
   B. Creation of the foregut.
   C. Differentiation of urogenital system.
   D. Establishment of primitive gut.
2. What structure arises from the ventral aspect of the hindgut?
   A. Allantoic diverticulum
   B. Primitive streak
   C. Notochord
   D. Cloacal membrane
3. What arises from the distal segment of the midgut?
   A. Foregut
   B. Hindgut
   C. Caecal bud
   D. Allantoic diverticulum
4. What is the defect in the ectoderm after lateral folding, where the vitello-intestinal duct passes?
   A. Buccopharyngeal membrane
   B. Proctodeum
   C. Umbilical opening
   D. Cloacal membrane
5. What structure does the endoderm form during mesodermal and endodermal fusion?
   A. Notochord
   B. Neural tube
   C. Primitive streak
   D. Endodermal tube
6. How many degrees of anticlockwise rotation does the midgut loop undergo within the umbilical cord?
   A. 45 degrees
   B. 90 degrees
   C. 180 degrees
   D. 360 degrees
7. What does the prearterial segment of the midgut elongate to form during development?
   A. Proximal duodenum
   B. Coils of jejunum and ileum
   C. Distal ileum
   D. Ascending colon
8. What structure arises from the postarterial segment, contributing to the formation of the caecum and appendix?
   A. Duodenal loop
   B. Caecal diverticulum
   C. Ascending colon
   D. Distal ileum
9. Which embryonic structure gives rise to the central tendon of the diaphragm?
   A. Pleuroperitoneal membranes
   B. Mesoderm of the body wall
   C. Oesophageal mesenchyme
   D. Septum transversum

10. What is the main nerve responsible for innervating the bulk of the diaphragm muscle?
    A. Vagus nerve
    B. Phrenic nerve
    C. Sciatic nerve
    D. Brachial plexus
11. Which part of the diaphragm muscle is predominantly innervated by thoracic spinal nerves (T7–T12)?
    A. Central tendon
    B. Left crus
    C. Right crus
    D. Outer rim
12. When is the process of midgut rotation typically finalized during embryonic development?
    A. 5th week
    B. 8th week
    C. 10th week
    D. 12th week

Answers

1. (C); 2. (A); 3. (C); 4. (C); 5. (D); 6. (B); 7. (B); 8. (B); 9. (D); 10. (B); 11. (D); 12. (C).

FURTHER READINGS

Bouzada J, Gemmell C, Konschake M, Tubbs RS, Pechriggl E, Sañudo J. New insights into the development of the anterior abdominal wall. *Front Surg.* 2022;9:863679. doi:10.3389/fsurg.2022.863679.

Kardon G, Ackerman KG, McCulley DJ, et al. Congenital diaphragmatic hernias: from genes to mechanisms to therapies. *Dis Model Mech.* 2017;10(8):955-970. doi:10.1242/dmm.028365.

Marques AT, Estevão-Costa J, Soares H, Fragoso AC. Short and medium-term outcomes of omphalocele and gastroschisis: a survey from a tertiary center. *Rev Bras Ginecol Obstet.* 2022;44(1):10-18. doi:10.1055/s-0041-1736299.

Patel N, Massolo AC, Kraemer US, Kipfmueller F. The heart in congenital diaphragmatic hernia: knowns, unknowns, and future priorities. *Front Pediatr.* 2022;10:890422. doi:10.3389/fped.2022.890422.

Ruschkowski B, Nasr A, Oltean I, Lawrence S, El Demellawy D. Examining the relationship between gastroschisis and placental fetal vascular malperfusion. *Pediatr Dev Pathol.* 2021;24(6):531-541. doi:10.1177/10935266211029629.

Placenta and Umbilical Cord 12

AN 80.2 Describe the formation and structure of umbilical cord.

AN 80.3 Describe the formation of placenta, its physiological functions, foetomaternal circulation and placental barrier.

AN 80.7 Describe the various types of umbilical cord attachments.

AN 80.5 Describe the role of placental hormones in uterine growth and parturition.

ANAMNESE

A 28-year-old primigravida, in her 32nd week of gestation, presented to the antenatal clinic with concerns about reduced foetal movements. Upon examination, an ultrasound revealed a case of umbilical cord anomaly. The umbilical cord was observed to have a true knot, a condition where the cord loops around itself, compromising blood flow. Foetal monitoring indicated occasional decelerations, raising concerns about foetal well-being. Continuous foetal monitoring was initiated to closely monitor the baby's heart rate. Given the risk of reduced oxygen supply, the medical team discussed the possibility of an earlier delivery, weighing the risks of preterm birth against the complications associated with the umbilical cord anomaly. The decision was made to schedule a caesarean section at 36 weeks to alleviate the risks. This case underlines the importance of antenatal monitoring and timely interventions in the presence of umbilical cord anomalies to improve foetal outcomes (Fig. 12.1).

Maternal human placentophagy describes the practice of ingesting one's own placenta during the postpartum period. This is done in different ways: either a piece of raw placenta is consumed immediately after parturition, or the tissue is heated, dried and then pulverized. **Placenta encapsulation** means the placenta is processed into capsules and this is a common practice in the Anglo-American world. It is done by the filling of placental tissue as a dried powder into gelatin capsules for everyday consumption. There are many studies to prove these facts. All these reveal the importance of placenta.

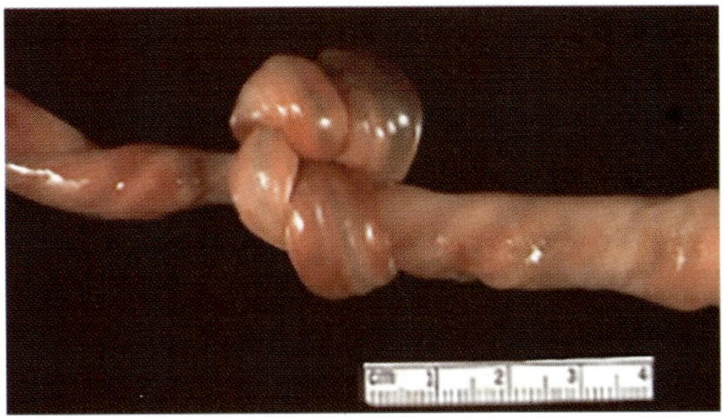

Fig. 12.1 Photograph of an umbilical cord showing a true knot. (From Figure 13.128 in the Robbins & Cotran Atlas of Pathology, 4th ed., published by Elsevier [Courtesy: Dr. E.C. Klatt, Department of Biomedical Sciences, Mercer University School of Medicine, Savannah, GA].)

PLACENTA (AN 80.3)

- Primary site of nutrient and gas exchange between mother and foetus.

- A foetomaternal organ consisting of two components:
  - Foetal part developed from **chorionic sac.**
  - Maternal part derived from **endometrium.**

FUNCTIONS

The placenta serves several vital functions during pregnancy:

- **Protection**—It acts as a protective barrier, shielding the developing foetus from potential harm.
- **Nutrition**—It plays an important role in providing essential nutrients to the growing foetus, ensuring its proper nourishment.
- **Respiration**—The placenta facilitates the exchange of gases, enabling the foetus to receive oxygen and expel carbon dioxide.
- **Excretion**—It serves as a mechanism for excretion, managing waste elimination.
- **Hormone production**—The placenta is involved in hormone production, contributing to the regulation of various physiological processes during pregnancy.

STRUCTURE OF PLACENTA

- By the beginning of the **fourth month**, the placenta exhibits the following components (Fig. 12.2):
  - The foetal portion is formed by the **chorion frondosum or chorionic plate** covered by the amnion.
  - The maternal portion originates from the **basal plate**.
  - **Villi** connect these foetal and maternal plates.
  - The **Intervillous space** is filled with maternal blood.
- Chorionic villi invade the decidua basalis, causing erosion of decidual tissue and enlarging the intervillous space.
- This erosion leads to the formation of wedge-shaped areas of decidua, known as **placental septa,** projecting towards the chorionic plate.
- Placental septa divide the maternal surface into rough, irregular convex areas called **Cotyledons,** ranging from 15 to 30 (Fig. 12.3).
- Each **Maternal cotyledon** consists of two or more **stem villi** (around 60 stem villi persist in human placenta) and **branching villi.**
- A **Foetal cotyledon** includes a major stem villus and the vessels formed from it.
- At **Full term**, the placenta has the following characteristics:
  - It is **discoid** in shape.
  - The diameter ranges from **15 to 25 cm.**
  - It occupies **30%** of the uterine wall.
  - Thickness measures **3 cm.**
  - The weight is about **500–600 g.**
  - The placenta-to-foetus ratio is **1:7.**

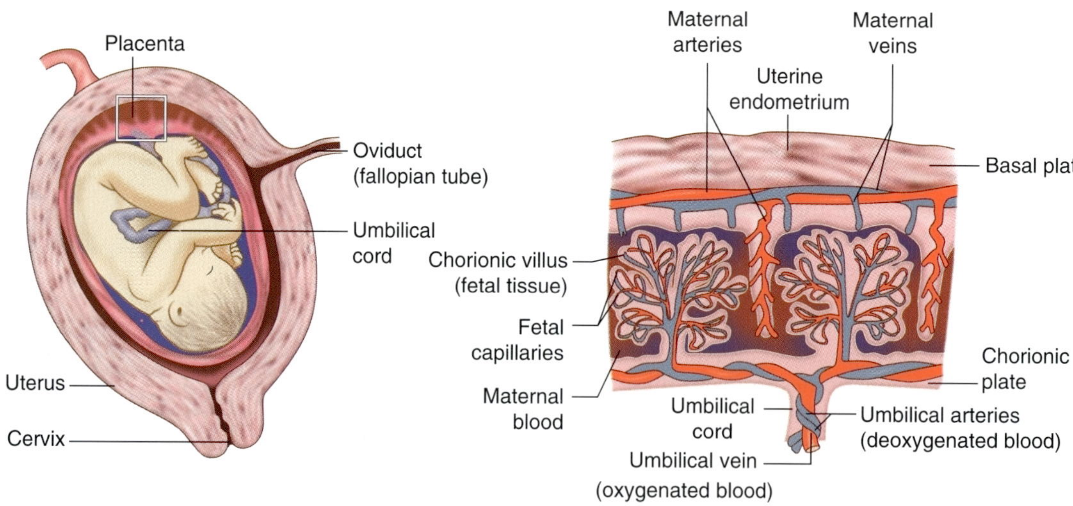

Fig. 12.2 Structure of placenta showing chorionic plate and basal plate. (Source: *Textbook of Anatomy and Physiology for Nurses*, 2017.)

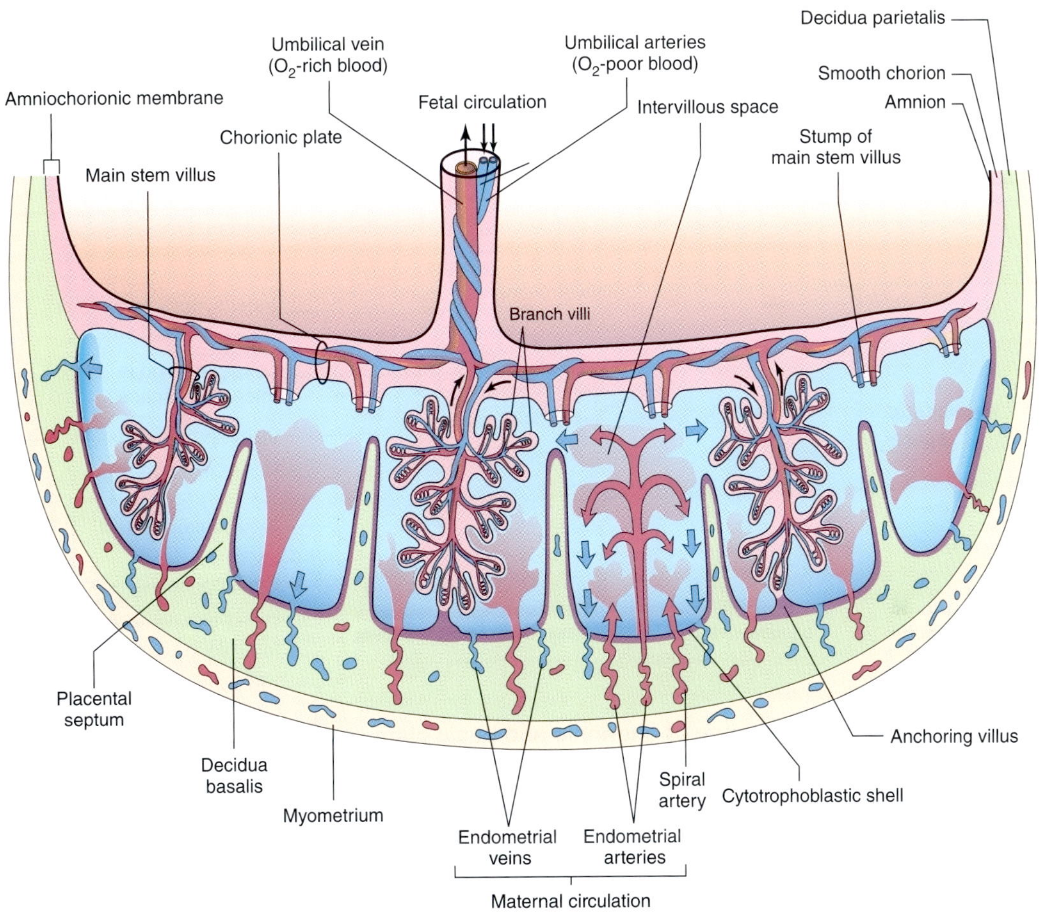

Fig. 12.3 The placenta with placental septa and cotyledons. Schematic drawing of a transverse section through a full-term placenta, showing the relation of the villous chorion (foetal part of placenta) to the decidua basalis (maternal part of placenta), the foetal placental circulation and the maternal placental circulation. Maternal blood flows into the intervillous spaces in spurts from the spiral arteries. Note that the umbilical arteries carry poorly oxygenated foetal blood (shown in *blue*) to the placenta and that the umbilical vein carries oxygenated blood (shown in *red*) to the foetus. Note that the cotyledons are separated from each other by placental septa, projections of the decidua basalis. Each cotyledon consists of two or more main stem villi and many branch villi. In this drawing, only one stem villus is shown in each cotyledon, but the stumps of those that have been removed are indicated. (Source: *The Developing Human: Clinically Oriented Embryology*, 11th ed. 2020.)

- At birth, it is separated from the uterine wall and expelled approximately 30 minutes after the child's birth, referred to as the **'Afterbirth'**.
- The **Chorionic plate** of the placenta is covered by the amnion (visible on the foetal side) and consists of:
  - **Primary mesoderm** with umbilical vessels (foetus).
  - **Cytotrophoblast**.
  - **Syncytiotrophoblast** lining the intervillous space.

  (This arrangement is as seen from **foetus to mother**.)
- On the maternal side, the **Basal plate** includes (Fig. 12.4):
  - **Decidua basalis** with maternal blood vessels **(stratum spongiosum)**.
  - **Syncytiotrophoblast** (outer layer or **Nitabuch's layer**).

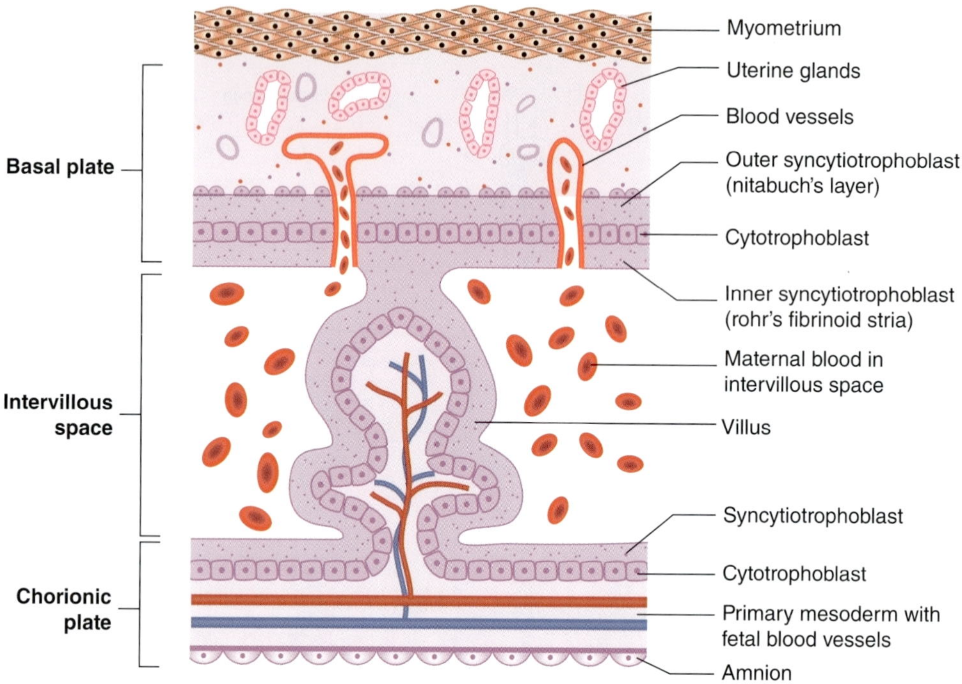

Fig. 12.4 Structure of chorionic and basal plate. (schematic diagram).

- **Cytotrophoblast** (outer shell).
- **Syncytiotrophoblast** (inner layer or **Rohr's fibrinoid stria**).

(The above structures are arranged from **mother to foetus**.)

- The attachment of the umbilical cord is usually central but can be eccentric or occasionally even marginal.
- The decidua basalis is responsible for forming the decidual plate, which firmly unites with the chorion, contributing to the establishment of a secure connection during embryonic development.

THE DECIDUA

Decidua refers to the endometrium after implantation (Fig. 12.5).

- Following implantation, stromal cells undergo enlargement and vacuolation, storing glycogen and lipids, a phenomenon known as the **decidual reaction**.
- The decidua can be categorized into three regions based on the implantation site:
  1. **Decidua basalis:** This is the part of the decidua located at the embryonic pole of the blastocyst.
  2. **Decidua capsularis:** This portion covers the abembryonic pole of the blastocyst.
  3. **Decidua parietalis:** The remaining part of the decidua lines the uterine cavity.

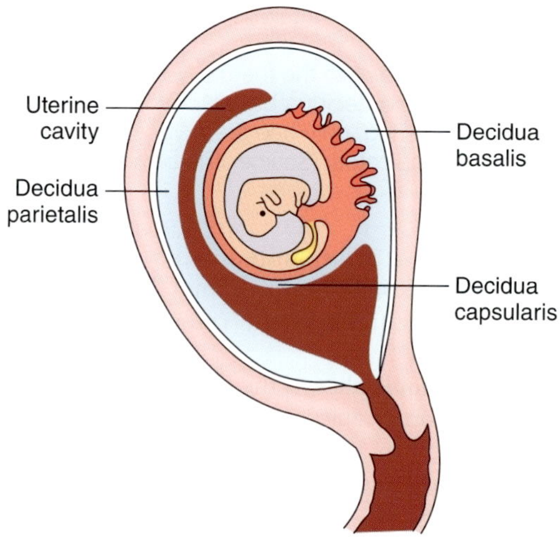

Fig. 12.5 The Decidua.

DEVELOPMENT OF PLACENTA

By the **eighth day** of development, the blastocyst begins partial embedding in the endometrial stroma.

- The **trophoblast** undergoes differentiation, particularly at the embryonic pole, forming two layers:
  a) **The Cytotrophoblast:**
    - **Mononucleated** pale-staining cells with distinct cell membranes.
    - Mitotically active, generating new cells that migrate into the syncytiotrophoblast layer.
  b) **The Syncytiotrophoblast:**
    - **Multinucleated** without a limiting cell membrane.
    - Rapidly expanding and deeply stained.
    - The erosive syncytiotrophoblast invades the endometrium, facilitating the gradual embedding of the blastocyst.
- The invasion is facilitated by the programmed cell death (apoptosis) of endometrial cells.
- **Lacunar spaces** appear in the syncytiotrophoblast, separated by trabeculae (syncytiotrophoblast) (Fig. 12.6). This developmental phase in the trophoblast is known as **the Lacunar stage**.
- The lacunae enlarge, eroding the spiral uterine vessels.
- As a result, the lacunar spaces fill with maternal blood—the first sign of establishing **Utero-placental circulation**.
- Maternal blood in the lacunar spaces (embryotroph; **'trophe'** means nourishment) reaches the embryonic disc via diffusion, providing nutrition to the embryo until placental circulation is established.
- Oxygenated blood passes into the lacunae from the spiral endometrial arteries, while poorly oxygenated blood is removed by endometrial veins.
- By the end of the second week, **Primary chorionic villi** form through the proliferation of cytotrophoblast as cellular extensions into the syncytiotrophoblast. The primary chorionic villi represent the **first stage** in the development of chorionic villi.
- At the beginning of the third week of development, the trophoblast consists of primary villi with a cytotrophoblastic core covered by the syncytiotrophoblast.
- Later, mesodermal cells (somatopleuric extra-embryonic mesoderm) penetrate into the primary villi, leading to the formation of **Secondary villi**. The secondary villi are then penetrated by foetal blood vessels, forming **Tertiary villi** (Fig. 12.7).
- According to development, there are three types of villi (Fig. 12.8):
  a) **Primary villi**—central core of cytotrophoblast covered by syncytiotrophoblast.
  b) **Secondary villi**—central core of primary mesoderm covered successively by cytotrophoblast and syncytiotrophoblast.
  c) **Tertiary villi**—central core of primary mesoderm with foetal blood vessels covered successively by cytotrophoblast and syncytiotrophoblast.
- The cytotrophoblastic cells extend through the syncytiotrophoblast to form an outer cytotrophoblastic shell that surrounds the chorionic sac and attaches it to the endometrium.
- By the end of the **fourth week**, maternal-foetal exchange of gases, nutrients and metabolic waste products occurs.

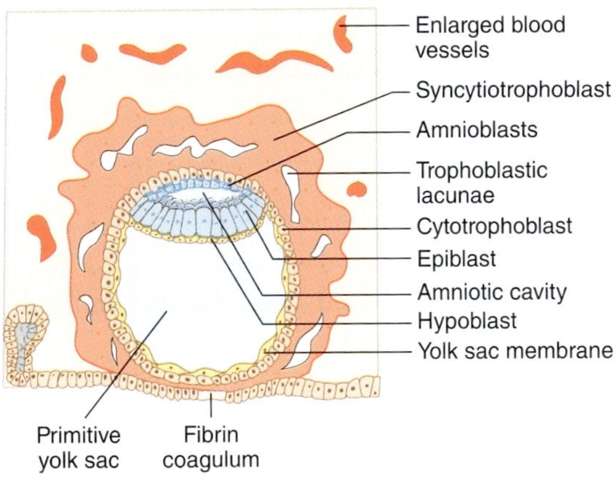

Fig. 12.6 The lacunar spaces getting filled with maternal blood.

FORMATION OF CHORIONIC VILLI

Chorionic villi are functional components of the placenta. They are surrounded by maternal blood and contains capillaries through which foetal blood circulates. They develop from the surface of the trophoblast.

- **Chorionic Villi:**
  - Villi arising from the chorion, where the chorion comprises trophoblast along with underlying extraembryonic mesoderm.

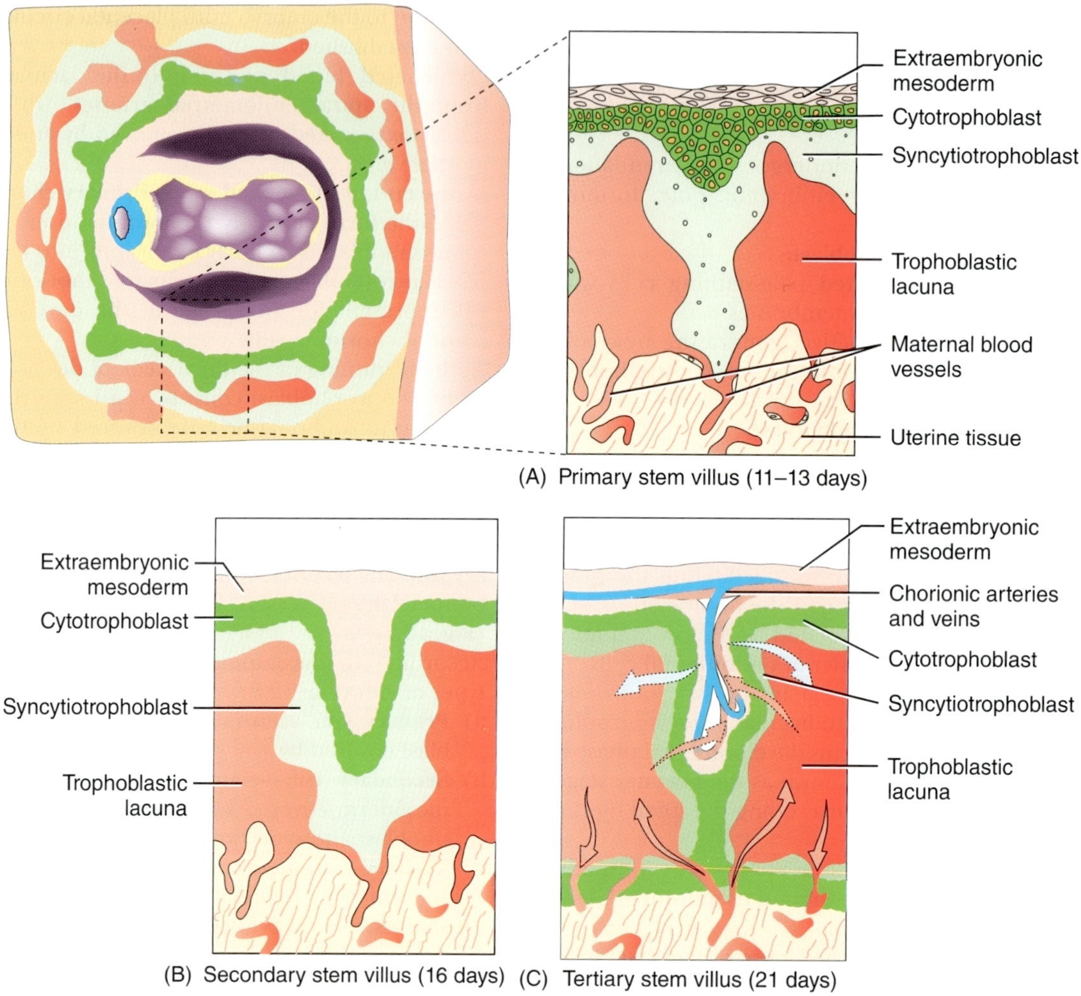

Fig. 12.7 The structures of primary, secondary and tertiary villus. Formation of chorionic villi. (A) Primary stem villi form on days 11–13 as cytotrophoblastic proliferations that bud into the overlying syncytiotrophoblast. (B) By day 16, the extraembryonic mesoderm begins to proliferate and invade the centre of each primary stem villus, transforming each into a secondary stem villus. (C) By day 21, the mesodermal core differentiates into connective tissue and blood vessels, forming the tertiary stem villi. (Source: *Larsen's Human Embryology,* 4th ed. 2008.)

- **Chorion Frondosum:**
  - The primary part of the chorion at the **embryonic pole** actively involved in the development of the placenta.
- **Chorion Laeve:**
  - Part of the chorion related to the **deciduas capsularis**, which undergoes degeneration and becomes smooth over time.
- The fully developed placenta covers 15%–30% of the decidua.

STRUCTURAL CLASSIFICATION OF VILLI

Anchoring Villi:

- First formed and connects the chorionic and basal plates.
- Consists of a stem called **truncus chorii**.
- The truncus chorii gives rise to a number of branches called **rami** (singular: ramus) **chorii**.
- Ramus chorii further divides into finer branches called **ramuli chorii**.

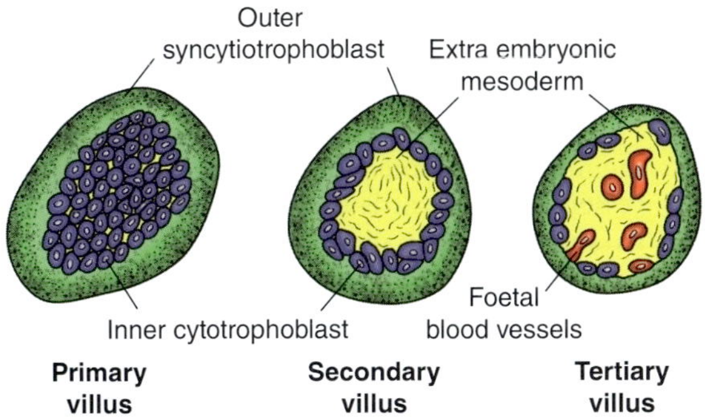

Fig. 12.8 Schematic representation of three types of villi (cross section).

Floating Villi:
- Anchoring villi give off numerous branches that extend into the **intervillous space** as free or floating villi (branch villi in Fig. 12.2).
- Eventually, the entire intervillous space becomes filled with villi, significantly increasing the surface area for exchange.

PLACENTAL CIRCULATION

- **Cotyledons and Spiral Arteries:**
  - Cotyledons receive blood through **80–100 spiral arteries** that penetrate the decidual plate and enter the intervillous space.
  - The volume of the intervillous space is approximately **140 mL**.
- **Maternal Blood Circulation:**
  - Around **500 mL** of maternal blood circulates through the intervillous space per minute, resulting in blood exchange occurring approximately **four times per minute**.
  - Pressure in the spiral arteries propels blood into the intervillous spaces, facilitating oxygenation of the entire villous tree.
  - As the pressure diminishes, blood flows back from the intervillous space towards the decidua and ultimately into the endometrial veins.

UMBILICAL CORD (AN 80.2)

- **Attachment**
  - Attaches the foetus to the placenta.
  - Formed from the **connecting stalk** attached to the caudal end of the germ disc.
  - Body folding of the embryo separates the umbilical cord from its extraembryonic membranes.
- **Amnion Expansion:**
  - As the embryo grows, the amnion expands, enclosing the entire embryo except for the umbilical area, where the connecting stalk and yolk sac emerge.
  - Increased production of amniotic fluid (fourth–eighth week) causes the amnion to swell until it entirely occupies the chorionic space.
  - When the amnion contacts the chorion, the layers of extraembryonic mesoderm covering the two membranes fuse loosely.
  - As a result, the chorionic cavity disappears except for a few rudimentary vesicles.
  - After embryonic folding, the amnion originates from the umbilical ring, surrounding the roots of the vitelline duct and connecting stalk.
- **Umbilical Cord Formation:**
  - The amnion expands, creating a tube of amniotic membrane enclosing the connecting stalk and the vitelline duct, known as the **umbilical cord**.
- **Vitelline Duct and Yolk Sac:**
  - The vitelline duct narrows, and the small yolk sac remains within the umbilical sheath.
  - Both the yolk sac and vitelline duct typically disappear by birth.
- **Dimensions:**
  - Length: **50 cm**, Diameter: **2 cm**.
- **Contents** (Fig. 12.9):
  - **Wharton's Jelly:**
    - **Mucoid connective tissue** derived from primary mesodermal cells.
    - Contains **mucopolysaccharides (hyaluronic acid), fibroblasts and macrophages.**
    - Protects the umbilical vessels.
  - **Umbilical Arteries:**
    - Two in number, originating from the ventral division of the **Internal iliac artery**.
    - Carries deoxygenated blood from the foetus to the mother.
    - After birth, the proximal part forms the **Superior vesical artery**, and the distal part obliterates (remnant seen as the **Medial umbilical ligament**).
  - **Umbilical Vein:**
    - **Left umbilical vein** persists, and the right disappears.

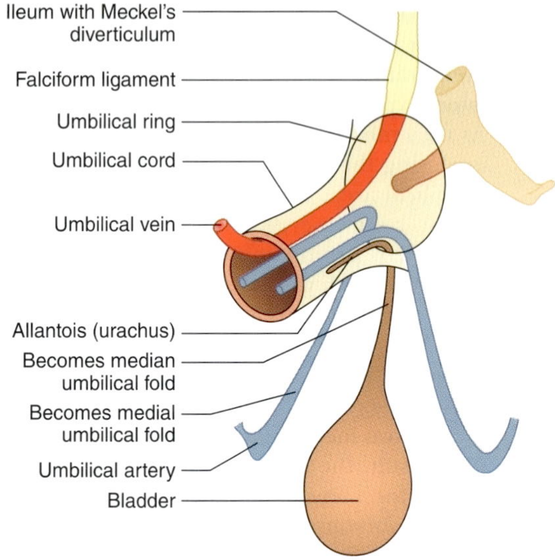

Fig. 12.9 Contents of umbilical cord.

- ➢ Carries oxygenated blood from the placenta to the foetus.
- ➢ Joins the left branch of the **Portal vein**.
- ➢ After birth, it persists as the **Ligamentum teres hepatis** (round ligament of the liver).

- **Vitellointestinal Duct:**
  - ➢ Connects **Midgut with yolk sac**.
  - ➢ Disappears during late foetal life, sometimes persisting after birth as **Meckel's diverticulum**.
- **Allantoic Diverticulum:**
  - ➢ Distal part forms **Urachus** in the late foetal period, and after birth, it forms the **Median umbilical ligament**.
  - ➢ Proximal part is attached to the apex of the urinary bladder.

PLACENTAL MEMBRANE/PLACENTAL BARRIER

- It consists of tissues which separate maternal and foetal blood.
- **Four layered** (up to third month).
  (Imagine as if you stand inside a foetal capillary and layers are numbered inside out.)
  1. **Endothelial lining** of foetal vessels and its basement membrane.
  2. **Connective tissue core** (primary mesoderm).
  3. **Basement membrane** with cytotrophoblastic layer.
  4. **Syncytiotrophoblast**.
- From fourth month onward, the placental membrane becomes **thin** as the foetal blood vessels move towards the periphery from centre for better exchange.
- As a result, the placental barrier is reduced to **two layers** (Fig. 12.10).
  1. **Endothelium** of foetal capillaries resting on basement membrane.
  2. **Syncytiotrophoblast**.
- At times, the **syncytium fuses** with the capillary wall forming **Vasculosyncytial membrane**.
- The **two zones** in the villi are:
  1) **Alpha zones** (membranous area)—site of exchange.
  2) **Beta zones** (nonmembranous)—hormone synthesis (cytotrophoblast and stroma persist).
- **Human placenta is haemochorial type**, separating maternal blood in intervillous space and foetal blood.

FOETAL MEMBRANE

- It consists of:
  - **Decidua parietalis.**
  - **Decidua capsularis.**
  - **Chorion laeve.**
  - **Amnion.**

AMNIOCHORIONIC MEMBRANE

- The amniotic sac undergoes rapid enlargement compared to the chorionic sac (Fig. 12.11).
- Consequently, fusion occurs between the amnion and chorion laeve, giving rise to the **Amniochorionic membrane**. This membrane further fuses with the decidua capsularis.
- Following the disappearance of the decidua capsularis, the amniochorionic membrane adheres to the decidua parietalis.
- **Role in Labour:**
  - During labour, it is the amniochorionic membrane that undergoes **rupture**.
  - Preterm rupture of this membrane is associated with premature labour.
- **Rupture and Fluid Release:**
  - When the membrane ruptures, amniotic fluid is released through the cervix and vagina.

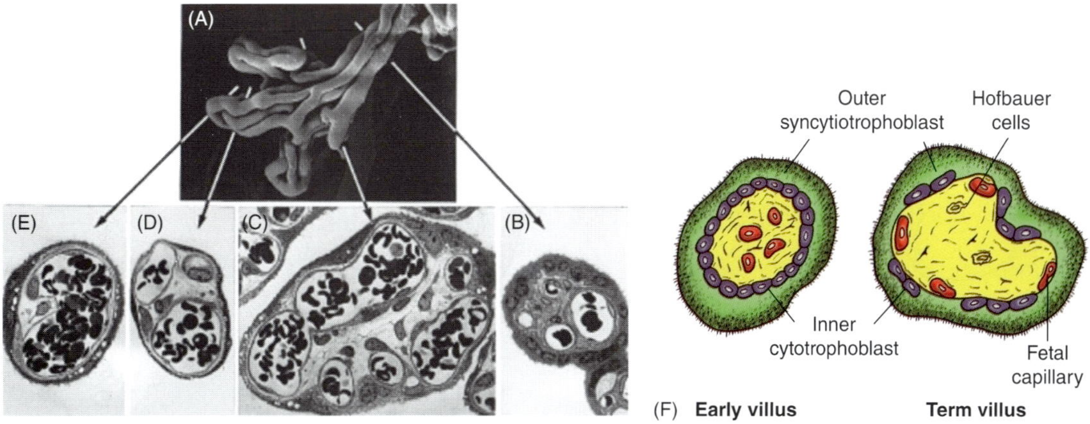

Fig. 12.10 Foetal vascularization of terminal villi. (A) Cast of vessels from a group of terminal villi. Corresponding semithin sections of the transition to a mature intermediate villus (B), the base of the branching terminal villi (C), a single terminal villus near its tip (D), and a flat section of the terminal villous tip (E). These pictures demonstrate the structural variability of terminal villi; they all have in common that foetal capillaries and the highly dilated sinusoids amount to more than 50% of the stromal volume as long as postpartal collapse can be avoided by early fixation. (F) Schematic representation of early and term villus. ×300. (With permission from Kaufmann et al. 146). (Source: *Fetal Medicine: Basic Science and Clinical Practice*, 2nd ed. 2009.)

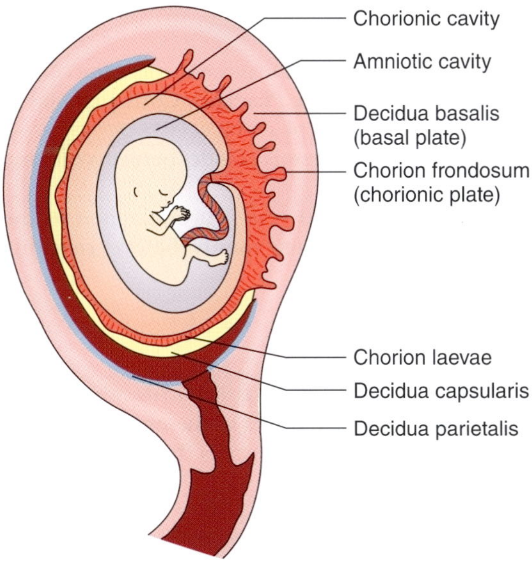

Fig. 12.11 Foetal membranes.

- Subsequently, the foetus follows this release.
- This process plays an important role in the progression of labour and shows the significance of the amniochorionic membrane in ensuring a timely and controlled release of amniotic fluid during childbirth.

NORMAL SITE OF IMPLANTATION

- The upper part of the uterus consisting of the fundus and the greater part of the body forms the **Upper uterine segment**.
- The lower part of the uterus consisting of the lower part of the body and the cervix constitutes the **Lower uterine segment**.
- Typically, the placenta attaches to the upper uterine segment during a normal pregnancy.

ABNORMAL SITE OF IMPLANTATION

PLACENTA PRAEVIA

- The attachment of the placenta extends partially or completely to the lower uterine segment. This condition may cause difficulties during childbirth and lead to severe bleeding.

Degrees of Placenta Praevia (Fig. 12.12):

1. **First Degree:** The attachment of the placenta **extends** to the lower uterine segment but does not reach the internal os.
2. **Second Degree:** The margin of the placenta **reaches** the internal os but does not cover it.
3. **Third Degree:** The edge of the placenta **covers** the internal os, but as the os dilates

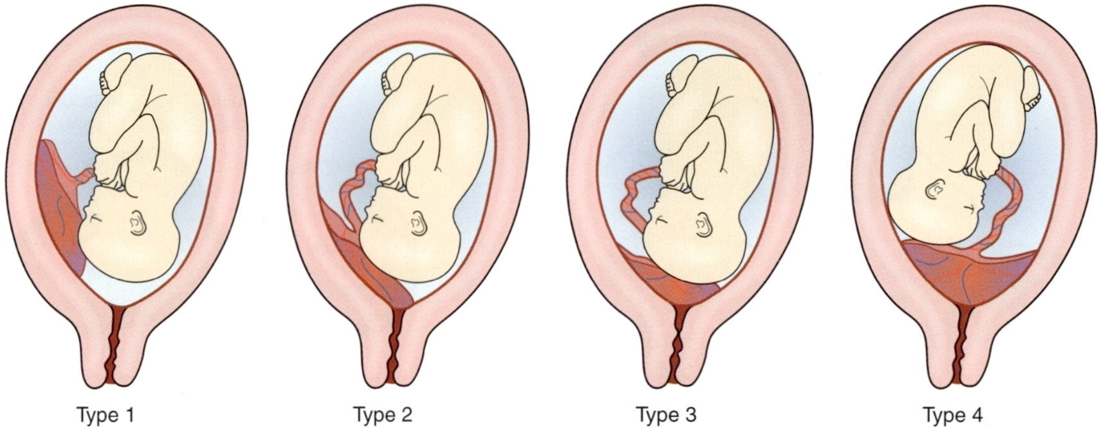

Fig. 12.12 Placenta praevia.

during childbirth, the placenta no longer occludes it.

4. **Fourth Degree:** The placenta **completely covers** the internal os and continues to occlude the os even after dilation.

ECTOPIC PREGNANCY

Extrauterine Pregnancy (Abnormal Implantation/ Ectopic):

1. **Ovary (Primary Ovarian Pregnancy):**
   - Implantation occurs in the ovary, leading to a primary ovarian pregnancy.
2. **Abdominal Cavity:**
   - Implantation can occur in the abdominal cavity, including the Pouch of Douglas or greater omentum.
3. **Uterine Tube (Tubal Pregnancy—95%):**
   - The majority of ectopic pregnancies occur in the uterine tube, known as tubal pregnancy.

Intrauterine Abnormal Implantation:

- The blastocyst attaches to the lower part of the uterine cavity, leading to a condition known as **Placenta praevia** (refer above).

CLASSIFICATION OF PLACENTA

According to Shape (Fig. 12.13)

- ***Bidiscoidal:*** Consists of two discs.
- ***Lobed:*** Divided into lobes.
- ***Diffuse (Placenta Membranacea):*** Chorionic villi persist all around the blastocyst, resulting in a thin placenta without a disc shape.
- ***Placenta Succenturiata:*** Small parts of the placenta are separated as accessory lobes.
- ***Fenestrated:*** Contains a hole in the disc.
- ***Circumvallate:*** The peripheral edge is surrounded by a sulcus covered by a circular fold of decidua.

According to the Insertion of the Umbilical Cord

- ***Normal:*** Attached to the placenta near the centre.
- ***Marginal (Battledore Placenta):*** Cord attached to the margin of the placenta.
- ***Furcate:*** Blood vessels divide before reaching the placenta.
- ***Velamentous:*** Blood vessels are attached to the amnion, where they ramify before reaching the placenta.

According to the Degree of Penetration Into the Uterine Wall

- ***Placenta Accreta:*** Adhered deep to decidua basalis.
- ***Placenta Increta:*** Adhered to the myometrium.
- ***Placenta Percreta:*** Penetrates the entire uterine wall.

According to Site of Implantation

- ***Placenta Praevia:*** Blastocyst implanted in the lower uterine segment; can be central or marginal, potentially leading to severe haemorrhage before parturition.
- ***Accessory Placenta (Placenta Succenturiata).***

According to the Branching Pattern of Umbilical Arteries

- ***Magistral Type:*** Umbilical arteries have the same caliber up to the periphery of the placenta.

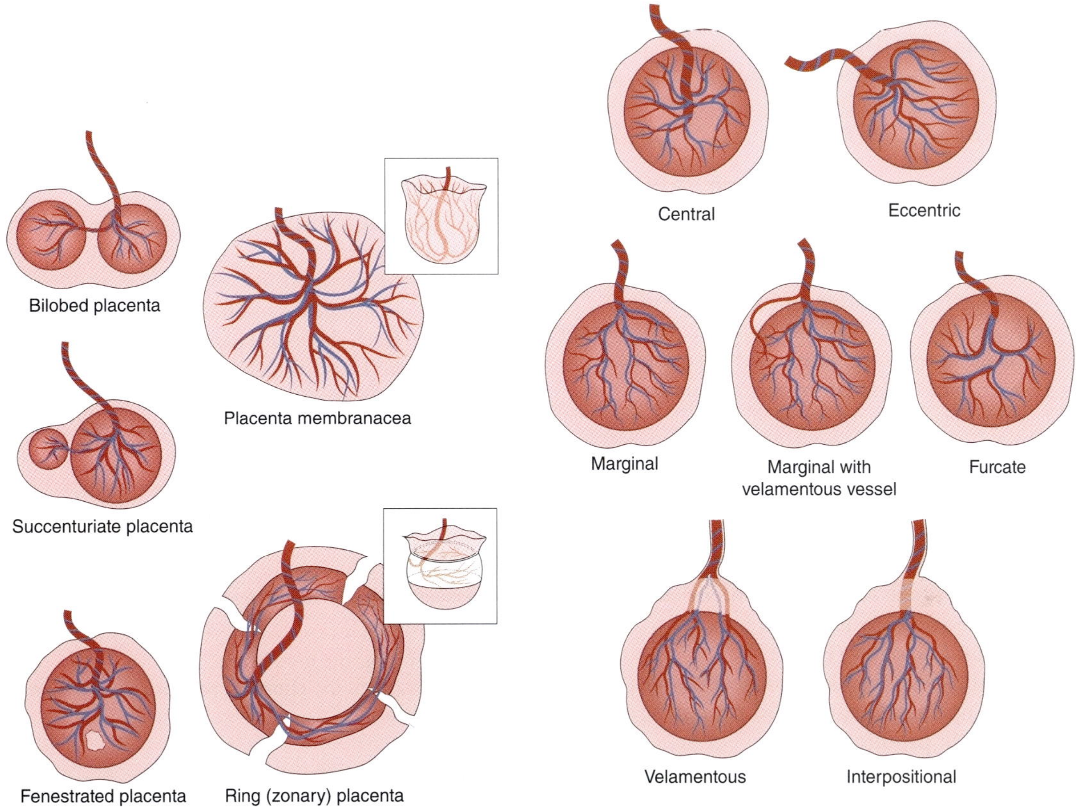

Fig. 12.13 Different types of placenta.

- ***Disperse Type:*** Umbilical arteries branch and undergo successive reduction in calibre.

CLINICAL NUGGETS

Transplacental therapeutics

- The placental barrier allows targeted treatment of foetal diseases.
- **Dexamethasone** is administered to pregnant mothers for foetal **Congenital adrenal hyperplasia** (CAH).
- Maternal use of **Digoxin** and Propranolol addresses foetal arrhythmias effectively.
- In multiple **Carboxylase** deficiency, vitamin **Biotin** is given to the mother.

Nutrient deficiency and IUGR

- **Placental insufficiency** contributes to inadequate nutrient delivery to the foetus.
- Conditions like drug abuse, preeclampsia, diabetes, impaired renal function and Rh incompatibility are implicated in placental insufficiency and intrauterine growth restriction (IUGR).

KLINISCHE PERLEN

AGENTS AND HORMONES CROSSING THE BARRIER

1. **Steroid Hormones and Thyroxine:**
   - Cross the placental barrier, influencing foetal development.
2. **Progestins (Masculinization):**
   - Impact foetal gender, potentially causing masculinization in female foetuses.
3. **Diethyl Stilbestrol (DES):**
   - Synthetic oestrogen linked to abnormalities in female genitalia and cervical **Clear cell carcinoma**.
   - Associated with testicular abnormalities in male foetuses.
4. **Viral Crossings:**
   - Viruses such as rubella, CMV (cytomegalovirus), coxsackie, varicella, variola, measles and polio can traverse the placental barrier.

5. **Substance Abuse Impact:**
   - **Cocaine and Heroin** can cross the placenta, affecting foetal development.

PLACENTAL HORMONES (AN 80.5)

- **Human Chorionic Gonadotropin (hCG):**
  - **Trophoblast** (syncytiotrophoblast and cytotrophoblast) synthesizes hCG.
  - **Pregnancy indicator**; detected in urine around 8 days after a missed period.
  - Maintains the **Corpus luteum**, supporting progesterone secretion and pregnancy.
  - Stimulates **Testosterone** production in foetal testes for scrotal descent.
- **Placental Oestrogen:**
  - Synthesized by syncytiotrophoblast, causing **uterine and breast** enlargement.
- **Placental Progesterone:**
  - Produced by syncytiotrophoblast, crucial for **decidual cell** development and breast preparation for **lactation**.
- **Placental Lactogen (HPL):**
  - Synthesized by syncytiotrophoblast, promoting **foetal growth** and preparing breasts for **milk production**.

ERYTHROBLASTOSIS FETALIS

- Maternal immune response to foetal blood cells crossing the placental barrier **(isoimmunization)**.
- Results in haemolysis, increased erythroblast production and, in severe cases, **Foetal hydrops**.
- Severity higher for CDE (rhesus) antigens than ABO blood group.
- **Rh-negative** mothers should receive Rh immunoglobulins postdelivery (if the child is Rh-positive) to prevent subsequent erythroblastosis.

AMNIOTIC BANDS

- Tears in the amnion that encircle foetal limbs and digits.
- May lead to **amputations or ring constrictions**.

AMNIOTIC FLUID

- **Production and Volume:**
  - Produced by amniotic cells, the volume changes during gestation:
    - **30 mL** at 10 weeks.
    - **450 mL** at 20 weeks.
    - **800–1000 mL** at 37 weeks.
  - Renewed every **3 hours**.
- **Foetal Contribution:**
  - Foetus starts swallowing by the fifth month (approximately 400 mL/day).
  - Foetal urine adds to amniotic fluid composition.
- **Polyhydramnios (Excessive Fluid):**
  - Defined as **>1500–2000 mL** and amniotic fluid index **(AFI) >25**.
  - **Causes:**
    - Maternal diabetes.
    - Congenital malformations.
    - CNS disorders (e.g. anencephaly).
    - GIT disorders (e.g. oesophageal atresia).
- **Oligohydramnios (Insufficient Fluid):**
  - Defined as **<400 mL** and **AFI <5**.
  - **Cause:**
    - Renal agenesis.

POINTS TO PONDER

Extraembryonic Membranes and Placental Development

- **Extraembryonic membranes:**
  - Consists of the **chorion, amnion, yolk sac and allantois.**
  - The amnion is a delicate ectodermal membrane with a mesodermal lining.
  - The yolk sac, lined with endoderm, lacks a prominent nutritive role in mammalian embryos.
  - The allantois, arising from the hindgut's ventral side, does not play a direct role in respiration or waste removal in humans.
- **Chorionic villi maturation:**
  - Chorionic villi, projections from the trophoblast, undergo maturation: **primary, secondary, tertiary and mature villi**.
  - Human placenta is termed **haemochorial** as chorionic villi float in maternal blood.
- **Decidual reaction and chorion maturation:**
  - Endometrial stromal cells undergo decidual reaction postimplantation.
  - The foetal chorion matures, with the part near the basal endometrium termed **chorion frondosum**, while regressing villi constitute **chorion laeve**.
  - Chorion frondosum eventually develops into the mature placenta.
- **Placental hormones and immunological tolerance:**
  - The first placental hormone released is **hCG,** forming the basis of pregnancy tests.
  - Despite immunological differences, foetal and placental tissues are not rejected.
- **Postulates** include reduced trophoblastic tissue antigenicity, temporary maternal immune system paralysis and local immunological barriers between the foetus and mother.

BRAIN TEASERS

1. At full term, what is the weight of the placenta?
   A. 100–200 g
   B. 300–400 g
   C. 500–600 g
   D. 700–800 g
2. Which layer of the trophoblast forms lacunae during placental development?
   A. Cytotrophoblast
   B. Syncytiotrophoblast
   C. Mesoderm
   D. Basal plate
3. What is the role of tertiary villi in placental development?
   A. Attach chorionic sac to endometrium.
   B. Form maternal-foetal exchange points.
   C. Initiate uteroplacental circulation.
   D. Increase the surface area of exchange.
4. What does the decidua capsularis cover?
   A. Embryonic pole
   B. Abembryonic pole
   C. Chorionic frondosum
   D. Chorionic laeve
5. What is the function of anchoring villi in the placenta?
   A. Increase surface area for exchange.
   B. Provide attachment to the endometrium.
   C. Form maternal blood vessels.
   D. Initiate uteroplacental circulation.
6. What is the primary mesoderm responsible for in the chorionic plate?
   A. Formation of maternal blood vessels.
   B. Development of umbilical vessels.
   C. Production of syncytiotrophoblast.
   D. Creation of cytotrophoblast.
7. What does the decidua capsularis degenerate into?
   A. Anchoring villi
   B. Free villi
   C. Smooth chorion laeve
   D. Cotyledons
8. At full term, what is the placenta's ratio to the foetus in terms of weight?
   A. 1:5
   B. 1:7
   C. 1:10
   D. 1:15
9. What term is used to describe a placenta with two discs?
   A. Lobed
   B. Diffuse
   C. Bidiscoidal
   D. Fenestrated
10. What is the characteristic feature of placenta succenturiata?
    A. Lobed appearance.
    B. Separation of a small part as an accessory lobe.
    C. Presence of a hole in the disc.
    D. Circular fold of decidua.
11. In a fenestrated placenta, what is the notable feature?
    A. Lobed appearance.
    B. Circular fold of decidua.
    C. Hole in the disc.
    D. Surrounding sulcus.
12. What happens at the end of the second week of placental development?
    A. Formation of primary chorionic villi.
    B. Penetration of spiral uterine vessels.
    C. Establishment of uteroplacental circulation.
    D. Formation of secondary villi.

Answers

1. (C); 2. (B); 3. (B); 4. (B); 5. (B); 6. (B); 7. (C); 8. (B); 9. (C); 10. (B); 11. (C); 12. (A).

FURTHER READINGS

Bohîlțea RE, Dima V, Ducu I, et al. Clinically relevant prenatal ultrasound diagnosis of umbilical cord pathology. *Diagnostics (Basel).* 2022;12(2):236. doi:10.3390/diagnostics12020236.

Ho A, Chappell LC, Story L, et al. Visual assessment of the placenta in antenatal magnetic resonance imaging across gestation in normal and compromised pregnancies: observations from a large cohort study. *Placenta.* 2022;117:29-38. doi:10.1016/j.placenta.2021.10.006. Epub 2021 Oct 14. Erratum in: Placenta. 2022;119:31.

Krzyżanowski A, Kwiatek M, Gęca T, Stupak A, Kwaśniewska A. Modern ultrasonography of the umbilical cord: prenatal diagnosis of umbilical cord abnormalities and assessement of fetal wellbeing. *Med Sci Monit.* 2019;25:3170-3180. doi:10.12659/MSM.913762.

Rosenfeld CS. The placenta-brain-axis. *J Neurosci Res.* 2021;99(1):271-283. doi:10.1002/jnr.24603.

Sherer DM, Al-Haddad S, Cheng R, Dalloul M. Current perspectives of prenatal sonography of umbilical cord morphology. *Int J Womens Health.* 2021;13:939-971. doi:10.2147/IJWH.S278747.

Yong HEJ, Chan SY. Current approaches and developments in transcript profiling of the human placenta. *Hum Reprod Update.* 2020;26(6):799-840. doi:10.1093/humupd/dmaa028.

13 Twinning

AN 80.4 Describe embryological basis of twinning in monozygotic and dizygotic twins.

ANAMNESE

A 32-year-old expectant mother arrived at the obstetric clinic for her routine prenatal checkup. Everything had been progressing smoothly until an unexpected twist emerged during an ultrasound examination. The initial joy of discovering she was pregnant with twins gave way to a reality—a **Vanishing twin**. The ultrasound revealed that one of the embryos had stopped developing, a phenomenon known as vanishing twin syndrome. She required sensitive counselling for the loss of one twin while simultaneously accepting the healthy pregnancy that remained.

Victorian scientist Francis Galton, a half-cousin of Charles Darwin, stands as a pioneer in recognizing the invaluable role of twins in trait heritability. In his seminal 1875 paper, '**The History of Twins**', Galton, credited with coining the term '**nature versus nurture**', utilized twins to gauge the relative influences of genetics and environment. To grasp the essence of contemporary twin studies, exploring the biology of twins is essential. As explained by Arseneault, twin studies serve as a tool to quantify the impact of genetic factors in comparison to environmental ones.

Twinning, the process where a mother gives birth to two offspring in a single pregnancy, occurs at an incidence of **1 in 80 births**, with a likelihood tied to the mother's age and fertility treatments.

Beyond twins, multiple births extend to triplets (three in single pregnancy), quadruplets (four in single pregnancy) and beyond.

- Twinning is classified into:
  - **Dizygotic (Fraternal twins).**
  - **Monozygotic (Identical twins).**

DIZYGOTIC TWINS (FRATERNAL TWINS) (AN 80.4)

More prevalent than monozygotic twins (Fig. 13.1):

- Approximately 70–90% of twins are dizygotic or fraternal twins.
- The incidence rises with advancing **maternal age** and **fertility treatments**.
- Dizygotic twins result from the concurrent release of **two oocytes** in a single ovarian cycle, each fertilized by a distinct sperm. This leads to the formation of two zygotes, each implanting separately in the uterine endometrial wall.
- These zygotes have entirely distinct genetic makeups, resulting in nonidentical appearances.
- Key features of dizygotic twins include:
  - Being of the **same or different sex** (with **twin boys** being the most common and twin girls the least common).
  - Each having a **separate placenta** and **chorionic sac**.
  - Possessing **different genetic constitutions**.

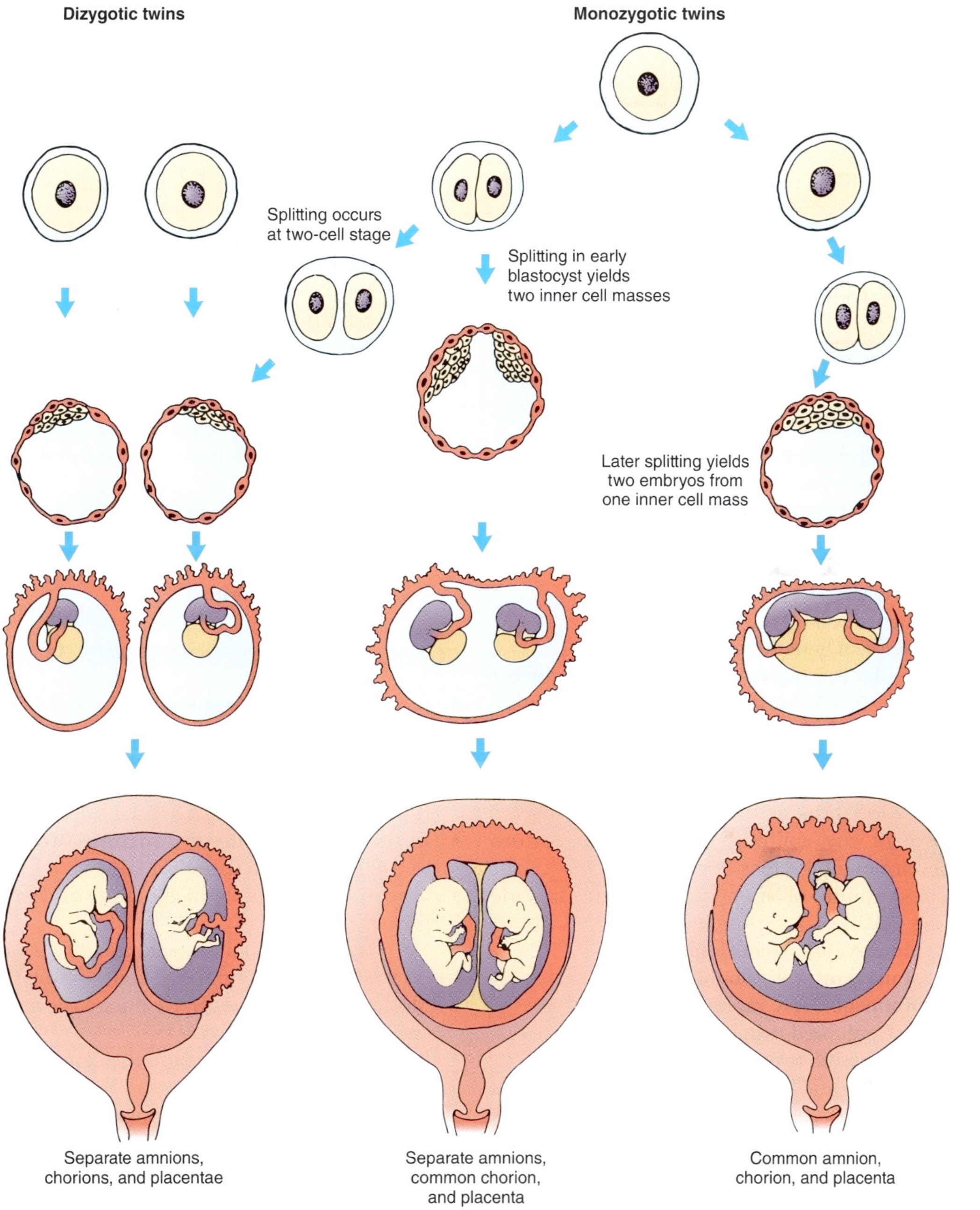

Fig. 13.1 Schematic diagram showing the formation of monozygotic and dizygotic twins. Foetal membrane development in various types of twins. The degree to which monozygotic twins share placental membranes depends on the stage of development at which the originally single embryo separates; if the splitting occurs at the two-cell stage of cleavage, the twins will develop as separately as dizygotic twins; if the splitting yields a blastocyst with two inner cell masses, then the embryos will share a single chorion and placenta but occupy separate amnions; if the splitting occurs after the formation of the inner cell mass, the embryos will occupy a single amnion. (Source: *Larsen's Human Embryology*. 4th ed. 2008.)

- In some instances, the placentas may be close and fuse together.
- There is potential for the exchange of genetically dissimilar cells between twins through the placenta.
- For instance, dizygotic twins may exhibit two types of RBCs (**erythrocyte mosaicism**), indicating the exchange of blood cells.
- The presence of genetically dissimilar cell groups within the bodies of nonidentical twins is termed **Chimera**.

MONOZYGOTIC TWINS (IDENTICAL/LIKE TWINS)

- Monozygotic twins account for approximately one-quarter (or 25%) of all twin births.
- The incidence of monozygotic twins is **3–4 per 1000 births**.
- Monozygotic twins originate from the fusion of **one Oocyte** and **one Sperm**.
- Characterized by the following traits:
  - **Identical genetic** makeup.
  - Similar in both **appearance** and **structure**.
  - Sharing the **same blood group** but exhibiting **different fingerprints** (with fingerprints influenced by the developing environment within the uterine cavity).
- The formation of monozygotic twins occurs through the splitting of zygotes at various developmental stages.
- **Classification** of monozygotic twins include (Fig. 13.2):
  - **Monozygotic bichorionic.**
  - **Monochorionic biamniotic.**
  - **Monochorionic monoamniotic.**
    - ➢ **Conjoined twins.**
    - ➢ **Parasitic twins.**
- Developmental separation occurs primarily at three stages:
  A. **At the two-celled stage (monozygotic, dichorionic and diamniotic)** (Fig. 13.3).
    - ➢ Earliest separation stage with an incidence of 25%–30%.
    - ➢ Cells formed can independently develop into complete embryos.
    - ➢ Two cells separate to develop independently, each with its own placenta, amniotic cavity and chorionic cavity (similar to dizygotic twins).

  B. **Splitting of inner cell mass (monozygotic, monochorionic and diamniotic).**
    - ➢ Incidence of 70%–75%.
    - ➢ Inner cell mass splits into two groups within the same blastocyst cavity.
    - ➢ Embryos share a common placenta and chorionic cavity but have separate amniotic cavities.

  C. **Splitting of bilaminar germ disc (monozygotic, monochorionic and monoamniotic).**
    - ➢ Very rare, with an incidence of 1%–2%.
    - ➢ Splitting occurs just before the appearance of the primitive streak or with two organizing centres.
    - ➢ Foetuses share a common chorionic and amniotic cavity, with a common placenta and typically balanced blood supply.
    - ➢ The complications during the formation of this type of twins are:
      - ○ **Conjoined twins.**
      - ○ **Parasitic twins.**

CONJOINED TWINS (DOUBLE MONSTERS)

- It is a type of **monozygotic** twins.
- Here the **two organizing centres** remain in the same germ disc during the time of division and the two embryos are incompletely separated from each other.
- In this condition, **the two foetuses are joined** to each other by a tissue bridge.
- Usually such twins are of equal size and receive proper blood supply.
- Conjoined twins **can be separated**, if they have no vital parts in common **(Siamese twins).**
- Most of them do not survive due to the complications during delivery.
- Based on the **level of fusion** they are classified as follows:
  - **Craniopagus**—fusion of head (Fig. 13.4).
  - **Thoracopagus**—fusion of thorax.
  - **Cephalothoracopagus**—fusion of head and thorax.
  - **Pygopagus**—fusion of sacral regions.
  - **Omphalopagus**—fusion at the abdomen and share a common umbilicus.
  - **Cephalopagus**—fusion at the head, the connection occurs at the level of the skull or face, and the twins often share a portion of the brain and other critical structures.

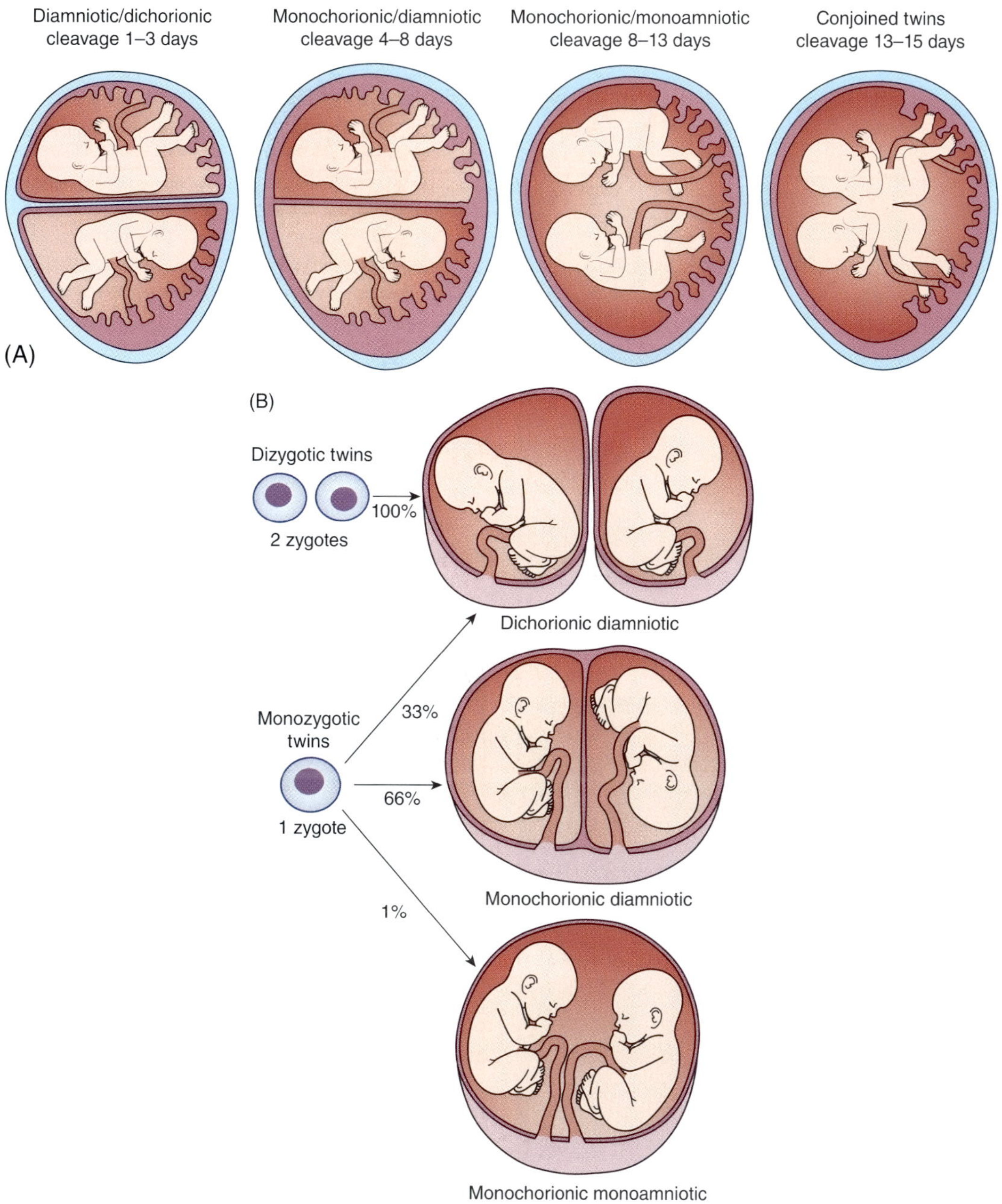

Fig. 13.2 Different types of monozygotic (A) and dizygotic twins (B). (B) Diagram illustrating zygosity and placentation in twins. Of all twins, 70% are dizygotic (from two sperm and two eggs) and 30% of twins are monozygotic (from one sperm and one egg). From all dizygotic twins, 100% form dichorionic diamniotic placenta. From all monozygotic twins, 33% are dichorionic diamniotic, 66% are monochorionic diamniotic and 1% are monochorionic monoamniotic. (Source: (Fig. B) *Diagnostic Ultrasound*, 5th ed.: Carol M. Rumack, Deborah Levine, Fig. 32.1, Elsevier Inc., 2018.)

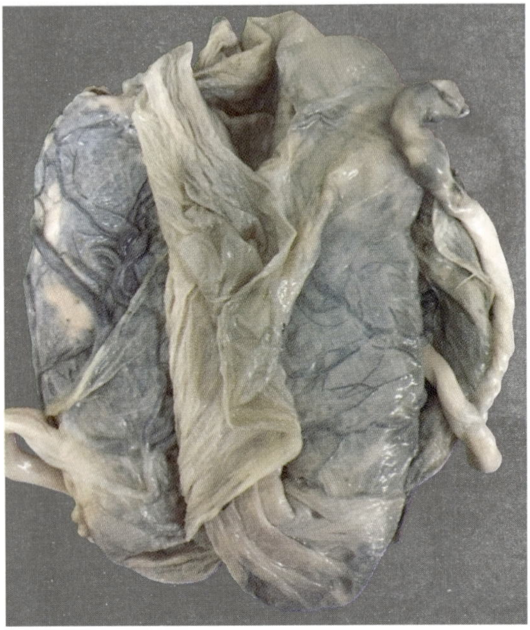

Fig. 13.3 Dichorionic diamniotic fused placenta. (Photo courtesy: Dr Nandagopalan.)

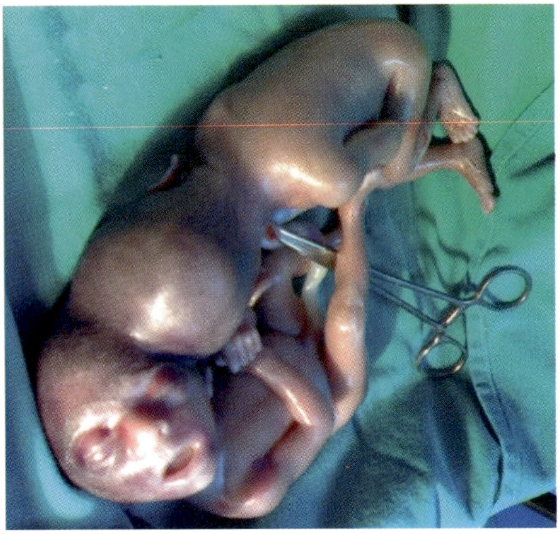

Fig. 13.4 Craniopagus (fusion of heads). (Photo courtesy: Dr Rema.)

- **Ischiopagus**—Fusion at the lower part of the spine, the sacrum and share some abdominal and pelvic organs.
- **Rachipagus**—Fusion along the back, and they may share vertebral structures or spinal cord segments.
- **Parapagus dicephalus**—twins have separate heads and necks but a fused or conjoined body.
- **Parapagus diprosopus**—extremely rare form of conjoined twins characterized by the presence of two heads (diprosopus) side by side on a single torso. In this condition, the twins may share facial features and cranial structures to varying degrees. The term 'diprosopus' is derived from the Greek words '**di**', meaning two and '**prosopon**', meaning face (Fig. 13.5).

PARASITIC TWINS

- One of the conjoined twins becomes rudimentary due to diminished blood supply.
- It grows like a parasite from the body of the well-developed cotwin. For example, dermoids, embryomata.
- **Foetus-in-foetu** is a condition where the parasitic twin is completely enclosed within the body of the cotwin.

CLINICAL NUGGETS

Twin-twin transfusion syndrome (TTTS)

- Primarily observed in **monochorionic twins**.
- Vascular anastomoses develop between the two placentae.
- The **donor twin** experiences oligohydramnios and growth restriction.
- The **recipient twin** suffers from polyhydramnios and cardiac failure.

Twin-reversed arterial perfusion (TRAP)

- Vascular anastomoses enable the **Pump twin** to supply blood to a second **Acardiac/Acephalic twin**.
- Cardiac overload leads to **cardiac failure in the pump twin**, resulting in its demise.
- Subsequently, the acardiac twin also succumbs as it relies on the pump twin for survival.
- Management involves performing a caesarean section once the healthy twin reaches viability to address these critical conditions.

KLINISCHE PERLEN

VANISHING TWINS

- Vanishing twins refer to a phenomenon in which one or more embryos, initially detected during early pregnancy, cease to develop

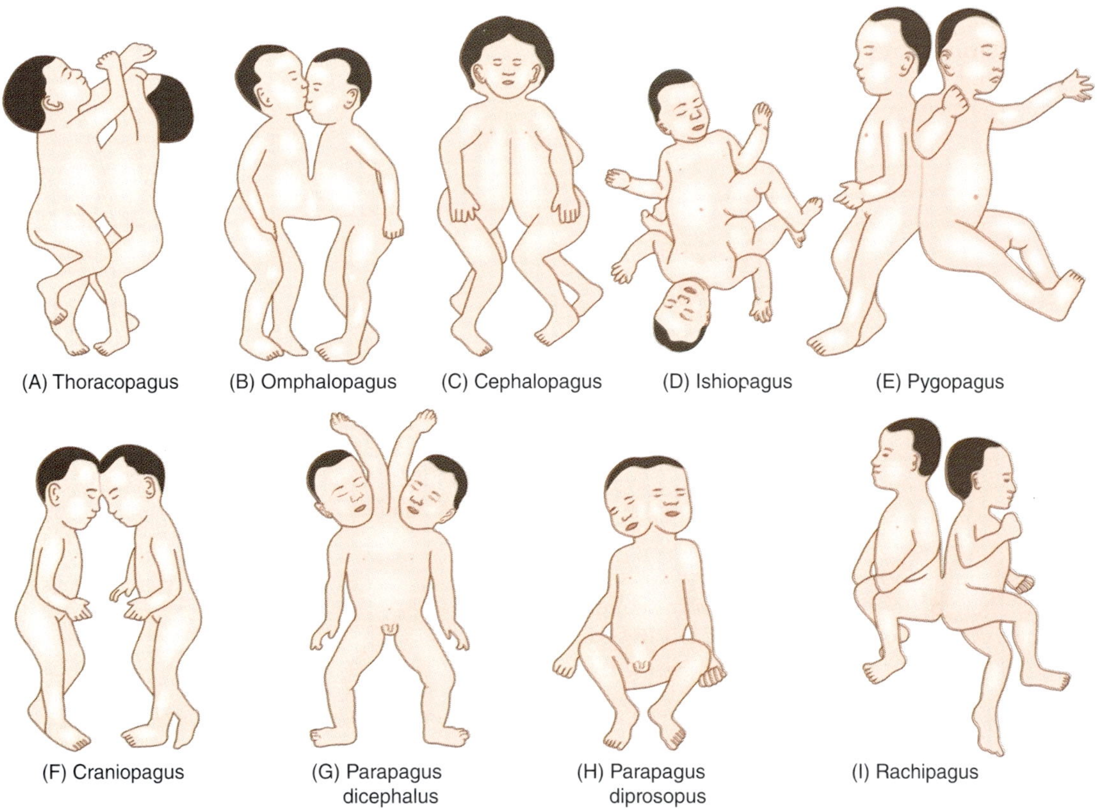

Fig. 13.5 Different types of conjoined twins.

(usually in the first trimester) and are eventually reabsorbed by the mother's body or remain as **Foetus papyraceus**.

- This occurrence is often discovered through ultrasound examinations, where a previously identified embryo is no longer detectable in subsequent scans.
- The reasons for vanishing twins can vary and may include **chromosomal abnormalities, developmental issues or natural selection processes**.
- While the surviving twin usually continues to thrive, the experience can evoke a range of emotions for the expectant parents, from initial excitement about the prospect of multiple births to the complex feelings surrounding the loss of one or more embryos.

SUPERFOECUNDATION

- Superfoecundation is a rare reproductive phenomenon where a woman conceives two or more foetuses from **separate acts of intercourse** within a short time frame.
- This occurrence leads to the fertilization of **multiple eggs** released during single ovarian cycle.
- As a result, the foetuses in a multiple pregnancy can have **different gestational ages** and, potentially, **different fathers**.
- This phenomenon is most commonly observed in certain polyovulatory mammals and not usually seen in humans.

SUPERFOETATION

- Superfoetation is an exceptional reproductive occurrence in which a woman conceives another foetus while already being pregnant.
- Unlike typical pregnancies, where a single egg is fertilized by a sperm and develops into a foetus, superfoetation involves the

fertilization of a second egg (**Aberrant ovulation during pregnancy**) during an ongoing pregnancy.

- This can lead to foetuses in the same womb with different gestational ages.
- These type of twin pregnancies have a high incidence of **perinatal mortality** and increased rate of **preterm delivery**.

POLAR BODY/HALF-IDENTICAL TWINS

- Following ovulation, the developing ovum undergoes division into two cells.
- Each cell possesses **an equal number of chromosomes** in the nucleus but **differs in cytoplasmic content**.
- The smaller cell, known as the polar body, typically undergoes degeneration and eventual demise.
- In the unique case of polar body twins, the **Polar body** is fertilized by one sperm concurrently with the ovum being fertilized by a different sperm.
- These twins share:
  - **Half of their genes** in common (inherited from the **mother**).
  - The remaining half of their genes differs since they originate from two distinct sperm cells.
- **Identical twins** share **100%** of genes in common.
- **Fraternal twins** share **50%** of genes in common.
- **Half-identical** twins share **75%** of genes in common.

POINTS TO PONDER

- Two distinct **blastocysts** originating from separate sperm and ova do not constitute identical twins.
- These **Non-identical twins** exhibit individual characteristics such as separate placentas (dichorionic), distinct amniotic sacs (diamniotic) and may share the same or different sexes—classified as **Dizygotic twins** (or fraternal).
- Conversely, if a single zygote undergoes division, it gives rise to identical twins.
- **Identical twins** stem from the same ovum and spermatozoon, resulting in **genetic uniformity**—referred to as **Monozygotic twins**.

BRAIN TEASERS

1. What is the term for twins that result from the concurrent release of two oocytes in a single ovarian cycle, each fertilized by a distinct sperm?
   A. Identical twins
   B. Fraternal twins
   C. Monozygotic twins
   D. Parasitic twins
2. What is the approximate percentage of twins that are dizygotic or fraternal?
   A. 25%
   B. 50%
   C. 65%
   D. 90%
3. What factor contributes to the increased incidence of dizygotic twins?
   A. Advancing maternal age
   B. Decreased maternal age
   C. Genetic factors
   D. Environmental factors
4. What is the key characteristic of dizygotic twins regarding their genetic makeup?
   A. Identical genetic constitution
   B. Similar appearance and structure
   C. Entirely distinct genetic makeups
   D. Shared blood group and fingerprints
5. In dizygotic twins, what is the potential term used for the exchange of genetically dissimilar cells between twins through the placenta?
   A. Mosaicism
   B. Fusion
   C. Chimera
   D. Conjoined
6. What is the term for twins that comprise approximately 25% of all twins and result from the fusion of one oocyte and one sperm?
   A. Fraternal twins
   B. Identical twins
   C. Monochorionic twins
   D. Parasitic twins
7. What is the classification of monozygotic twins that share a common placenta but have separate amniotic cavities?
   A. Monozygotic bichorionic
   B. Monochorionic biamniotic
   C. Monochorionic monoamniotic
   D. Conjoined twins
8. At what stage of development does splitting occur in monozygotic twins with a common placenta and common chorionic cavity but separate amniotic cavities?
   A. Two-celled stage
   B. Inner cell mass splitting
   C. Bilaminar germ disc stage
   D. Blastocyst cavity stage

9. What type of twins are conjoined twins?
   A. Dizygotic twins
   B. Fraternal twins
   C. Monozygotic twins
   D. Parasitic twins
10. What determines the classification of conjoined twins into types such as Craniopagus, Thoracopagus, Cephalothoracopagus and Pygopagus?
   A. The level of blood supply.
   B. The level of fusion.
   C. The number of organs in common.
   D. The type of genetic makeup.

Answers

1. (B); 2. (D); 3. (A); 4. (C); 5. (C); 6. (B); 7. (B); 8. (B); 9. (C); 10. (B).

FURTHER READINGS

Baijal N, Sahni M, Verma N, Kumar A, Parkhe N, Puliyel JM. Discordant twins with the smaller baby appropriate for gestational age—unusual manifestation of superfoetation: a case report. *BMC Pediatr.* 2007;7:2. doi:10.1186/1471-2431-7-2.

Hankoff LD. Why the healing gods are twins. *Yale J Biol Med.* 1977;50(3):307-319.

Ito A, Furukawa T, Nakaoka K, et al. Heterotopic pregnancy with suspicion of superfetation after the intrauterine insemination cycle with ovulation induction using clomiphene citrate: a case report. *Clin Pract.* 2019;9(1):1129. doi:10.4081/cp.2019.1129.

Mogollón F, Casas-Vargas A, Rodríguez F, Usaquén W. Twins from different fathers: a heteropaternal superfecundation case report in Colombia. *Biomedica.* 2020;40(4):604-608. doi:10.7705/biomedica.5100.

Morong JJ, Janssen J, Morgan JC, Rodriguez SM. Heterotopic triplet pregnancy after clomiphene citrate. *Ochsner J.* 2021;21(4):416-418. doi:10.31486/toj.20.0150.

14 The Pharyngeal (Branchial) Apparatus

AN 43.4 Describe the development of branchial apparatus.
AN 43.4 Describe the development of thyroid gland.
AN 43.4 Describe the development of tongue.
AN 43.4 Describe the development basis of congenital anomalies of branchial apparatus, tongue and thyroid gland.

ANAMNESE

A 3-day-old infant was admitted to the neonatal intensive care unit (NICU) with a diagnosis of **Pierre Robin Sequence (PRS)**. The child presented with a triad of characteristic features, including **micrognathia** (undersized lower jaw), **glossoptosis** (posterior displacement or retraction of the tongue) and **cleft palate**. The micrognathia led to a compromised airway due to the posteriorly positioned tongue, resulting in respiratory distress. The newborn underwent immediate interventions to manage airway obstruction, including prone positioning and continuous positive airway pressure (CPAP). Further assessment also revealed a U-shaped cleft palate. The sequence of anomalies is depicted in Fig. 14.1.

The oral or pharyngeal apparatus serve the dual functions of respiration and feeding. It develops from structures called pharyngeal arches, which are a series of outgrowths on the lateral side of the head. The structural organization of the pharyngeal arches involve contributions from each of the three—primary endoderm, mesoderm and ectoderm germ layers. The endoderm is important for pharyngeal arch formation. The ectoderm gives rise to **Neural crest cells (NCC)**. The pharyngeal arches give rise to most of the neurovasculature and musculoskeletal systems in the head and neck. The complexity of development results in series of birth defects.

- In a 4-week-old embryo, the neck is indistinct.
- Between the fourth and fifth week, pharyngeal (branchial) arches emerge on the lateral wall of the primitive pharynx (Fig. 14.2).

PHARYNGEAL ARCHES

- There are **five pairs** of pharyngeal arches numbered 1, 2, 3, 4 and 6.
- Arch 5 never forms or remains rudimentary or regresses over time.
- Each arch is arranged in the craniocaudal direction and consists of a core of mesenchymal tissue covered externally by ectoderm and internally by endoderm.
- Mesenchyme is derived from paraxial mesoderm, supplemented by NCC migration.

ARCH COMPONENTS

- **Ectodermal cleft.**
- **Mesodermal core.**
- **Endodermal pouch.**
- **Closing membrane.**

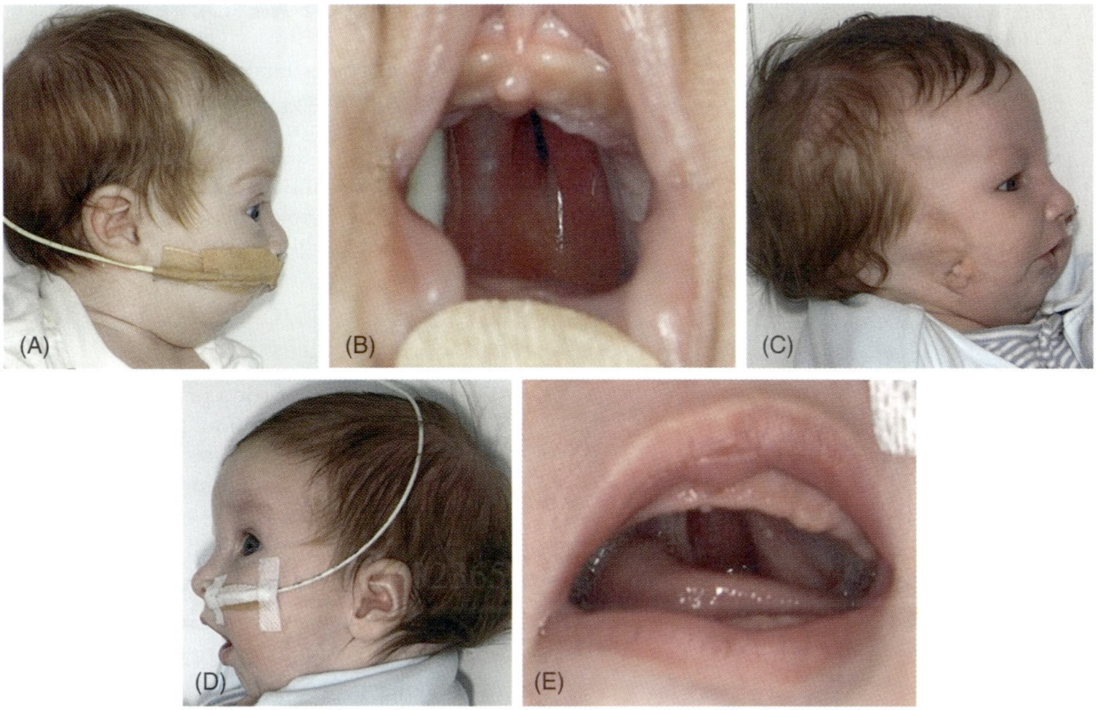

Fig. 14.1 Pierre Robin sequence. (Source: Plastic Surgery Principles and Practice, Sabrina Cugno, Babak J. Mehrara, Neil W. Bulstrode, Rostam Farhadieh, Fig. 17.4, Elsevier Inc., 2022.)

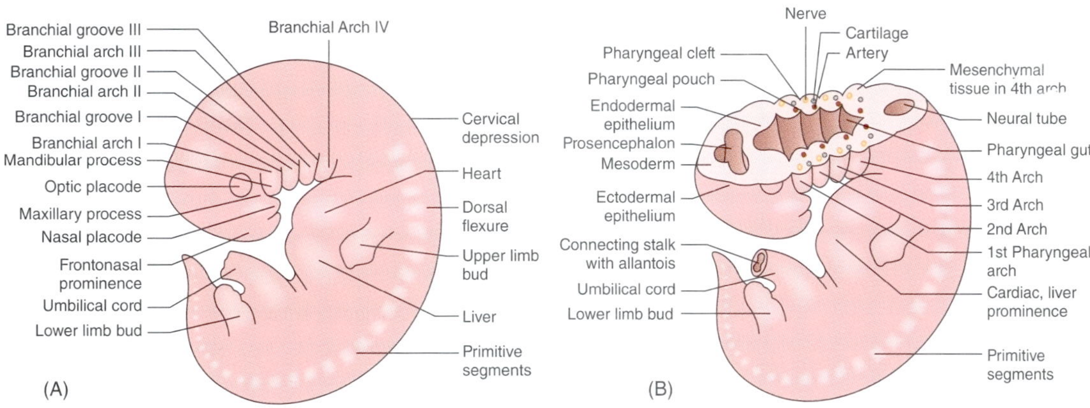

Fig. 14.2 Development of pharyngeal arches. (A) Lateral view. (B) Cross-section through the arches.

- **Formation of Clefts and Pouches:**
  - Ectoderm of pharyngeal arches dips inward, creating pharyngeal clefts or grooves.
  - Endoderm extends outward as pharyngeal pouches situated between the arches.
  - The meeting point of ectoderm and endoderm forms **closing membranes**.
  - **Four clefts**, **five pouches** (with the fifth being rudimentary), **four closing membranes** and **five arches** constitute the structural elements.
  - Pharyngeal arches become visible on the ventral floor of the primitive pharynx and they meet from two sides converging towards the midventral line.

- The **Branchial apparatus** forms: (AN 43.4)
  - **Face.**
  - **Neck.**
  - **Definitive mouth.**
  - **Pharynx.**
  - **Larynx.**
- The derivatives of apparatus are discussed under the following headings (Fig. 14.3):
  - **Derivatives of Mesoderm.**
  - **Derivatives of Ectoderm.**
  - **Derivatives of Endoderm.**

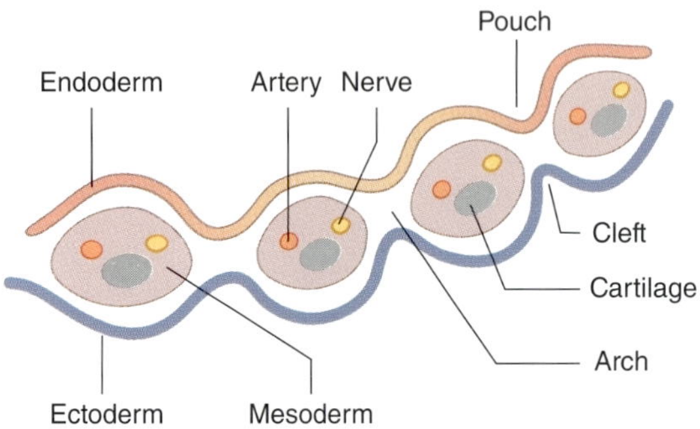

Fig. 14.3 Pharyngeal arch components.

DERIVATIVES OF MESODERM

- Mesodermal cells exhibit pluripotency, with the arch mesoderm, derived from NCC, specializing in the formation of skeletal elements and connective tissue.
- Simultaneously, the paraxial mesoderm contributes to the development of muscles in the head and neck regions (Fig. 14.3).

SKELETAL ELEMENTS/CARTILAGES OF THE PHARYNGEAL ARCHES

- The cartilaginous portion of the mesodermal core undergoes ossification, giving rise to the skeletal elements, including both bone and cartilage. Certain components may disappear, while others, such as the perichondrium, may persist and transform into ligaments (Fig. 14.4).

First Arch/Mandibular Arch

- The ventral portion of the first arch is called **Mandibular process** and the dorsal portion is called the **Maxillary process**.

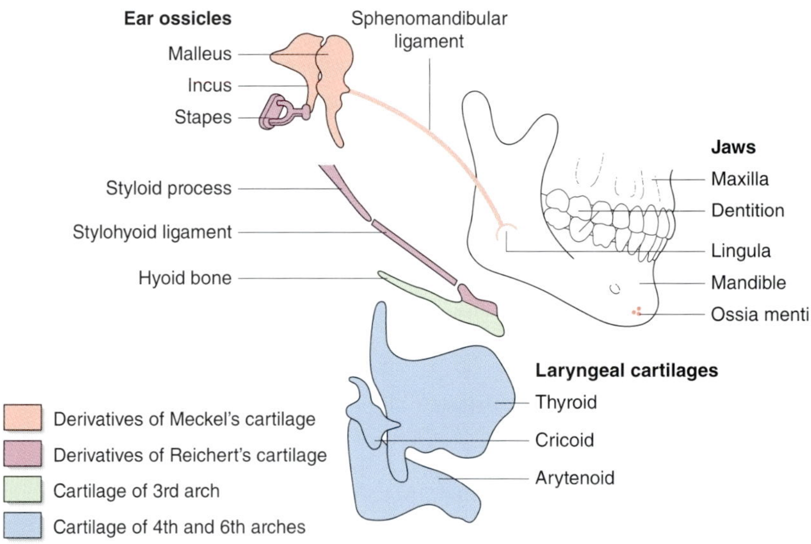

Fig. 14.4 Skeletal derivatives of the pharyngeal arches. The first arch gives rise to the upper and lower jaws, the dentition, the malleus, incus (middle ear ossicles) and sphenomandibular ligament. The second arch gives rise to the styloid process, stylohyoid ligament, stapes (middle ear ossicle) and the lesser cornu and upper part of the body of the hyoid bone. The third arch gives rise to the greater cornu and lower part of the body of the hyoid bone. The fourth arch gives rise to the laryngeal cartilages. Those structures formed by the pharyngeal arch cartilages are indicated in colour. (Source: Redrawn from Wendell-Smith CP, Williams RL, Treadgold S. *Basic Human Embryology*, 3rd ed. London: Pitman Publishing, 1984; *Handbook of Orthodontics*, 2nd ed. 2016.)

- The cartilage of the first arch called **Meckel's cartilage** is formed in the ventral portion. The Meckel's cartilage has got a dorsal end and a ventral end. The dorsal end which lies close to the middle ear forms **Malleus** and **Incus**. The ventral end acts as a mould for the mandible and the mesenchyme surrounding it undergoes membranous ossification to form **Mandible**.
- After the formation of mandible, the cartilage disappears. The part of the cartilage persisting between mandible and ear ossicles form the **Anterior ligament of malleus** and **Sphenomandibular ligament**.
- The dorsal portion of the arch called the maxillary process gives rise to **Premaxilla, Maxilla, Temporal bone** and **Zygomatic bone** by membranous ossification.

Second Arch/Hyoid Arch

- The cartilage of the arch is called **Reichert's cartilage**. It has got a dorsal end and ventral end.
- The dorsal end ossifies to form **Stapes** and **Styloid process** of temporal bone and the ventral end forms **small/lesser cornu** and **superior/upper part of the body of Hyoid bone**.
- The perichondrium of the cartilage persists as the **Stylohyoid ligament**. (Note all structures start with the letter **'S'** which stands for the **Second arch**.)

Third Arch

- The cartilage located at the ventral aspect of the arch has got a ventral and dorsal part. The ventral part ossifies to form the **greater horn** and **lower part** of the body of **Hyoid bone**. The dorsal part disappears.

Fourth and Sixth Arches

- Fourth and sixth arch cartilages fuse to form the cartilages of the larynx namely **thyroid, cricoid, arytenoid, corniculate** and **cuneiform** except epiglottis which develop from the caudal part of hypobranchial eminence (Fig. 14.5).

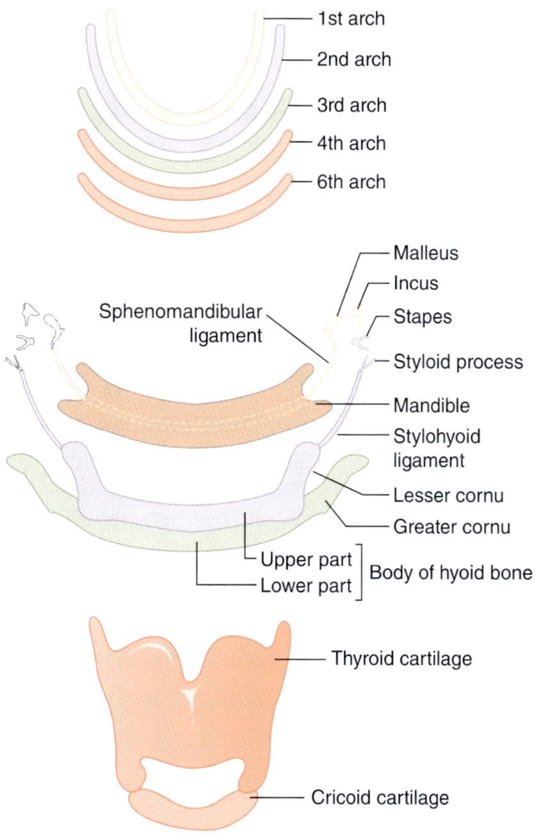

Fig 14.5 Schematic representation of the skeletal derivatives of the pharyngeal arches.

MUSCLES OF THE PHARYNGEAL ARCHES (Table 14.1)

- The mesoderm originating from the paraxial mesoderm gives rise to the muscles associated with the arch, and these muscles are innervated by the corresponding nerves of the arch.

First Arch/Mandibular Arch

- The muscles originating from the first arch include the muscles of **Mastication** (temporalis, masseter, medial pterygoid and lateral pterygoid), the anterior belly of the digastric, tensor tympani and tensor palatini.
- These muscles are innervated by the nerve of the arch, the **Mandibular nerve**.

Second Arch/Hyoid Arch

- The muscles originating from the second arch include the muscles of **Facial expression**, posterior belly of digastric, stylohyoid and stapedius. They are supplied by **Facial nerve**.

Third Arch

- **Stylopharyngeus** muscle is the only muscle derived from the third arch, and it is supplied by **Glossopharyngeal nerve**.

Table 14.1 Musculoskeletal Derivatives of Pharyngeal Arches

Pharyngeal Arch	Nerve	Skeleton	Muscle	Ligaments
First arch or Mandibular arch	Mandibular nerve	**Meckel's** cartilage, mandible, malleus, incus, premaxilla, maxilla, zygomatic bone, part of temporal bone	Muscles of mastication, anterior belly of digastric, tensor tympani, tensor palatini	Anterior ligament of malleus, sphenomandibular ligament
Second arch or Hyoid arch	Facial nerve	**Reichert's** cartilage, stapes, styloid process, lesser horn and upper portion of body of hyoid bone	Muscles of facial expression, stapedius, posterior belly of digastric, stylohyoid	Stylohyoid ligament
Third arch	Glossopharyngeal nerve	Greater horn and lower part of body of hyoid bone	Stylopharyngeus	
Fourth–sixth arches	• Superior laryngeal nerve–fourth • Recurrent laryngeal nerve–sixth	Laryngeal cartilages	Cricothyroid, levator palatine, constrictors of larynx, intrinsic muscles of larynx	

First arch–Mandibular-M is the key letter; **Second arch** can be easily remembered with the letter S; **Third arch**–glossopharyngeal-stylopharyngeus.

Fourth Arch

- The muscles originating from the fourth arch include cricothyroid, levator veli palatini and constrictors of the **Pharynx**. They are supplied by **Superior laryngeal nerve**.

Sixth Arch

- The muscles originating from the fourth arch include intrinsic muscles of the **Larynx**, and they are supplied by **Recurrent laryngeal nerve** (Table 14.1).

ARTERIES OF THE PHARYNGEAL ARCHES

- A sequence of aortic arch arteries running through the pharyngeal arches establishes connections between the **dorsal and ventral Aortae** (Fig. 14.6).
- The ventral aorta and dorsal aorta are arterial structures derived from the ventral and dorsal regions of the foregut, respectively. They are discussed in detail in development of cardiovascular system.

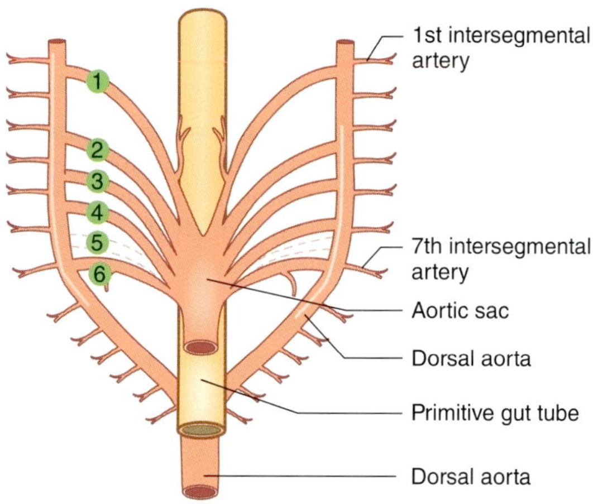

Fig. 14.6 Arteries of the pharyngeal arches.

NERVES OF THE PHARYNGEAL ARCHES (FIG. 14.7)

- The nerve running along the cranial border of the arch is termed the **Posttrematic nerve** of the arch (Fig. 14.8).

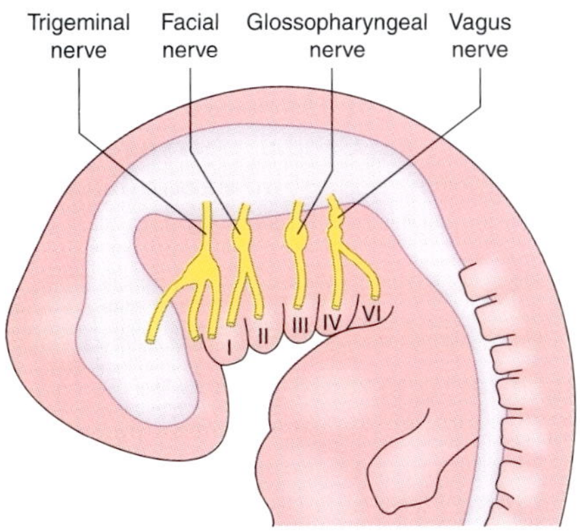

Fig. 14.7 Nerves of the pharyngeal arches.

- On the caudal border, the nerve is referred to as the **Pretrematic** nerve.
- In humans, the first pharyngeal arch exhibits double innervation.
- The **Mandibular nerve** serves as the post-trematic nerve for the first arch, while the **Chorda tympani** (a branch of the facial nerve) functions as the pretrematic nerve.
- Additional components such as the **tympanic branch of Glossopharyngeal** and **auricular branch of the Vagus** are sometimes recognized as pre-trematic remnantstof the corresponding arches.
- **Trigeminal nerve** with its maxillary and mandibular divisions supply the first arch. Sensory branches from maxillary and mandibular nerve supply the skin of the face, mucous membranes, soft palate and tongue. Motor branches of mandibular nerve supplies the muscles of the first arch. The chordae tympani supplies taste fibres to the anterior two-thirds of the tongue.
- **Facial nerve** supplies motor branches to the muscles of the second arch.
- Motor branches of **Glossopharyngeal** supplies stylopharyngeus muscle, and its sensory branches supply the mucous membrane of the pharynx.
- **Vagus nerve** supplies the fourth arch and sixth arch through superior and recurrent laryngeal nerves, respectively. Motor branches of **Superior laryngeal nerve** supplies cricothyroid muscle and sensory branch supplies mucous membrane above vocal cords. Motor branches of **Recurrent laryngeal nerve** supplies rest of the intrinsic muscles of larynx, and sensory branches supply mucous membrane below the vocal cords.

CLINICAL NUGGETS

In addition to the derivatives of the pharyngeal apparatus, structures associated with this apparatus receive innervation from specific cranial nerves:

- **Six extraocular muscles:**
  - Inferior oblique, medial rectus, superior rectus and inferior rectus are innervated by the **Oculomotor nerve**, originating from the mesencephalon.
  - Superior oblique is innervated by the **Trochlear nerve**, originating from the hindbrain.
  - Lateral rectus is innervated by the **Abducens nerve**, originating from the hindbrain.
- **Neck muscles:**
  - The sternocleidomastoid and Trapezius muscles receive innervation from the **Accessory nerve**.
- **Three sensory organs:**
  - The **Olfactory nerve**, originating from the nasal placode in the telencephalon, innervates the olfactory epithelium.
  - The **Optic nerve**, originating from the sensory layer of the optic cup in the diencephalon, innervates the developing retina.
  - The **Vestibulocochlear nerve**, originating from the otic placode in the hindbrain, innervates the developing inner ear.

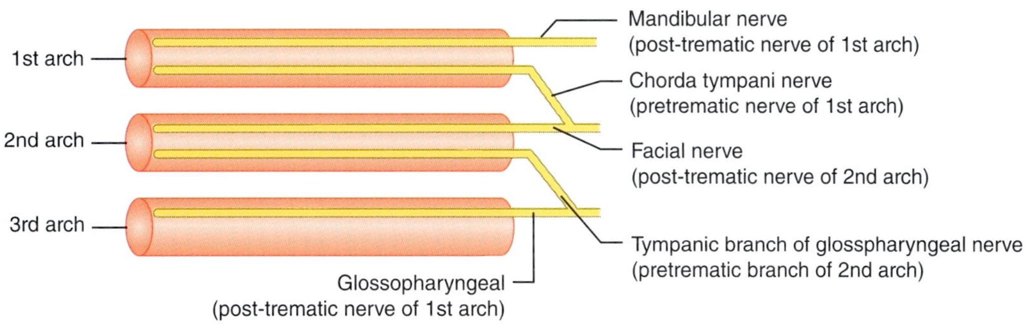

Fig. 14.8 Pretrematic and posttrematic nerves.

DERIVATIVES OF ENDODERM (PHARYNGEAL POUCHES; Table 14.2)

The endoderm lining the primitive pharynx undergoes evagination between adjacent arches, forming pharyngeal pouches. There are five pharyngeal pouches, with the fifth pouch (**Ultimobranchial pouch**) fusing with the fourth pouch immediately upon formation, giving rise to the **Caudal pharyngeal complex**. The distribution of the pouches is as follows: the first pouch lies between the first and second arch, the second pouch between the second and third arch, the third pouch between the third and fourth arch, and the fourth pouch merges with the fifth pouch, situated between the fourth and sixth arches (Fig. 14.9).

1. **First Pouch:**
   - The dorsal part of the first pouch, along with the dorsal part of the second pouch, forms a diverticulum known as the **Tubotympanic recess** (Table 14.2).
   - The **Pharyngotympanic tube** (eustachian/auditory tube) develops from the proximal portion, and the middle ear cavity, including the tympanic/mastoid antrum, develops from the distal part.
2. **Second Pouch:**
   - The ventral part of this pouch forms the **Palatine tonsil**. The remaining part in adults forms the crypta magna/intratonsillar cleft.
   - The dorsal part combines with the first pouch to form the **Tubotympanic recess**.
3. **Third Pouch:**
   - The third pouch elongates to form a dorsal bulbar and ventral tubular portion.
   - The dorsal bulbar part gives rise to the **Inferior parathyroid glands** (parathyroid iii), and the ventral tubular portion contributes to the **Thymus**.
   - As the thymus grows downward, the inferior parathyroid is positioned below the superior parathyroid, even though it develops from a higher pouch. Eventually, the thymus and parathyroid glands lose their connection with the pharynx.
4. **Fourth Pouch:**
   - This pouch contributes to the formation of the **Superior parathyroid glands** (parathyroid iv) and the **Thyroid gland**.
5. **Fifth Pouch (rudimentary):**
   - Also known as the **Ultimobranchial pouch**.
   - This pouch combines with the fourth pouch to form the **Caudal pharyngeal complex**, which gives rise to the **Parafollicular cells** of the thyroid gland (Fig. 14.10).

CLINICAL NUGGETS

Congenital hypoparathyroidism

- This condition results from the failure of the development of one or more parathyroid glands.
- It leads to the secretion of **Parathyroid hormone (PTH) at low levels**.
- Symptoms typically manifest **after 2 years** of age.
- Clinical presentation includes seizures and poor growth.
- Treatment involves the administration of vitamin D and calcium supplements.

Ectopic parathyroid tissue

- Ectopic parathyroid tissue arises due to the failure of the migration of cells from the third pouch. This condition is usually asymptomatic.
- It commonly affects the **Inferior parathyroid gland**.

DERIVATIVES OF ECTODERM (PHARYNGEAL CLEFTS)

The surface ectoderm undergoes invagination between the pharyngeal arches, giving rise to four pharyngeal clefts or grooves. The developmental fate of these clefts includes:

- The dorsal part of the first cleft evolves into the **External acoustic meatus** (Fig. 14.10). The meeting point of first cleft and first pouch is called the **First pharyngeal membrane** which is very thin and consists of three layers from superficial to deep, namely ectoderm mesoderm and endoderm. This three-layered embryonic disc acts as a primordium for the **Tympanic membrane**.
- The ventral portion of the cleft undergoes obliteration.
- The second, third and fourth clefts are obliterated by the overgrowth of the mesenchyme of the **second arch**. Consequently, these three clefts become buried under the surface, forming a slit-like space referred to as the **Cervical sinus**, which is lined by ectoderm. As the neck develops, the cervical sinus also disappear.

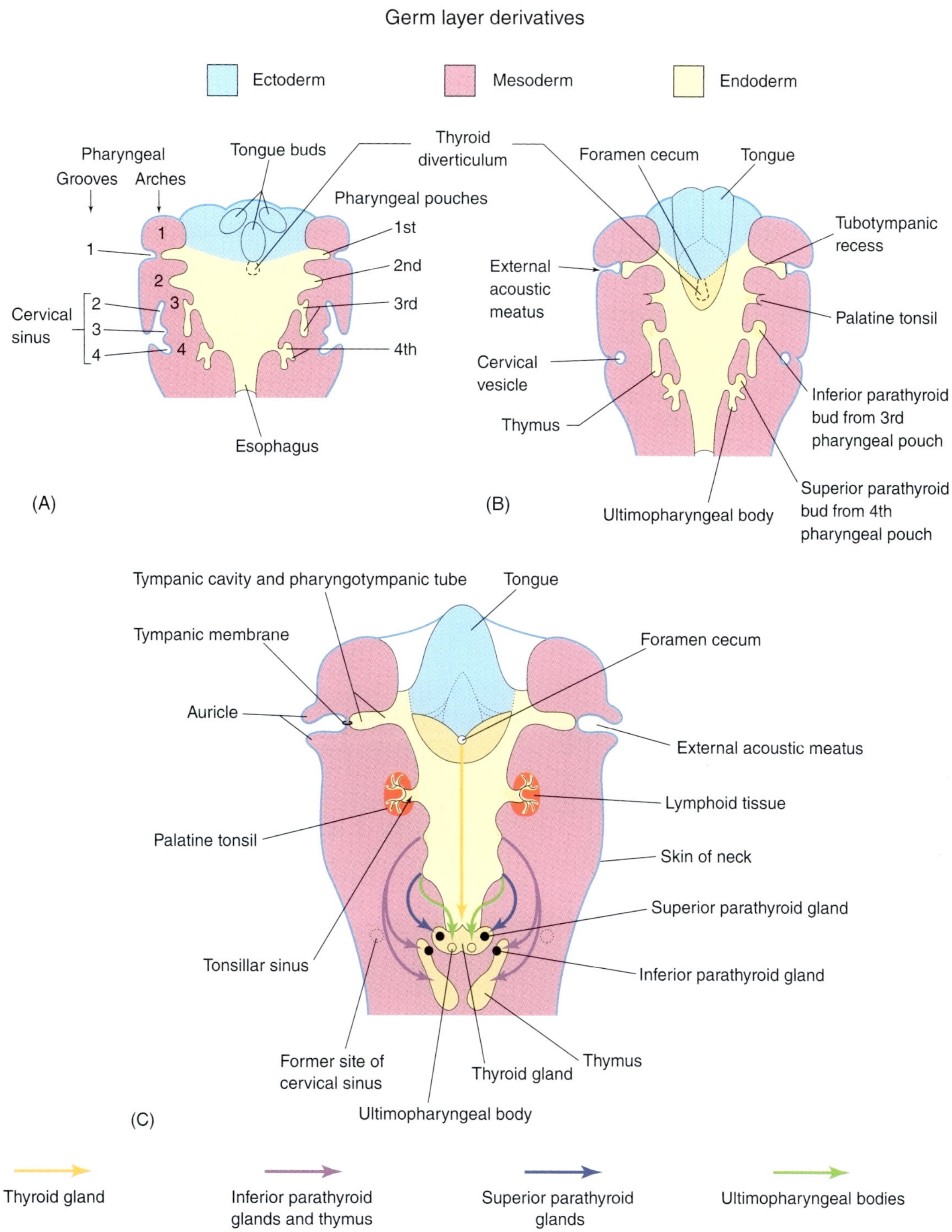

Fig. 14.9 Derivatives of pharyngeal pouches. (A) At 5 weeks, the second arch grows over the third and fourth arches, burying the second to fourth grooves in the cervical sinus. (B) Development at 6 weeks. (C) At 7 weeks, the developing thymus, parathyroid and thyroid glands migrate into the neck (*arrows*). (Source: *The Developing Human: Clinically Oriented Embryology*. 11th ed. 2020.)

Table 14.2 Derivatives of Pharyngeal Pouches

Pouch	Derivatives
1. **First pouch**	• Dorsal part forms **Tubotympanic recess.** • **Pharyngotympanic tube** (eustachian/auditory tube) develops from proximal portion. Middle ear cavity, including tympanic/mastoid antrum, develops from distal part.
2. **Second pouch**	• Ventral part forms **Palatine tonsil**. Remaining part in adults forms crypta magna/intratonsillar cleft. • Dorsal part combines with the first pouch to form **Tubotympanic recess**.
3. **Third pouch**	• Elongates to form dorsal bulbar and ventral tubular portions. • Dorsal bulbar part gives rise to **Inferior parathyroid glands** (parathyroid iii). Ventral tubular portion contributes to the **Thymus**.
4. **Fourth pouch**	• Contributes to the formation of **Superior parathyroid glands (parathyroid iv)** and the **Thyroid gland**.
5. **Fifth pouch (rudimentary)**	• **Ultimobranchial pouch.** Combines with the fourth pouch to form **Caudal pharyngeal complex**. Gives rise to **Parafollicular cells** of the thyroid gland.

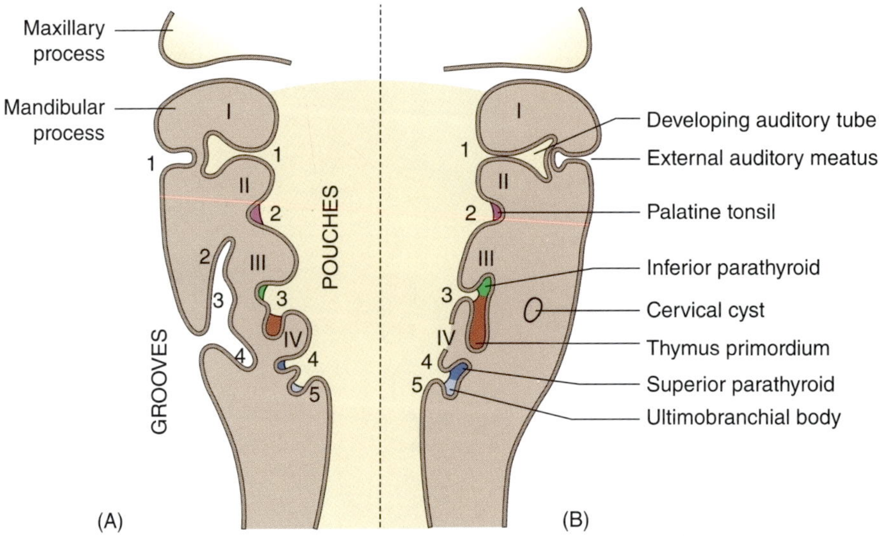

Fig. 14.10 Pharyngeal clefts and pouches.

DEVELOPMENT OF THYROID GLAND (AN 43.4)

- The thyroid gland initiates development during the third week of intrauterine life as an endodermal thickening, forming a diverticulum known as the **Thyroglossal duct** in the pharyngeal floor. The thyroid gland primarily develops from the thyroglossal duct.
- The **Caudal pharyngeal complex**, arising from the fourth and fifth pharyngeal pouches, gives rise to **Parafollicular cells or C-cells** that produce calcitonin in humans.
- Thyroid function begins in the **fourth month** of intrauterine life, with follicular

cells producing thyroxine and triiodothyronine.

FORMATION OF THYROGLOSSAL DUCT

- The medial ends of two mandibular arches are separated by a midline swelling called the **Tuberculum impar**.
- Behind the tuberculum, the endoderm forms a thickening that depresses to create a bilobed diverticulum connected to the tongue through a canal called the thyroglossal duct.
- The site of origin is now seen as a depression called the **Foramen caecum** (Fig. 14.11).

FATE OF THYROGLOSSAL DUCT

- The cranial end, indicated by the foramen caecum, sees the diverticulum growing along the midline into the neck.
- In the neck, it passes in front of the hyoid bone, winds back at the lower border of the hyoid as retrohyoid and then descends below the hyoid with an inclination towards the left.
- The duct's tip becomes a solid mass, bifurcates, and the proliferation of parafollicular and NCC develops them into two lobes of the thyroid gland. NCC migrate into the **Ultimobranchial body (Caudal pharyngeal complex)**, contributing to the parafollicular or C cells. The lobes are connected by the isthmus, lying against the second and third tracheal rings (Fig. 14.12).
- The solid mass of endoderm splits into epithelial cords due to invasion by surrounding mesenchyme. These cords then form clusters with a central lumen, creating **Thyroid follicles**.
- The thyroid gland reaches its final position in front of the trachea by the seventh week.
- The cystic remnant of the thyroglossal duct is known as a **Thyroglossal cyst** (Fig. 14.13).
- When the thyroglossal cyst is connected to the outside by a fistulous canal, it is termed a **Thyroglossal fistula**.
- **Aberrant thyroid tissue** may be observed along the descent path, commonly at the base of the tongue as **Lingual thyroid**.
- The thyroglossal duct may persist, giving rise to an occasional **Pyramidal lobe** (present in 10%–30% of individuals) and the **Levator glandulae thyroideae**, a fibro-muscular band connecting the pyramidal lobe or isthmus to the hyoid bone.

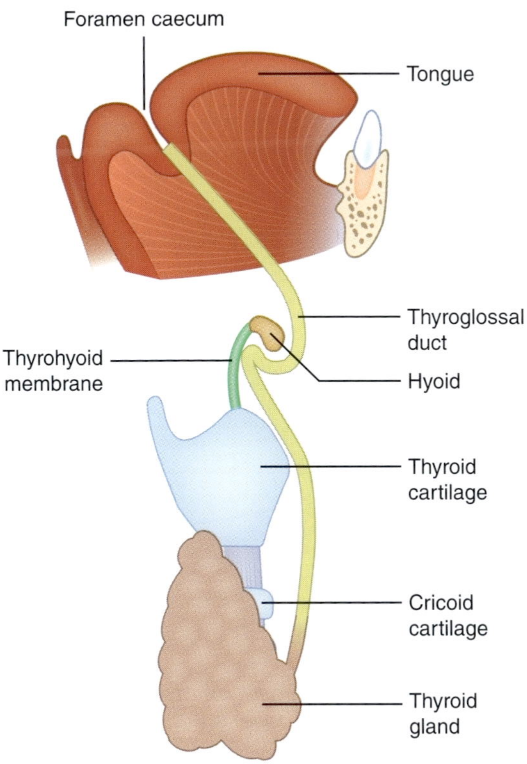

Fig. 14.11 Thyroglossal duct.

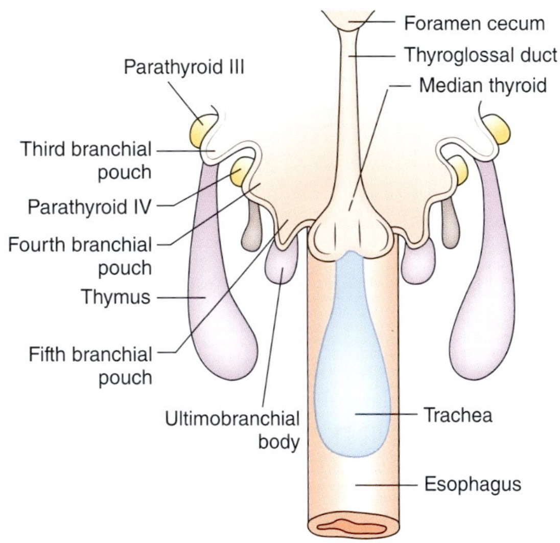

Fig. 14.12 Thyroid gland development.

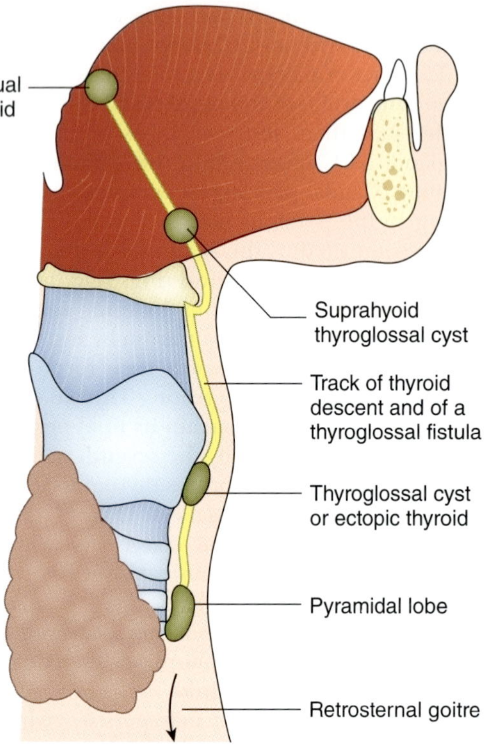

Fig. 14.13 Anomalies of thyroid gland formation.

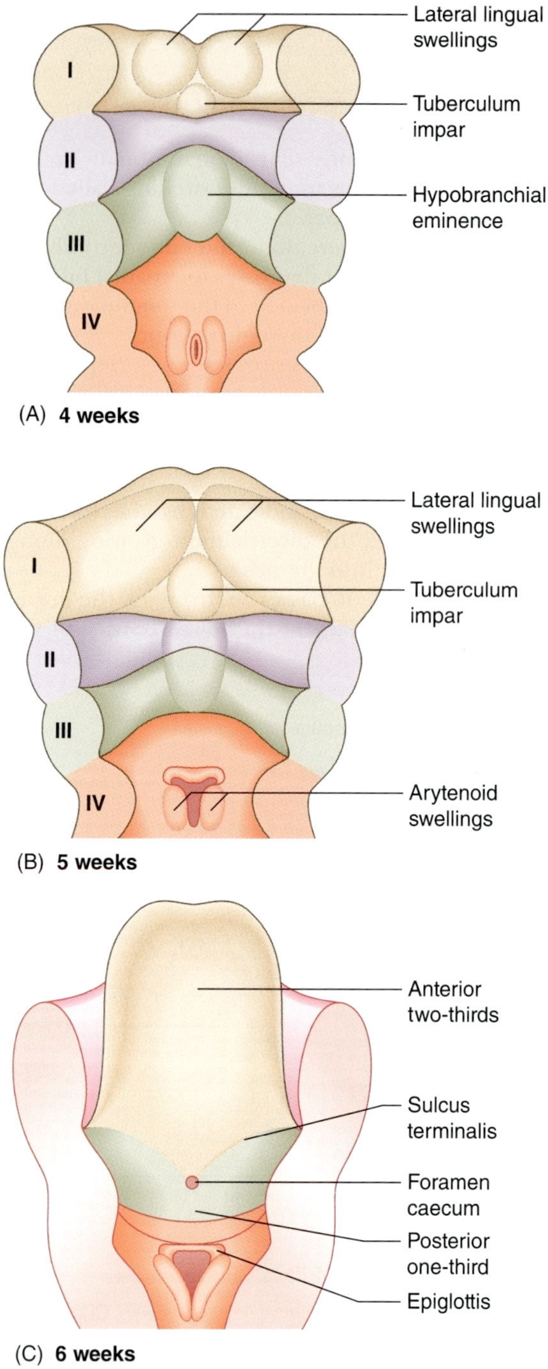

Fig. 14.14 Development of the tongue on the pharyngeal floor at 4 weeks (A), 5 weeks (B), and 6 weeks (C). (Source: *Embryology: An Illustrated Colour Text.* 2nd ed. 2009.)

DEVELOPMENT OF TONGUE (AN 43.4)

- The tongue is anatomically divided into the anterior two-thirds (oral part) and the posterior one-third (pharyngeal part) by the **Sulcus terminalis**.
- Tongue development commences during the fourth month of intrauterine life. The process of development is related to the pharyngeal arches in the floor of the pharynx.

LINGUAL SWELLINGS AND TUBERCULUM IMPAR

- The medial end of the first arch proliferates, forming two lateral lingual swellings (Fig 14.14).
- Lingual swellings are partially separated by a midline swelling called tuberculum impar and the fusion of lingual swellings results in the formation of a **Median sulcus** on the dorsum of the tongue.

HYPOBRANCHIAL EMINENCE

- Another midline swelling, the hypobranchial eminence, develops from the second, third and fourth arches.

REGIONAL DIFFERENTIATION

- The **anterior two-thirds** of the tongue develops from tuberculum impar and lingual swellings.
- The **posterior one-third** of the tongue, including circumvallate papillae, originates from the cranial part of the hypobranchial eminence.
- Mesoderm of the **third arch** grows over the buried mesoderm of the second arch, fusing with the mesoderm of the **first arch** (Fig. 14.15).
- The first arch and third arch lie in close proximity, with their corresponding nerves supplying the dorsum of the tongue.

SULCUS TERMINALIS

- A **V-shaped groove**, known as the sulcus terminalis, distinctly separates the anterior two-thirds of the tongue from the posterior one-third.

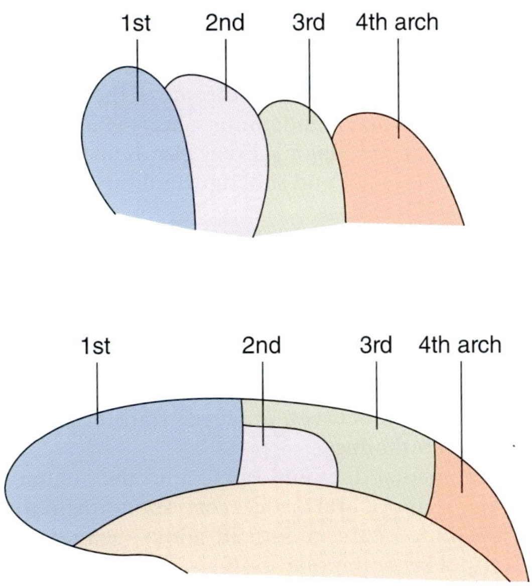

Fig. 14.15 Development of tongue lateral view.

LATE DEVELOPMENTAL STAGES

- The posterior-most part of the tongue and epiglottis develop from the caudal part of the hypobranchial eminence.
- Musculature of the tongue originates from myoblasts of **Occipital myotomes**, migrating to the developing tongue.

ADULT POSITIONING

- Initially, the entire tongue resides in the oral cavity at birth. By approximately 4 years of age, it descends to attain its adult position, with the posterior part of the tongue in the oropharynx forming the anterior wall of the oropharynx.

CORRELATION WITH INNERVATION (TABLE 14.3)

- **Anterior Two-Thirds:** Derived from the first arch, supplied by the **Lingual nerve** (branch of the mandibular nerve), serving as the post-trematic nerve of the first arch.
  Special Sensations: Carried by the **Chorda tympani nerve**, functioning as the pretrematic nerve of this arch (Table 14.3).
- **Posterior One-Third:** Innervated by the **Glossopharyngeal nerve**, the nerve of the third arch, and the posterior-most part by the **Superior laryngeal nerve**, the nerve of the fourth arch.
- **Muscles:** Developed from occipital myotomes and innervated by the **Hypoglossal nerve**.

Table 14.3 Correlation of Development With Innervation

Motor	Sensory
• **Hypoglossal nerve** Occipital myotomes	• **Anterior two-thirds** General-Lingual N Special-Chorda tympani N **(First arch)** • **Posterior one-third (including circumvallate papillae)** General and sensory-Glossopharyngeal N **(Third arch)** • **Posterior most part** General and sensory-Superior laryngeal N **(Fourth arch)**

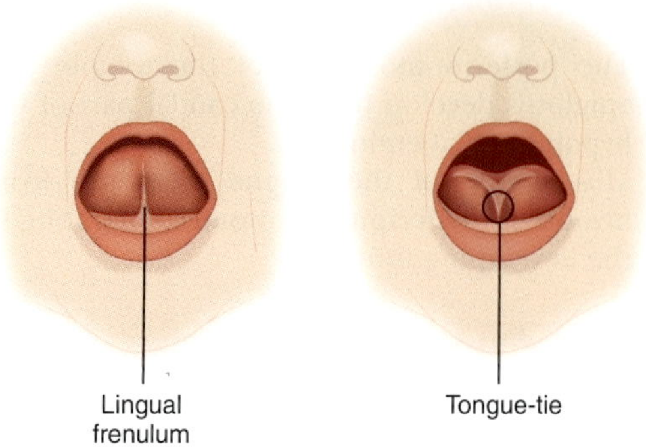

Fig. 14.16 Ankyloglossia.

CLINICAL NUGGETS

Ankyloglossia (tongue-tie)

- Most common malformation of the tongue (Fig. 14.16).
- Caused by the failure of the normal regression of the **Frenulum**, resulting in restricted movements of the tongue. The frenulum extends up to the tip of the tongue.
- Leads to difficulty in articulation for speech and tongue protrusion.

Macroglossia

- Hyperplasia of lingual tissue, characterized by an unusually **large tongue**.

Microglossia

- Hypoplasia of lingual tissue, characterized by a **small tongue**.

Bifid tongue

- Failure of fusion of **lingual swellings** results in the splitting of the tongue into two parts.

Fissured tongue

- A characteristic feature of **Down syndrome** where lingual papillae get hypertrophied, and the surface of the tongue appears fissured.

DEVELOPMENT OF SALIVARY GLANDS

Salivary glands develop as outgrowths of buccal epithelium near the junction of the ectoderm of the stomodeum and endoderm of the foregut. The development involves the following steps (Fig. 14.17):

- **Epithelial Cord Formation:**
  - Outgrowths invade the surrounding mesenchyme, forming epithelial cords of cells.

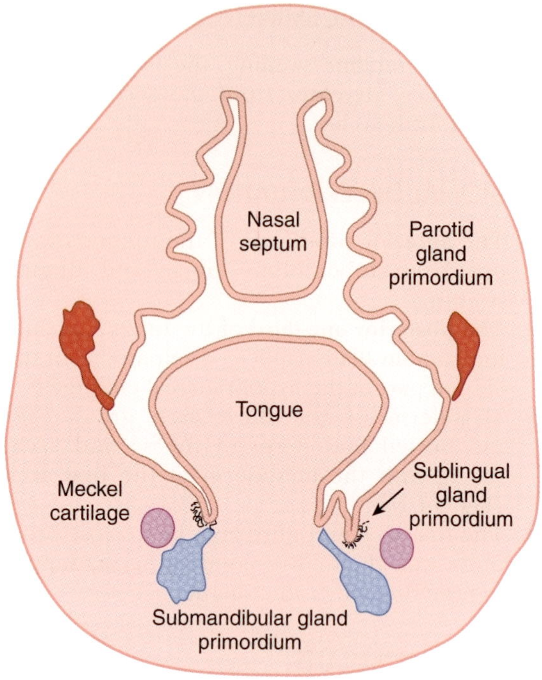

Fig. 14.17 Salivary glands development.

- **Acini and Duct Formation:**
  - Terminal ends of cords differentiate into secretory acini, while the remaining part canalizes to form the ducts of the gland.
- **Connective Tissue and Capsule:**
  - Surrounding mesenchyme contributes to the connective tissue and capsule of the glands.
- There are major and minor salivary glands. The three pairs of **Major salivary glands** are parotid submandibular and sublingual salivary glands.

PAROTID GLAND

- Arises as an **Ectodermal outgrowth** where maxillary and mandibular processes fuse to form the cheek around the fifth week of intrauterine life (IUL).
- The furrow between processes transforms into the **Parotid duct**.
- The medial duct end opens into the angle of the primitive oral orifice, corresponding to the vestibule of the mouth in adults, against the upper second molar tooth.
- Ectodermal cells at the lateral end proliferate into surrounding mesoderm, forming **epithelial cords**.

- These cords canalize to create ducts and acini within the gland.

SUBMANDIBULAR GLAND

- Develops as an **Endodermal outgrowth** during the sixth week from the floor of the oral cavity (linguogingival sulcus), lateral to the developing tongue.
- The linear furrow on the surface fuses, forming the **Submandibular duct**, which opens onto the sublingual papilla.

SUBLINGUAL GLANDS

- Arise in relation to the linguogingival sulcus, emerging 2 weeks later than other glands (eighth week).
- Develop as **Endodermal outgrowths** that later canalize, opening at the summit of the sublingual fold.

MINOR SALIVARY GLANDS

- Distributed throughout the oral cavity except the gingivae.
- Develop similarly to major salivary glands, opening on the surface with minimal branching.

CLINICAL NUGGETS

Branchiootorenal (BOR) syndrome (Fig. 14.18)

- Autosomal dominant disorder with varied clinical manifestations.
- **Branchial arch anomalies**
  - Includes abnormalities such as branchial clefts, fistulae and cysts.
- **Anomalies of the ear**
  - Malformation of the auricle.
  - Presence of **Preauricular sinuses**.
  - Hearing impairment can be conductive, sensorineural or mixed.
- **Renal malformations**
  - Urinary tract malformation.
  - Renal hypoplasia or agenesis.
  - Formation of renal cysts.

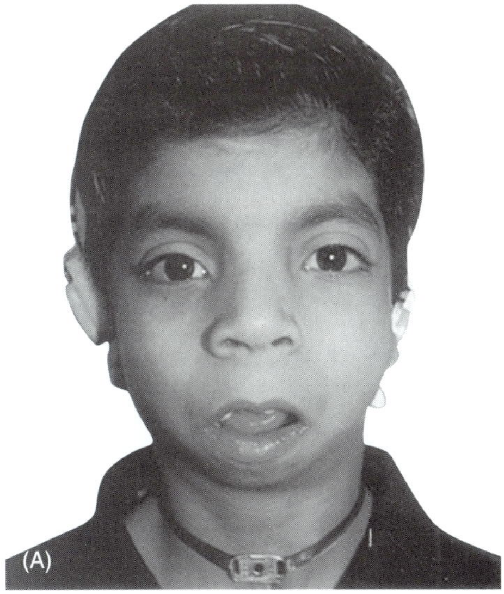

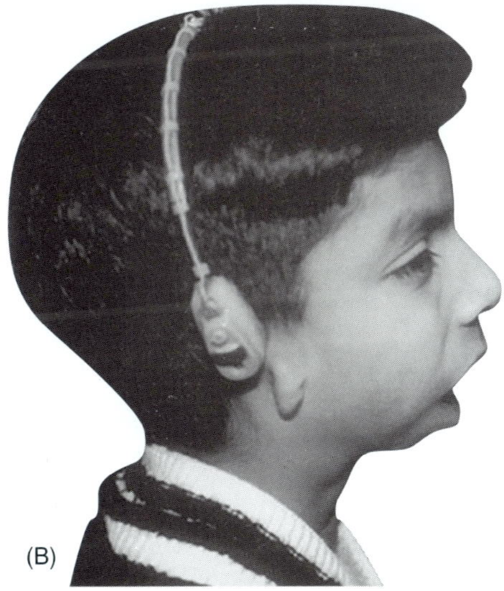

Fig. 14.18 Branchiootorenal syndrome. (Source: *Smith's Recognizable Patterns of Human Deformation*, 5th ed.: Pedro A. Sanchez-Lara, John M. Graham Jr.: Fig. 23.4, Elsevier Inc. 2024.)

KLINISCHE PERLEN (AN 43.4)

BRANCHIAL FISTULA

- Occurs when the **Second pharyngeal arch** fails to grow caudally. Results in the persistence of the second, third and fourth clefts, making contact with the surface (Fig. 14.19).
- Persistence of the cervical sinus, which may rupture onto the surface, can also result in a **Fistula** (Fig. 14.20).
- Two types:
  - **External branchial fistula** (lateral cervical cyst in front of sternocleidomastoid at the

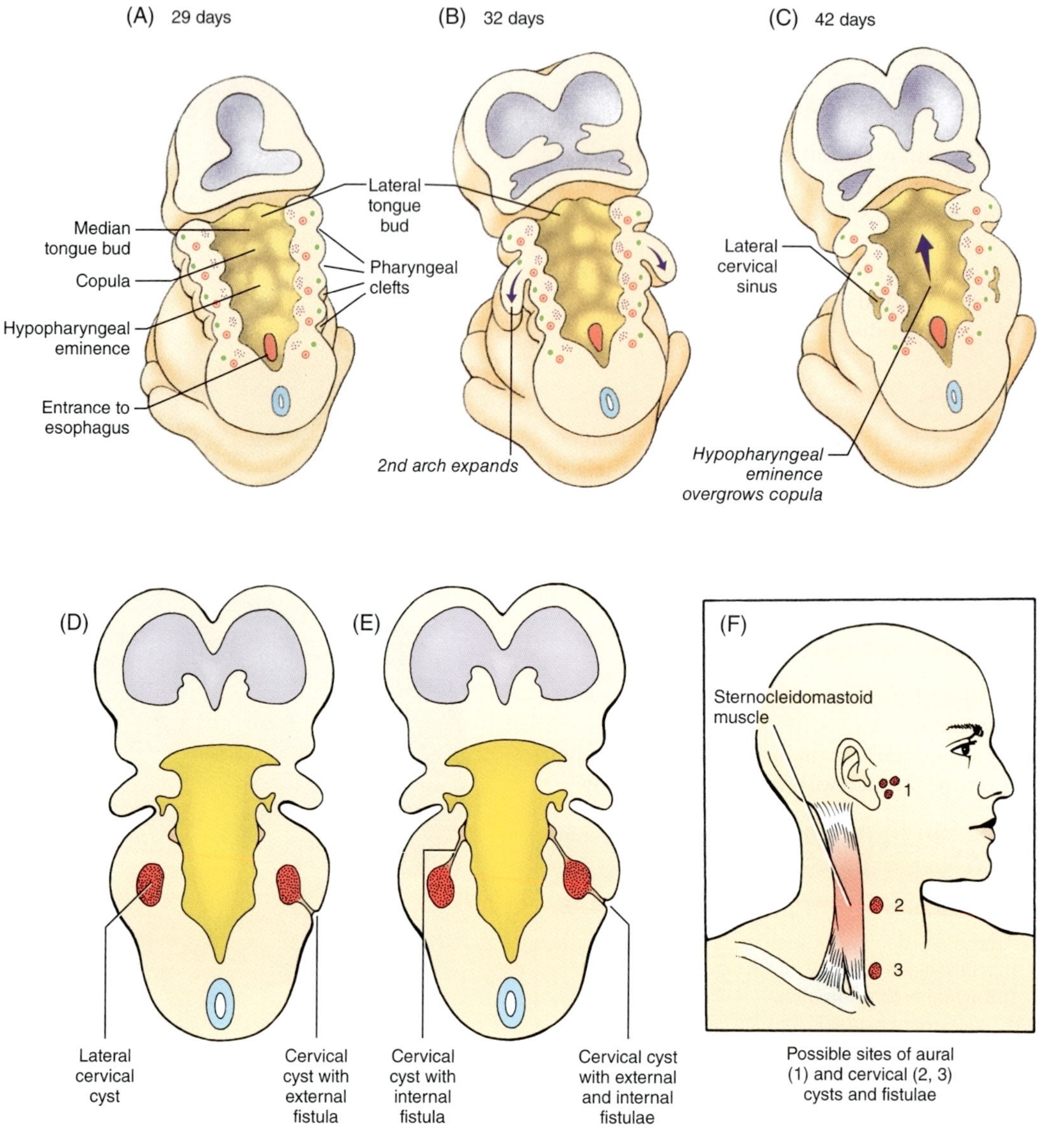

Fig. 14.19 Normal and abnormal fates of the pharyngeal clefts. (A–C) Three stages in normal development. The first pharyngeal cleft forms the external auditory meatus. The second pharyngeal arch expands and fuses with the cardiac eminence to cover the remaining pharyngeal clefts, which form the transient lateral cervical sinus. (D–F) Formation of cysts. (D and E) Sections through the pharynx and pharyngeal arches show that cervical cysts may be isolated or may connect to the skin of the neck by an external cervical fistula, or to the pharynx by an internal fistula, or both. (F) Lateral cervical cysts (2, 3) are located just medial to the anterior border of the sternocleidomastoid muscle. Anomalous derivatives of the first pharyngeal cleft, known as aural (or preauricular) cysts, may form anterior to the ear (1). (Source: *Larsen's Human Embryology*. 5th ed. 2014.)

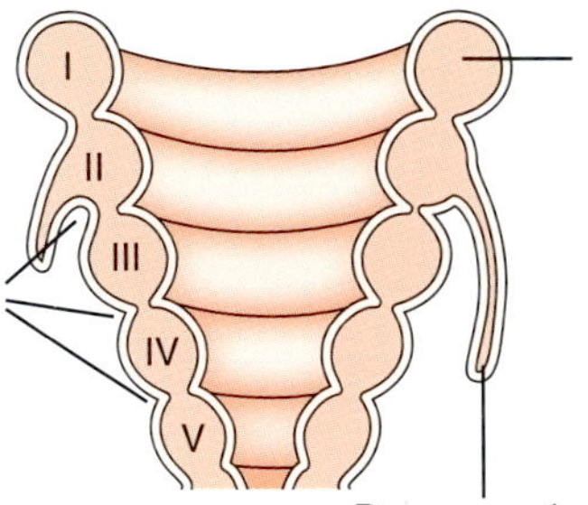

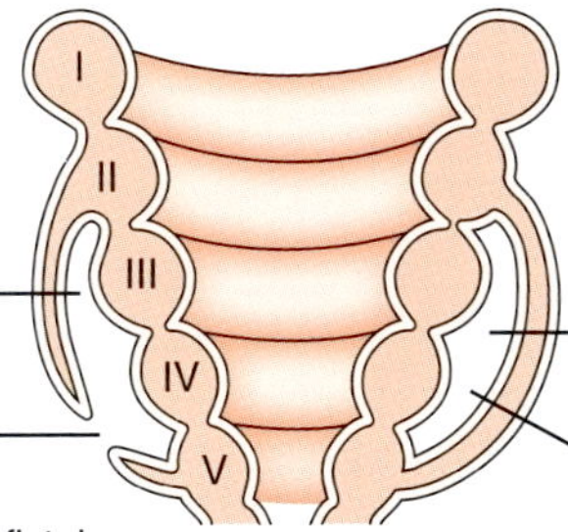

Fig. 14.20 Brachial cyst and fistula schematic diagram.

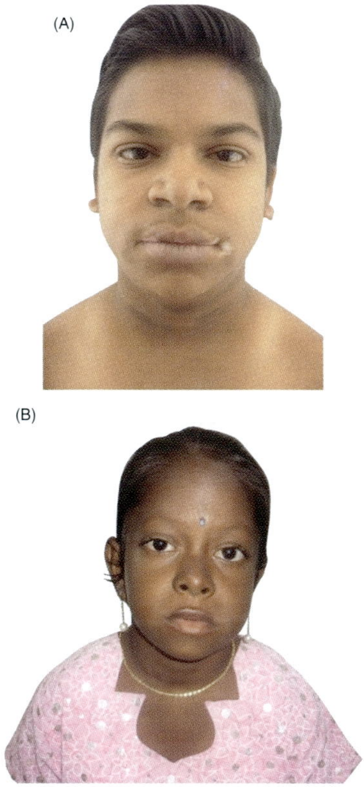

Fig. 14.21 Congenital hypothyroidism. (A) 25-year-old male with puffy dull face, hypopigmentation and periorbital oedema. (B) 32-year-old female with retarded growth. (Photo courtesy: Dr Suja.)

junction of upper one-third and lower two-thirds).

- **Internal branchial fistula** (cervical sinus opens in the tonsillar region).

CONGENITAL HYPOTHYROIDISM

- A condition of thyroid hormone deficiency present at birth (Fig. 14.21).
- If untreated for several months after birth, it can lead to growth failure and permanent intellectual disability.

THYROGLOSSAL CYST

- Cystic remnant of the thyroglossal duct.
- **Thyroglossal fistula:** A cyst opening to the exterior.

LINGUAL THYROID

- A specific type of ectopic thyroid resulting from the lack of normal caudal migration of the thyroid gland (Fig. 14.22).

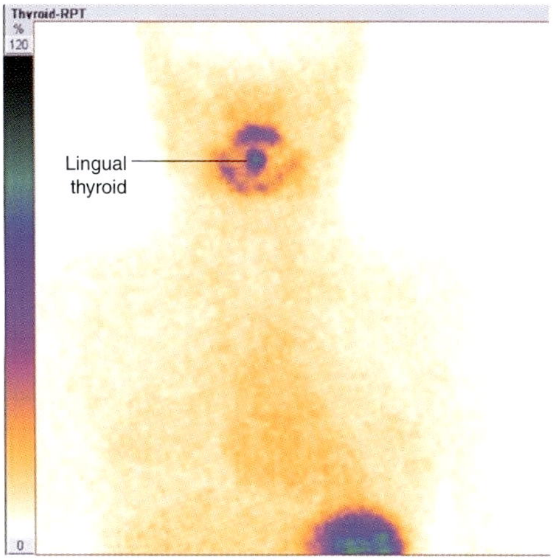

Fig. 14.22 Thyroid scan showing lingual thyroid. (Photo courtesy: Dr Suja.)

FIRST ARCH SYNDROMES

Sometimes the **NCC** fail to migrate into the first pharyngeal arch and result in facial anomalies known as **First arch syndromes**.

1. **Treacher Collins Syndrome (Mandibulofacial Dysostosis):**
   - **Autosomal dominant.**
   - Involves the nucleolar protein **Treacle**.
   - Features include malar (zygomatic) hypoplasia, mandibular hypoplasia, lower eyelid coloboma, malformed external ear and down-slanting palpebral fissures.
2. **Pierre Robin Sequence:**
   - **Autosomal recessive** disorder.
   - Triad of micrognathia, cleft palate and a posteriorly placed tongue.
3. **DiGeorge Syndrome:**
   - Microdeletion of the long arm of **chromosome 22**.
   - Features include absent thymus and parathyroid glands, fish mouth deformity, low-set ears.

GOLDENHAR SYNDROME (OCULOAURICULOVERTEBRAL SPECTRUM)

- Involves ocular tumours, auricular microtia and vertebral anomalies, such as spina bifida and hemivertebrae.

POINTS TO PONDER

- In humans, a total of six pairs of pharyngeal arches (branchial arches) develop on either side of the pharyngeal foregut.
- The fifth arch regresses, and the remaining arches are numbered 1, 2, 3, 4 and 6.
- Each arch consists of outer ectoderm, inner endoderm and a core of mesenchyme derived from paraxial, lateral plate mesoderm and neural crest cells (NCC).
- **Components** of each arch include:
  - **A Cartilaginous element.**
  - **An Aortic arch artery.**
  - **Cranial nerve (V, VII, IX and X).**
- Ectodermal clefts separate the pharyngeal arches externally, while endodermal pouches separate them internally.
- Skeletal elements originate from NCC, while muscles and endothelial cells are derived from the mesoderm.

BRAIN TEASERS

1. What is the fate of the dorsal part of the first pharyngeal cleft?
   A. Develops into the external acoustic meatus
   B. Forms the palatine tonsil
   C. Obliterated
   D. Connects to the tongue through a canal
2. Which nerve supplies the muscles derived from the first pharyngeal arch?
   A. Oculomotor nerve
   B. Trochlear nerve
   C. Abducens nerve
   D. Mandibular nerve
3. What is the primary function of the accessory nerve in the pharyngeal region?
   A. Innervates sternocleidomastoid
   B. Innervates trapezius
   C. Innervates the olfactory epithelium
   D. Innervates the developing inner ear
4. Which nerve is associated with lingual swelling in the development of the tongue?
   A. Lingual nerve
   B. Oculomotor nerve
   C. Glossopharyngeal nerve
   D. Trochlear nerve
5. What structures arise from the tubotympanic recess?
   A. External acoustic meatus
   B. Middle ear cavity
   C. Palatine tonsil
   D. Inferior parathyroid glands
6. Which clinical condition is associated with failure of migration of the cells of the third pharyngeal pouch?
   A. Lingual thyroid
   B. Thyroglossal cyst
   C. Thyroglossal fistula
   D. Ectopic parathyroid tissue
7. Which structure is a remnant of the thyroglossal duct and may be present in 10%–30% of individuals?
   A. Thyroglossal fistula
   B. Lingual thyroid
   C. Pyramidal lobe
   D. Aberrant thyroid
8. What is the embryonic origin of the anterior two-thirds of the tongue?
   A. First pharyngeal arch
   B. Second pharyngeal arch
   C. Third pharyngeal arch
   D. Fourth pharyngeal arch
9. In the development of the tongue, what is the role of the hypobranchial eminence?
   A. Forms lingual swellings

   B. Develops the posterior one-third of the tongue
   C. Separates lingual swellings
   D. Innervates the tongue muscles
10. Which nerve supplies the posterior one-third of the tongue?
   A. Lingual nerve
   B. Trochlear nerve
   C. Glossopharyngeal nerve
   D. Hypoglossal nerve
11. What is the main function of the chorda tympani nerve in tongue development?
   A. Innervates sternocleidomastoid
   B. Innervates trapezius
   C. Carries special sensations
   D. Innervates the olfactory epithelium
12. At what stage does the thyroid gland start functioning during intrauterine life?
   A. Second month
   B. Fourth month
   C. Sixth month
   D. Eighth month

Answers

1. (A); 2. (D); 3. (A); 4. (A); 5. (B); 6. (D); 7. (C); 8. (A); 9. (B); 10. (C); 11. (C); 12. (B).

FURTHER READINGS

Li Y, Mashhood A, Mamlouk MD, Lindan CE, Feldstein VA, Glenn OA. Prenatal Diagnosis of Third and Fourth Branchial Apparatus Anomalies: Case Series and Comparison with Lymphatic Malformation. *AJNR Am J Neuroradiol.* 2021;42(11):2094-2100. doi:10.3174/ajnr.A7293.

Stefanicka P, Profant M. Branchial cleft cyst and branchial cleft cyst carcinoma, or cystic lymph node and cystic nodal metastasis? *J Laryngol Otol.* 2023;137(1):31-36. doi:10.1017/S0022215122001293.

Vrînceanu D, Sajin M, Dumitru M, Mogoantă CA, Cergan R, Georgescu MG. Current approach to branchial remnants in the neck. *Rom J Morphol Embryol.* 2022;63(3):485-490. doi:10.47162/RJME.63.3.02.

Alarfaj AA. Coexistence of thyroglossal duct cyst and second branchial cleft cyst in a young woman: A case report and literature review. *Int J Surg Case Rep.* 2022 Jun;95:107192. doi:10.1016/j.ijscr.2022.107192.

Ortiz WJ, Ahumada EC, Paz-Moreno OL, McKowen RL, Cervantes M. Posterior mediastinal mass: an uncommon presentation of a branchial cleft cyst. *Cureus.* 2022:31;14(10):e30924. doi:10.7759/cureus.30924.

SECTION 3

SYSTEMIC EMBRYOLOGY

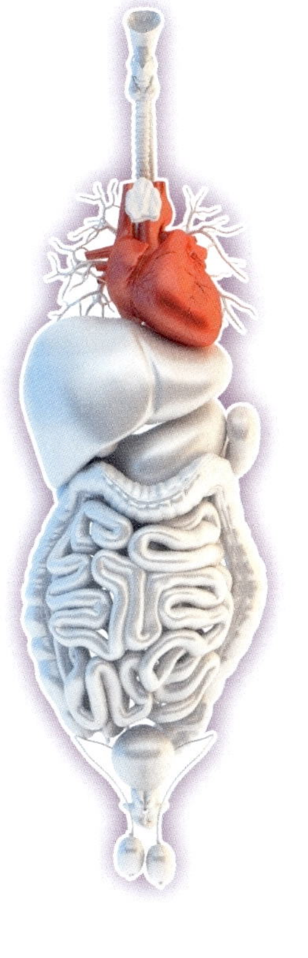

Cardiovascular System 15

AN 25.2 Describe development of heart.
AN 25.3 Describe foetal circulation and changes occurring at birth.
AN 25.4 Describe embryological basis of atrial septal defect.
AN 25.4 Describe embryological basis of ventricular septal defect.
AN 25.4 Describe embryological basis of Fallot's tetralogy.
AN 25.5 Describe developmental basis of coarctation of aorta.
AN 25.5 Describe developmental basis of transposition of great vessels.
AN 25.5 Describe developmental basis of dextrocardia.
AN 25.5 Describe developmental basis of patent ductus arteriosus.
AN 25.6 Mention development of SVC.
AN 25.6 Mention development of IVC.
AN 25.6 Mention development of coronary sinus.
AN 25.6 Mention development of aortic arch arteries.

ANAMNESE

A 3-year-old female presented with complaints of persistent respiratory distress and inadequate weight gain, prompting her parents to seek medical attention. The child's medical history revealed an uneventful birth and normal antenatal ultrasounds. Clinical examination disclosed a continuous machinery-like murmur and bounding pulses in the femoral arteries. Further investigations, including an echocardiogram and chest X-ray, confirmed the diagnosis of Patent ductus arteriosus (PDA). The persistent opening between the Pulmonary artery and Aorta was causing increased blood flow to the lungs, contributing to the respiratory difficulties (Fig. 15.1).

The first cardiac contractions start at the straight tube stage approximately **22 days** in humans and the blood begin to circulate throughout the embryo by **24th day**. The first heart beats are irregular and do not propel blood through the circulation. It quickly becomes coordinated and primitive blood starts to circulate through the embryo, thus enabling its further growth. The postnatal period differs from childhood, as there is a time-window during which cardiomyocytes are still capable of proliferation. In humans, it lasts to about 6 months, and surgical interventions, such as biventricular repair for hypoplastic left heart syndrome, are most successful during this window. The cardiovascular system is the major system to function in an embryo.

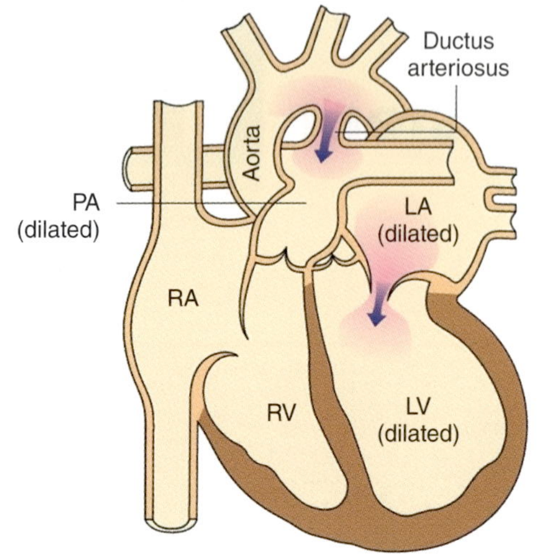

Fig. 15.1 Patent ductus arteriosus. (Source: Davidson's Principles & Practice of Medicine. 22nd ed. Edinburgh: Churchill Livingstone; 2014 [Fig. 18.96/pp. 631].)

EARLY NUTRITION TO THE EMBRYO

Prior to the establishment of the cardiovascular system, the embryo receives nutrition through distinct phases:

- At the **Morula** stage: from the cytoplasm of the ovum.
- At the **Blastocyst** stage: via secretions from the uterine glands.
- During **Implantation**: through diffusion from the maternal blood within the lacunar spaces.
- In subsequent stages (post-third week): through the **Placenta**.
- Continued nourishment of the embryo involves the participation of two categories of vessels:
  - **Extraembryonic vessels.**
  - **Intraembryonic vessels.**

EXTRAEMBRYONIC VESSELS

By third week of development, the mesenchyme of yolk sac, connecting stalk and chorion differentiate to form the angioblasts, which ultimately give rise to the extraembryonic blood vessels and blood cells.

- The vessels arising in the extraembryonic mesoderm are of two types (Fig. 15.2):

  A) **Vitelline vessels:**
  - Formed from the capillary plexus in the wall of the **Yolk sac**.

  B) **Umbilical vessels:**
  - Formed in the **Chorion** and **Connecting stalk**.

INTRAEMBRYONIC VESSELS

The intraembryonic blood cells and blood vessels are formed from the angioblasts of the intraembryonic mesoderm.

- The intraembryonic vessels establish secondary connections with the extraembryonic vessels.
- The two longitudinal intraembryonic vessels known as the **dorsal aortae** arise on each side of the notochord.
- In the cardiogenic area, the dorsal aortae become continuous with the **endothelial heart tubes** from which the heart is formed.
- At the caudal end, the dorsal aortae extend into the connecting stalk as the **umbilical arteries** which divides into capillaries of the chorionic villi.
- The returning venules from the chorion form two **umbilical veins**.
- The lateral branches of the dorsal aorta form a **plexus** in the wall of the yolk sac.
- Two **vitelline veins** arise from this plexus and along with **umbilical veins** join the venous end of the endothelial tubes of primitive heart.
- The veins of the body wall, that is the **cardinal veins**, also join the venous end of the primitive heart.
- The **oxygenation** status of veins (Fig. 15.2).
  - **Vitelline veins**: poorly oxygenated blood from **umbilical vesicle**.
  - **Umbilical veins**: well-oxygenated blood from the **chorion**.
  - **Common cardinal veins**: poorly oxygenated blood from the **body** of the embryo.

THE DEFINITIVE HEART (AN 25.2)

- As a result of the cephalic and lateral folding of the embryo, the two paramedian endothelial tubes are brought closer in the thoracic region and they fuse in the craniocaudal direction to form a single **Primitive heart tube** (Fig. 15.3). (The primitive heart is separated from the ventral wall of foregut by the **myoepicardial mantle**. The developing myocardium secretes **cardiac jelly**

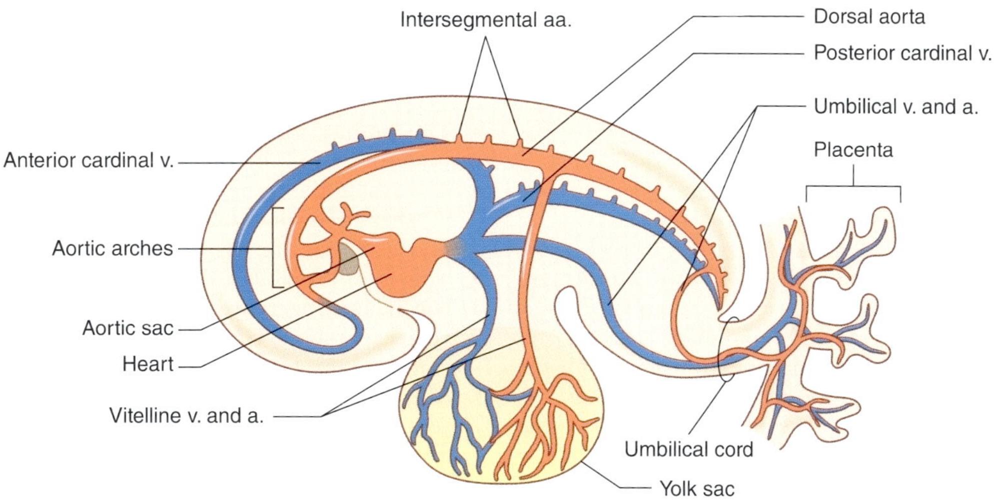

Fig 15.2 Vitelline and umbilical vessels.

which is seen between the myoepicardial mantle and the heart tube. Later this jelly is replaced by the myocardium formed from the myoepicardial mantle. It is also believed that the myoepicardial mantle gives rise to epicardium as well.)

- Three layers of heart:
  - **Endocardium:** from the endothelial tube.
  - **Myocardium:** from the primordial myocardium derived from **splanchnic mesoderm** surrounding the pericardial coelom.
  - **Epicardium:** mesothelial cells arising from the surface of sinus venosus.
- After the folding, **the heart** and **the pericardial cavity** lie ventral to the foregut and caudal to buccopharyngeal membrane. As a result, the cardiogenic area is bounded by the pericardial sac ventrally, by the foregut dorsally, by the stomodeum and buccopharyngeal membrane at the cephalic side and by the septum transversum at the caudal end.
- The **cranial** end of the primitive heart is the **arterial end** and is called **bulbus cordis.** This end forms the **first pair of aortic arch** which pass along the sides of the pharynx to become continuous with the dorsal aortae. Later **five** more pairs of aortic arches develop connecting the cranial end of the primitive heart tube with the dorsal aortae.
- The caudal end is the venous end and is called **Sinus venosus**. It is embedded in the septum transversum and has right and left horns.

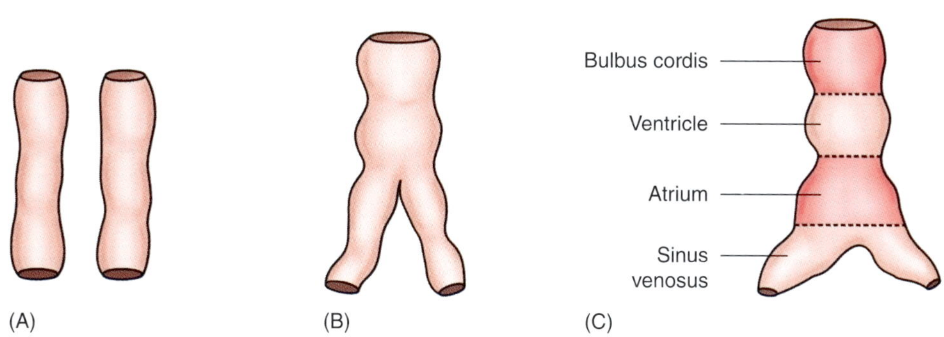

Fig. 15.3 Formation of primitive heart tube.

- Thus, the heart tube presents four dilatations craniocaudally as follows:
  - **Bulbus cordis.**
  - **Primitive ventricle.**
  - **Primitive atrium.**
  - **Sinus venosus.**
- The first constriction is seen between the bulbus cordis and the primitive ventricle.
- The **bulbus cordis** is further subdivided into:
  - **Truncus arteriosus**—which is continuous cranially with the aortic sac and form the roots of aorta and pulmonary arteries. This end bifurcates and get connected with the dorsal aortae through six aortic arches.
  - **Conus cordis**—the mid portion forms the outflow tract of both ventricles.
  - **Proximal portion**—which forms the trabeculated inflow part of right ventricle.
- **Bulboventricular sulcus** indicates the junction between ventricle and bulbus cordis. This forms the interventricular foramen.
- The trabeculated primitive ventricle forms the **primitive left ventricle**.
- So, the **right ventricle** is formed from the bulbus cordis and **left ventricle** from primitive ventricle.
- The primitive heart starts beating on **22nd** day and circulation of blood throughout the embryo on **24th** day.

FORMATION OF THE BULBOVENTRICULAR LOOP

- The bulbus cordis and ventricle grow faster than the rest of the regions.
- As a result, the heart bends on itself forming a **'U'-shaped cardiac loop** and bulges into the pericardial sac which is lying ventrally (Fig. 15.4).
- This loop is mainly contributed by **the bulbus cordis** and the **ventricle**, hence called **bulboventricular loop**. The cardiac loop formation is completed by fourth week of intrauterine life.
- After the formation of loop, the atrium and sinus venosus lie dorsal to bulbus cordis and ventricle. The sinus venosus after folding possess two horns, roof, floor and a dorsal wall.
- The sinus venosus ventrally communicates with the primitive atrium. This loop is suspended from the dorsal wall of pericardial cavity by a mesentery, the **dorsal mesocardium**.
- The central part of the mesocardium later degenerates forming the **transverse pericardial sinus** which communicates between the right and left pericardial cavities and lies between the arterial and venous ends of the cardiac loop.
- Meanwhile the **pleuropericardial canals** are closed and the cells from the upper part of

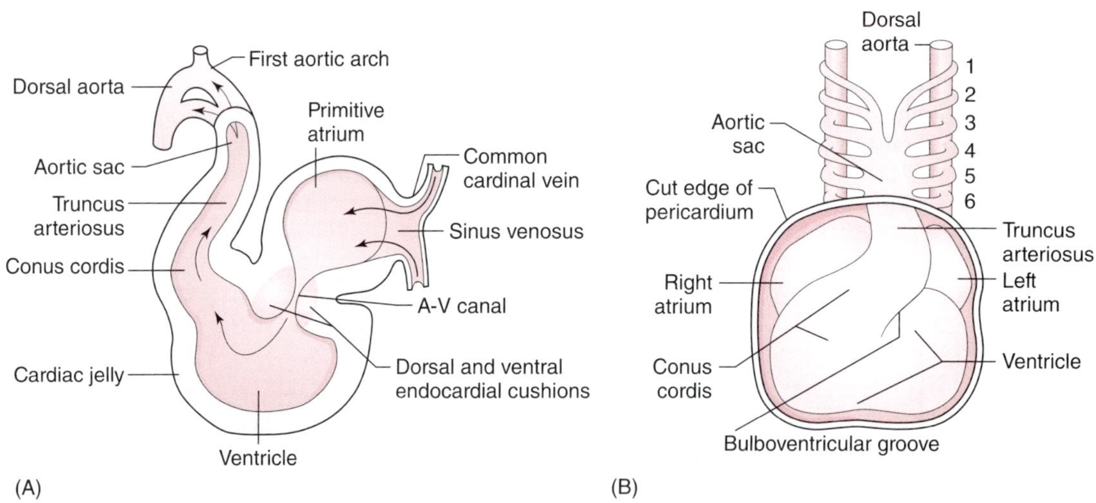

Fig. 15.4 Formation of bulboventricular loop. (A) Blood flow through the primordial heart (week 4). (B) Ventral view of the heart and aortic arches (week 5). Not all aortic arches are present at the same time. The heart tube forms the bulboventricular loop consisting of five dilatations: sinus venosus, primitive atrium, ventricle, conus cordis and truncus arteriosus. All except sinus venosus are subsequently partitioned. *Arrows*, blood flow. *Numbers*, aortic arches. (Source: *Rapid Review Gross and Developmental Anatomy*. 3rd ed. 2011.)

septum transversum forms the fibrous pericardium over the pericardial sac. The **parietal** layer of serous pericardium is formed from somatopleuric layer of the pericardial sac and the **visceral** layer of serous pericardium is formed from the myoepicardial mantle.

THE PRIMORDIAL HEART

- Blood enters the sinus venosus through common cardinal veins, umbilical veins and vitelline veins and then to the primordial atrium through **Sinoatrial (SA) valves**.
- Then the blood reaches the primordial ventricle through the **Atrioventricular canal**.
- From the ventricle, blood is pumped into the aortic sac through bulbus cordis.
- The dorsal aorta then carries the blood to the embryo, umbilical vesicle and placenta.
- The specification of structures in the cardiac tube is by the **Retinoic** the **acid (RA)** produced by the mesoderm. Hence, RA can produce a variety of cardiac defect.
- The septations of the chambers of the definitive heart is completed by eighth week of intrauterine life.

CHANGES IN THE HEART TUBE

- Changes in the heart tube are discussed under the following headings (Fig. 15.5):
  A) **Sinus venosus.**
  B) **Primitive atrium.**
  C) **Primitive ventricle.**
  D) **Bulbus cordis.**

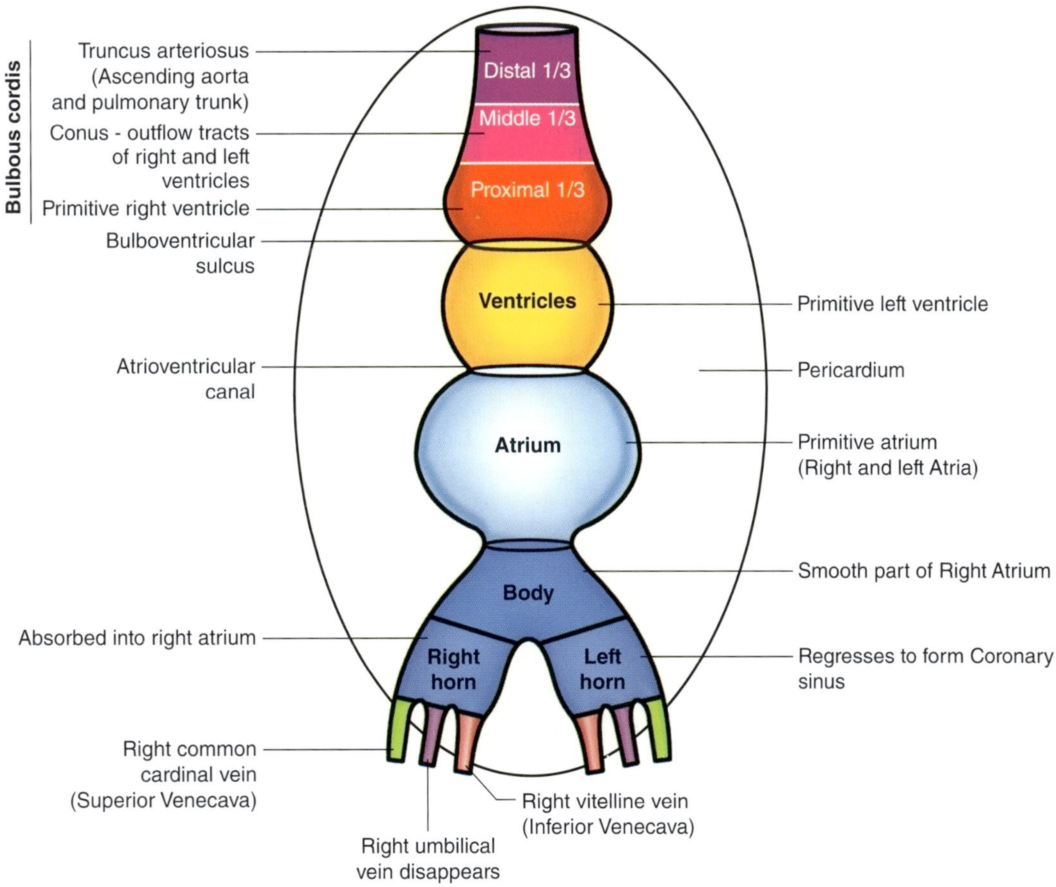

Fig. 15.5 Derivatives of heart tube.

SINUS VENOSUS (AN 25.6)

- The sinus venosus after folding possess two horns, roof, floor and a dorsal wall. The sinus venosus ventrally communicates with the primitive atrium through the sinoatrial orifice. Sinoatrial fold which arises from the left side of the orifice shifts the orifice to the right side of the primitive atrium. Right and left sinus valves guard the sinoatrial opening. Apart from the two horns, the sinus venosus thus possess a body as well and the blood from sinus venosus reach the right half of primitive atrium because of the shift of the sinoatrial orifice to the right side.
- Sinus venosus receives venous blood from right and left sinus horns:
- **Three pairs** of veins (one parietal/somatic and two visceral) join sinus venosus.
  1) The **Vitelline** (omphalomesenteric) veins from umbilical vesicle enters the floor of sinus venosus.
  2) The **Umbilical** veins from chorion enters the floor of sinus venosus lateral to the vitelline veins.
  3) The **Common cardinal veins (duct of Cuvier)** from body of the embryo which is formed by the union of anterior and posterior cardinal veins draining the cranial and caudal parts of the body wall, respectively. The common cardinal veins join the horn of sinus venosus.
- With the formation of the **hepatic bud** in the septum transversum, the right and left umbilical veins above the hepatic bud (suprahepatic) and the left vitelline vein disappears.
- The suprahepatic part of **right vitelline** persists as the common hepatic vein and forms **inferior vena cava (terminal portion)**. The **caudal** part of left umbilical vein forms umbilical vein proper.
- Umbilical vein is connected to the inferior vena cava (IVC) through **Ductus venosus (DV)**. Thus, DV shunts oxygenated blood directly to the heart from umbilical vein bypassing the liver.
- The right and left anterior cardinal veins make an oblique communication so that the blood from the cranial end of the left side of the body reaches the right horn of sinus venosus.
- The **left brachiocephalic (innominate) vein** is thus formed by the anastomoses of anterior cardinal veins, and the left anterior cardinal vein distal to the anastomoses obliterates to form the **ligament of left vena cava** (Fig. 15.6).
- The **Superior vena cava** is formed from (Fig. 15.7):
  - **Right anterior cardinal vein** (caudal/extrapericardial part).
  - **Right common cardinal vein** (intrapericardial part).
- The left and right posterior cardinal veins degenerates except for the cephalic part of right

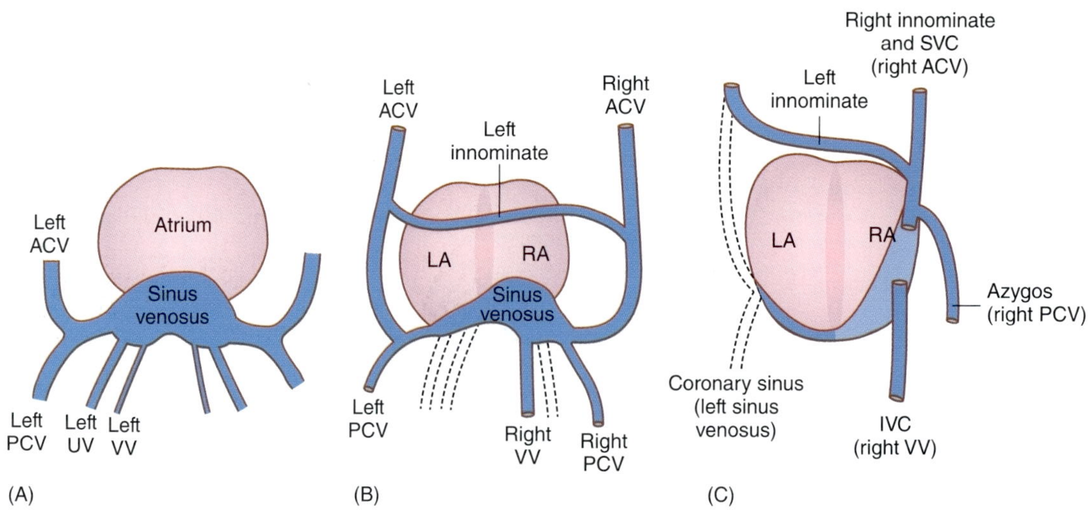

Fig. 15.6 Fate of sinus venosus. (*ACV,* anterior cardinal vein; *PCV,* posterior cardinal vein; *UV,* umbilical vein; *VV,* vitelline vein; *IVC,* inferior vena cava; *SVC,* superior vena cava).

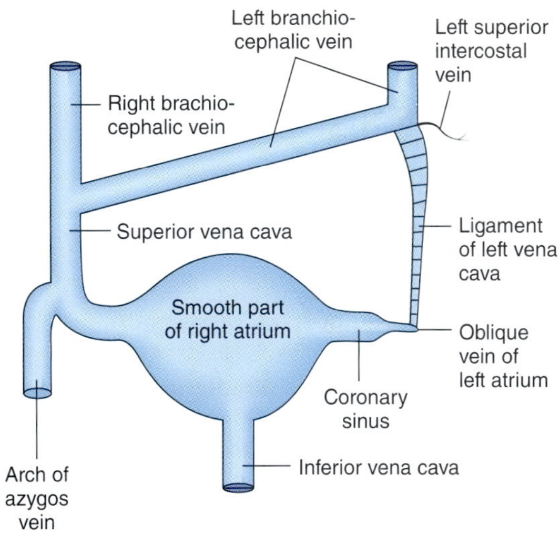

Fig. 15.7 Formation of superior vena cava.

posterior cardinal vein which forms the **arch of azygos vein**.

- Venous return usually occurs through common cardinal veins into the right and left sinus horns.
- Later, the venous flow shifts to the right through the superior and inferior vena cava.
- The **right sinus** horn becomes **larger** than the left.
- The **left sinus** horn stops to grow and gets transformed into a small venous sac on the posterior wall of the heart. This sac gives rise to the **coronary sinus** and the **oblique vein** of the left atrium.
- The **sinoatrial orifice** moves to the right and opens into future right atrium.
- The right horn then gets incorporated as the posterior wall of right atrium **(sinus venarum)**.
- The rough anterior part is derived from primitive atrium.
- The sinoatrial (SA) valves fuse at the cephalic end to form **septum spurium**.
- The sinoatrial valves right and left have different fates.
- The **right SA valve** forms (Fig. 15.8):
  - **Crista terminalis** (from cranial part).
  - **Valves of IVC and coronary sinus** (from caudal part).
- The **left SA valve**:
  - Fuses with septum secundum to form **Interatrial septum**.

FATE OF THE VEINS

THE VITELLINE VEINS

The presence of hepatic bud in the septum transversum divides the vitelline veins into three parts:

1) **Suprahepatic part**—Suprahepatic part of left vitelline vein disappears. Right vitelline vein enlarges to form common hepatic vein, which later persist as the terminal part of **Inferior vena cava**.
2) **Intrahepatic part**—This part of vitelline veins are broken down into afferent and efferent capillary networks. The afferent vessels form the intrahepatic branch of **Portal vein** and efferent forms the tributaries of **Hepatic veins**
3) **Infrahepatic part**—This part gives rise to the **Portal vein** which is mentioned in detail below.

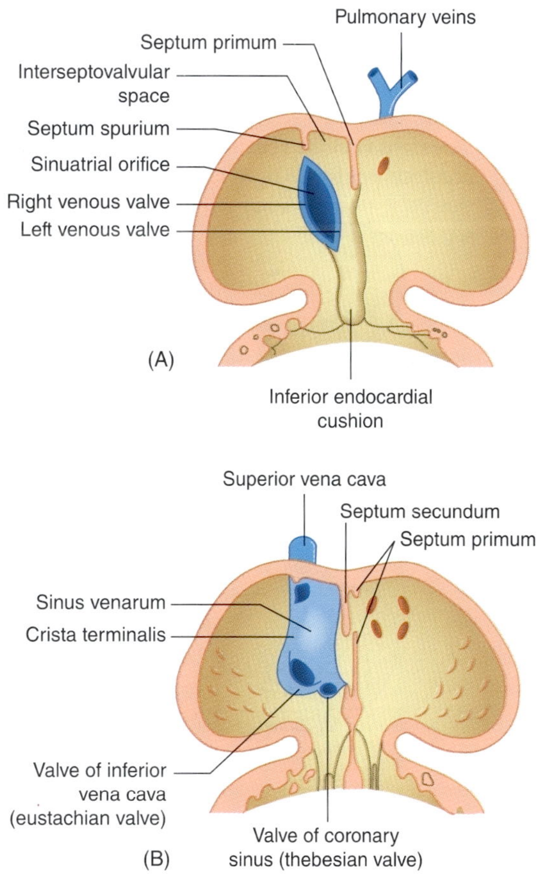

Fig. 15.8 Fate of sinus valve.

PORTAL VEIN

- The **two vitelline veins** which lie on either side of the duodenum are connected by three anastomotic channels to give a **figure of 8** appearance (Fig. 15.9).
- **Ventral** → (1) proximal and (2) distal.
  - **Dorsal** → middle.
- The **Splenic vein** joins the left end of dorsal anastomoses.
- The **left umbilical** vein joins the left end of proximal ventral anastomoses.
- With the rotation of gut, the right vitelline vein becomes posterior and left vitelline vein becomes anterior.
- The following changes happen:
  - The **posterior limb** below dorsal anastomoses disappear.
  - The **anterior limb** below dorsal anastomoses form **Superior mesenteric vein**.
  - The posterior limb above the dorsal anastomoses along with the dorsal anastomoses forms the **trunk** of **the portal vein.**
  - The anterior limb above dorsal anastomoses disappear.
  - The **right vitelline vein** above proximal ventral anastomoses forms right branch of portal vein.
  - The proximal ventral anastomoses along with remaining part of left vitelline vein forms the **left branch of portal vein** (hence it is longer than the right).

THE CARDINAL VEINS

- The **common cardinal vein** is formed by the fusion of anterior cardinal veins (draining head and neck, brain and upper limb) and posterior cardinal veins (draining the rest of the body).
- By eighth week of intrauterine period, an oblique connection develops between the anterior cardinal veins distal to the termination of subclavian veins. This oblique channel later forms the **left brachiocephalic vein.**
- The right anterior cardinal vein between subclavian vein and the oblique anastomosis forms the **right brachiocephalic vein.**
- The anterior cardinal veins cephalic to the subclavian veins form the **internal jugular veins.**

SUPERIOR VENA CAVA

- It has got two parts. The **extrapericardial** part and the **intrapericardial** part. The extrapericardial

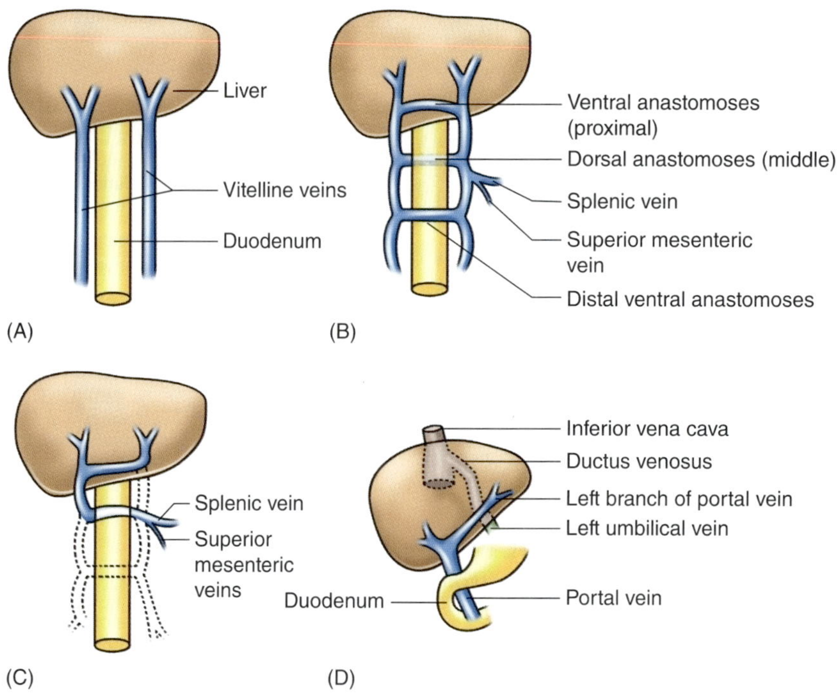

Fig. 15.9 Formation of portal vein. (See the text for description.)

part develops from the caudal part of the **right anterior cardinal vein** and the intrapericardial part from the **right common cardinal vein**.

- The **right common cardinal vein** opens into the right horn of sinus venosus which later gets absorbed into the right atrium. As a result, the superior vena cava finally opens into the right atrium.
- On the **left side**, the following changes occur:
  - **Left anterior cardinal vein**—the caudal part of this vein mostly regresses to form left superior intercostal vein and ligament of the left vena cava.
  - **Left common cardinal vein**—forms the oblique vein of left atrium.
- The **posterior cardinal veins** receive the iliac veins, the intersegmental veins and the veins of mesonephros. Before the regression of posterior cardinal veins, four pairs of **longitudinal veins** are formed.
  1) **Subcardinal veins**—These veins receive blood from the mesonephros and the preaortic anastomoses between them persist as a part of the **left renal vein**. The subcardinal veins are connected to the posterior cardinal veins cranially caudally and in between. The right subcardinal vein after receiving right suprarenal vein makes a communication with common hepatic vein to form the hepatic part of **inferior vena cava**. The common hepatic vein forms the terminal part of inferior vena cava. The remaining right subcardinal vein forms the renal part of inferior vena cava. Most of the left subcardinal vein forms the **left renal vein**.
  2) **Supracardinal veins**—These veins join with the corresponding posterior cardinal veins cranially and caudally. They also anastomose with the subcardinal veins of the same side. The anastomosis between the supra and subcardinal veins receives gonadal veins and they form postrenal part of **inferior vena cava** on the right side and a part of **left renal vein** on the left side. The right supracardinal vein caudal to the anastomosis also contribute to the formation of inferior vena cava.
  3) **Azygos veins**—The intersegmental veins are received by the azygos veins after the regression of cranial part of supracardinal veins. The right azygos venous channel forms the vertical part of azygos vein, and the cephalic part of right posterior cardinal vein persist as arch of azygos vein. The left azygos venous channel forms the superior and inferior **hemiazygos veins**.
  4) **Subcentral veins**—These develop dorsal to dorsal aorta. Anastomotic veins connecting subcentral and azygos veins form a renal collar around dorsal aorta. The preaortic renal collar forms **left renal vein** and postaortic forms **third** and **fourth lumbar veins** and the communication between azygos and hemiazygos veins. Left common iliac vein is formed by the anastomosis between caudal end of right and left posterior cardinal veins.

INFERIOR VENA CAVA

The following sources contribute to the formation of inferior vena cava (Fig. 15.10):

- Caudal part of **posterior cardinal vein**.
- **Right supracardinal vein** (third and fourth lumbar veins join here).
- **Right supracardinal subcardinal anastomosis** (right gonadal veins join here).
- Upper **right subcardinal vein** (renal veins and right suprarenal vein join here).
- **Communication** between right subcardinal and common hepatic vein.
- **Common hepatic vein** formed from suprahepatic part of right vitelline vein.

CLINICAL NUGGETS

Anomalies of vena cava

- **Double inferior vena cava** (Fig. 15.11):
  - The caudal portion of the **left supracardinal system** fails to regress.
  - It results in an abnormal left IVC.
  - The blood from this left IVC drains into the right IVC via the left renal vein or into the hemiazygos vein.
- **Double superior vena cava** (Fig. 15.12):
  - The **left anterior cardinal** vein persists and maintains its connection with the left sinus venosus.
  - In this case, the **left brachiocephalic vein** will be missing or very small.
  - Blood from the left side of the head and neck and from the left upper extremity drains through the abnormal left superior vena cava into the coronary sinus.
- **A single left superior vena cava:**
  - The **left anterior cardinal vein** persists and the right is obliterated.
  - The blood from the head and neck, both upper extremities, and the azygos system, usually reaches right atrium through coronary sinus.

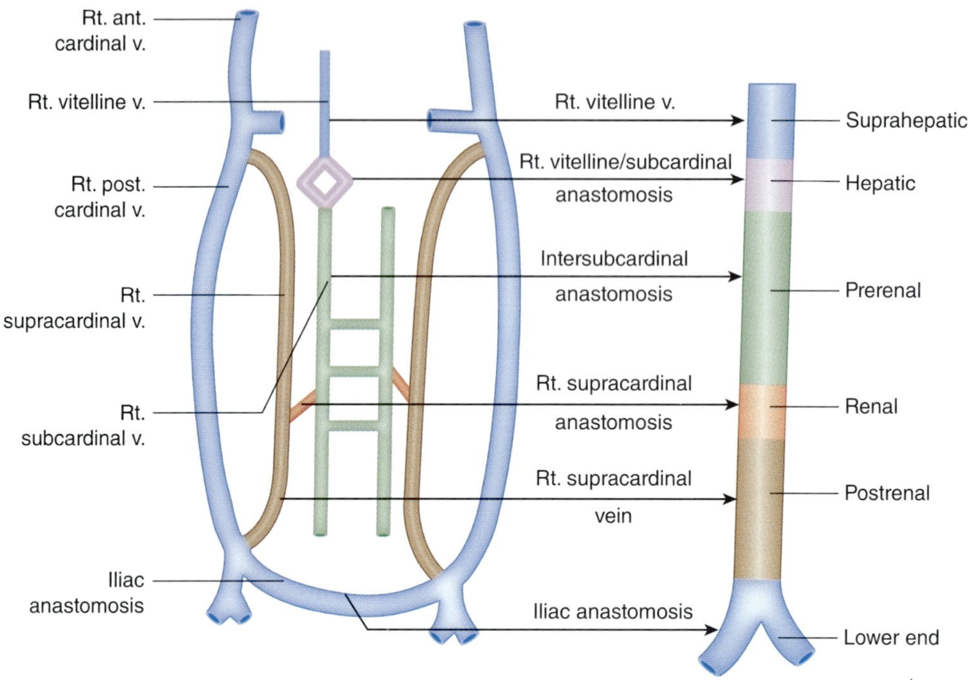

Fig. 15.10 Formation of inferior vena cava. (*Rt,* right; *v,* vein; *ant,* anterior; *post,* posterior).

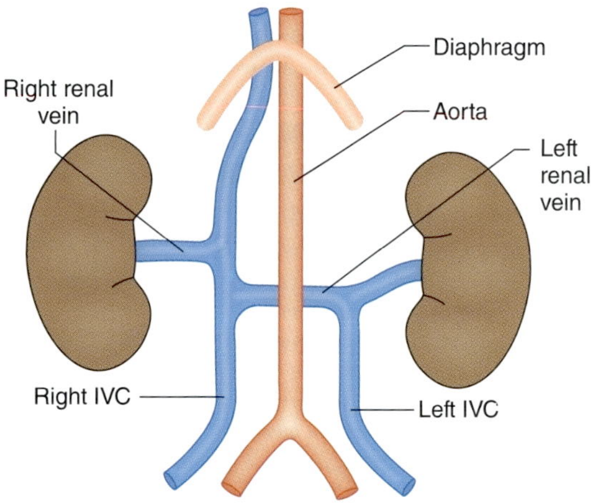

Fig. 15.11 Double inferior vena cava.

PRIMITIVE ATRIUM

- The common atrial chamber communicates with the bulboventricular cavity through **atrioventricular canal**.
- **Left atrium** including the left auricle is formed from **primitive atrium**. The smooth part is formed by the absorption of **pulmonary veins**.
- Formation of interatrial septum divides the atria into right and left chambers.
- The first formed septum from the roof of atria is called **Septum primum** (sickle-shaped) (Fig. 15.13).
- The **Endocardial cushions** are formed on the anterior and posterior wall of the atrioventricular (AV) canal.
- The AV cushions fuse to form **Septum intermedium** which divides the AV canal into right and left AV canals.
- The opening at the lower end of septum primum between septum primum and endocardial cushion is called **Ostium primum**.
- Further development of the septum primum and endocadial cushions close the ostium primum. (Before the complete closure of ostium primum, perforations appear in the upper part of septum primum by programmed cell death [**apoptosis**].) So, the secondly formed foramen is called **Ostium secundum**.
- Ostium primum and ostium secundum maintains the transfer of oxygenated blood from the inferior vena cava to the left atrium.

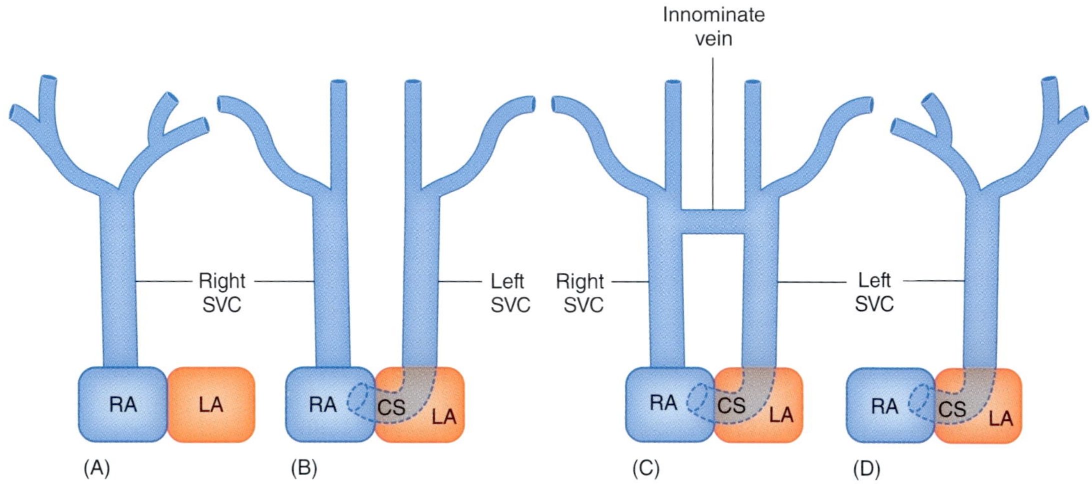

Fig. 15.12 Anomalies of superior vena cava. (*RA,* right atrium; *LA,* left atrium; *CS,* coronary sinus; *SVC,* superior vena cava).

- The **Septum secundum** grows down on the right side of septum primum from the roof of right atrium.
- The **left venous valve** and **septum spurium** are incorporated on to the septum secundum. The part of the right venous valve along with septum spurium becomes rudimentary and forms the **Crista terminalis**. The intermediate part of venous valve below crista terminalis forms **valve of the inferior vena cava** and the caudal part of the venous valve forms the **valve of coronary sinus**.
- Once the caudal end of the septum secundum overlaps the septum primum, the

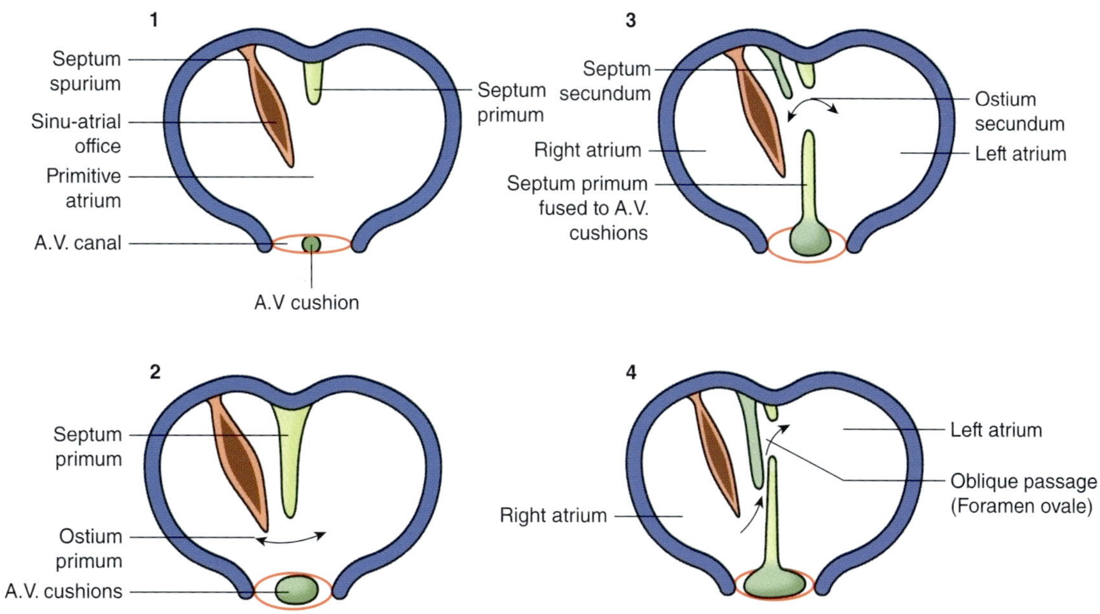

Fig. 15.13 Formation of interatrial septum. (*AV,* Atrioventricular) **(See the text for description.)**

ostium secundum gets transformed as **foramen ovale**.
- Septum secundum is **rigid** and septum primum acts like a **flap valve**.
- When the pulmonary circulation sets in after the birth, the left atrial pressure increases and septum primum is pushed against septum secundum. Thus, **foramen ovale** is closed both structurally and functionally.
- **The probe patency of foramen** ovale means, the foramen is closed only functionally (in 20%).
- Remnants are as follows:
  - **Limbus fossa ovalis**—caudal edge of septum secundum (right atrium).
  - **Fossa ovalis**—septum primum (right atrium).
  - **Semilunar fold**—cephalic-free edge of septum primum on the left side of the interatrial septum.
  - **Fossa lunata**—semilunar depression on the surface of the atrial septum in the left atrium formed by septum secundum.
- To summarize, the **Right atrium** is formed from the following sources:
  - **Sinus venarum (smooth part):** This part is behind crista terminalis and is formed from the absorbed portion of **right horn of sinus venosus**. Upper part of right venous valve with septum spurium forms the crista terminalis and the lower part forms the valves of inferior vena cava and coronary sinus.
  - **Trabeculated part:** The rough part anterior to crista terminalis and the right auricle is developed from the right half of **primitive atrium**.
- **Left atrium** is developed as follows:
  - **The smooth part:** The posterior aspect of left atrium between the openings of **pulmonary veins** are formed from the absorbed endocardial cushions of pulmonary veins.
  - **Trabeculated part:** The trabeculated anterior part including the left auricle is formed from the left half of primitive atrium.

PRIMITIVE VENTRICLE

- Along with the formation of interatrial septum, the interventricular septum also develops by around sixth week of intrauterine period. The atrioventricular canal is divided into right and left atrioventricular orifice by the fusion of dorsal and ventral endocardial cushions to form **Septum intermedium**.
- The ventricular septum grows cranially between the ventricular part of bulbus cordis and primitive ventricle.
- The upper margin is free and concave with dorsal and ventral horns. The **dorsal horn** fuses with the right edge of dorsal AV cushion and **ventral horn** fuses with the left edge of ventral AV cushion.
- As a result, a **ventricular foramen** is formed in the upper part between the two ventricles. This foramen is closed by around **eighth week** by the contribution from interatrial septum and proximal bulbar septum.
- The **proximal bulbar septum** is formed by the fusion of right and left bulbar ridges. The **right bulbar ridge** is formed in the dorsal wall of bulbus cordis in line with the dorsal horn of ventricular septum, and the **left bulbar ridge** is formed in the ventral wall of the bulbus cordis in line with the ventral horn of the ventricular septum. These ridges fuse to form the proximal bulbar septum which closes a part of the interventricular foramen.
- The remaining part of the interventricular foramen is closed by the endocardial cushion cells which proliferate from the right edge of septum intermedium.
- The **Right ventricle** is formed from:
  - Proximal part of the **bulbus cordis** and right part of **primitive ventricle** (inflow part).
  - **Conus cordis** (outflow part).
- The **Left ventricle** is formed from:
  - Left part of **primitive ventricle** (inflow part).
  - **Conus cordis** (outflow part).
- **The Interventricular septum** consists of three parts (Fig. 15.14):
  - **Muscular part.**
  - **Membranous part.**
  - **Bulbar part.**
- **Muscular part** arises from the floor of the ventricle towards the AV cushion.
- **Bulbar part** arises from the right and left bulbar ridges in the bulbus cordis which fuse together in a spiral manner.
- The gap between the muscular and bulbar part is closed by the **membranous part** of the interventricular septum. The membranous part closes this interventricular foramen by the proliferation of:

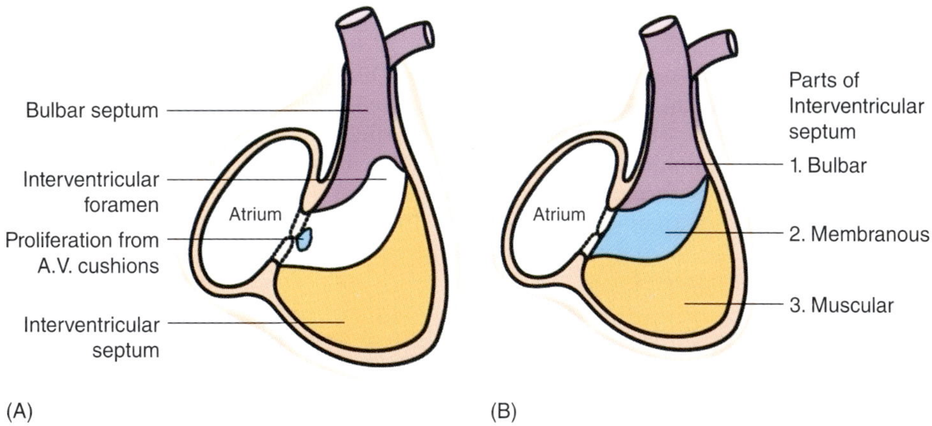

Fig. 15.14 Formation of interventricular septum. (See the text for description.)

  - **Right and left bulbar ridges.**
  - **AV cushion.**
- The presence of interventricular foramen is essential in the embryonic period until the septation of bulbus cordis and truncus arteriosus is complete.

BULBUS CORDIS

- **Truncus arteriosus** forms the cephalic end of bulbus cordis.
- Truncus dilates to form an **aortic sac** which divides to form right and left limbs.
- These limbs are connected to the dorsal aortae by **six pairs of aortic arches.**
- Each aortic arch passes through the mesodermal core of the pharyngeal arch.
- The truncus is divided by a spiral aorticopulmonary septum into:
  - **Ascending aorta.**
  - **Pulmonary trunk.**
- The **position** of the septum decides the relation between aorta and pulmonary trunk.
- In the proximal part, pulmonary trunk lies in front of the aorta because septum is **coronally oriented**.
- In the middle portion, the pulmonary trunk lies on the left side of aorta because septum is in **anteroposterior** direction.
- In the distal part, aorta lies in front of the pulmonary trunk because septum is again **coronally** aligned.

DEVELOPMENT OF THE CONDUCTING SYSTEM OF HEART

- The **myoepicardial mantle** around the endothelial heart tube replaces the cardiac jelly with cardiac muscle fibres, and the myocardium begins to beat by around fourth week of intrauterine period.
- The ventricular muscles appear first and begins to beat followed by the atrial musculature. The **AV node** and bundle appear in the dorsal endocardial cushion by sixth week of intrauterine period. The **SA node** is formed by around third month in the sinus venarum part of right atrium close to the superior vena cava.

AORTIC ARCHES (AN 25.6)

- Aortic arches arise from the **aortic sac** (distal portion of truncus arteriosus). The aortic sac has a right limb and a left limb.
- Each aortic arch passes through pharyngeal arches and they end in dorsal aortae.
- There are **five arches**, namely **I, II, III, IV and VI** (fifth arch disappears).
- By 27th day, most of the **first** aortic arch disappears followed by **second** aortic arch, leaving **maxillary** artery as remnant of first and **hyoid and stapedial** arteries as remnant of second arch.
- The **third** arch is larger and its ventral part forms the **common carotid artery**. The internal carotid artery is formed from the dorsal

part of the third arch along with the dorsal aorta cranial to ductus caroticus.

- The fourth and sixth arches are in the process of formation, and **sixth arch** is known as **pulmonary arch** since it gives off an important branch to the developing lung bud.
- **Right subclavian artery** is formed from the right fourth arch, part of right dorsal aorta and right seventh intersegmental artery. Left seventh intersegmental artery forms the **left subclavian artery**.
- Right limb of the aortic sac forms the **brachiocephalic trunk** and the left limb along with the left fourth arch and left dorsal aorta forms the **definitive arch of aorta**. A portion of dorsal aorta between third and fourth aortic arches known as ductus caroticus disappears on both sides.
- The fifth arch never forms completely and usually regresses.
- The **sixth aortic arch** has got a dorsal and ventral part. The dorsal part of right arch disappears and this causes the **right recurrent laryngeal nerve** to hook the right subclavian artery which is formed from the right fourth arch. The left arch forms the ductus arteriosus which persist as **ligamentum arteriosum** after birth. As a result, the **left recurrent laryngeal nerve** hooks ligamentum arteriosum around the caudal part of arch of aorta. The ventral part forms the right and left **pulmonary arteries**.
- Right dorsal aorta distal to the origin of right seventh intersegmental artery regresses completely.
- The derivatives of aortic arches are (Fig. 15.15):
  - **I**-Maxillary artery.
  - **II**-Hyoid and Stapedial arteries.
  - **III**-Common carotid and first part of Internal carotid arteries.
  - **IV**-
    - **Left side**—Arch of Aorta (the portion between left subclavian and left common carotid).
    - **Right side**—the proximal portion of Right Subclavian artery.
  - **VI**-
    - **Right side**—Right Pulmonary artery.
    - **Left side**—Left Pulmonary artery and Ductus arteriosus.
    - Right (a part) and left subclavian arteries arise from the **seventh intersegmental artery**.
- **Arch of Aorta:**
  - **Proximal**—Left horn of aortic sac.
  - **Distal**—Fourth arch (left side).
- **Brachiocephalic artery**—right horn of the aortic sac.
- **External carotid artery** bends from the third aortic arch.
- **Internal carotid artery**
  - **Proximal**—Third arch.
  - **Distal**—Dorsal aorta.

DEVELOPMENT OF HEART VALVES

- **Tricuspid and mitral valves** are developed by the proliferation of subendocardial mesenchyme.
- Mesenchymal tissue later degenerates and is replaced by the connective tissue.
- **Pulmonary and Aortic valves** are formed from the endocardial cushions. They are developed at the junction of truncus arteriosus and conus.
- **Four cushions** are formed first (Fig. 15.16):
  - **Anterior.**
  - **Posterior.**
  - **Right.**
  - **Left.**
- The **Aorticopulmonary septum** divides the right and left cushions into two equal parts. Now each opening (aortic and pulmonary) has three cushions from which three cups develop.
- **Pulmonary trunk** first lies anterior to the aortic opening. With the rotation of the heart, it lies lateral and to the left of the aortic opening.

THE PERICARDIUM

- The intraembryonic coelom which lies in the midline cranial to the prechordal plate forms the pericardial cavity.
- **The Somatopleuric mesoderm** lining the pericardial cavity forms:
  - **Fibrous** pericardium.
  - **Parietal layer** of serous pericardium.
- **The Splanchnopleuric mesoderm** lining the pericardial cavity forms:
  - **Visceral layer** of the serous pericardium.
- As the heart tube folds, the dorsal mesogastrium suspending the heart tube disappears to form the **Transverse sinus** of the pericardium.

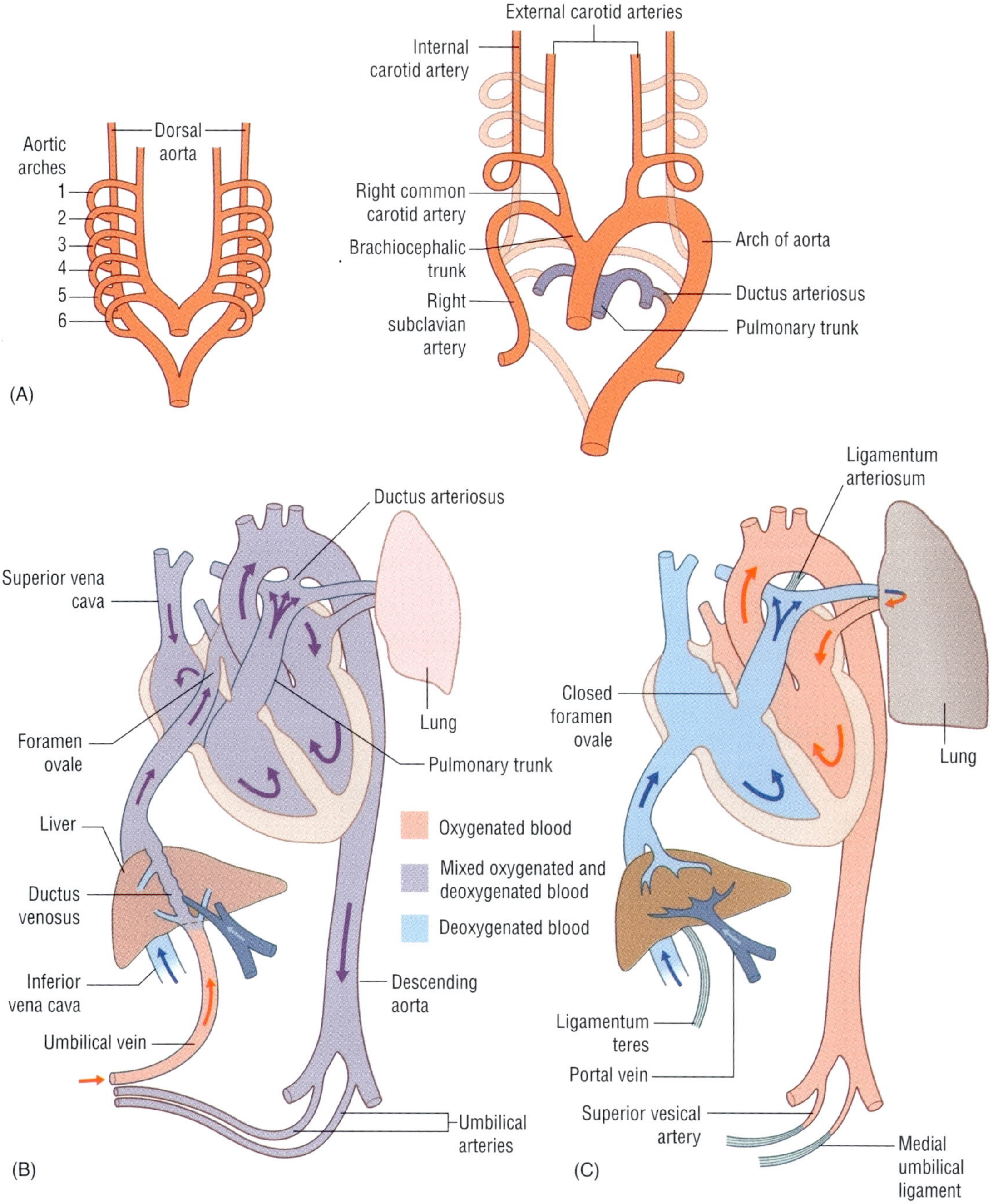

Fig. 15.15 Derivatives of aortic arches. (A) The six pairs of aortic arches and their derivatives: the pattern of blood flow through the heart before (B) and after (C) birth. (Source: *Anatomy and Human Movement: Structure and Function*. 7th ed. 2019.)

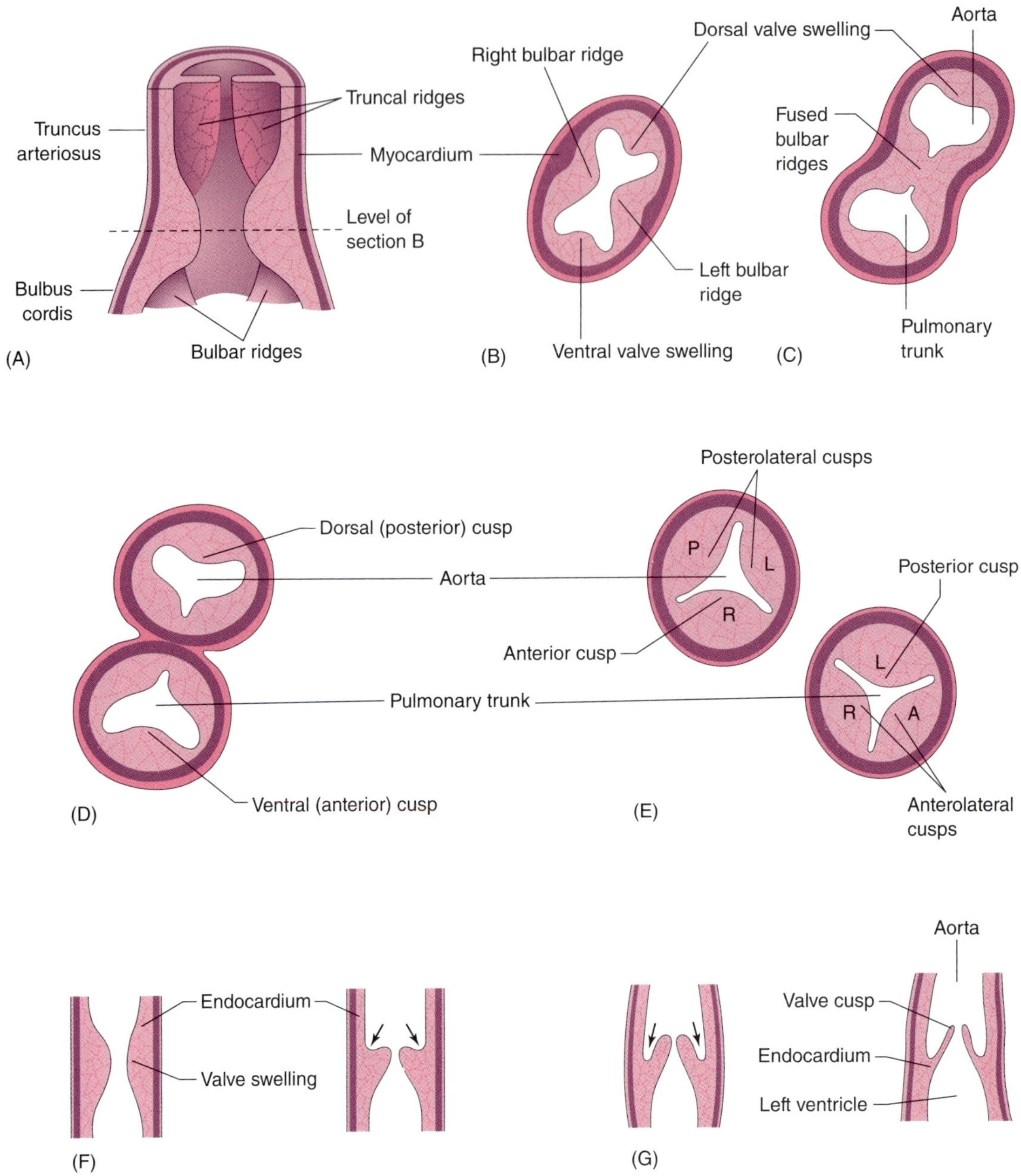

Fig. 15.16 Development of the semilunar valves of the aorta and pulmonary trunk. (A) Sketch of a section of the truncus arteriosus and bulbus cordis showing the valve swellings. (B) Transverse section of the bulbus cordis. (C) Similar section after fusion of the bulbar ridges. (D) Formation of the walls and valves of the aorta and pulmonary trunk. (E) Rotation of the vessels has established the adult positions of the valves in relation to each other. (F and G) Longitudinal sections of the aorticoventricular junction illustrating successive stages in the hollowing *(arrows)* and thinning of the valve swellings to form the valve cusps. (*A*, Anterior; *L*, left; *P*, posterior; *R*, right.) (Source: *Before We Are Born: Essentials of Embryology and Birth Defects*, First South Asia ed. 2016.)

- Once the arrangement of vena cava and pulmonary veins are finalized, the isolated pouch of pericardium formed behind the left atrium is called **Oblique sinus**.

FOETAL CIRCULATION (AN 25.3)

- In foetus, there is **no gas exchange** in lungs (Fig. 15.17). Hence, pulmonary vessels are constricted
- The **placenta** serves as the organ of respiration, and the gaseous exchange occurs by diffusion through the placental barrier.
- The three important structures in foetal circulation are:
  - **Ductus venosus.**
  - **Foramen ovale.**
  - **Ductus arteriosus.**
- The oxygenated blood from the mother (placenta) reaches the foetus through left **umbilical vein** (Fig. 15.18).
- Once the blood in the umbilical vein reaches the portal vein, it has two ways to reach IVC.
  - Through **ductus venosus**, it bypasses the liver and reaches the IVC.
  - Through the **sinusoids** of liver enter the IVC through hepatic veins.
- When the blood reaches the right atrium through IVC, most of it is directed through foramen ovale into the left atrium by the inferior border of **Septum secundum (crista dividens).** The blood in the inferior vena cava is guided by the **valve of inferior vena cava** to the foramen ovale.
- In the left atrium, the oxygenated blood from IVC will get mixed with a minimal amount of poorly oxygenated blood (oxygenated blood is used up by the foetal lungs for nutrition) returning from the lungs through **pulmonary veins**.
- The blood from the left atrium flows to the left ventricle and comes out through the ascending aorta.
- The blood in the **Ascending aorta** (though mixes up with deoxygenated blood in atria) is well oxygenated compared to the rest of the body (except umbilical vein) and it supplies:
  - **Heart.**
  - **Head (developing brain).**
  - **Neck.**
  - **Upper limbs.**
- The main function of **Foramen ovale** is to shunt maximum amount of oxygenated blood into the ascending aorta so that the **developing brain** will get well-oxygenated blood.
- The remaining blood in the right atrium along with the blood from SVC and coronary sinus flow to the right ventricle and then to the pulmonary trunk. The right ventricle pumps the blood against a higher resistance since the lungs is inactive. To counteract this, the right ventricle acts more than the left ventricle and hence the **right ventricle is muscular in foetal life** compared to the left ventricle.
- After birth, the aortic resistance is more and the left ventricle has to work more and becomes more muscular compared to the right ventricle.
- The blood in the **pulmonary trunk** goes in two directions:
  - 90% of blood passes through the **Ductus arteriosus (DA)** into the descending aorta.
  - Only 10% of blood flows to the **Lungs** (because of increased pulmonary resistance).

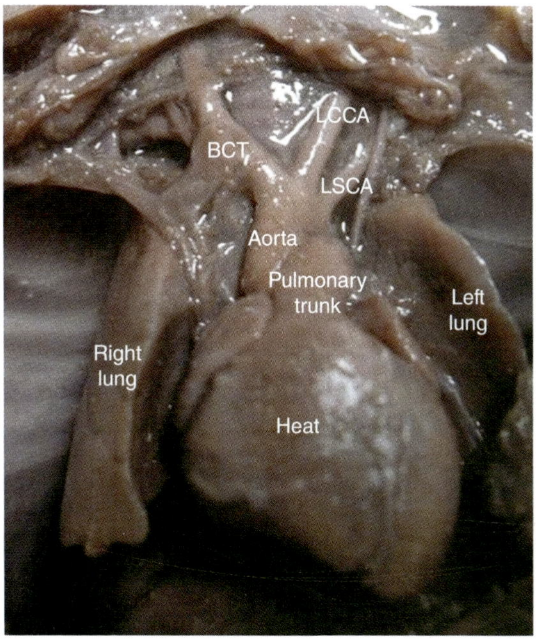

Fig. 15.17 Foetal heart with major blood vessels. (Photo courtesy: Dr Rose.)

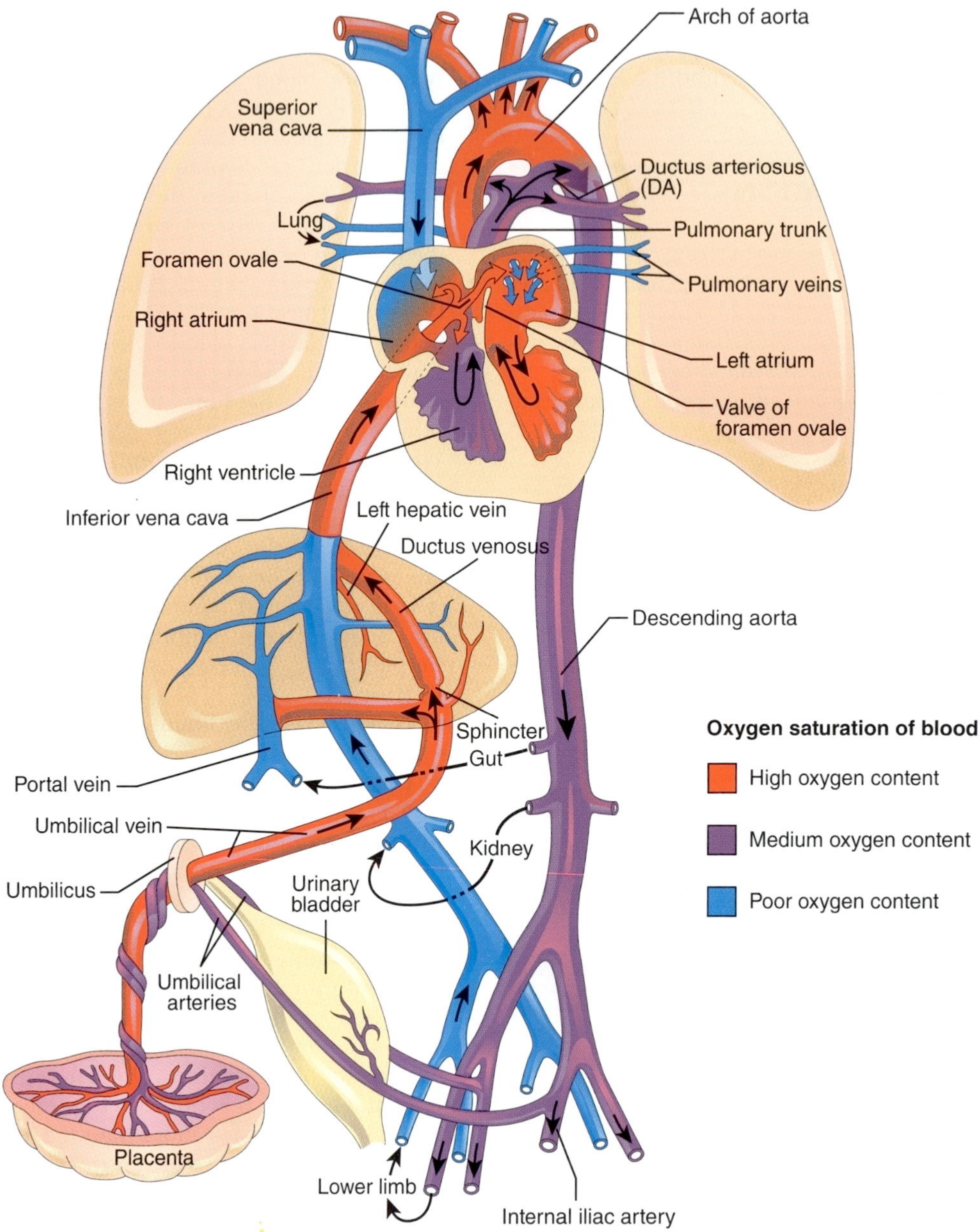

Fig. 15.18 Foetal circulation. The *colours* indicate the oxygen saturation of the blood, and the *arrows* show the course of the blood from the placenta to the heart. The organs are not drawn to scale. A small amount of highly oxygenated blood from the inferior vena cava remains in the right atrium and mixes with poorly oxygenated blood from the superior vena cava. Blood with medium oxygenation then passes into the right ventricle. Observe that three shunts permit most of the blood to bypass the liver and lungs: (1) ductus venosus, (2) foramen ovale and (3) ductus arteriosus. The poorly oxygenated blood returns to the placenta for oxygenation and nutrients through the umbilical arteries. (Source: *The Developing Human: Clinically Oriented Embryology*. 11th ed. 2020.)

- **The patency** of ductus arteriosus is controlled by:
  - **Low oxygen content.**
  - **Prostaglandins** (PGE2, PGI2 [prostacyclin]).
- **Indomethacin,** which is an inhibitor of PG synthesis, constricts PDA in premature infants. So, the blood in the descending aorta is from DA (90%) and ascending aorta (10%).
- The blood in the **Descending aorta** flows in two directions:
  - **35%** enters the body of Foetus.
  - **65%** through the umbilical arteries reaches the Placenta.

CHANGES AFTER BIRTH

- **After birth:**
  - Circulation of blood through placenta stops.
  - Lungs begin to function.
- The following structures confined to foetal circulation are no longer needed:
  - **Umbilical vessels.**
  - **Ductus venosus.**
  - **Foramen ovale.**
  - **Ductus arteriosus.**
- As the placenta gets detached from the mother after birth, no blood flows through the umbilical vessels.
- The **umbilical arteries** constrict soon after birth to prevent blood loss.
- The **umbilical veins** remain patent for a few minutes so that the maximum amount of blood can be drained from placenta to infant.
- The sphincter of ductus venosus contracts so that whole blood now enters the liver and then into hepatic sinusoids.
- When the **lungs** started functioning:
  - Pulmonary resistance decreased.
  - Blood flow to the lungs increased.
  - The walls of the pulmonary vessels get stretched.
  - The pressure in the left atrium increased (blood from pulmonary veins).
- The increased pressure in the left atrium **closes the foramen ovale** by pushing the septum primum, which is flap like, against the rigid septum secundum. As a result, blood reaching the right atrium passes to the right ventricle, then to the pulmonary trunk.
- Since the pulmonary resistance is low as compared to systemic resistance, blood will stop flowing through the ductus arteriosus to the descending aorta.
- **Ductus arteriosus** closes as follows:
  - 20% by 24 hours.
  - 82% by 48 hours.
  - 100% by 96 hours.
- Factors controlling functional closure of ductus arteriosus:
  - High **oxygen** content.
  - **Bradykinin** (released by lung constricts smooth muscle).
  - **Nervous reflex**.
- Anatomical closure of ductus arteriosus is by **Transforming Growth Factor-beta (TGF-beta)**.
- The closure of ductus arteriosus is primary which is followed by the closure of foramen ovale.
- **Patent ductus arteriosus** is seen in:
  - **Premature infants.**
  - **Persistent hypoxia.**
- In **foetus**, the wall of the **right ventricle** is thicker since it has been working against resistance.
- In **adults**, the wall of the **left ventricle** is thicker due to increased work load.

FOETAL REMNANTS

- The umbilical vein transforms into the **Ligamentum teres/round ligament of the liver**.
- The ductus venosus evolves into the **Ligamentum venosum**.
- The umbilical arteries persist proximally as the **Superior vesical arteries**. Distally, they transform into the **Medial umbilical ligament**.
- The foramen ovale is present in the interatrial septum. On the right side, it corresponds to the **Fossa ovalis**. On the left side, it is marked by the **lunate impression** within the interatrial septum.
- The septum primum forms the **floor of the fossa ovalis**.
- The septum secundum (lower border) contributes to the **limbus fossa ovalis**.
- The ductus arteriosus undergoes changes, becoming the **Ligamentum arteriosum** in the adult anatomy.

Foetal remnants	Adult structures
• Umbilical vein	• Ligamentum teres/round ligament of liver
• Ductus venosus	• Ligamentum venosum
• Umbilical arteries	• Proximal—superior vesical arteries
	• Distal—medial umbilical ligament
• Foramen ovale	• Fossa ovalis (right side of interatrial septum)
	• Lunate impression (left side of interatrial septum)
• Septum primum	• Floor of fossa ovalis
• Septum secundum (lower border)	• Limbus fossa ovalis
• Ductus arteriosus	• Ligamentum arteriosum

DEVELOPMENT OF LYMPHATIC SYSTEM

- Lymphatic channels arise by vasculogenesis and angiogenesis from **mesoderm**.
- By fifth week, the lymphatics of upper limbs, upper trunk, head and neck are collected by a pair of **Jugular lymph sacs** formed at the junction of the subclavian and anterior cardinal veins.
- By sixth week, the lymph from the trunk and lower extremities are collected by the retroperitoneal lymph sac, cisterna chyli and paired posterior lymph sacs related with the junctions of the external and internal iliac veins.
- The **Cisterna chyli** drains into a pair of thoracic lymphatic ducts that empty at the junctions of the internal jugular and subclavian vein. Two main ducts, the right and the left lymphatic ducts, connect the jugular sacs with the cisterna chyli. These ducts are later connected in the midthoracic region.
- The **definitive Thoracic duct** is derived from the caudal portion of the right duct, the cranial portion of the left duct and a median anastomosis. The **right lymphatic duct** is formed from the cranial part of right duct.
- The part of the ducts which are not forming definitive thoracic duct gets obliterated.

KLINISCHE PERLEN

AXIS ARTERIES

- **Upper limb**—The axis artery of the upper limb is formed from the lateral branch of the seventh intersegmental artery (subclavian artery).
  - **Axillary artery.**
  - **Brachial artery.**
  - **Anterior interosseous artery, Median artery.**
  - **Deep palmar arch.**
- **Lower limb**—The axis artery of the lower limb is formed from the dorsal root of the umbilical artery (fifth lumbar intersegmental artery).
  - **Inferior gluteal artery.**
  - **Arteria nervi ischiadici.**
  - **Popliteal artery.**
  - **Peroneal artery.**
  - **Plantar arch.**

HOLT–ORAM SYNDROME (HEART–HAND SYNDROME)

- **Autosomal dominant.**
- **Atrial septal defects.**
- **Preaxial (radial) limb anomalies.**

ATRIAL SEPTAL DEFECTS (ASD) (AN 25.4)

- Atrial septal defect results in communication between **right and left atria** through an opening in the interatrial septum as a result of defective fusion.
- It can be classified as:
  - **Morphologic defects** where the right and left atria directly communicate through interatrial septum as in—ostium primum ASD, endocardial cushion defects, ostium secundum ASD and cor triloculare biventriculare.
  - **Physiological defects** where there is no anatomical defect in the interatrial septum but behave like interatrial septal defects as in sinus venosus ASD and unroofed coronary sinus.
    a) **Ostium secundum (most common):**
      - It accounts to **80%–90% of ASDs**.
      - It is seen as a direct communication between the two atria (patent foramen ovale is seen as a tunnel between the two atria).

- It is located at the region of **fossa ovalis**.
- In this defect, the **septum secundum** fails to overgrow the opening of ostium secundum, thus allowing a direct communication between right and left atria.
- The size of the defect varies and is usually larger than patent foramen ovale.

b) **Ostium primum (endocardial cushion defect):**
- It is the **mildest form** of endocardial cushion defects (2%–3% of the ASDs).
- The **Endocardial cushions** form:
  - The medial aspects of the **Mitral and Tricuspid valves**.
  - The portion of the **Atrial septum** adjacent to the atrioventricular valves.
  - The inlet portion of the **ventricular septum**.
- The failure of fusion between the free edge of the septum primum and the endocardial cushion is termed as ostium primum ASD.
- If this defect is associated with abnormal development of the atrioventricular valves or ventricular septum, it is known as **Endocardial cushion defects**.
- Seen commonly associated with **Down syndrome**.

c) **Cor triloculare biventriculare:**
- Complete absence of septum resulting in **single atrium** (so three chambers, one atrium and two ventricles, hence the name).

EBSTEIN ANOMALY

- **Tricuspid valve** displaced towards the apex of right ventricle (anterior leaflet enlarged).
- Hypertrophy of **right atrium**.
- ASD/patent foramen ovale (50%).

VENTRICULAR SEPTAL DEFECT (VSD) (AN 25.4)

- Most common congenital cardiac malformation where there is a direct communication between the two ventricles.
- It is more commonly seen in **males**.
- The different types of VSD are as follows:

a) **Perimembranous VSD:**
- **Most common** type of VSD.
- It lies in the LV outflow tract just below the aortic valve.
- It occurs in the membranous septum with defects in the adjacent muscular portion of the septum.
  - **Perimembranous inlet.**
  - **Perimembranous outlet.**
  - **Perimembranous muscular.**

b) **Supracristal VSD:**
- It lies beneath the pulmonic valve and communicate with the RV outflow tract above the supraventricular crest.
- Usually associated with **Aortic regurgitation**.

c) **Muscular VSD:**
- It is entirely bounded by the muscular septum.
- They are often multiple **(Swiss-cheese septum).**
- Classified as:
  - **Central muscular.**
  - **Midmuscular.**
  - **Apical.**
  - **Marginal.**

d) **Posterior VSD:**
- Atrioventricular canal/septal type.
- It lies posterior to the septal leaflet of the tricuspid valve.

FALLOT'S TETRALOGY (FIG. 15.19) (AN 25.4)

- Louis Arthur Etienne Fallot in 1888 described Fallot's tetralogy as **La Maladie Bleue** (the blue disease).
- It is a **cyanotic congenital heart disease** with decreased pulmonary blood flow.
- It occurs in 3 of every 10,000 live births.
- **Fallot's tetralogy** is a combination of following malformations:
  1) **VSD (perimembranous or muscular).**
  2) **Pulmonary stenosis.**
  3) **Right ventricular hypertrophy.**
  4) **Overriding of Aorta.**
- The combination of these lesions results in the characteristic **right ventricular outflow tract obstruction** of tetralogy of Fallot.
- It is seen associated with untreated maternal diabetes, phenylketonuria and intake of retinoic acid.
- Associated chromosomal anomalies are trisomies **21 (Down), 18 (Edward) and 13 (Patau).**

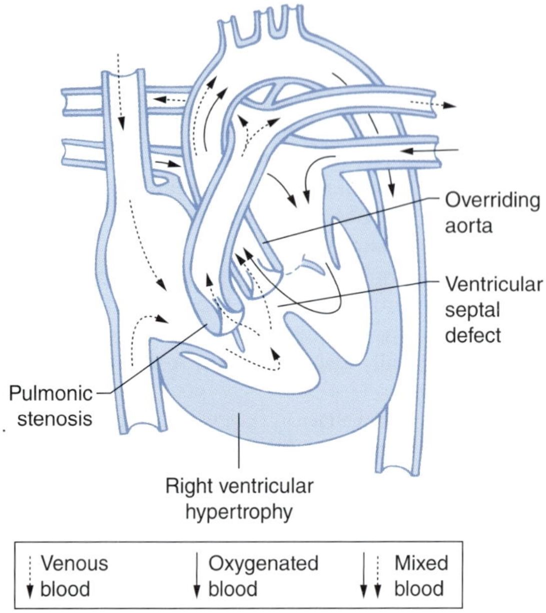

Fig. 15.19 Fallot's tetralogy-schematic representation. Blood flow through the heart with Fallot's tetralogy. (Source: Adapted with permission from Whaley LF, Wong DL. *Nursing Care of Infants and Children*, 4th ed. St Louis, MO: CV Mosby, 1991; *Children in Intensive Care: A Survival Guide*, 3rd ed. 2019.)

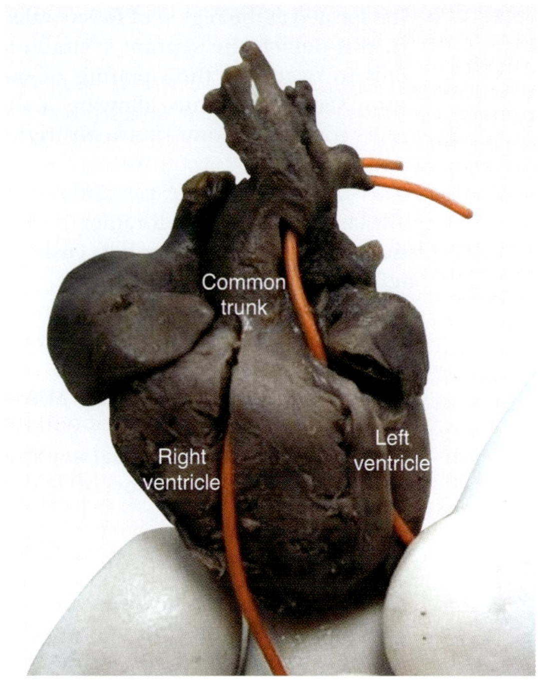

Fig. 15.20 Foetal heart showing common truncus arteriosus. (Photo courtesy: Dr Rose.)

- **Tet spell**—When affected babies cry or strain, they turn **blue,** have difficulty breathing and occasionally lose consciousness.
- The **hypercyanotic spell** is characterized by a sudden and striking decrease in the saturation of oxygen due to acute obstruction of the subpulmonary outflow tract.
- **Fallot's pentalogy** is tetralogy with **ASD/patent foramen ovale.**
- **Trilogy** of Fallot:
  1) **Pulmonary stenosis.**
  2) **Right ventricular hypertrophy.**
  3) **Atrial septal defect.**

COMMON (PERSISTENT) TRUNCUS ARTERIOSUS (FIG. 15.20)

- Conotruncal ridges fail to develop.
- Outflow tract remains as a **single tract**.
- Associated with **VSD** (due to contribution from ridges to form ventricular septum).

TRANSPOSITION OF GREAT VESSELS (AN 25.5)

- Aorta from right ventricle and pulmonary arteries from left ventricle.
- Conotruncal septum develops straight down instead of spiral pattern.

COARCTATION OF AORTA (AN 25.5)

- Congenital narrowing of the aorta in the region of attachment of ductus arteriosus. Based on the attachment, it is classified as two types:
  - **Preductal** (patent ductus arteriosus).
  - **Postductal** (ductus arteriosus obliterated, more common).

DEXTROCARDIA (AN 25.5)

- In this condition, the heart lies on the right, whereas **the apex** of the left ventricle points to the **right** instead of the left.

- This happens when there is **abnormal looping** of the heart tube.
- Usually associated with **Situs inversus**.

PATENT DUCTUS ARTERIOSUS (AN 25.5)

- During the time of birth, the ductus arteriosus constricts as a response to increased oxygen tension.
- The ductus is kept patent during foetal life by **Prostaglandins**.
- Increased oxygen tension decreases circulating levels of prostaglandins.
- This results in the release of **endothelins** which promote contraction of vascular smooth muscle in the ductus arteriosus.
- Failure of the ductus arteriosus to close after birth occurs in pregnancies complicated by **Rubella or hypoxia**.
- The flow of blood from the higher-pressure aortic circulation into the pulmonary circulation results in **pulmonary hypertension and heart failure**.
- Pulmonary hypertension causes a **reversal** of flow of blood through the persistent ductus and results in cyanosis in the lower body parts (**Eisenmenger syndrome**).
- In **premature** infants, the ductus arteriosus may not constrict spontaneously and are treated with **prostaglandin inhibitors like indomethacin**.

POINTS TO PONDER

- The vascular system develops from **mesoderm** in the wall of the yolk sac.
- Blood cells and vascular endothelial cells are derived from **hemangioblasts**.
- The **three mechanisms** by which the embryonic blood vessels are formed are:
  - **Vasculogenesis**.
  - **Migration of angioblasts**.
  - **Angiogenesis**.
- **Aortic arches:**
  - The **first three** pairs—arteries that supply the head.
  - The **fourth** pair—the left arch forms part of the aortic arch.
  - The **fifth** pair—never forms.
  - The **sixth** pair—the distal part of the left sixth arch forms the ductus arteriosus.
  - The larger arteries of adults arise from three sets of aortic branches:
    - The **dorsal** intersegmental.
    - The **lateral** segmental.
    - The **ventral** segmental.
- The venous system arises from the **cardinal vein system**.
- Anterior and posterior cardinal veins form the **common cardinal veins** which drain into the sinus venosus of the heart.
- Paired extraembryonic umbilical and vitelline veins pass through the liver and drains into the sinus venosus.
- The **Pulmonary veins** arise separately and drains into the left atrium.
- The heart arises from **splanchnic mesoderm.**
- The fused endocardial tubes undergo an **S-shaped** looping.
- It starts with the **inflow tract → the sinus venosus → the atria → the ventricles → the outflow tract (bulbus cordis)**.
- The left and right atria are separated by the development of the **Septum primum** and **Septum secundum**.
- The ventricles are divided by the **Interventricular septum**.
- **Spiral ridges** partition the outflow tract into pulmonary and aortic trunks.
- The **foetal circulation** carries oxygenated blood from the placenta through the umbilical vein into the right atrium.
- From the right atrium, considerable amount is shunted into the left atrium.
- The remaining blood entering the right atrium passes into the right ventricle and from there into the pulmonary trunk.
- Blood coming out of the right ventricle enters the pulmonary trunk.
- From the pulmonary trunk, some blood goes to the lungs and a major portion to the aorta via the **Ductus arteriosus**.
- Blood in the left atrium voids into the left ventricle and aorta through which it supplies the rest of the body.
- Poorly oxygenated blood is carried by the **Umbilical arteries** to the placenta for oxygenation.

BRAIN TEASERS

1. What are the two longitudinal intraembryonic vessels known as?
   A. Ventral aortae
   B. Lateral aortae
   C. Dorsal aortae
   D. Extraembryonic vessels
2. Where do the dorsal aortae arise in relation to the notochord?
   A. Above the notochord

B. Below the notochord
C. On each side of the notochord
D. Anterior to the notochord

3. What is the caudal extension of the dorsal aortae called?
   A. Umbilical arteries
   B. Vitelline veins
   C. Connecting stalk
   D. Bulbus cordis
4. Which vessels join the venous end of the primitive heart along with the umbilical veins?
   A. Vitelline veins
   B. Umbilical arteries
   C. Cardiac veins
   D. Pulmonary veins
5. What is the oxygenation status of the umbilical veins?
   A. Poorly oxygenated
   B. Well-oxygenated
   C. Deoxygenated
   D. Hypoxic
6. What layer of the heart is derived from splanchnic mesoderm surrounding the pericardial coelom?
   A. Endocardium
   B. Myocardium
   C. Both
   D. None
7. Which part of the primitive heart is continuous cranially with the aortic sac?
   A. Bulbus cordis
   B. Primitive ventricle
   C. Sinus venosus
   D. Primitive atrium
8. What marks the junction between the ventricle and bulbus cordis?
   A. Bulboventricular sulcus
   B. Interventricular foramen
   C. Sinus venosus
   D. Septum spurium
9. When does the primitive heart start beating?
   A. 20th day
   B. 22nd day
   C. 24th day
   D. 26th day
10. Blood enters the primordial atrium through which valves?
    A. Semilunar valves
    B. Atrioventricular valves
    C. Sinoatrial valves
    D. Pulmonary valves
11. Which structure shunts oxygenated blood directly to the heart from the umbilical vein?
    A. Foramen ovale
    B. Ductus arteriosus
    C. Ductus venosus
    D. Interventricular foramen
12. What controls the patency of ductus arteriosus in foetal circulation?
    A. High oxygen content
    B. Low oxygen content
    C. Prostaglandins
    D. Bradykinin
13. What controls the anatomical closure of ductus arteriosus?
    A. Oxygen content
    B. Prostaglandins
    C. Transforming growth factor-beta
    D. Bradykinin
14. What foetal structure becomes the ligamentum teres/round ligament of the liver?
    A. Umbilical vein
    B. Ductus venosus
    C. Foramen ovale
    D. Ductus arteriosus
15. What is the remnant of the ductus arteriosus called after birth?
    A. Ligamentum venosum
    B. Ligamentum arteriosum
    C. Fossa ovalis
    D. Ligamentum teres
16. What structure divides the atrioventricular canal into right and left AV canals?
    A. Septum primum
    B. Septum secundum
    C. Endocardial cushions
    D. Bulbar part

Answers

1. (C); 2. (C); 3. (A); 4. (A); 5. (B); 6. (B); 7. (A); 8. (A); 9. (B); 10. (C); 11. (C); 12. (C); 13. (C); 14. (A); 15. (B); 16. (C).

FURTHER READINGS

de Klerk JCA, Engbers AGJ, van Beek F, et al. Spontaneous closure of the ductus arteriosus in preterm infants: a systematic review. *Front Pediatr.* 2020;8:541. doi:10.3389/fped.2020.00541.

Ganni E, Ho SY, Reddy S, et al. Tetralogy of Fallot across the lifespan: a focus on the right ventricle. *CJC Pediatr Congenit Heart Dis.* 2023;2(6 Part A): 283-300. doi:10.1016/j.cjcpc.2023.10.009.

Giblett JP, Williams LK, Kyranis S, Shapiro LM, Calvert PA. Patent foramen ovale closure: state of the art. *Interv Cardiol.* 2020;15:e15. doi:10.15420/icr.2019.27.

Li SJ, Lee J, Hall J, Sutherland TR. The inferior vena cava: anatomical variants and acquired pathologies. *Insights Imaging.* 2021;12(1):123. doi:10.1186/s13244-021-01066-7.

Wang Z, Zhan Y, Jin J, et al. Individualized experience with percutaneous transcatheter closure of multiple atrial septal defects: a single-center study. *Front Cardiovasc Med.* 2021;8:628322. doi:10.3389/fcvm.2021.628322.

Respiratory System 16

AN 25.2 Describe development of pleura and lung.
AN 25.4 Describe embryological basis of tracheo-oesophageal fistula.

ANAMNESE

A newborn was diagnosed with tracheal stenosis, a condition characterized by the narrowing of the trachea. The newborn exhibited symptoms such as noisy breathing, respiratory distress and difficulty in feeding shortly after birth. The medical team conducted diagnostic imaging, revealing a significant constriction in the trachea, impairing normal airflow (Fig. 16.1). Tracheal stenosis can result from various causes, including congenital abnormalities or acquired factors such as trauma or prolonged intubation. The baby needs surgical intervention to alleviate the stenosis and ensure proper airflow.

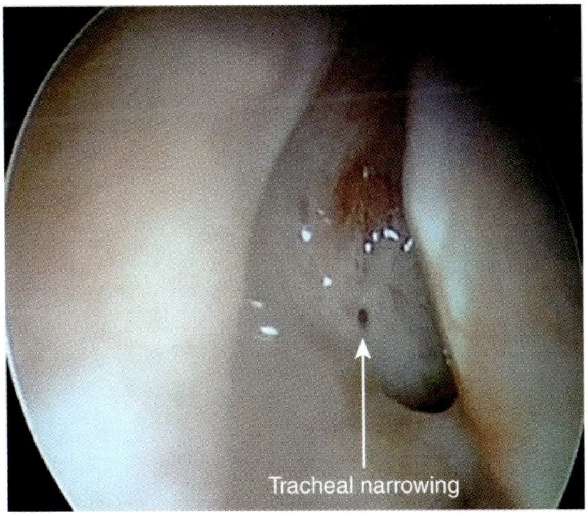

Fig. 16.1 Tracheal stenosis. (Source: Hagberg and Benumof's Airway Management, 5th ed.: Carin Hagberg, Fig. 24.7, Elsevier Inc., 2023.)

LUNG DEVELOPMENT

Lung development is divided into three distinct periods: embryonic, foetal and postnatal.

- **Embryonic Period:**
  - The lungs and trachea originate from the anterior foregut endoderm.
- **Foetal Period:**
  - The foetal period consists of pseudoglandular, canalicular and saccular stages, marking the milestones in lung maturation.
- **Postnatal Period:**
  - Postnatal lung development involves continued alveolarization, ensuring the completion of the lung structure.

LARYNGOTRACHEAL DIVERTICULUM

- At around 28 days (fourth week), **the laryngotracheal diverticulum**, or lung bud, emerges from the ventral wall of the pharyngeal part of the foregut, positioned caudal to the fourth pair of pharyngeal pouches (Fig. 16.2).
- As the diverticulum grows, the groove between it and the foregut deepens. Initially, the diverticulum maintains an open communication with the foregut.
- Later in development, the **tracheo-oesophageal septum** forms through the fusion

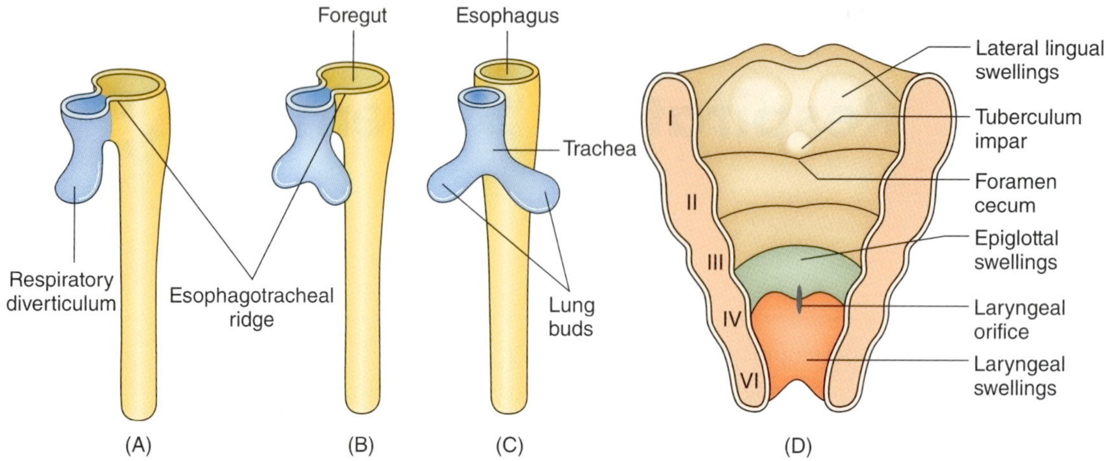

Fig. 16.2 Showing how respiratory diverticulum separates from foregut.

of **tracheo-oesophageal folds**, segregating the cranial portion of the foregut (Fig. 16.3).

- The septum divides the cranial portion of the foregut into the ventral part, known as the **laryngotracheal tube** (the primordium of larynx, trachea, bronchi and lungs), and the dorsal part, representing the primordium of oropharynx and oesophagus.
- The primordial laryngeal inlet, marking the opening of the laryngotracheal tube into the pharynx, is established during this developmental stage.

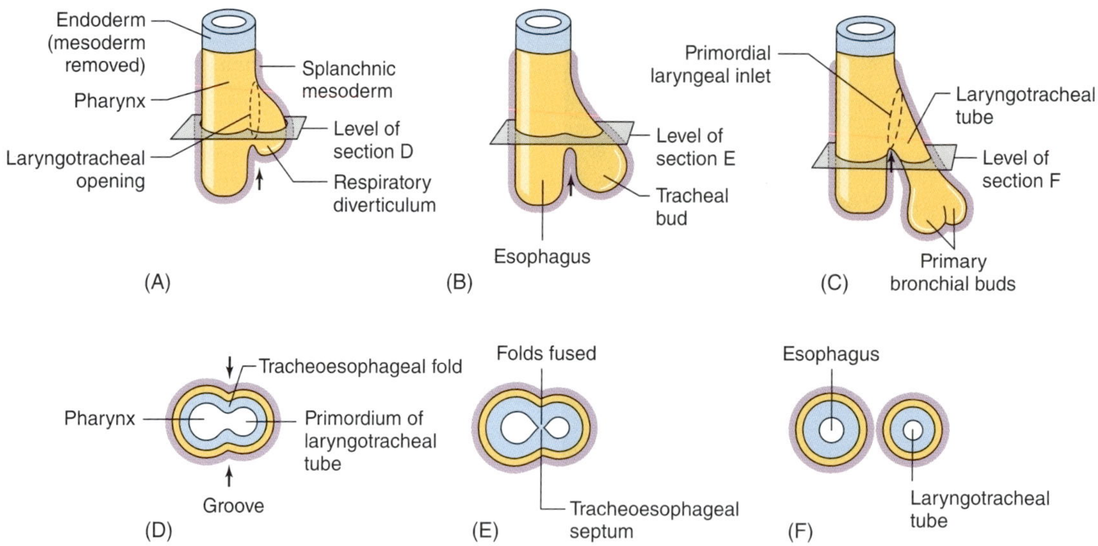

Fig. 16.3 Formation of tracheo-oesophageal septum. Successive stages in the development of the respiratory system from the primitive foregut. (A–C) Lateral views of the caudal part of the primordial pharynx showing the respiratory diverticulum and partitioning of the foregut into the oesophagus and laryngotracheal bud. (D–F) Transverse sections illustrating the formation of the tracheo-oesophageal septum and showing how it separates the foregut into the laryngotracheal bud and oesophagus. (Source: *Egan's Fundamentals of Respiratory Care*. 11th ed. 2017; Credit line: Moore KL, Persaud TVN. The respiratory system. In: Moore KL, Persaud TVN, eds. *The Developing Human: Clinically Oriented Embryology*. 8th ed. Philadelphia, 2008, WB Saunders.)

- The mucus membrane of the respiratory passages, including lung alveoli, develops from the foregut **endoderm**. Simultaneously, the musculature, cartilage and fibroareolar stroma are derived from the **splanchnic mesoderm**, contributing to the overall lung structure.

DEVELOPMENT OF THE LARYNX

- Larynx develops from the cranial end of laryngotracheal tube. It communicates with the pharynx through the laryngeal inlet (Fig. 16.4
- The epithelial lining of the larynx has its developmental roots in the endoderm.
- The cartilages and muscles within the larynx are derived from the mesenchyme of fourth and sixth pharyngeal arches.
- Distinctive arytenoid swellings emerge from mesenchymal proliferation at the cranial end of the laryngotracheal tube. This process converts the primordial **U-shaped furcula** (laryngeal inlet) into a **T-shaped**, narrow laryngeal inlet.
- Proliferation of laryngeal epithelium leads to the temporary occlusion of the lumen, a crucial phase in laryngeal development. By the **10th week**, recanalization occurs, ensuring the proper formation of the laryngeal structure.
- The **laryngeal ventricles** thus formed are surrounded by mucosal folds and their subsequent differentiation yields vestibular and vocal folds.
- **Cartilaginous Derivatives: Thyroid, Cricoid, Arytenoid and Corniculate:**
  - Distinct cartilaginous elements originate from specific pharyngeal arches. The thyroid cartilage, along with the epiglottis and cuneiform cartilages, stems from the **fourth arch**. In contrast, the cricoid, arytenoid and corniculate cartilages trace their lineage to the **sixth arch**.
- **Innervation and Muscular Development:**
  - The network of laryngeal muscles takes shape through the contribution of the fourth and sixth pharyngeal arches. The innervation of these muscles is by the branches of the **10th cranial nerve** (vagus): the **superior laryngeal nerve** from the 4th arch and the **recurrent laryngeal nerve** from the 6th arch.

TRACHEA, BRONCHI AND LUNGS (AN 25.2)

- The epithelium and glands of the trachea and pulmonary epithelium are derived from the **endodermal** lining of laryngotracheal tube.
- The cartilage, connective tissue and muscles of trachea are derived from the **splanchnopleuric mesoderm** surrounding the laryngotracheal tube.

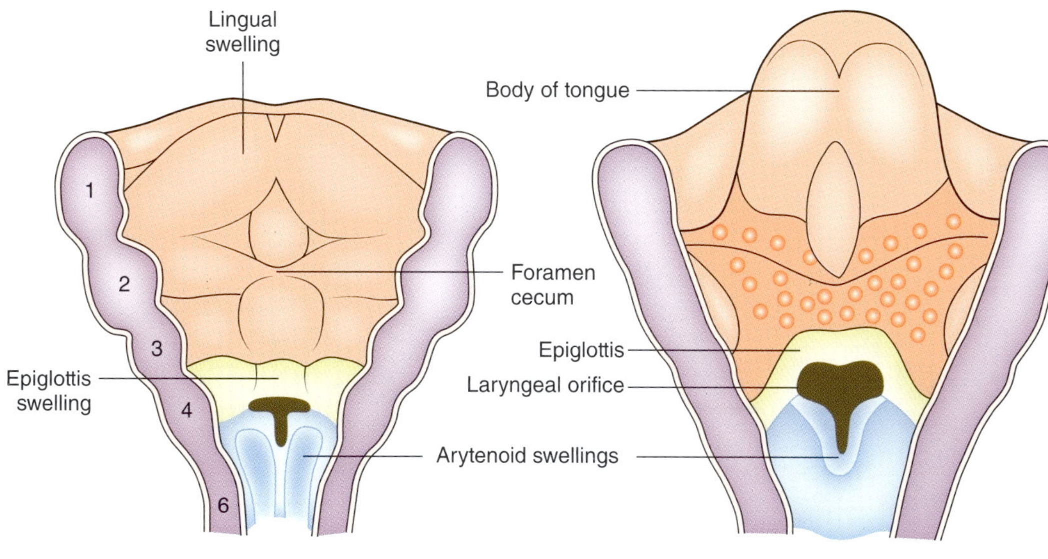

Fig. 16.4 Formation of larynx.

- The process of lung development begins with the caudal end of the laryngotracheal diverticulum forming the respiratory bud or lung bud around the fourth week (Fig. 16.5).
- **Primary Bronchial Buds:**
  - The respiratory bud then undergoes division into primary bronchial buds, projecting into the pericardioperitoneal canals.
- **Pleural Cavities:**
  - The enlargement of the bud transforms the canals into pleural cavities.
  - Each pleural cavity establishes communication with the pericardial cavity through the **pericardiopleural** opening and with the peritoneal cavity through the **pleuroperitoneal** opening. Over time, these openings are closed by pericardiopleural and pleuroperitoneal membranes, ensuring the separation of the pleural cavity from the pericardial and peritoneal cavities.
- **Parietal and Visceral Pleura:**
  - Distinct layers of the coelom contribute to the formation of pleura. The somatopleuric layer, lining the body wall, forms the **parietal pleura**. Simultaneously, the splanchnopleuric layer, investing each bud, persists as the **pulmonary or visceral pleura**.
- Foetal differentiation of the lung pleura consists of two critical stages:
  - The **Early stage**, spanning up to 17 weeks of gestation.
  - The **Late stage**, extending up to birth.
- The mesothelium undergoes membranous differentiation, microvillus covering, the emergence of a vesicular system and intercellular contacts. The late stage witnesses the appearance of the elastic membrane and the differentiation of components within the submesothelial connective tissue layer, including fibroblasts, collagen, elastic fibres, blood vessels and lymph vessels.

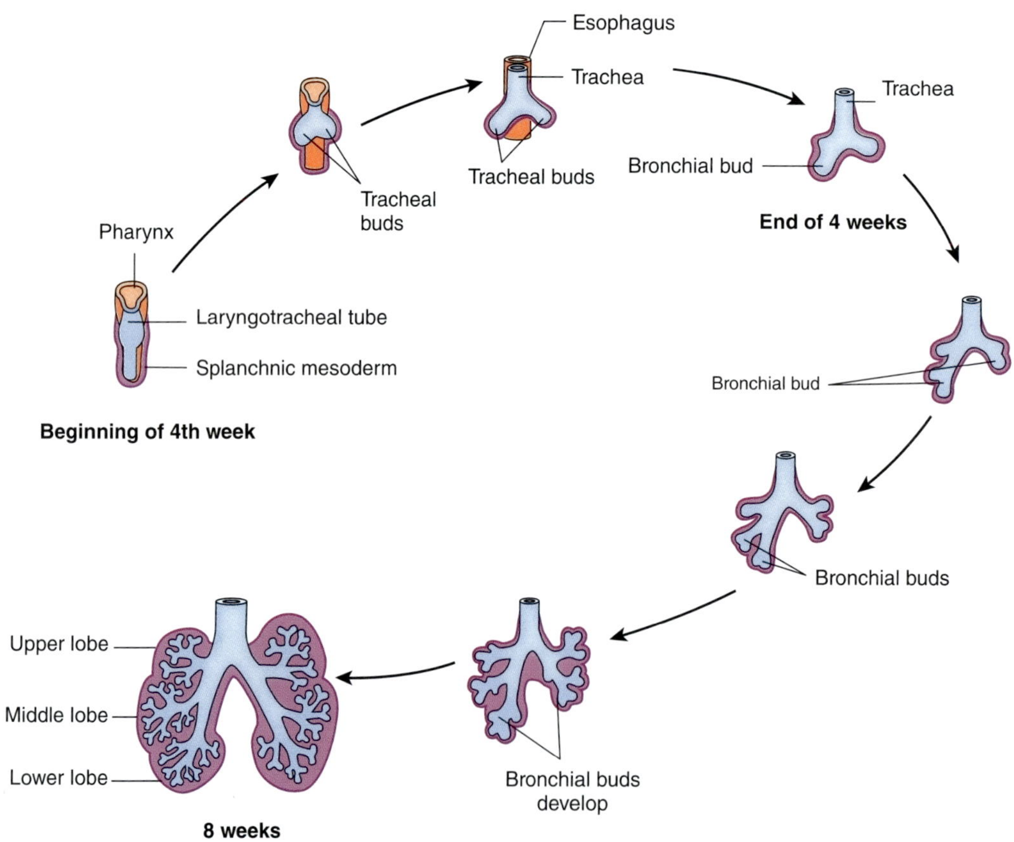

Fig. 16.5 Development of lung buds into primary bronchial buds and secondary bronchi.

- By fifth week of development, the buds enlarge to form right and left main bronchi.
- The **right** principal bronchus divides into **three secondary bronchi** and the **left** principal bronchus divides into **two secondary bronchi**; around which the lobes of lung are differentiated.

MATURATION THROUGH FOUR DISTINCT STAGES

The maturation of the lung progresses through four distinct stages (Fig. 16.6, Table 16.1):

1. **Pseudoglandular Stage (6–16 weeks):** The airways are lined by columnar and cuboidal epithelium, resembling a **tubuloacinar gland**.
2. **Canalicular Stage (16–26 weeks):** Lumina of bronchi and terminal bronchioles enlarge, accompanied by increased vascularity.
3. **Terminal Sac Stage (26 weeks–birth):** Numerous terminal sacs or saccules develop, and their epithelium becomes exceptionally thin.
4. **Alveolar Stage (up to 8 years):** Extending from 32 weeks until around 8 years, this stage witnesses the transformation of respiratory bronchioles into alveolar saccules, representing future alveolar ducts.

PSEUDOGLANDULAR STAGE (6–16 WEEKS)

- During the pseudoglandular stage, the airways exhibit a distinctive epithelial composition. Proximally and distally, the airways are lined by a layer of high columnar and cuboidal epithelium.
- This specific epithelial arrangement bears a striking resemblance to a **tubuloacinar gland**. Hence, this developmental phase is termed the pseudoglandular stage (Fig. 16.6B).
- The mesenchymal cells around the epithelium differentiates into smooth muscle, cartilages and other connective tissue cells.

CANALICULAR STAGE (16–26 WEEKS)

- In the canalicular stage, notable changes occur within the developing lung. The lumina of bronchi and terminal bronchioles undergo considerable enlargement. Simultaneously, the lung tissue undergoes vascularization, facilitating the exchange of gases as the respiratory system matures.
- Respiratory bronchioles further subdivide, giving rise to **primordial alveolar ducts**.
- The cuboidal respiratory epithelium differentiates into simple squamous **type I pneumocytes**. Meanwhile, undifferentiated portions of the epithelium contribute to the formation of **type II pneumocytes**. Type II pneumocytes act as **stem cells** for the developing alveolar epithelium.
- An important event occurring in this stage is the **storage of Surfactants** by type II pneumocytes, a process initiated around the **sixth month** of gestation. Surfactants play a vital role in reducing surface tension within the alveoli, ensuring their stability and preventing collapse during the respiratory cycle (Fig. 16.6B).

TERMINAL SAC STAGE (26 WEEKS–BIRTH)

- During the terminal sac stage from 26 weeks until birth, a significant progression occurs in the lung's structural maturation:
  1. **Terminal Sac and Saccule Formation:** Numerous terminal sacs or saccules undergo development, contributing to the structure of lungs.
  2. **Epithelial Thinning:** The epithelium of these structures becomes notably thin, an important adaptation for efficient gas exchange.
- **Establishment of the Blood–Air Barrier**
  - During this stage, the blood–air barrier is established between the epithelial cells and the endothelial cells, which facilitates optimal gas exchange between the respiratory and circulatory systems (Fig. 16.6B).

ALVEOLAR STAGE (UP TO 8 YEARS)

- It extends from 32 weeks till birth and continues up to 8 years.
- The **respiratory bronchiole** terminates as alveolar saccules, which represent future alveolar ducts.
- For optimal gas exchange capabilities, several changes unfold during this period:
  1. **Surfactant Production in Alveolar Sacs:** Alveolar sacs, integral for gas exchange, actively produce surfactants. These substances play a vital role in lowering surface tension within the alveoli, preventing their collapse during expiration.

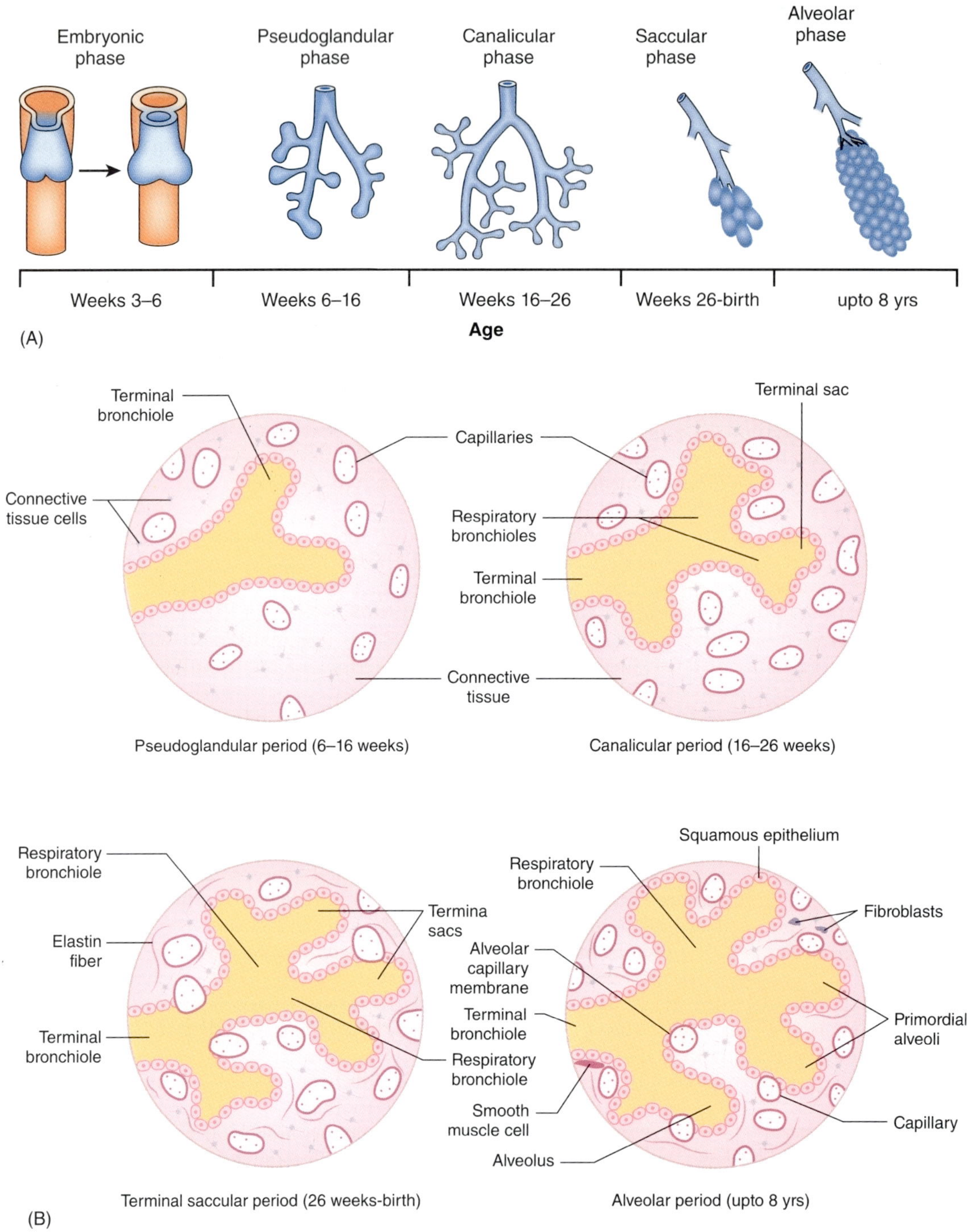

Fig. 16.6 Developmental Progression of Pulmonary Maturation Across Various Stages and Correlation with GestationaL Age.

Table 16.1 Maturation stages of lungs

Developmental Stages	Description
Pseudoglandular stage (6–16 weeks)	The airways are lined by high columnar and cuboidal epithelium proximally and distally, resembling a tubuloacinar gland.
Canalicular stage (16–26 weeks)	Lung tissue becomes highly vascular, and respiratory bronchioles divide into primordial alveolar ducts. Cuboidal respiratory epithelium differentiates into simple squamous type I pneumocytes, while undifferentiated portions form type II pneumocytes, acting as stem cells. Type II pneumocytes store surfactants from the sixth month of gestation.
Terminal sac stage (26 weeks–birth)	Terminal sacs or saccules develop, and their epithelium becomes thin for efficient gas exchange. The blood–air barrier is established between epithelial and endothelial cells, facilitating optimal gas exchange.
Alveolar stage (up to 8 years)	Several changes occur for optimal gas exchange, including surfactant production in alveolar sacs, transformation into gas exchange organs and the establishment of pulmonary and systemic circulation. The appearance of surfactants ensures foetal lung maturity, marking the seventh month as the point of foetal viability.

2. **Transformation to Gas Exchange Organs:** The lungs undergo a transformative shift from primarily secretory organs to specialized structures optimized for gas exchange.
3. **Establishment of Pulmonary and Systemic Circulation:** As the lungs mature, the establishment of both pulmonary and systemic circulation becomes crucial for the efficient transport of oxygen and removal of carbon dioxide.

- Surfactant and Foetal Lung Maturity
  - The appearance of surfactants, particularly those produced by type II alveolar cells, ensures foetal lung maturity. This is significant for the **viability** of the foetus, with the **seventh month** commonly regarded as the point of foetal viability.
- Regulation of Lung Maturation
  - Lung fibroblasts in the surrounding connective tissue play a role in maturation. **Fibroblast pneumocyte factor (FPF)**, secreted by these fibroblasts, stimulates type II pneumocytes to produce surfactants. In instances of preterm births, the administration of **cortisol (hydrocortisone)** serves to release FPF, accelerating lung maturation. Conversely, androgens can delay foetal lung maturation by inhibiting the maturation of lung fibroblasts.

CLINICAL NUGGETS

VACTERL

- VACTERL is an acronym for a diverse range of congenital anomalies affecting multiple organ systems.
- The components of the acronym include:
  - **V**ertebral anomalies.
  - **A**nal atresia.
  - **C**ardiac defects.
  - **T**racheo-oesophageal fistula.
  - **E**sophageal atresia.
  - **R**enal anomalies.
  - **L**imb defects.
- The estimated frequency of VACTERL association ranges from 1 in 10,000 to 1 in 40,000 live-born infants, with a higher prevalence observed in males.
- Several risk factors contribute to the development of VACTERL association.
- **Maternal risk factors:**
  - Maternal diabetes.
  - Assisted reproductive techniques.
  - Chronic lower obstructive pulmonary disorders.
- **Genetic risk factors:**
  - Various gene mutations.
- **Chromosomal anomalies**, including deletions of 5q11.2, duplication of 9q and 22q11.21, supernumerary der (22) syndrome and mosaicism for supernumerary ring chromosome 12 or 18.

KLINISCHE PERLEN

LARYNGOMALACIA

- It is a congenital condition characterized by the softening of the tissues of the larynx above the vocal cords. It is the most common cause of stridor in infants and is typically present at birth.
- Laryngomalacia occurs due to the structural immaturity of the laryngeal cartilages, leading to their collapse during inhalation.

LARYNGEAL WEB

- A laryngeal web/glottic web is a congenital or acquired abnormality in the larynx where there is a membrane or tissue that partially obstructs the airway within the laryngeal inlet. This condition can affect individuals of all ages, and its severity can vary.

Types of Laryngeal Web:

- **Congenital:** Some laryngeal webs are present from birth and may be associated with other congenital anomalies.
- **Acquired:** Others may develop later in life due to trauma, inflammation or surgical procedures involving the larynx.

TRACHEO-OESOPHAGEAL FISTULA (TEF) (AN 25.4)

- It is one of the most frequently seen congenital anomalies in paediatrics. TEF arises from a specific developmental anomaly characterized by a defective tracheo-oesophageal septum. This defect leads to an abnormal connection between the trachea and the oesophagus.
- Infants diagnosed with TEF typically manifest distinctive clinical signs, including:
  - **Respiratory Distress:** A hallmark feature, reflecting the compromised respiratory function.
  - **Feeding Difficulties:** Challenges in swallowing and feeding due to the anatomical abnormality.
  - **Choking Episodes:** Occasional episodes of choking affecting the upper respiratory tract.
  - **Aspiration Risk:** Predisposition to aspiration because of the aberrant communications.
- **Association With Other Anomalies:**
  - TEF often coexists with other congenital anomalies, with cardiac defects being particularly common.
- **Blind Oesophageal Pouch With Tracheo-oesophageal Fistula:**
  - Occurring in approximately 84% of cases, this variant features a blind oesophageal pouch along with a fistula connecting the trachea to the distal oesophagus.
  - The fistula typically enters the trachea in close proximity to the carina.
  - The proximal oesophageal pouch often undergoes **hypertrophy** and dilation due to the foetus's attempts to swallow amniotic fluid.
  - Muscular pouch compression may contribute to **tracheal compression**, potentially leading to **tracheomalacia**.
- **Pure Atresia Without Tracheo-oesophageal Fistula:**
  - This variant represents the second most common anomaly.
  - It involves pure atresia, lacking a tracheo-oesophageal fistula, and is associated with an underdeveloped distal oesophageal remnant.
- **H-Type Fistula:**
  - The H-type fistula is the third most common variation.
  - This variant is characterized by a tracheo-oesophageal fistula without oesophageal atresia. The other variants are depicted in Fig. 16.7.

OESOPHAGEAL ATRESIA

- Oesophageal atresia, a congenital malformation closely related to TEF, shares a similar clinical presentation.
- Oesophageal atresia may occur independently or along with a fistula.
- The proximal end of the oesophagus ends in a blind-ending segment, creating a gap in the continuity of the oesophageal tube. Simultaneously, the distal segment establishes a connection with the trachea, forming a tracheo-oesophageal fistula. This particular presentation represents the most common type of **Oesophageal atresia–TEF combination**.

HYALINE MEMBRANE DISEASE (RESPIRATORY DISTRESS SYNDROME)

- Hyaline membrane disease, also known as respiratory distress syndrome (RDS) in newborns, primarily occurs due to the insufficient production of surfactant in the lungs.
- Waxy layers of **hyaline membrane** line the collapsed alveoli of the lung blocking gas exchange.
- The aetiology of hyaline membrane disease is primarily associated with the immaturity of the premature infant's lungs. The condition is most commonly observed in premature infants, especially those born before 28 weeks of gestation.

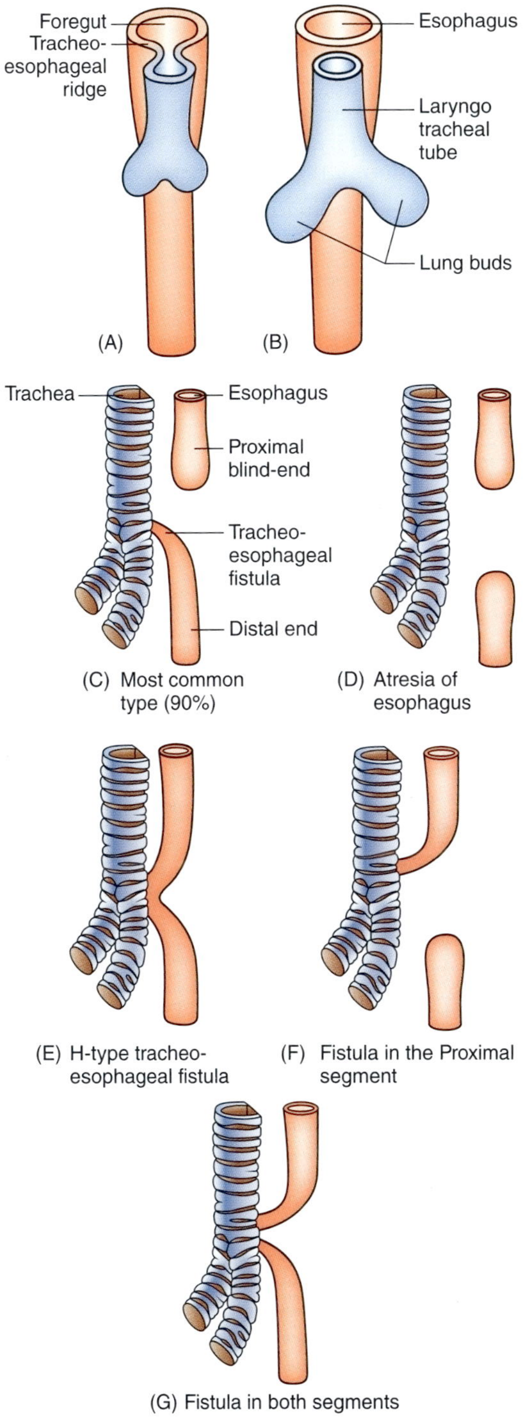

Fig. 16.7 Different types of tracheo-oesophageal fistula. (A and B) Successive stages in the development of the respiratory system. The tracheo-oesophageal ridges form a septum that separates the trachea from the oesophagus. (C–G) are various types of tracheo-oesophageal fistula.

- Surfactant production usually begins around **28–32 weeks** of gestation. Premature infants born before this period often lack sufficient surfactant, leading to RDS.
- Maternal diabetes is considered a potential risk factor for hyaline membrane disease. Poorly controlled diabetes in the mother may contribute to delayed foetal lung maturity.

ABNORMAL LOBES OF LUNGS (FIGS 16.8–16.11)

Azygos Lobes

- Azygos lobes are **supernumerary** structures observed in the lungs.

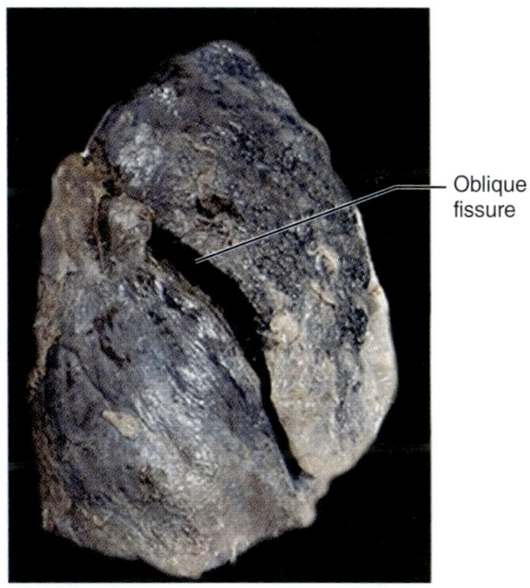

Fig. 16.8 Right lung showing single oblique fissure. (Photo courtesy: Dr Rose.)

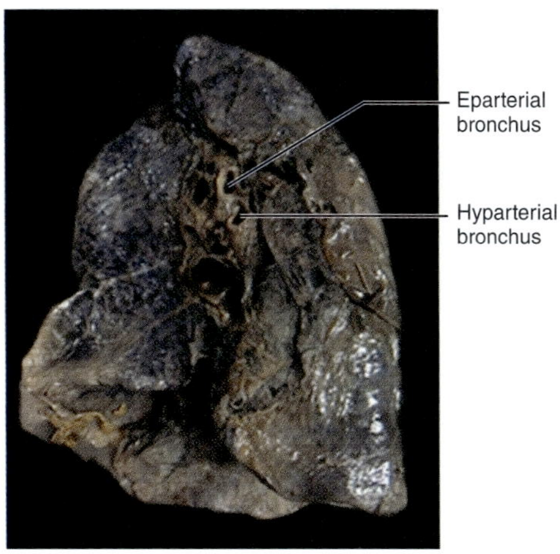

Fig. 16.9 Hilum of right lung showing the bronchi. (Photo courtesy: Dr Rose.)

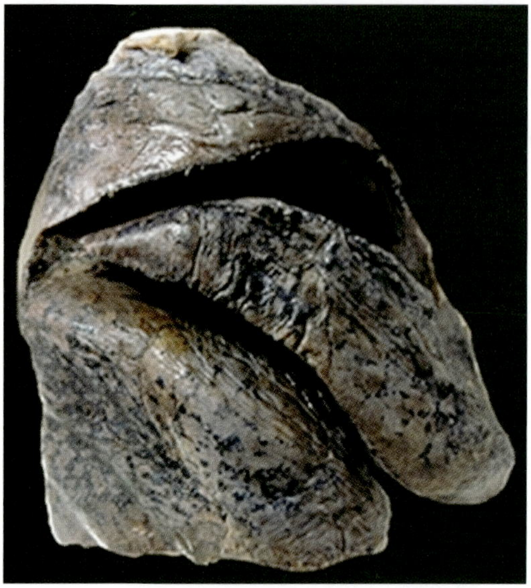

Fig. 16.10 Costal surface of right lung showing two oblique fissures and three lobes. (Photo courtesy: Dr Rose.)

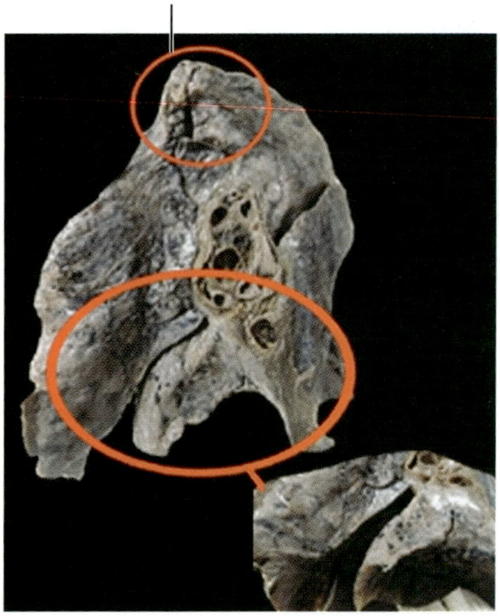

Fig. 16.11 Gross specimen of right lung showing lobe of azygos vein and inferior accessory lobe—a case of pentalobed lung. (Photo courtesy: Dr Rose.)

Lobe of Azygos Vein

- Formed by the arching of the **Azygos vein** over the upper lobe of the right lung.
- The azygos vein courses within a groove created in the **apical lobe.**
- The portion of the lung situated medial to the azygos vein is termed the **lobe of the azygos vein.**

Ectopic Lung Lobes

- Ectopic lung tissue originates from respiratory buds arising from the foregut, which includes the trachea and oesophagus.

Tracheal Lobe

- Refers to a **lung segment** aerated by a bud or diverticulum emerging from the trachea.

POINTS TO PONDER

Initiation of respiratory system

- The respiratory system originates as a ventral diverticulum from the gut, situated caudal to the pharynx.
- The tip of the respiratory diverticulum undergoes dichotomous branchings, with up to 23 sets of divisions.
- Developmental stages
  - **Pseudoglandular stage.**
  - **Canalicular stage.**
  - **Terminal sac stage.**
- **Alveolar stage.**
- These represent crucial phases in the maturation of the respiratory system.
- Common respiratory malformations include **Tracheo-oesophageal fistulas, Atresia and Hyaline membrane disease**.
- The **definitive diaphragm** is formed from the following structures:
  - **Septum transversum.**
  - **Pleuroperitoneal membrane.**
  - **Ingrowths from the body wall.**
  - **Oesophageal mesentery.**
- **Division of coelom:**
- The septum transversum plays a key role in dividing the coelom into thoracic and abdominal regions, establishing connectivity through pleural canals.

BRAIN TEASERS

1. What is the origin of the epithelial lining of the larynx?
   A. Ectoderm
   B. Mesoderm
   C. Endoderm
   D. Neural crest cells
2. From which pharyngeal arches do the cartilages and muscles of the larynx develop?
   A. First and second
   B. Third and fourth
   C. Fourth and sixth
   D. Fifth and seventh
3. What forms the T-shaped narrow laryngeal inlet during development?
   A. Arytenoid swellings
   B. Thyroid cartilage
   C. Vocal folds
   D. Epiglottis
4. When does the recanalization of the laryngeal lumen occur?
   A. 8th week
   B. 10th week
   C. 12th week
   D. 14th week
5. What is the precursor of vestibular and vocal folds in the larynx?
   A. Thyroid cartilage
   B. Laryngeal ventricles
   C. Arytenoid swellings
   D. Cricoid cartilage
6. Which cranial nerve innervates the laryngeal muscles derived from the fourth and sixth pharyngeal arches?
   A. Facial nerve (VII)
   B. Glossopharyngeal nerve (IX)
   C. Vagus nerve (X)
   D. Accessory nerve (XI)
7. From which pharyngeal arch is the thyroid cartilage derived?
   A. First
   B. Second
   C. Third
   D. Fourth
8. What does the caudal end of the laryngotracheal diverticulum form during the fourth week?
   A. Oesophagus
   B. Primary bronchial buds
   C. Respiratory bud or lung bud
   D. Trachea
9. Which layer of the coelom forms the parietal pleura?
   A. Somatic mesoderm
   B. Splanchnic mesoderm
   C. Ectoderm
   D. Endoderm
10. What is the early stage of foetal lung development known as?
    A. Canalicular stage
    B. Pseudoglandular stage
    C. Terminal sac stage
    D. Alveolar stage
11. Which stage of foetal lung development involves the establishment of the blood–air barrier?
    A. Canalicular stage
    B. Pseudoglandular stage
    C. Terminal sac stage
    D. Alveolar stage
12. At what age is the foetus considered viable due to sufficient lung maturity?
    A. Sixth month
    B. Seventh month
    C. Eighth month
    D. Ninth month
13. What stimulates type II pneumocytes to produce surfactants during foetal lung development?
    A. Progesterone
    B. Cortisol (hydrocortisone)
    C. Androgens
    D. Estrogens
14. Which cells act as stem cells for the alveolar epithelium in the developing lungs?
    A. Type I pneumocytes
    B. Type II pneumocytes
    C. Fibroblasts
    D. Smooth muscle cells

Answers

1. (C); 2. (C); 3. (A); 4. (B); 5. (B); 6. (C); 7. (D); 8. (C); 9. (A); 10. (B); 11. (C); 12. (B); 13. (B); 14. (B).

FURTHER READINGS

Clark DC. Esophageal atresia and tracheoesophageal fistula. *American Fam Phys.* 1999;59(4):910-920.

McGowan NA, Grosel J. An overview of esophageal atresia and tracheoesophageal fistula. *JAAPA.* 2022;35(6):34-37. https://doi.org/10.1097/01.JAA.0000830180.79745.b9.

Minuye Birihane B, Alebachew Bayih W, Yeshambel Alemu A, Belay DM, Demis A. The burden of hyaline membrane disease, mortality and its determinant factors among preterm neonates admitted at Debre Tabor General Hospital, North Central Ethiopia: a retrospective follow up study. *PloS One.* 2021;16(3):e0249365. https://doi.org/10.1371/journal.pone.0249365.

Pariza PC, Stavarache I, Dumitru VA, et al. VACTERL association in a fetus with multiple congenital malformations – case report. *J Med Life.* 2021;14(6):862-867. https://doi.org/10.25122/jml-2021-0346.

Reed MF, Mathisen DJ. Tracheoesophageal fistula. *Chest Surg Clin N Am.* 2003;13(2):271-289. https://doi.org/10.1016/s1052-3359(03)00030-9.

Zhang W, Chen J. Prenatal diagnosis of VACTERL association in the first trimester. *Prenat Diagn.* 2022;42(4):482-483. https://doi.org/10.1002/pd.6100.

17 Digestive System

AN 52.6 Describe the development and congenital anomalies of foregut, midgut and hindgut.

ANAMNESE

A 32-year-old male presented with recurrent episodes of abdominal pain and vomiting. Upon investigation, a rare congenital anomaly was identified—**Annular pancreas**. The patient had experienced chronic discomfort, especially after meals, with episodes of bilious vomiting. Imaging studies revealed a ring of pancreatic tissue encircling the second part of the duodenum, causing partial obstruction. Surgical intervention was recommended to relieve the obstruction and alleviate symptoms. The patient underwent a successful bypass procedure, resulting in a significant improvement in his quality of life (Fig. 17.1).

At birth there is a dramatic switch in the supply of nutrients from the placenta to the gut. After the first feeding, the gastrointestinal system is exposed to something different from amniotic fluid. This transition makes it necessary to digest the nutrients prior to their absorption from the gut. The intestine is a site of rapid cellular turnover, mediated by a population of **Intestinal stem cells (ISCs)** that reside at the base of intestinal crypts. The fate of the cells according to the specific regions they are intended to is a complicated task to be undergone in course of development.

- The digestive system extends from mouth to anus. It also includes associated glands and organs.
- During the fourth week, the gut has a head, caudal eminence (tail) and lateral folds in the dorsal part of the yolk sac. With the folding of

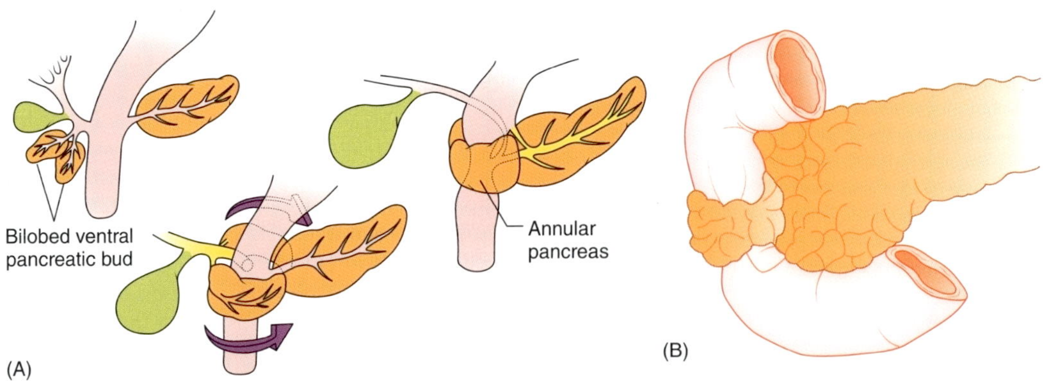

Fig. 17.1 Annular pancreas. (Source: (A) from Schoenwolf GC, Bleyl SB, Brauer PR, Francis-West PH. *Larsen's Human Embryology*. 4th ed. Philadelphia: Elsevier; 2008. (B) from Carlson B. *Human Embryology and Developmental Biology*. 4th ed. Philadelphia: Elsevier; 2008.)

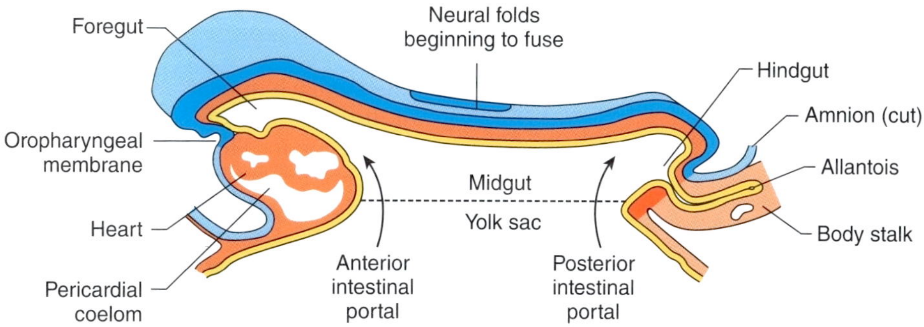

Fig. 17.2 The different parts of primordial gut.

the embryo, the yolk sac is incorporated into the body of the embryo which later develops into the gastrointestinal system.

- The primordial gut is closed cranially by **Oropharyngeal membrane** and caudally by the **Cloacal membrane**.
- Most of the gut epithelium and glands are formed from the **endoderm of primordial gut** (except the epithelium of the cranial and caudal ends which is derived from the ectoderm of the stomodeum and proctodeum).
- The primordial gut is divided in to three parts (Fig. 17.2):
  - **Foregut.**
  - **Midgut.**
  - **Hindgut.**

FOREGUT (AN 52.6)

- The part of the yolk sac which is incorporated into the **headfold** of the embryo is known as the **foregut**.
- The foregut is separated from the primitive oral cavity/stomodeum at the cephalic end by the **Oropharyngeal/buccopharyngeal membrane** and caudally by the **Anterior intestinal portal** (corresponds to the opening of bile duct into the second part of duodenum), which marks the junction between foregut and midgut.
- **Laryngotracheal groove** bulges from the foregut at the ventral aspect of pharyngo-oesophageal junction. Laryngotracheal groove later forms the respiratory system.
- The derivatives of foregut are broadly classified into two parts based on the position of laryngotracheal groove:
  - **Prelaryngeal.**
  - **Postlaryngeal.**
- **Prelaryngeal** or cephalic part develops into:
  - Floor of oral cavity.
  - Tongue.
  - Pharynx.
  - Palate.
  - Submandibular and sublingual glands.
  - Palatine tonsils, middle ear and auditory tubes.
  - Respiratory passages.
  - Some of the structures mentioned above are derived from the branchial arches and their development is discussed in Chapter 14.
- **Postlaryngeal:**
  - Oesophagus and stomach.
  - Duodenum, up to the opening of bile duct.
  - Liver, biliary apparatus and pancreas.
  - Spleen.
- The endodermal part of the primitive gut forms the mucous lining of the gut, and the rest of the wall of the gut including the musculature, stroma and serosa are formed from the splanchnopleuric layer of the lateral plate mesoderm.
- The primitive dorsal mesentery which suspends the primitive gut from the dorsal body wall is formed by the fusion of splanchnopleuric mesoderm and it is through this mesentery the blood vessels reach the gut tube.
- The foregut derivatives (the abdominal part) are supplied by the **Coeliac trunk**, the **artery of foregut** (except pharynx, lower respiratory tract and most of the oesophagus).

PHARYNX

- After the development of the pharyngeal apparatus, the primitive pharynx develops into the **definitive pharynx**.
- The pharynx communicates with the **stomodeum** (which develops into nasal and oral

cavities) by the rupture of oropharyngeal membrane by around fourth week of development.

- The caudal end of the pharynx communicates with the laryngotracheal tube and oesophagus. Thus the pharynx is divided into nasal, oral and laryngeal parts.
- The nasopharynx is connected to the notochord dorsally and later it persists as a mucous diverticulum known as **Pharyngeal bursa or pouch of Luschka**.
- The contribution of endoderm lining of pharyngeal arches to the pharynx are as follows:
  - **First arch**—mucous membrane of lateral wall of nasopharynx.
  - **Second arch**—palatoglossal arch.
  - **Third arch**—pharyngoepiglottic fold.
  - **Fourth arch**—mucous lining of epiglottis.
  - **Sixth arch**—aryepiglottic fold.

OESOPHAGUS

- Develops from foregut immediately caudal to pharynx below the laryngotracheal groove.
- Respiratory diverticulum formed during the fourth week is separated from the oesophagus by the **tracheo-oesophageal septum.** The oesophagus extends from the laryngeal diverticulum cranially to the rudimentary stomach caudally.
- At first the oesophagus is short, but with the descent of the heart and lungs, it lengthens rapidly. Dorsal mesentery or **meso-oesophagus** suspends the oesophagus from the vertebral bodies, and its root contains fused dorsal aortae.
- The oesophagus reaches its final relative length by the **seventh week**. The lining epithelium proliferates and the lumen is narrowed in the beginning and later the central epithelial cells degenerate by a process called **recanalization** and the lumen of the oesophagus is thus restored.
- Its **epithelium and glands** are derived from endoderm. The epithelium gets transformed from ciliated columnar to simple columnar epithelium and finally into stratified squamous epithelium by a process called as **metaplasia**.
- The **muscular coat** is derived from mesenchyme in the **fourth and sixth arch**.
- The muscle layer is **striated** in its upper two-thirds and innervated by the **Vagus**.
- The muscle coat derived from splanchnic mesenchyme is **smooth** in the lower one-third and is innervated by the **Splanchnic plexus**.

STOMACH

- The stomach appears as a fusiform dilatation of distal part of foregut in the fourth week of development. Then the primordial stomach enlarges dorsoventrally.
- The dorsal border of stomach grows faster than ventral border and forms the fundus and **greater curvature of stomach.** The ventral border is concave and forms the **lesser curvature.**

ROTATION OF STOMACH

- Rotation of the stomach is contributed by the rapid enlargement of right lobe of liver, extension of omental bursa dorsal to the stomach and the active growth process of the stomach. Stomach rotates **90 degrees to the right** around a vertical axis (Fig. 17.3).
- Due to this:
  - The **ventral border** (lesser curvature) moves to the right and the **dorsal border** (greater curvature) moves to the left.
  - The left surface of the stomach becomes the **ventral surface** and the right surface becomes **dorsal surface**.
- Its cranial region moves to the left and slightly inferiorly, and its caudal region moves to the right and slightly superior to the median plane.
- **Left vagus nerve** supplies anterior wall of the stomach, and the **right vagus** supplies the posterior wall of the stomach.

MESENTERIES OF STOMACH

DORSAL MESENTERY

- The **Primordial dorsal mesogastrium** is a part of dorsal mesentery of primitive gut and it suspends the stomach from the posterior abdominal wall (Fig. 17.4).
- It also attaches the duodenum with the liver and the abdomen.
- Dorsal mesogastrium is divided by the spleen which develops in its mesenchyme into:
  - **Gastrosplenic ligament** (between spleen and stomach).
  - **Lienorenal ligament** (between spleen and dorsal body wall).

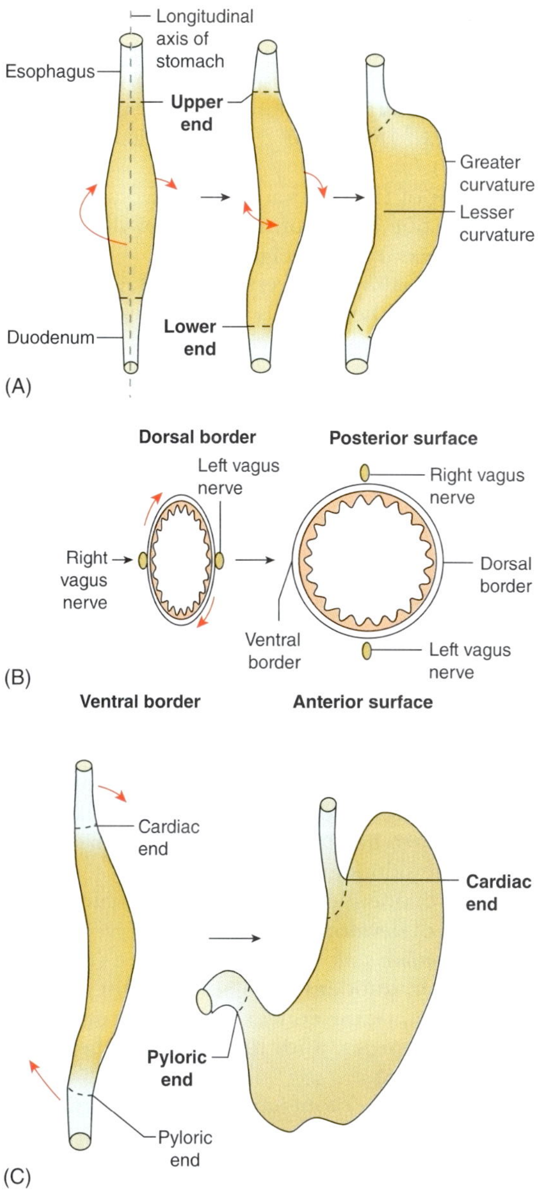

Fig. 17.3 Development of stomach.

VENTRAL MESENTERY

- The ventral mesentery/the ventral mesogastrium is a double-layered membrane which suspends the ventral border of the stomach from the anterior abdominal wall. It is derived from the **Septum transversum**.
- The **hepatic bud** which develops in the ventral mesogastrium divides it into two parts:

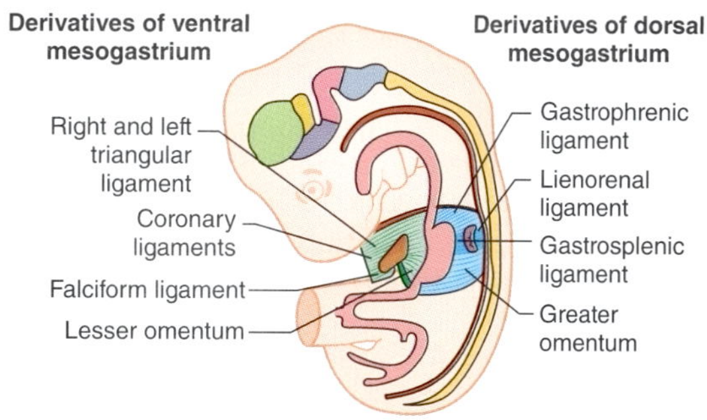

Fig. 17.4 Derivatives of mesentery of stomach.

(a) Lesser omentum, (b) Falciform and coronary ligament.

- **The Lesser omentum.**
  - It consists of two parts:
    - ➢ **Hepatogastric part** (from liver to the lesser curvature of the stomach).
    - ➢ **Hepatoduodenal part** (from liver to the duodenum).
- **The Falciform and Coronary ligaments:**
  - Extending from liver to the anterior abdominal wall.
  - **Umbilical vein** passes in the free border of the falciform ligament.

OMENTAL BURSA

- Isolated clefts develop in the mesenchyme (between the cells of dorsal mesogastrium) which fuse to form a single cavity, the omental bursa or **lesser peritoneal sac**, which communicates with greater peritoneal sac through **Epiploic foramen or foramen of Winslow**.
- Bursa allows the movement of the stomach. This sac pushes dorsal mesogastrium caudally to form **greater omentum**.

CLINICAL NUGGETS

Hypertrophic pyloric stenosis (HPS)

- The **pylorus** (the distal sphincteric region of the stomach) is markedly thickened.
- The circular muscles in the pyloric region are hypertrophied.
- It results in the **obstruction** of the passage of the food.
- As a result, stomach will be distended.
- Presents **3–5** days after birth and boys are usually affected.

DUODENUM

- Duodenum is a **C**-shaped loop.
- It begins to develop in the fourth week (Fig. 17.5).
- It has got **two origins**:
  - Cranial part including the hepatopancreatic ampulla from the terminal part of the **Foregut**.
  - Caudal part from the proximal part of the **Midgut**.

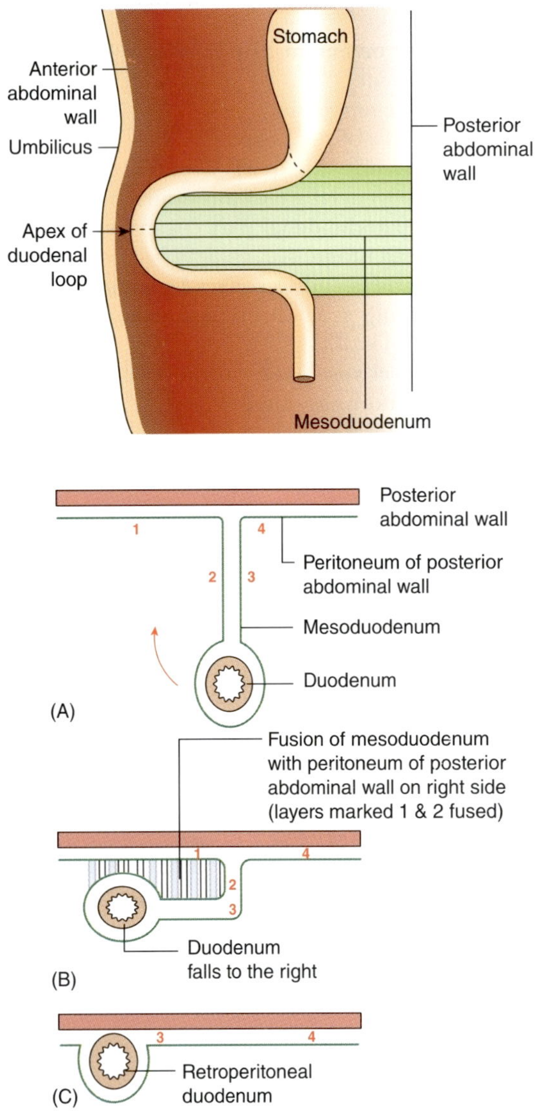

Fig. 17.5 Development of duodenum.

- The junction of these two parts is just distal to the opening of the bile duct. So, it is supplied by both **Coeliac (superior pancreaticoduodenal artery)** and **Superior mesenteric arteries (inferior pancreaticoduodenal artery)**.
- Lumen of the duodenum is temporarily obliterated due to the proliferation of the epithelial cells during the **eighth week.**
- It is recanalized as a result of the degeneration of the epithelial cells by the end of **third month**.
- By the end of the embryonic period, most of the ventral mesentery of the duodenum disappears.
- Musculature is from **splanchnic layer** of lateral plate mesoderm.
- Primitive duodenum presents loop with convexity directed ventrally and in median plane.
- Convex margin attached to anterior abdominal wall by **ventral mesogastrium. Hepatopancreatic bud** arises from this margin at the junction of foregut and midgut and extends into ventral mesogastrium.
- Concave margin is attached to posterior abdominal wall by **mesoduodenum**. From this margin, dorsal **pancreatic bud** arises slightly cephalic to hepatic bud and extends backward into mesoduodenum.
- Then duodenum undergoes **three successive stages** of development:
  - ***Rotation***: along with rotation of stomach, duodenum rotates to right side, so that anterior convex border becomes lateral border and right surface becomes posterior.
  - ***Fixation***: peritoneum of posterior surface of duodenum disappears by **zygosis**. Developing transverse mesocolon pushes duodenum to posterior aspect, making it retroperitoneal **except the proximal 2.5 cm** of the first part (Fig. 17.5).
  - ***Axial rotation***: second part of duodenum undergoes axial rotation due to difference in rate of growth of its wall.
- **Hepatopancreatic bud** comes in posteromedial aspect of second part and dorsal pancreatic bud shifts more ventrally. As a result of the axial rotation, head of the pancreas joins with the rest of the pancreas and the duct system gets established.

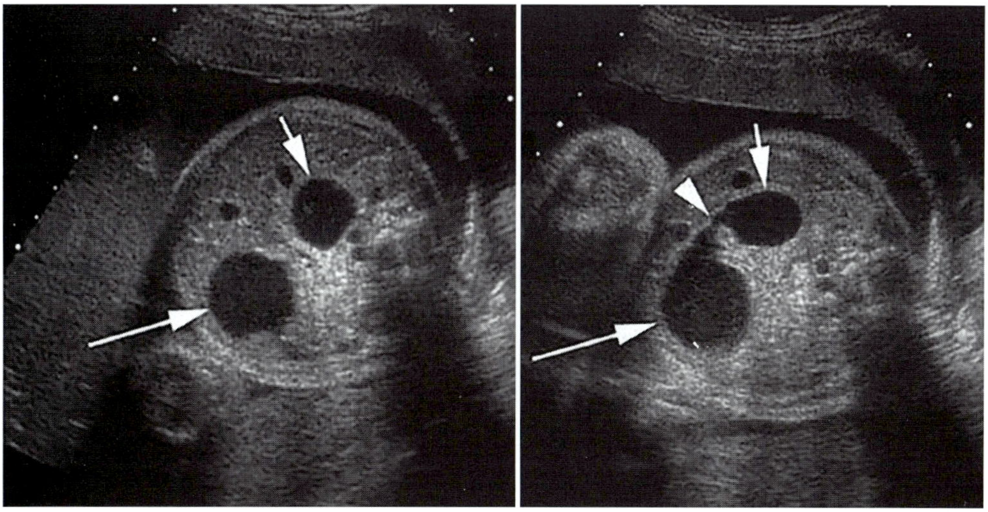

Fig. 17.6 Duodenal atresia. (Source: Rumack CM, Levine D. *Diagnostic Ultrasound*, 5th ed. Elsevier; 2018.)

CLINICAL NUGGETS

Duodenal stenosis

- **Partial** occlusion of the duodenal lumen.
- Due to the **incomplete recanalization** of the duodenum.
- The stomach contents are vomited out due to the duodenal obstruction.

Duodenal atresia

- The **complete** occlusion of the lumen.
- In this, the recanalization of the lumen fails to occur.
- A short segment of the duodenum is occluded.
- Blockage usually occurs at the junction of the bile duct and the pancreatic duct.
- Annular pancreas and ischaemia of duodenum in foetal life can also result in duodenal atresia.
- This condition is diagnosed as **double bubble (distension of stomach and first part of duodenum) sign** in ultrasound (Fig. 17.6).

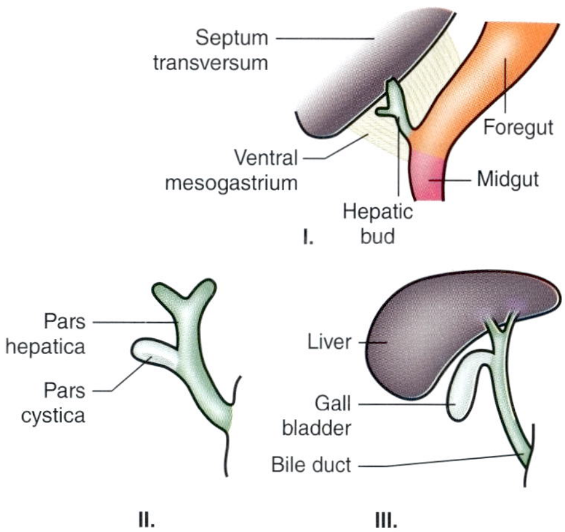

Fig. 17.7 Schematic diagram showing formation of hepatic bud.

DEVELOPMENT OF THE LIVER AND THE BILIARY APPARATUS

- In the beginning of fourth week, the liver, gallbladder and the biliary duct system arise as a ventral outgrowth known as the **hepatic bud** from the distal part of the foregut (Fig. 17.7). Both the hepatic bud and the ventral bud of the pancreas are developed from the **embryonic endoderm**.
- The hepatic bud extends into the **Septum transversum**, a mass of the splanchnic mesoderm separating the pericardial and peritoneal cavities.
- The bud enlarges and divides into two parts: Pars hepatica and pars cystica.
- **Pars hepatica** is large and forms the liver. **Pars cystica** is small and forms the gallbladder.
- The pars hepatica forms the hepatic bud which divides into right and left branches. The liver cells cluster around each branch forming two solid

masses which later differentiate as the right and left lobes of the liver. The proliferating endodermal cells form interlacing cords of **hepatocytes** (parenchyma of the liver) and also form the epithelial lining of the intrahepatic part of the biliary apparatus. The mesenchyme of the **Septum transversum** forms the stroma of the liver.

- The hepatic cords anastomose around the endothelium lined spaces forming the **hepatic sinusoids. The vitelline and umbilical veins** thus break up and join with the hepatic sinusoids.
- First, the **right** and **left lobes** of the liver are of the same size, but later the right lobe becomes larger. The stalk of the hepatic bud forms the bile duct and its two branches persist as the right and left **hepatic ducts.**
- **Haematopoiesis** begins in the liver by **sixth week.**
- **Bile secretion** usually begins in the fifth month of intrauterine life.
- The distal part of the pars cystica forms the gallbladder and the stalk of the diverticulum forms the cystic duct.
- The extrahepatic biliary apparatus is later canalized.

DEVELOPMENT OF THE PANCREAS

- Pancreas develops from the **dorsal** and **ventral pancreatic buds** arising from the caudal part of the foregut (Fig. 17.8). Most of the pancreas develop from the dorsal bud.
- During the rotation of the duodenum to the right, it also carries the ventral bud with it (90 degrees) (Fig. 17.9). The dorsal bud now lies on the left side.

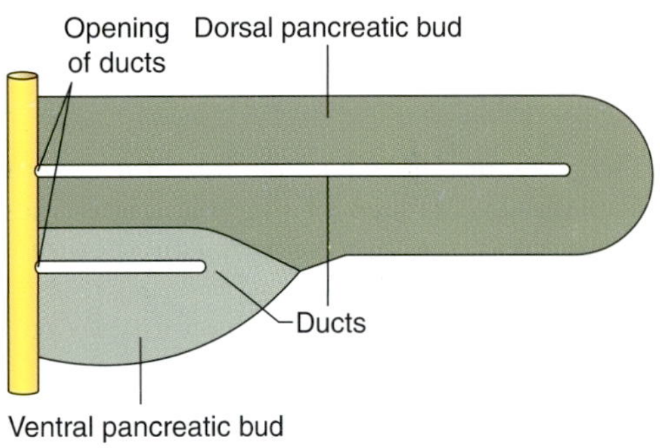

Fig. 17.8 Schematic diagram showing the formation of pancreas from the dorsal and ventral pancreatic buds.

- The ventral bud which is now lying on the right side makes a **180 degree rotation** (total-**90 + 180 = 270 degrees**) so that it comes and lie on the left side below the dorsal bud. It lies posterior to the dorsal bud and fuses with it.
- The **Ventral pancreatic bud** forms:
  - The **Uncinate** process.
  - A part of the **Head** of the pancreas.
- The **Dorsal pancreatic bud** forms:
  - The **entire pancreas** except the lower part of head.
- As the pancreatic buds fuse, their ducts also anastomose.
- The **Main pancreatic duct** is formed by the fusion of:
  - Duct of the **Ventral pancreatic bud.**
  - The distal part of the duct of the **Dorsal pancreatic bud.**
  - The communication between the two ducts.
- The main pancreatic duct opens in to **the Major Duodenal papilla.**
- The proximal part of the duct of the dorsal pancreatic bud sometimes persists as the **Accessory Pancreatic duct**, that opens into the **Minor Duodenal papilla**, located approximately 2 cm cranial to the main duct (Fig. 17.10). The two ducts often communicate with each other.

HISTOGENESIS OF THE PANCREAS

- **Parenchyma** of the pancreas is formed from the endoderm of the pancreatic bud.
- The **pancreatic acini** develop from the cell clusters around the ends of primordial pancreatic tubules.
- The cells lying between the tubules and the acini form **the Islet of the Langerhans.**
- During the 10th week, it starts secreting **Insulin.**
- The cells that secrete **Glucagon** and **Somatostatin** begin to develop before the formation of the beta cells.
- In the case of maternal diabetes mellitus, beta cells get exposed to high level of glucose and these cells undergo hypertrophy.

DEVELOPMENT OF SPLEEN

- Spleen is a haematolymphoid organ. It develops during the **fifth week.**

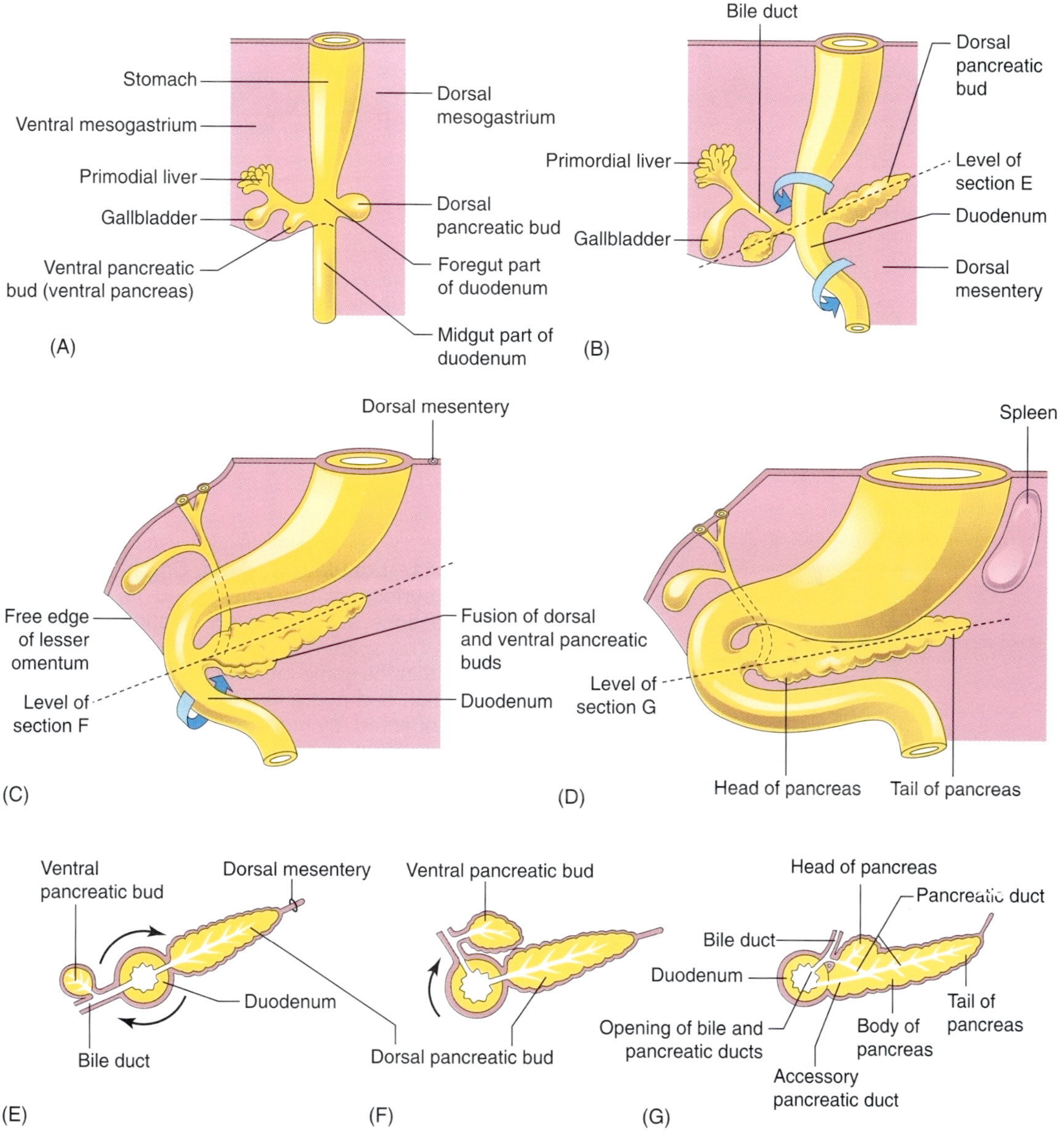

Fig. 17.9 Rotation of duodenum and development of pancreas. (A–C) Illustrations of successive stages in the development of the pancreas from the fifth to the eighth weeks. (D–G) Transverse sections through the duodenum and the developing pancreas. Growth and rotation (arrows) of the duodenum bring the ventral pancreatic bud towards the dorsal bud; these two structures subsequently fuse. Note that the bile duct initially attaches to the ventral aspect of the duodenum and is carried around to the dorsal aspect as the duodenum rotates. The pancreatic duct is formed by the union of the distal part of the dorsal pancreatic duct (duct of Santorini) and the entire ventral pancreatic duct (duct of Wirsung). The proximal part of the dorsal pancreatic duct usually is obliterated, but it may persist as an accessory pancreatic duct, as labelled in the figure. (Source: Moore KL, Persaud TVN. The alimentary or digestive system. In: Moore KL, Persaud TVN, eds. *Before We Are Born: Essentials of Embryology and Birth Defects*. 7th ed. Philadelphia: Saunders Elsevier; 2008.)

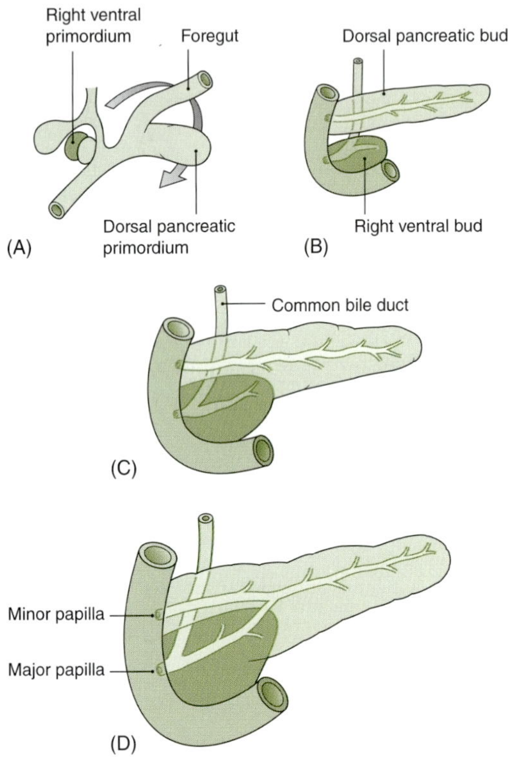

Fig. 17.10 Schematic diagram showing the formation of pancreatic ducts. (A) Four weeks of gestation: formation of the dorsal and ventral pancreatic buds. (B) Six weeks of gestation: rotation of the ventral bud bringing it alongside the dorsal bud. (C) Seven to eight weeks of gestation: fusion of the dorsal and ventral pancreatic buds. (D) Final arrangement of the pancreatic ducts with the accessory duct draining part of the head of the pancreas via the minor papilla *(above)*. The common bile duct meets the main pancreatic duct, which drains the majority of the pancreas via the main papilla *(below)*. (Source: *Pediatric Gastrointestinal and Liver Disease*, 5th ed. 2016.)

- Spleen is developed from a mass of mesenchymal cells **(Splenunculi)** located between the layers of the dorsal mesogastrium.
- The spleen is first lobulated, but the lobules disappear after the birth.
- **Lienorenal ligament** is formed by the fusion of the left surface of the mesogastrium with the peritoneum over the left kidney.
- Lienorenal (splenorenal) ligament contains the **Splenic artery**.
- Presence of **splenic notches** on superior border indicates lobulated origin of spleen (Fig. 17.11).

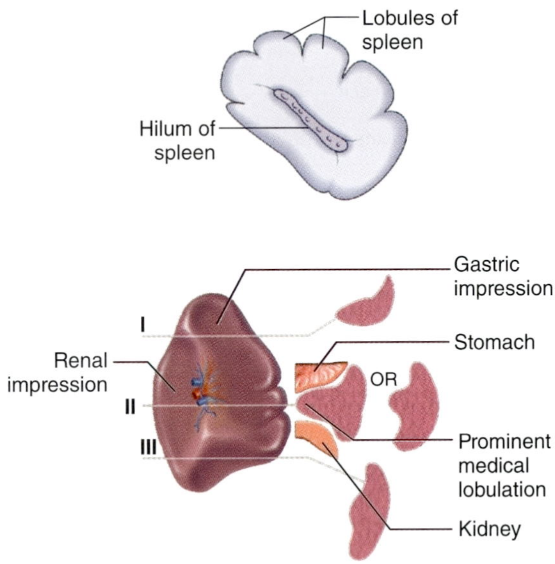

Fig. 17.11 Lobulated spleen. Graphic shows the medial surface of the spleen and representative axial sections at three levels through the parenchyma. The spleen is of variable shape and size, even within the same individual, varying with states of nutrition and hydration. It is a soft organ that is easily indented by adjacent organs. The medial surface is often quite lobulated as it is interposed between the stomach and the kidney. (Source: *Diagnostic Ultrasound for Sonographers*, 2019.)

MIDGUT

- The primitive gut is that part of the gut tube lying between the **Anterior and Posterior intestinal portals**.
- It is suspended by the primitive dorsal mesentery from the dorsal body wall and the **Superior mesenteric artery** which is known as the artery of midgut passes through this dorsal mesentery.
- The **derivatives** of the midgut are:
  - Small intestine, including the duodenum distal to the opening of the bile duct.
  - Cecum, appendix, ascending colon and right two-thirds of the transverse colon.
- Since the coelomic cavity is filled with developing liver and kidneys, there is no space for the coils of intestine inside the abdominal cavity.
- So the elongated midgut forms a ventral **'U'-shaped loop/primary intestinal loop (the Midgut loop)** and projects into the extraembryonic coelom in the proximal part of the

umbilical cord as **umbilical sac**, and the loop remains there from 5th week to 10th week **(Physiological umbilical hernia).**

- **The Superior mesenteric artery** divides the loop into (a) **Cephalic/prearterial segment** (b) **Caudal/postarterial segment**.
- **Cephalic limb** gives rise to duodenum distal to the opening of bile duct, jejunum and major portion of ileum. **Caudal limb** gives rise to terminal part of ileum, caecum, appendix, ascending colon and proximal two-thirds of transverse colon.
- The dorsal end of the cephalic limb forms the duodenojejunal flexure and the dorsal mesentery condenses at this point to form the **Superior retention band** which later forms the **suspensory ligament of duodenum/ligament of Treitz.**
- The dorsal end of the caudal limb forms the colic angle and the **inferior retention band** at this point forms the **phrenicocolic ligament.**
- The loop is connected to the yolk sac at the apex through the **Omphaloenteric duct** Vitellointestinal duct) until the 10th week.

ROTATION OF THE MIDGUT LOOP

- Around the axis of superior mesenteric artery, the midgut loop rotates **90 degrees anticlockwise when viewed from the front** (Fig. 17.12).
- The small intestine (**cranial limb** of the loop) is now on the right and the large intestine (**caudal limb** of the loop) on the left.
- The **cranial limb** elongates and forms the intestinal loops.

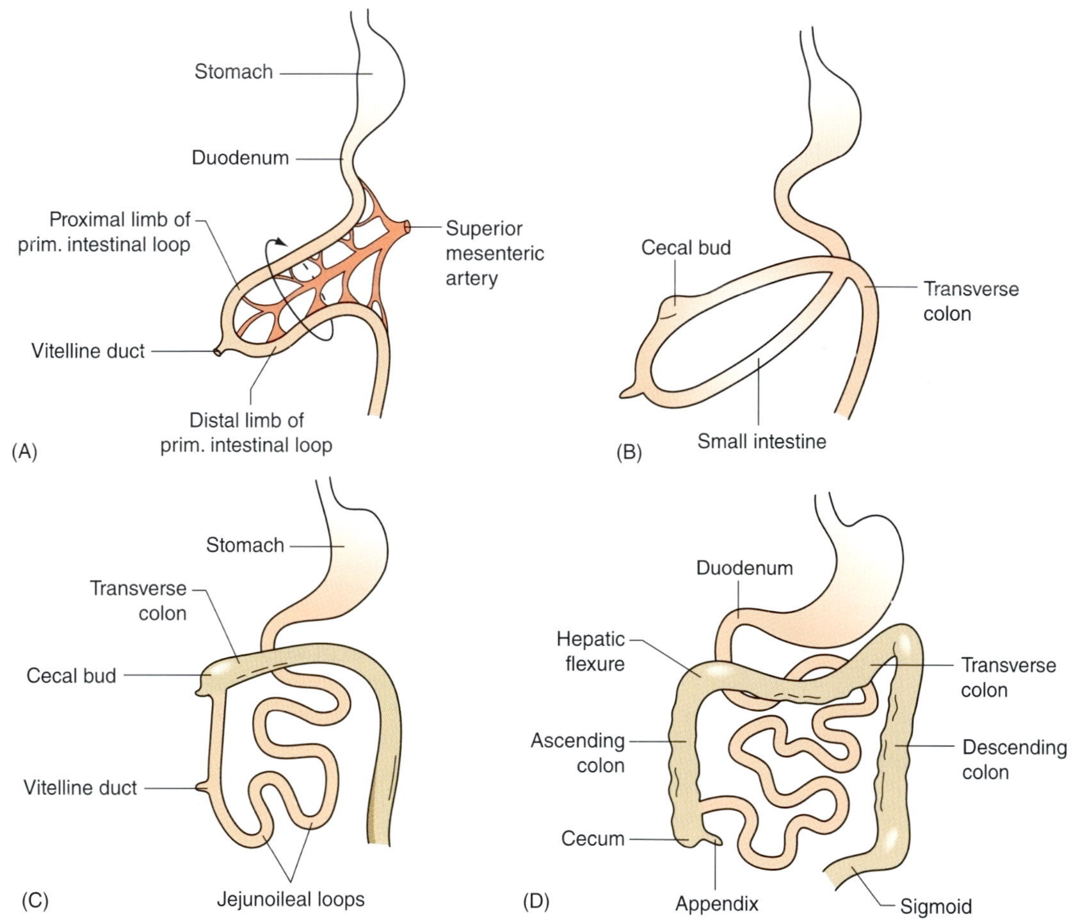

Fig. 17.12 Schematic diagram showing midgut loop and rotation of the loops around the axis of superior mesenteric artery.

RETRACTION OF THE INTESTINAL LOOPS

- The coils of intestines return in to the abdominal cavity during **the 10th week** (reduction of the midgut hernia).
- The factors favouring this are:
  - The enlargement of the **abdominal cavity**.
  - The relative decrease in the size of the **Liver and the Spleen**. But the exact cause is still not known.
- First, the **right limb** or small intestine returns and occupies the central and the right part of the abdomen. The **left limb** including caecum and ascending colon enters last.
- During the return of the large intestine, it undergoes a further **180-degree anticlockwise rotation** upwards and to the right over the small gut around the **axis of the Superior mesenteric artery.** During this rotation, caecum passes through the **left iliac, umbilical and subhepatic regions,** and this explains the reason for abnormal positions of the caecum in rotational anomalies.
- The total rotation by caecum around the axis of superior mesenteric artery is around **270 degrees**. The initial 90 degrees during the phase of **Physiological umbilical hernia** and remaining 180 degrees occurs within the **abdominal cavity** after the reduction of physiological hernia.

CLINICAL NUGGETS

Rotational defects of midgut

- These defects arise when the primary intestinal loop fails to undergo the normal 180-degree anticlockwise rotation while it returns into the abdominal cavity.
- As a result, **the cranial limb** of the primary intestinal loop (jejunum and ileum) ends up on the right side of the body, and **the caudal limb** (colon) ends up on the left side.
- This condition is called **left-sided colon**.

Volvulus of intestines

- In this condition, a part of small intestine or large intestine twists around itself causing an **obstruction** (Fig. 17.13).
- Sometimes, duodenum may be held against the dorsal body wall by **Ladd's band** (bands of abnormal mesentery), resulting in constriction and obstruction.

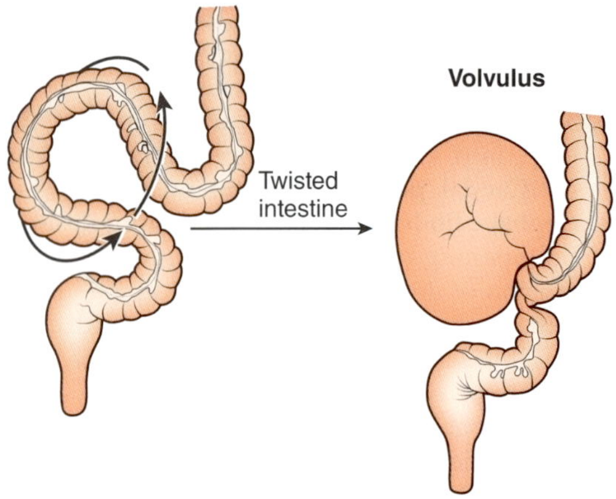

Fig. 17.13 Volvulus.

FIXATION OF THE INTESTINE

- The enlarged colon pushes the duodenum and the pancreas against the posterior abdominal wall.
- Most of the duodenal mesentery gets absorbed. **Prearterial segment** of the dorsal mesentery forms the **mesentery proper** and suspends jejunum and ileum. **Postarterial segment** of dorsal mesentery persists for the transverse colon as **transverse mesocolon**.
- As a result, the following structures become **retroperitoneal**:
  - Major portion of the **Duodenum** (except for the initial 2 cm).
  - The head of the **Pancreas**.
  - The **Ascending colon**.
- Other derivatives of the midgut loop retain their mesentery.

CAECUM AND APPENDIX

- During the sixth week, the caecal swelling appears as an elevation on the antimesenteric border of the caudal limb of the midgut loop. After rotation and fixation, caecum lies in its normal position in the right iliac fossa.
- In case of malrotation, caecum can occupy any position along its course, that is **left iliac fossa, lumbar or subhepatic region.**
- According to the **shape**, the Caecum is classified as follows:
  - **Foetal:** The shape of the caecum is conical and appendix arises as a tube from the apex.

   - **Infantile:** At the base of the appendix, two sacs of equal size develop and the caecum attains a quadrate form.
   - **Adult/normal type (90%):** The right sac enlarges more than the left and the appendix is positioned 2 cm below the ileocaecal junction.
   - **Exaggerated:** In this condition, the right sac enlarges and the left sac gets atrophied. As a result, the appendix lies very close to the ileocaecal junction.
- Initially, the appendix is a small pouch opening from the caecum.
- The appendix increases rapidly in length, so that at birth it is relatively a long-tube arising from the distal end of the caecum.
- After birth, appendix moves to its medial side due to the unequal growth of the caecum.
- There are **various positions** for the Appendix:
   - **Retrocaecal** (appendix may pass posterior to the caecum).
   - **Retrocolic** appendix (posterior to the colon).
   - **Paracolic** (ascends along the sides of ascending colon).
   - **Splenic** (points towards the spleen in front or behind ileum - pre ileal/post ileal).
   - **Pelvic** (appendix may descend over the pelvic brim).
   - **Promontoric** (towards sacral promontory).
   - **Mid-inguinal** (tip vertically downward).
- Most common type is **Retrocaecal** (64%). Most dangerous is **Splenic** (preileal).

HINDGUT

Hindgut lies between the **Posterior intestinal portal** and the **Cloacal membrane** and occupies the tailfold of the embryo.

- The derivatives of **Hindgut** are:
   - Left one-third of transverse colon, the descending colon, the sigmoid colon, the rectum and the superior part of the anal canal.
   - Epithelium of urinary bladder and most of the urethra.
- All hindgut derivatives are supplied by **Inferior mesenteric artery** through the primitive dorsal mesentery.
- The junction between the midgut and hindgut origin of transverse colon is indicated by the change in blood supply **(superior mesenteric artery for right two-thirds and inferior mesenteric artery for left one-third)**.
- The **descending colon** is a retroperitoneal organ.
- The **Allantois** extends as a diverticulum from the ventral wall of the hindgut and divides the hindgut into a narrow tubular **Preallantoic** part and dilated **Postallantoic** part.
- The **Preallantoic** part forms the distal third of transverse colon, descending colon and sigmoid colon. The dorsal mesentery disappears in the descending colon and persists in the sigmoid colon as sigmoid mesocolon. The inferior retention band at the colic angle forms the **Phrenicocolic ligament**.
- The **Postallantoic part** or the endodermal cloaca forms the rectum, upper part of the anal canal, mucous lining of the urinary bladder and the urethra.
- Mucous membrane of rectum above the **Houston's third valve** is developed from preallantoic part of hindgut and below the valve is formed from the dorsal part of endodermal cloaca (see below). The rest of the wall of the rectum is formed from **splanchnopleuric mesoderm**.

CLOACA

- Cloaca is the expanded terminal part of hindgut.
- It is a chamber into which the hindgut and allantois empty.
- It is an endoderm lined chamber and is continuous with the surface ectoderm of cloacal membrane.
- Therefore, cloacal membrane is made up of:
   - **Endoderm** of the Cloaca.
   - **Ectoderm** of the Anal pit.

PARTITIONING OF CLOACA

- The **Urorectal septum** (which develops in the angle between the hindgut and the allantois as the fold of Tourneux) divides the cloaca into **dorsal** and **ventral** parts (Fig. 17.14).
- Infoldings of lateral walls of the cloaca (**folds of Rathke**) grows towards each other and fuse with the **Tourneux fold** to form a partition known as the urorectal septum. The Rathke's fold contain **mesonephric** and **paramesonephric ducts**.
- This partition divides the cloaca into:
   - **Dorsal**—Primitive rectum.
   - **Ventral**—Primitive urogenital sinus.

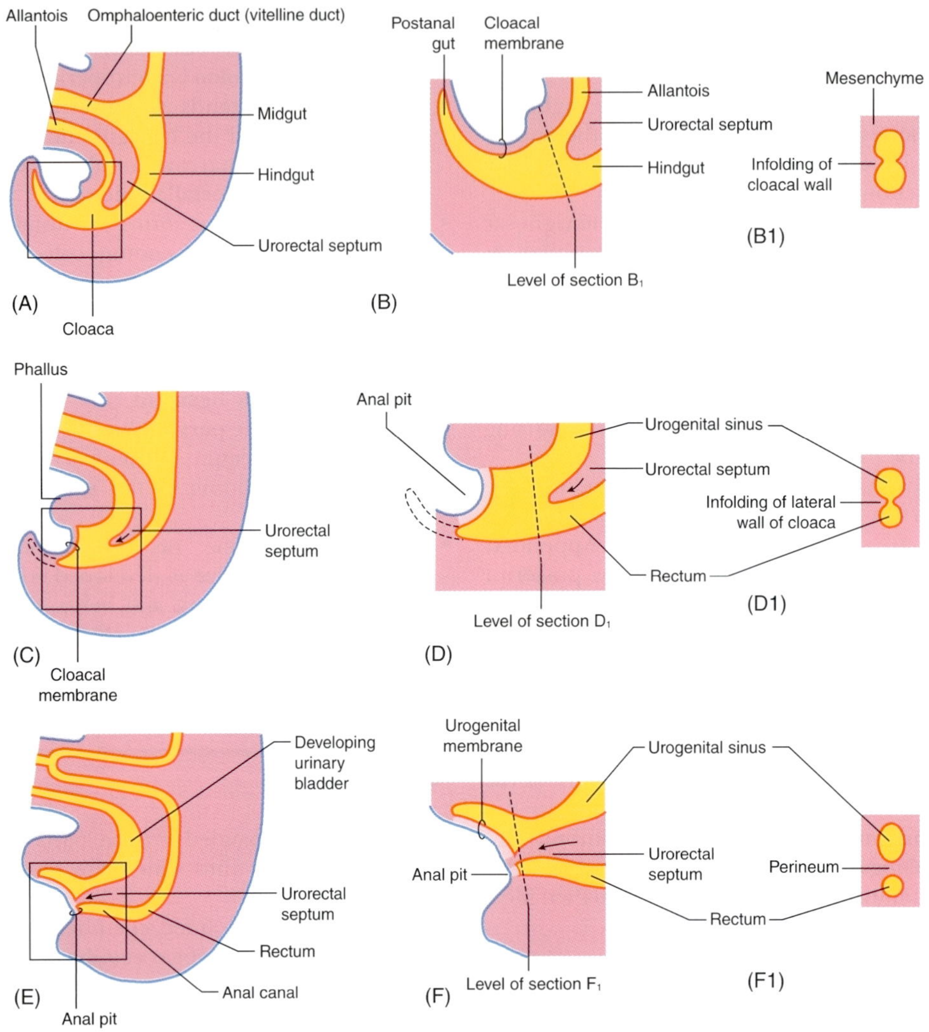

Fig. 17.14 Partitioning of cloaca. Successive stages in the partitioning of the cloaca into the rectum and urogenital sinus by the urorectal septum. (A, C and E) Views from the left side at 4, 6 and 7 weeks, respectively. (B, D, and F) Enlargements of the cloacal region. (B1 and D1) Transverse sections of the cloaca at the levels shown in B and D. Note that the postanal portion (*shown in B*) degenerates and disappears as the rectum forms. (Source: *Pathophysiology*. 6th ed. 2018; Credit line: Moore KL et al, editors: *The Developing human: Clinically Oriented Embryology*. 10th ed. Philadelphia: Saunders, 2016.)

- **Cloacal duct** is a gap between the caudal end of the urorectal septum and the cloacal membrane. Till seventh week, the primitive rectum communicates with the primitive urogenital sinus through the cloacal duct and later the urorectal septum fuses with the cloacal membrane.
- As a result, the cloacal duct is closed and the cloacal membrane is divided into **Urogenital membrane** anteriorly and the **Anal membrane** posteriorly. The point of fusion forms the **Perineal body**.
- The ectodermal cloaca behind the perineal body has a surface depression known as **Proctodeum/Anal pit**.
- **Anorectal lumen** is temporarily closed by an epithelial plug after the degeneration of the cloacal membrane.

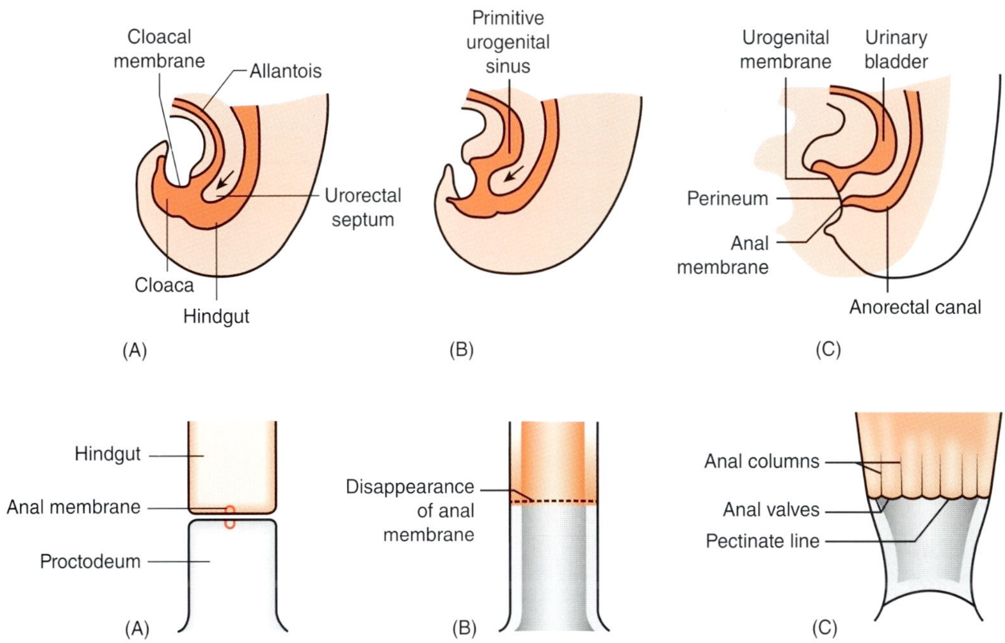

Fig. 17.15 Development of rectum and anal canal. (Source: *Clinical Manual of Surgery*. 2014.)

- Recanalization of anorectal canal results in communication of the rectum with the exterior.

ANAL CANAL

- Upper two-thirds of the anal canal is formed from the hindgut (**Endodermal cloaca**) (Fig. 17.15). The lower part is from the **Anal pit/Ectodermal proctodeum**.
- The junction between the two parts is indicated by the irregular **Pectinate line**, located in the inferior limit of the anal valves.
- Anocutaneous line (**white line of Hilton**) is where the anal epithelium changes from columnar to **stratified squamous cells** (located 2 cm above the anus).
- Epithelium is keratinized and continuous with the skin around the anus.
- **Upper two-thirds** of the Anal canal:
  - Supplied by **Superior rectal artery** (continuation of the inferior mesenteric artery).
  - Venous drainage is to the corresponding vein.
  - Lymphatic drainage to the inferior mesenteric nodes.
- **Lower one-third** of the Anal canal:
  - Supplied by **Inferior rectal artery** (branch of the internal pudendal artery).
  - Venous drainage is through inferior rectal vein.
  - Lymphatic drainage to the superficial inguinal nodes.

HISTOGENESIS OF MIDGUT AND HINDGUT

- The mucous membrane and glands are of **Endodermal origin.**
- The submucosa, muscularis externa and serosa are derived from the **Splanchnic mesoderm**.
- Peristaltic movements begin by fourth month of intrauterine life.

KLINISCHE PERLEN

OESOPHAGEAL ATRESIA

- Blockage of the oesophageal lumen (Fig. 17.16). **Polyhydramnios** is usually present.
- Occurs mainly (one-third) in the infants born prematurely.

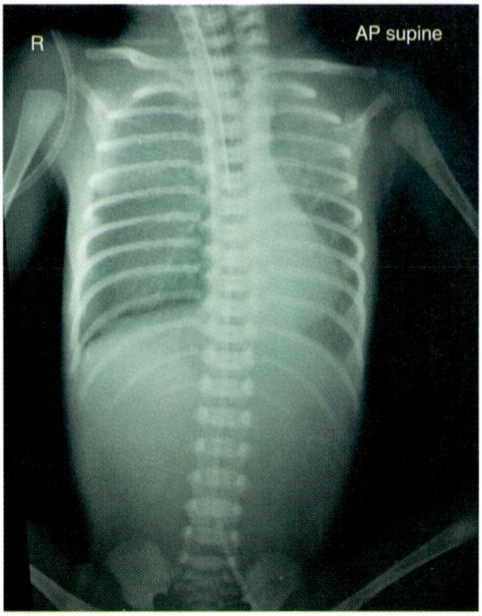

Fig. 17.16 X-ray of a newborn with oesophageal atresia. The nasaogastric tube failed to proceed beyond a point behind the sternum. (Photo courtesy: Dr Nithya.)

- Associated with **tracheo-oesophageal fistula** in more than 90% cases.
- Atresia results due to:
  - The deviation of **Tracheo-oesophageal septum** posteriorly.
  - Incomplete separation of oesophagus from the **Laryngotracheal tube**.

OESOPHAGEAL STENOSIS

- Narrowing of the lumen of oesophagus.
- Can occur anywhere (usually in the **lower one-third**).
- Due to:
  - **Incomplete recanalization** of oesophagus during eighth week.
  - Failure of **blood vessels** to develop in the affected area.

LIVER ANOMALIES

- Liver lobulations (not common).
- Variations of the hepatic duct, bile duct and cystic duct.
- Accessory hepatic ducts are also present.

EXTRAHEPATIC BILIARY ATRESIA

- It is the obliteration of the bile ducts between porta hepatis and duodenum.

ECTOPIC PANCREAS

- It is located other than the normal position of the pancreas.
- It may be present in:
  - The mucosa of the **Stomach**.
  - Proximal **Duodenum**.
  - **Jejunum.**
  - **Pyloric antrum.**
  - **Meckel's diverticulum.**
- This is usually asymptomatic.

ANNULAR PANCREAS

- Seen around the **second part of the Duodenum** (Fig. 17.17). It may cause obstruction of the duodenum.
- This defect is also associated with:
  - **Down syndrome.**
  - **Intestinal malrotation.**
  - **Cardiac defects.**
- It results from the **bifurcation** of the ventral pancreatic bud around the duodenum.
- As a result, the ventral bud fuses with the dorsal bud forming a **ring**.
- **Pancreatic divisum** is a congenital anomaly in which a single pancreatic duct is absent, instead two distinct dorsal and ventral ducts are seen.

ACCESSORY SPLEENS

- Development of one or more small functional spleens other than the main spleen.
- Found in:
  - The **hilum of Spleen**.
  - Tail of **Pancreas**.
  - Within the **Gastrosplenic ligament**.
- In **Polysplenia** multiple small spleens are formed without a main spleen.

CONGENITAL OMPHALOCELE

- The **physiological herniation** of the abdominal contents into the proximal part of the umbilical cord persists.
- Intestine and liver commonly herniated and are covered by a peritoneal sac.
- Associated with **chromosomal anomalies**.

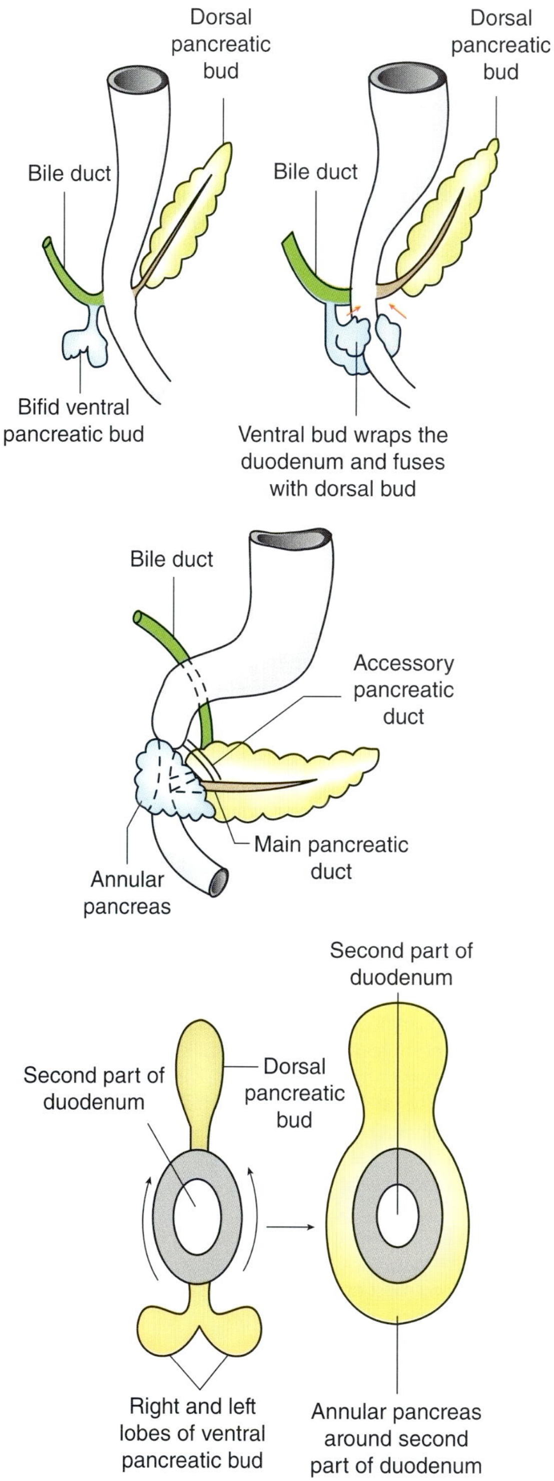

Fig. 17.17 Annular pancreas.

UMBILICAL HERNIA

- Herniation of the intestine after the return of the intestine into the abdominal cavity during the **10th** week.
- Presents as a soft swelling near the umbilicus.
- Seen in **premature babies** and low birth weight babies.
- It becomes more evident when the infant cries or strains.
- 95% of umbilical hernias **close spontaneously** by the age of 5 years.
- It is seen associated with **Beckwith-Wiedemann** syndrome.

GASTROSCHISIS

- It is a defect lateral to the median plane of the **anterior abdominal wall**.
- Through this defect the abdominal viscera herniate.
- **Not associated** with chromosomal anomalies.

ANORECTAL ANOMALIES

- It results from the incomplete separation of the cloaca into the urogenital and anorectal parts due to the abnormal development of the **Urorectal septum** (Fig. 17.18).

CONGENITAL MEGACOLON

- Congenital megacolon (**Hirschsprung disease**) is dominantly inherited multigenic disorder (**RET** gene coding **tyrosine kinase** receptor on chromosome **10q11**).
- **Rectum** most commonly involved.
- It is the absence of parasympathetic ganglion cells in the distal colon due to the failure of **neural crest cells** to migrate.
- Colon is **dilated** above the affected region (Fig. 17.19).

MECKEL'S DIVERTICULUM (ILEAL DIVERTICULUM)

- Usually presents before **2 years** of age.
- It is the persistent vitellointestinal duct seen in **2%** of the population.
- **Two inches** in length.
- Two types of heterotopic mucosa (**Pancreatic or Gastric mucosa**).

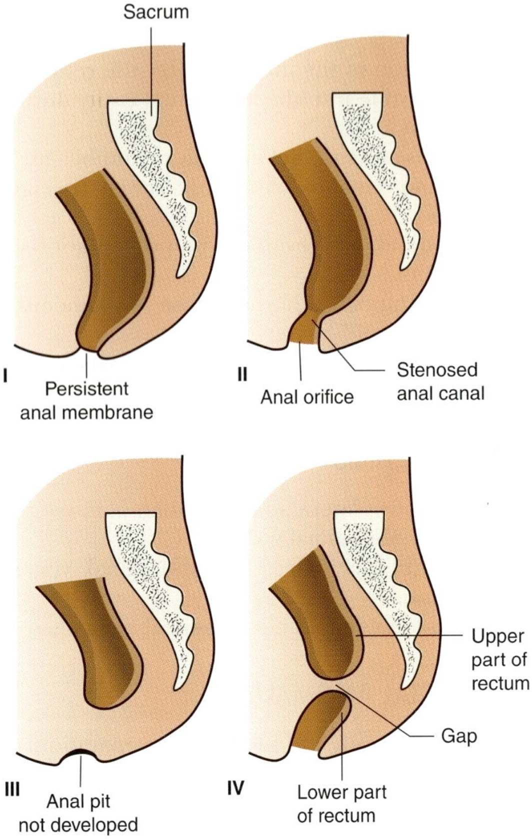

Fig. 17.18 Various types of imperforate anus.

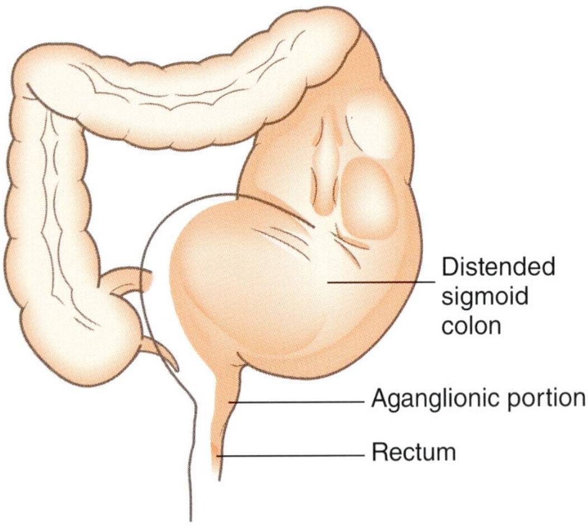

Fig. 17.19 Congenital aganglionic megacolon. (Source: *Radiographic Pathology for Technologists*, 7th ed. 2018.)

- **Two feet** away from ileocaecal valve on the antimesenteric border of ileum.

APPLE-PEEL ATRESIA

- Atresia of proximal **Jejunum**,
- The affected portion is coiled around a mesenteric remnant like an apple-peel.

POINTS TO PONDER

- The endodermal gut tube consists of a cranial foregut, caudal hindgut and a midgut, which opens into the yolk sac through the **vitelline duct**.
- The arterial supply to the gut develops from ventral branches of the **Dorsal aortae**.
- Five of these vitelline artery derivatives supply the thoracic foregut, and three arterial trunks—the **coeliac, superior mesenteric and inferior mesenteric arteries** supply the abdominal gut.
- The **Primary intestinal loop** herniates and rotates around its long axis by **90 degrees** anticlockwise.
- As a result, the future ileum lies in the right abdomen and the future large intestine lies in the left abdomen.
- After 10 weeks, the intestinal loop is retracted into the abdominal cavity and rotates through an additional **180 degrees anticlockwise** to reach the final destination.

BRAIN TEASERS

1. What are the two broad classifications of derivatives of the foregut?
   A. Preoral and postoral
   B. Prelaryngeal and postlaryngeal
   C. Prepharyngeal and postpharyngeal
   D. Preoesophagus and postoesophagus
2. Which part of the foregut develops into the floor of the oral cavity, tongue, pharynx and palate?
   A. Prelaryngeal
   B. Postlaryngeal
   C. Sublaryngeal
   D. Infraglottic
3. What is the primary artery supplying the derivatives of the foregut, excluding the pharynx, lower respiratory tract and most of the oesophagus?
   A. Superior mesenteric artery
   B. Common carotid artery
   C. Inferior vena cava
   D. Celiac trunk
4. During the development of the oesophagus, what separates it from the respiratory diverticulum?
   A. Tracheo-oesophageal septum
   B. Broncho-oesophageal septum

C. Pulmo-oesophageal septum
D. Laryngo-oesophageal septum

5. Which nerve innervates the upper two-thirds of the oesophagus?
   A. Phrenic nerve
   B. Vagus nerve
   C. Sympathetic trunk
   D. Glossopharyngeal nerve
6. What is the purpose of the omental bursa (lesser peritoneal sac)?
   A. Allows stomach movement
   B. Aids in digestion
   C. Stores nutrients
   D. Facilitates gas exchange
7. Which condition is characterized by the marked thickening of the pylorus, resulting in obstruction of food passage?
   A. Gastritis
   B. Hiatal hernia
   C. Hypertrophic pyloric stenosis (HPS)
   D. Peptic ulcer disease
8. What temporary process occurs during the eighth week concerning the duodenal lumen?
   A. Fusion
   B. Obliteration
   C. Dilation
   D. Recanalization
9. Which bud gives rise to the uncinate process and a part of the head?
   A. Ventral pancreatic bud
   B. Dorsal pancreatic bud
   C. Hepatopancreatic bud
   D. Splenopancreatic bud
10. What is the role of the urorectal septum in the development of the cloaca?
    A. Forms the anal canal
    B. Divides the cloaca into dorsal and ventral parts
    C. Initiates recanalization
    D. Develops into the urethra
11. Where does the upper two-thirds of the anal canal originate from?
    A. Foregut
    B. Midgut
    C. Hindgut
    D. Urogenital sinus
12. What is the embryonic origin of the venous drainage for the upper two-thirds of the anal canal?
    A. Inferior vena cava
    B. Inferior mesenteric vein
    C. Superior mesenteric vein
    D. Hepatic portal vein
13. What vessels supply the derivatives of the hindgut?
    A. Celiac artery
    B. Superior mesenteric artery
    C. Inferior mesenteric artery
    D. Hepatic artery
14. What structure divides the cloaca into dorsal-rectum and ventral-urogenital sinus?
    A. Omphaloenteric duct
    B. Urorectal septum
    C. Tracheo-oesophageal septum
    D. Mesentery

Answers

1. (B); 2. (A); 3. (D); 4. (A); 5. (B); 6. (A); 7. (C); 8. (B); 9. (A); 10. (B); 11. (C); 12. (B); 13. (C); 14. (B).

FURTHER READINGS

Ali Almoamin HH, Kadhem SH, Saleh AM. Annular pancreas in neonates; Case series and review of literatures. *Afr J Paediatr Surg.* 2022;19(2):97-101. doi:10.4103/ajps.AJPS_180_20.

Devi GK, Goei AHY, Ragavendra K, et al. Meckel's diverticulum – clinical presentation and pitfalls in diagnosis in the pediatric age group in Singapore. *J Indian Assoc Pediatr Surg.* 2022;27(3):340-344. doi:10.4103/jiaps.JIAPS_392_20.

Ma S, Yu Y, Pan A, et al. The classification and surgical treatments in adult Hirschsprung's disease: a retrospective study. *Front Med.* 2022;9:870342. doi: 10.3389/fmed.2022.870342.

Sapkota A, Batajoo A, Lamichhane S, Shrestha A, Bhatt N. Twists and turns: a case report of cecal volvulus. *Clin Case Rep.* 2023;11(9):e7936. doi:10.1002/ccr3.7936.

18 Urogenital System

AN 52.7 Describe the development of urinary system.
AN 52.8 Describe the development of male and female reproductive system.

ANAMNESE

A newborn was diagnosed with **Urachal fistula**, a rare congenital anomaly involving the persistence of the urachus, a structure that connects the bladder to the umbilicus during foetal development. Concerned about persistent drainage near the umbilicus, the parents sought medical attention, leading to a thorough examination and diagnostic imaging. The presence of urachal fistula was identified, which caused urine to drain through an abnormal opening. Prompt surgical intervention was done to prevent complications, such as infections (Fig. 18.1).

The intermediate mesoderm, a region that lies between the somites and lateral plate in the developing embryo, is the source of all vertebrate kidney tissue. The **Intermediate mesoderm** is highly patterned along the anterior-posterior axis. Organs and structures arise at particular locations along the anterior-posterior embryonic axis. The kidney is an example of an organ that develops in a specific position along this axis. In humans, the definitive kidney is the metanephros, whereas the pronephros- and mesonephros largely degenerate or are incorporated into the developing reproductive system. The pronephros appears to arise *de novo* from cells in the intermediate mesoderm, the mesonephros arises along the course of the nephric duct and the metanephros is generated by mutual inductions between duct and mesenchyme.

- **Urogenital system** consists of **urinary system** and **genital system** which are developed from intermediate mesoderm. Urinary system appears first compared to the genital system.
- The mesonephric ridge of the developing kidney induces the formation of genital ridge from which the gonads are developed.

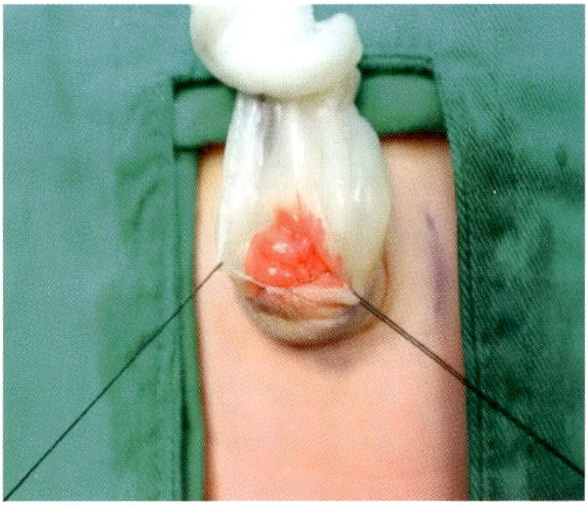

Fig. 18.1 Urachal fistula. (Source: *EUCR*: An-Shine Chao, Chih-Wei Chien, Jin-Yao Lai, et al., Fig. 3, Volume 39, ISSN 2214-4420, Copyright Authors, 2021.)

URINARY SYSTEM (AN 52.7)

Urinary system consists of:
- **Kidneys**
- **Ureters**

- **Urinary bladder**
- **Urethra**

KIDNEY (RENAL SYSTEM)

- The intermediate mesoderm in the cervical and upper thoracic region forms segments known as **Nephrotome**. The remaining unsegmented region is known as **Nephrogenic cord** (Fig. 18.2).
- Renal system develops from the **Intermediate mesoderm** in the cranio caudal direction. Pronephric and mesonephric kidneys are temporary, whereas metanephric kidney persist as the permanent kidney.
  - **Pronephros** (rudimentary and nonfunctioning—seen in fish).
  - **Mesonephros** (functioning during early foetal period—seen in fish and amphibians).
  - **Metanephros** (forms permanent kidney).

PRONEPHROS

- Formed in the cervical region and upper thoracic region of the intermediate mesoderm at the beginning of fourth week. It consists of **Pronephric tubules** (seven to eight) and a single **Pronephric duct**. The duct opens into the ventral part of cloaca.
- By the end of **fourth week**, all pronephric tubules disappear and the pronephric duct persists. The duct is utilized as the duct of mesonephric kidney in later course of development.

MESONEPHROS

- Mesonephros is formed in the **upper thoracic** and **lumbar region** (up to L3) as mesonephric tubules (70–80) and its lateral end opens into the pronephric duct (Fig. 18.3).
- The excretory tubules appear first which give rise to **Glomerulus and Bowman's capsule (Renal corpuscle)**.
- The excretory tubules enter the collecting duct known as **Mesonephric duct/Wolffian duct (Primitive Pronephric duct)**.
- By eighth week only 26 tubules and a single duct persist in the upper three lumbar region.
- The mesonephros forms an ovoid mass and projects into the coelomic cavity as

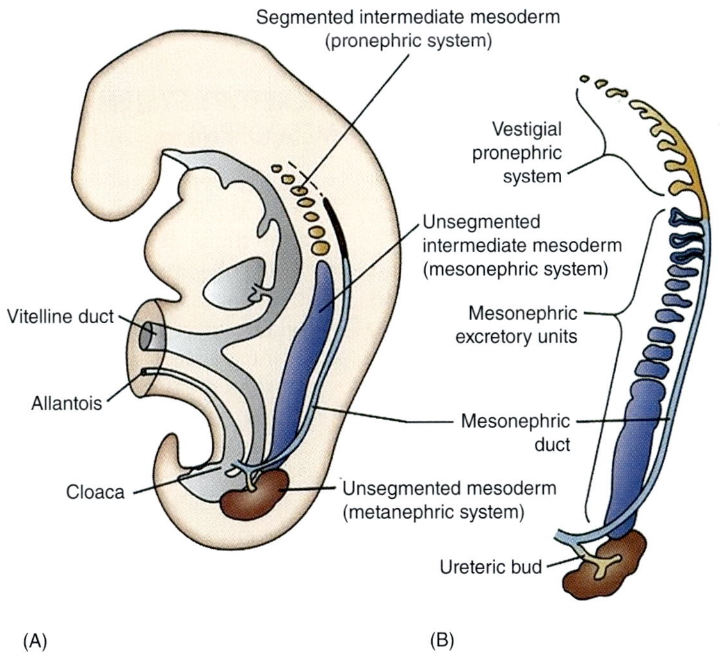

Fig. 18.2 Nephrotome (segmented) and nephrogenic cord (unsegmented). (Source: Fanaroff and Martin's Neonatal-Perinatal Medicine, 2-Volume Set: Diseases of the Fetus and Infant, 11th ed.: Richard J. Martin, Avroy A. Fanaroff, Michele C. Walsh, Fig. 93.1, Elsevier Inc., 2020.)

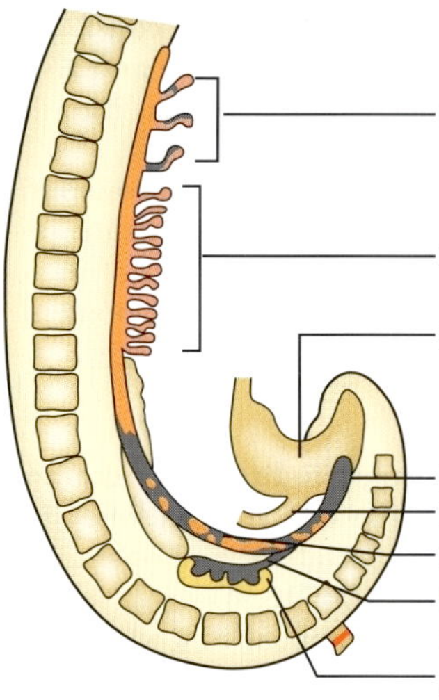

Fig. 18.3 The developing duct system of kidney.

Mesonephric ridge on each side of the dorsal mesentery.

- The mesothelium covering the medial side of the mesonephric ridge forms the **Genital ridge** from which male and female gonads develop.
- The remaining mesonephric tubules form efferent ductules of testes (proximal two persist as **Ductus superior aberrant**, distal tubules persist as **Ductus inferior aberrant** and **Paradidymis** and the middle tubules form the **efferent ductules of testes**) in males. The **Mesonephric duct** forms the canal of epididymis, vas deferens, seminal vesicle and ejaculatory duct.
- Most of the tubules disappear in females and some persist as tubules of **Epoophoron** and **Paroophoron**. Mesonephric duct also disappear and sometimes persist as the duct of **Gartner** or duct of epoophoron in the broad ligament.
- **Ureteric bud** develops from the mesonephric duct before its complete disappearance.

METANEPHROS

- It gives rise to the permanent excretory system—the **Kidney**. It appears in the lumbosacral segment.
- The kidney consists of
  - **Collecting system** (develops earlier).
  - **Excretory system**.

COLLECTING SYSTEM (MESONEPHRIC DUCT)

- It consists of ureter, pelvis, major and minor calyces, and collecting tubules.
- The mesonephric duct (caudal part) close to cloaca forms the **Ureteric bud** dorsomedially in the fifth week of intrauterine life.
- **Common excretory duct** is the portion of the mesonephric duct between ureteric bud and cloaca.
- The ureteric bud dilates and shifts to the dorsolateral aspect of the mesonephric duct and penetrates the **nephrogenic cord dorsal to the mesonephric ridge.**
- The nephrogenic cord forms a cap known as **Metanephric blastema** around the dilated end of ureteric bud.
- The stalk of the ureteric bud forms the **Ureter**. It presents two fusiform dilatations known as **Pelvic** and **Lumbar** dilatations. The ends of these dilatations persist as **three constrictions** of the ureter.
- The dilated end persists as the **Pelvis** of ureter.
- The branches from the ureteric bud form the **Major** and **Minor calyces** and collecting tubules.
- The common excretory duct blends with the mucous membrane of the **Internal trigone** (Fig. 18.4).

EXCRETORY SYSTEM (METANEPHRIC MESODERM)

- The excretory portion consists of nephrons and is derived from the metanephric blastema formed from the mesenchyme of the nephrogenic cord.
- The collecting tubules are covered by metanephric tissue like a cap made of solid mass of bilaminar cells (Fig. 18.5).
- Some of the cells from the solid mass form clusters on the sides of the collecting tubules. These cell clusters form hollow renal vesicles which later forms **s-shaped** tubules.
- **Nephrons or excretory units** are derived from s-shaped tubules.
- The proximal end of the tubules forms the **Bowman's capsule.**
- Capillaries formed from the angiogenic mesenchyme of the nephrogenic cord grow into the capsule forming **Glomeruli**. Distal end communicates with the collecting tubules.
- The rest of the tubules elongates to form:
  - **Proximal convoluted tubule**

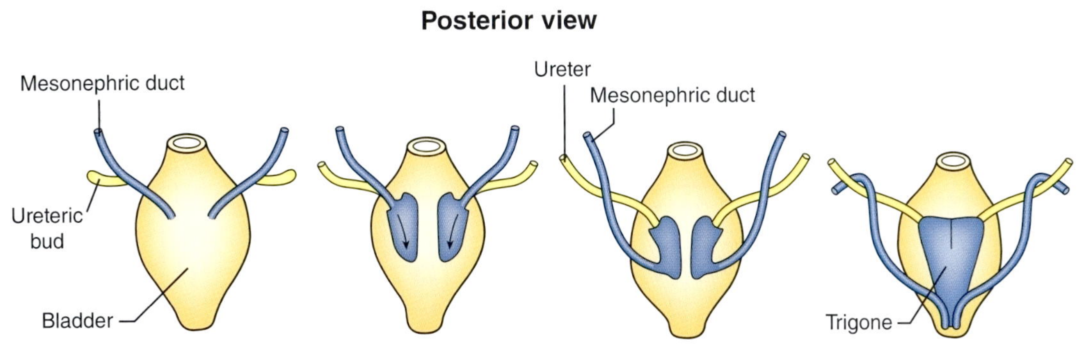

Fig. 18.4 Mesonephric duct and trigone of bladder.

- **Loop of Henle**
- **Distal convoluted tubule**

- The first formed nephrons (juxtamedullary) occupy the corticomedullary junction of kidney.
- The tubular function begins by around **9th week** and kidney becomes **functional** by the **12th week**.
- During the development process, the kidneys are **lobulated** and this persists till first year of life.

ASCENT AND ROTATION OF THE KIDNEY

- The kidney at first lies at the level of **Sacral segments** in the pelvic cavity and is supplied by the **Median sacral artery** (Fig. 18.6).
- Later it ascends into the **Iliac fossa** where it receives blood supply from **Common and Internal iliac arteries**.
- Finally it reaches the adult position under the **diaphragm** where its ascent is arrested by the already developed suprarenal gland.

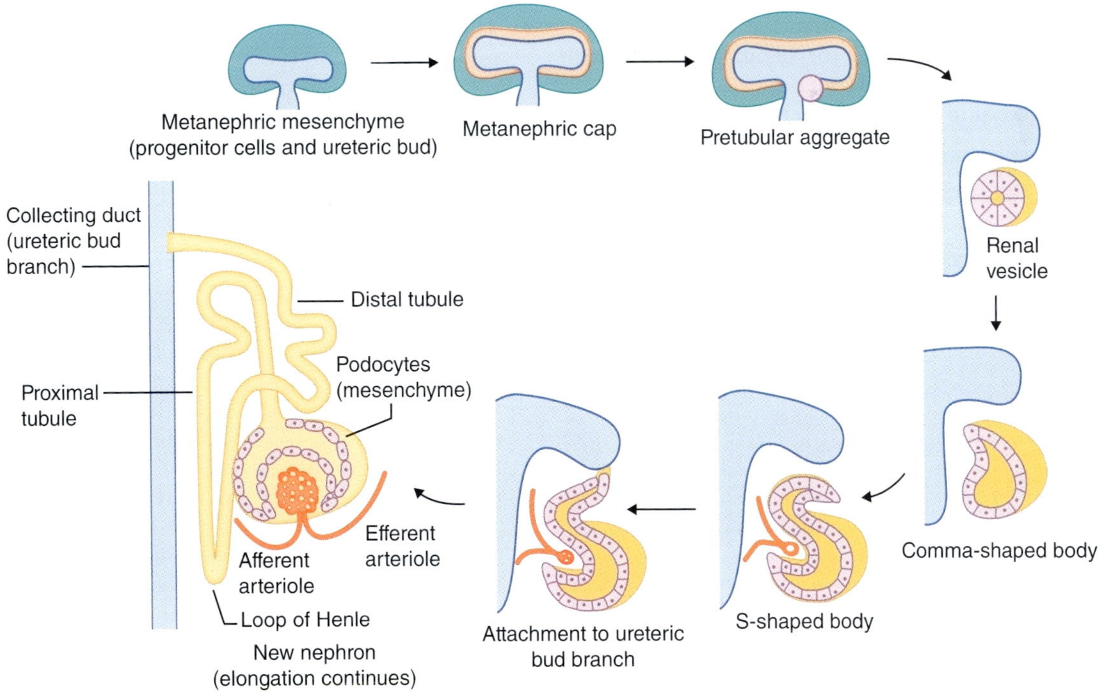

Fig. 18.5 Development of nephron.

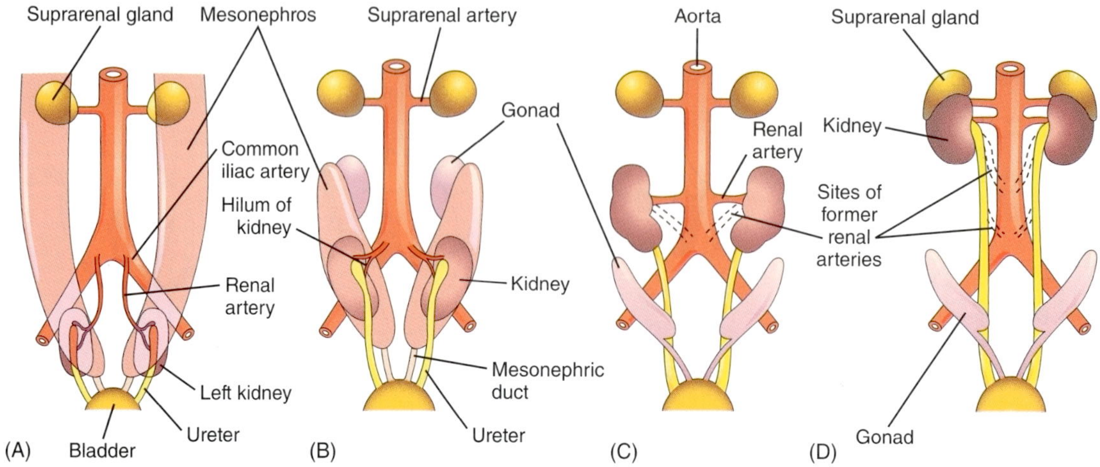

Fig. 18.6 Ascent of kidney and descent of gonads. Embryology of the kidneys between the critical sixth and ninth weeks of gestation. Ventral views of the abdominopelvic region of embryos and foetuses (sixth to ninth weeks) showing medial rotation and 'ascent' of the kidneys from the pelvis to the abdomen. (A and B) Observe also the decrease in size of the mesonephroi. (C and D) Note that as the kidneys 'ascend', they are supplied by arteries at successively higher levels, and that the hilum of the kidney (where the vessels and nerves enter) is eventually directed anteromedially. (Source: *The Science of Paediatrics: MRCPCH Mastercourse,* 2017; With permission from: Moore KL, Persaud TVN, Torchia MG. *Before We Are Born*, 8th ed. Saunders, 2013.)

- There it receives blood supply from the lowest **Suprarenal artery** which later persist as the permanent **Renal artery**.
- In the initial phase, the hilum of kidney is directed ventrally and later it rotates medially along the vertical axis and attain the adult position.

CLINICAL NUGGETS

- Incomplete division of the ureteric bud results in **supernumerary Kidneys** and **supernumerary Ureters**.
- When the developing nephrons fail to connect to a collecting tubule or if the collecting ducts fail to develop, **Polycystic Kidneys** are formed (dominant/recessive). It is usually bilateral and is the commonest of all anomalies. Abnormal dilatation of different parts of uriniferous tubules also result in polycystic kidney.
- **Accessory renal arteries** (enter the kidney through the superior or inferior poles) occur mostly on the left and are often asymptomatic.

URINARY BLADDER AND URETHRA

- The **Allantoic diverticulum** attached to the hindgut divides the hindgut into **preallantoic** and **postallantoic** part. The preallantoic part is tubular and the postallantoic part is dilated to form the endodermal cloaca.
- The cloaca is bounded by the cloacal membrane on the ventral and caudal aspect. The mesodermal cells from the primitive streak migrate on either side of the cloacal membrane forming the **genital folds** which converge on the cephalic end of the cloacal membrane to form the **genital tubercle** (which elongates to form **Phallus**).
- The cloaca divides into (Fig. 18.7).
  - **Primitive urogenital sinus** (anteriorly).
  - **Rectum** (posteriorly).
- The mesoderm separating the two is known as **Urorectal septum**, which is formed by the fusion of vertical fold of **Tourneux** from the ventral wall of hindgut cephalic to allantois and two lateral folds of **Rathke**. The urorectal septum contains a pair of **Mesonephric duct** and a pair of **Paramesonephric duct**.
- The **cloacal duct** connects the primitive urogenital sinus and primitive rectum. At about **seventh week**, the duct is closed when the urorectal septum fuses with the cloacal membrane dividing it into anterior **Urogenital membrane** and posterior **Anal membrane**. The area of fusion of urogenital septum forms the **Perineal body**.

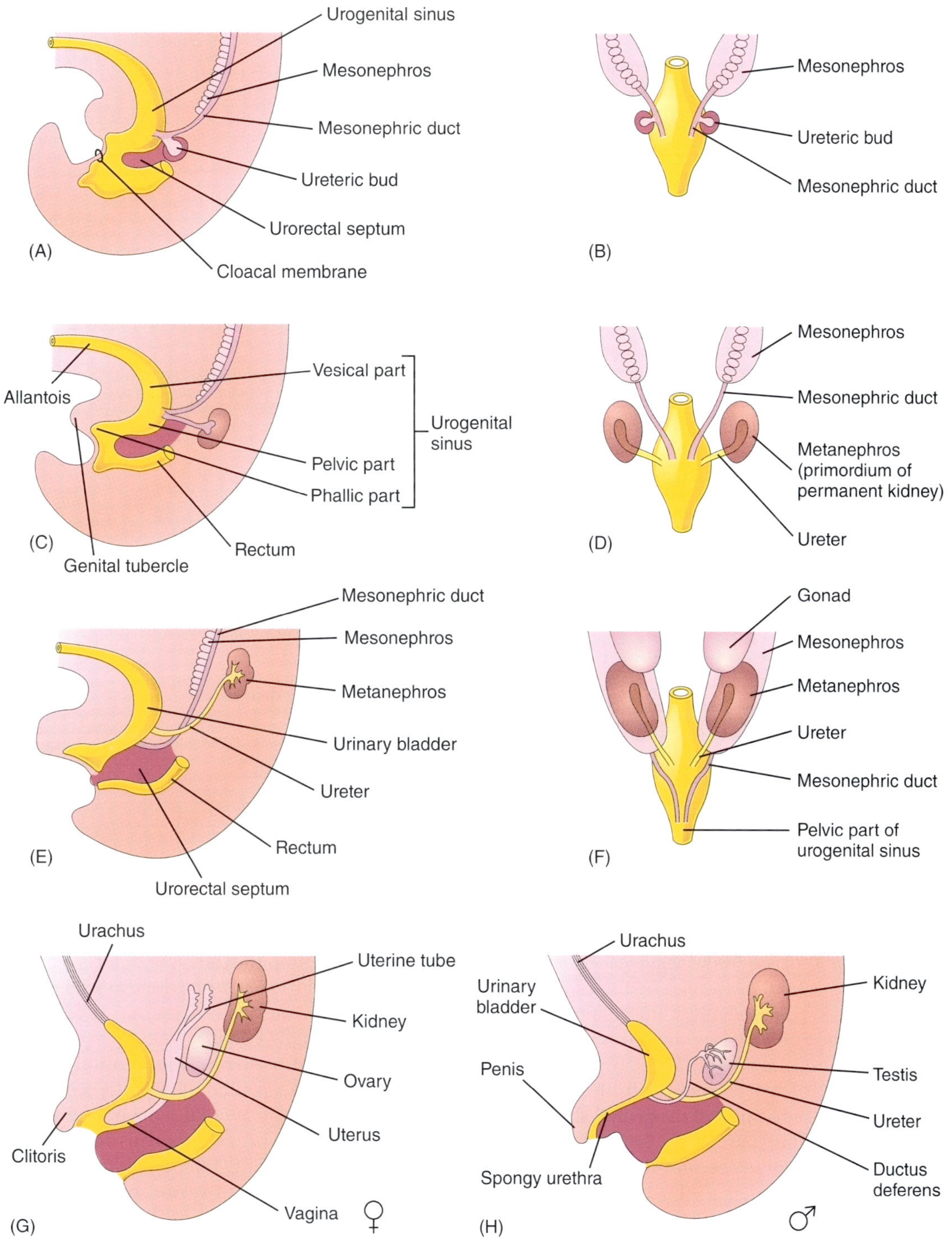

Fig. 18.7 Formation of definitive urogenital sinus. (A) Lateral view of 5-week embryo showing division of the cloaca by the urorectal septum into the urogenital sinus and rectum. (B, D and F) Dorsal views showing the development of the kidneys and bladder and changes in the location of the kidneys. (C, E, G and H) Lateral views. The stages shown in G and H are reached by the 12th week. (Source: *The Developing Human: Clinically Oriented Embryology*, 11th ed. 2020.)

- **Urogenital sinus** is further divided into:
  - Largest upper part is known as the **Vesicourethral part** which communicates with the allantoic diverticulum to form the urinary bladder.
  - The lower part is the **Definitive urogenital sinus** which is further subdivided into narrow upper **Pelvic part** (in males—prostatic and membranous urethra) and dilated lower **Phallic part**.
- The **Pelvic part** receives mesonephric duct which persist as **Ejaculatory ducts** in males but disappear in females. The **Phallic part** presents Müllerian eminence on the dorsal aspect formed by the fusion of the caudal end of paramesonephric duct. In males, it corresponds to the **Colliculus seminalis of Prostatic urethra**, and in females, it corresponds to the **Hymenal membrane** which later ruptures in the centre to form the hymenal orifice.
- The **Urachus** is a fibrous cord which connects the apex of the bladder with umbilicus.
- The lumen of the allantois gets obliterated to form the **Urachus**.
- Urachus is replaced by the **Median umbilical ligament** in adults.
- The caudal portion of mesonephric ducts are absorbed into the bladder. As a result, the ureters which bud from mesonephros are also incorporated into the bladder.
- Thus, the **Trigone of the bladder** is mesodermal in origin due to the incorporation of the ducts (Fig. 18.8). The mesoderm lining is later replaced by **Endodermal epithelium**. The musculature of the bladder is derived from the **Splanchnic layer** of lateral plate mesoderm surrounding the cloaca.
- **Male urethra** is developed as follows:
  A) **Prostatic part**—Above the ejaculatory duct, the dorsal wall is formed by the caudal part of the two **mesonephric ducts** and the ventral wall is formed by the endoderm of the vesicourethral part of **cloaca**. Below the ejaculatory duct, it is formed from the endoderm of pelvic part of **urogenital sinus**.
  B) **Membranous part**—It is formed from the pelvic part of **urogenital sinus**.
  C) **Spongy part**—Up to the base of the glans penis, it is developed from the endoderm of the phallic part of **urogenital sinus**. The part of the urethra within the glans penis is developed from the ectodermal groove which appears on the undersurface of glans penis.
- **Female urethra** is developed from the **vesicourethral part** of the endodermal cloaca.
- In males, the mesonephric ducts which enter the prostatic urethra forms the **Ejaculatory ducts**.
- In **Urethra** (both males and females):
  - **Epithelium**—Endodermal in origin.
  - **Smooth muscle**—Mesoderm (visceral).
- The epithelium of urethra proliferates as outgrowths into the surrounding mesenchyme:
  - **In males**—Buds from the prostatic urethra form **Prostate gland**.
  - **In females**—Urethra buds from the cranial part forming **Urethral and Paraurethral glands**.

CLINICAL NUGGETS

Wilms tumour

- Cancer of the kidneys.
- Children below 5 years usually affected.
- Mutation of **WT1 gene on 11p13**.

WAGR syndrome

- **W**ilms tumor.
- **A**niridia.
- **G**onadoblastoma.
- **R**etardation (mental).

Denys–Drash syndrome

- Wilms tumour.
- Renal failure.
- **Ambiguous genitalia.**

GENITAL SYSTEM (AN 52.8)

- Genital system consists of the **gonads** (testes and ovaries), the **ducts** (efferent ductules of testes, canal of epididymis, vas deferens, seminal vesicle and ejaculatory duct in males and uterine tubes, uterus and vagina in females) and the **external genitalia**.
- By around fifth week, the genital ridges are formed by the proliferation of the coelomic epithelium on the medial side of the mesonephric ridges. The gonads thus formed are called the **Indifferent gonads**.
- Sex differentiation involves genes on the **Y chromosome** (at the time of fertilization) which are essential for male development. In the absence of Y chromosome, female development occurs by the expression of genes on X chromosome and autosomes.

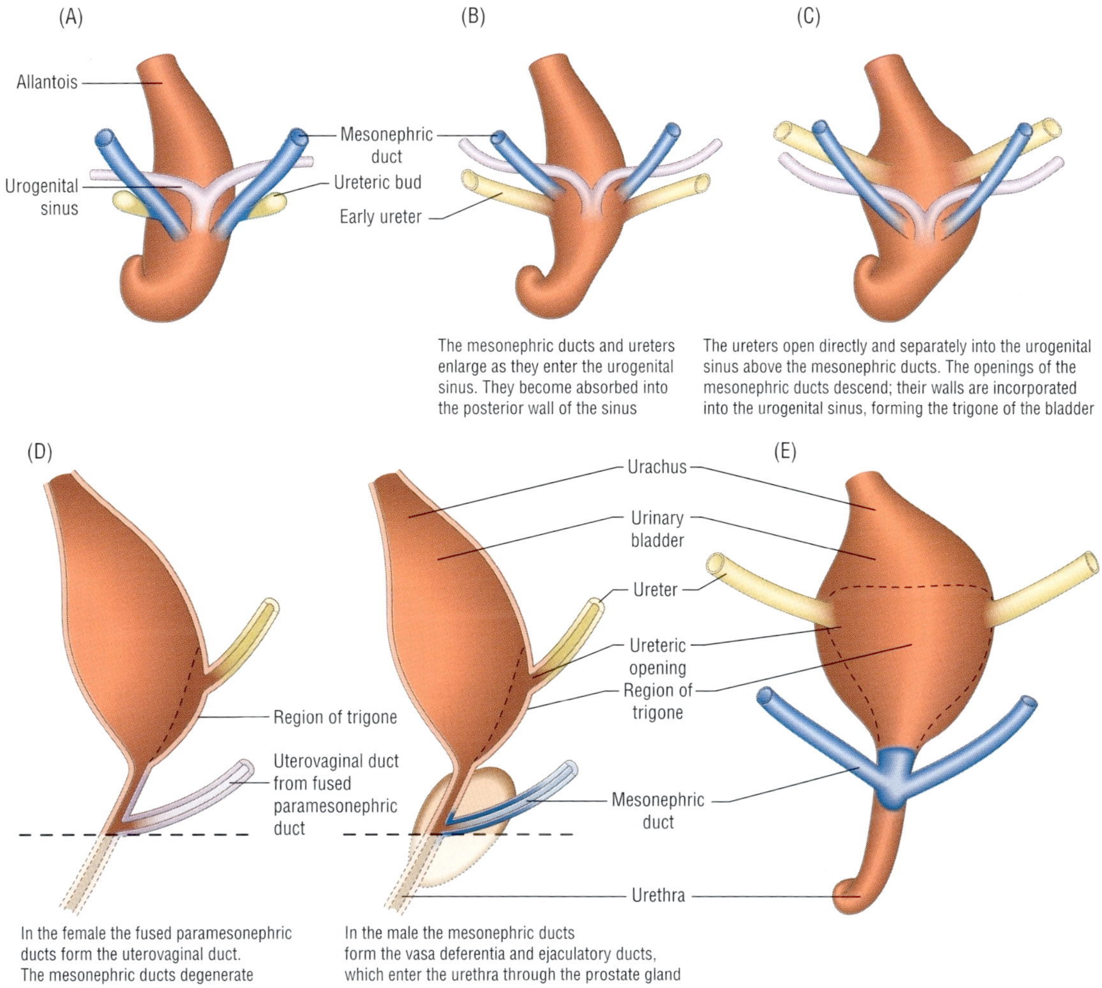

Fig. 18.8 The development of the urinary part of the urogenital sinus and formation of the trigone of the bladder. (A–C, E) Posterior views. (D) Male and female, median sagittal sections. (Source: Tuchmann-Duplessis H, Haegel P. *Illustrated Human Embryology*. Vol 2 Organogenesis. London: Chapman and Hall, 1972. With kind permission of Springer Science+Business Media; *Gray's Anatomy: The Anatomical Basis of Clinical Practice*, 2016.)

- Y chromosome contains **SRY** (sex-determining region on Y) gene on its short arm (Fig. 18.9) SRY protein is the **Testis-Determining Factor (TDF)**.
- Its **presence** influence male development by inducing the differentiation of sex cords into Sertoli cells which then results in the differentiation of Leydig cells and other cells of the testes.
- Its **absence** results in female development by the conversion of sex cords into follicular cells of ovaries. Two genetically active X chromosomes are necessary for the formation of primary ovarian follicles and later one X chromosome becomes heterochromatic and forms genetically inactive **Barr body**.

DEVELOPMENT OF GONADS

- **Genital or gonadal ridges** are longitudinal ridges formed by the proliferation of coelomic epithelium on the medial side of the mesonephric

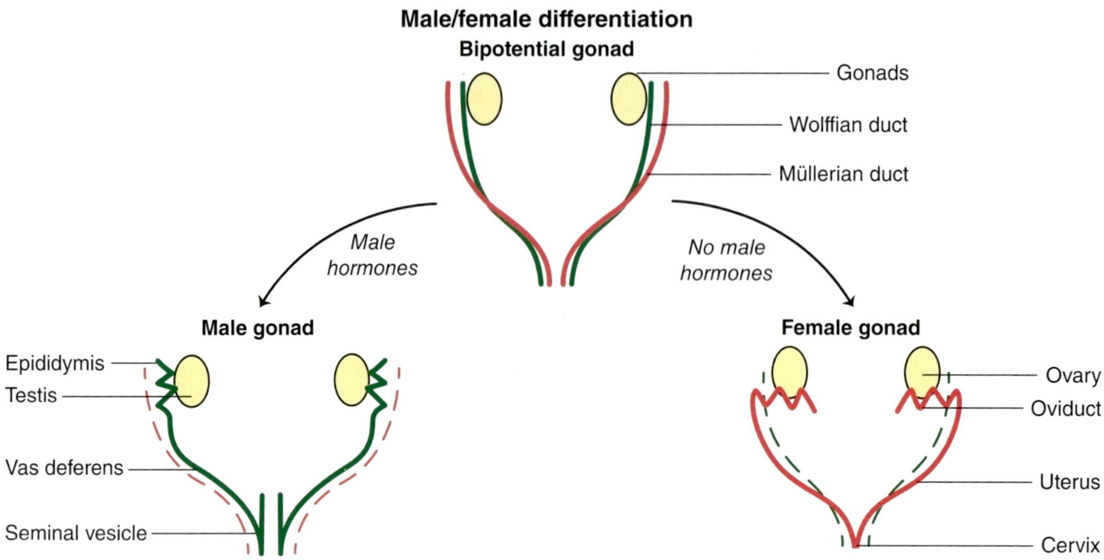

Fig. 18.9 Fate of genital ducts.

ridge by around fifth week of development. The genital ridge consists of an **outer cortex** and **inner medulla**.

- The primitive gonad is attached to the diaphragm by a **Suspensory ligament**. It disappears in males but persist as the **suspensory ligament of Ovary** in females.
- **Primordial germ cells** originate in the epiblast. They reach the wall of the yolk sac close to the allantois through primitive streak.
- Through the dorsal mesentery of the hindgut, they reach the **Genital ridges** by around fifth week.
- When the primitive cells appear in the medulla, the cortex degenerates and the primitive cells are converted into **Spermatogonia** and finally **Testes** is formed.
- When the primitive cells appear in the cortex, the medulla degenerates and the cells in the cortex form **Oogonia** and the cortex finally forms the **Ovary**.
- The epithelial cells of the genital ridge penetrate the underlying mesenchyme and form **Primitive sex cords** before the arrival of the primordial germ cells (Fig. 18.10).

TESTES

- The **SRY gene** influence the primitive sex cords to proliferate into the deeper aspect to form the medullary cords of testis. **Sertoli cells** are differentiated in the medullary portion of the genital ridge by the testes determining factor of Y chromosome (Fig. 18.11).
- Sertoli cells inhibit further mitosis of primordial germ cells in the medullary cords and hence male gametogenesis is delayed till puberty. Sertoli cells secrete **Müllerian regression factor (MRF)** which inhibits Müllerian ducts in males. MRF induces differentiation of **Leydig cells**.
- At the hilum of the gland, the cords breakup to form the **Rete testis**. Lumen is formed in rete testis by sixth month of intrauterine life.
- The fibrous connective tissue **(Tunica albuginea)** separates the cords from surface epithelium by around seventh week.
- **Sustentacular cells of Leydig** are derived from the mesenchyme of the gonadal ridge.
- **Testosterone** is produced by Leydig cells and influence sexual differentiation of external genitalia.
- After puberty, lumen is developed in the cords, transforming the cords into **Seminiferous tubules**. Sex cells in the walls of the tubules persist as the Spermatogonia. Seminiferous tubules join the rete testis.
- Mesonephric duct or Wolffian duct after linking with rete testis form the **Ductus deferens** (Table 18.1).

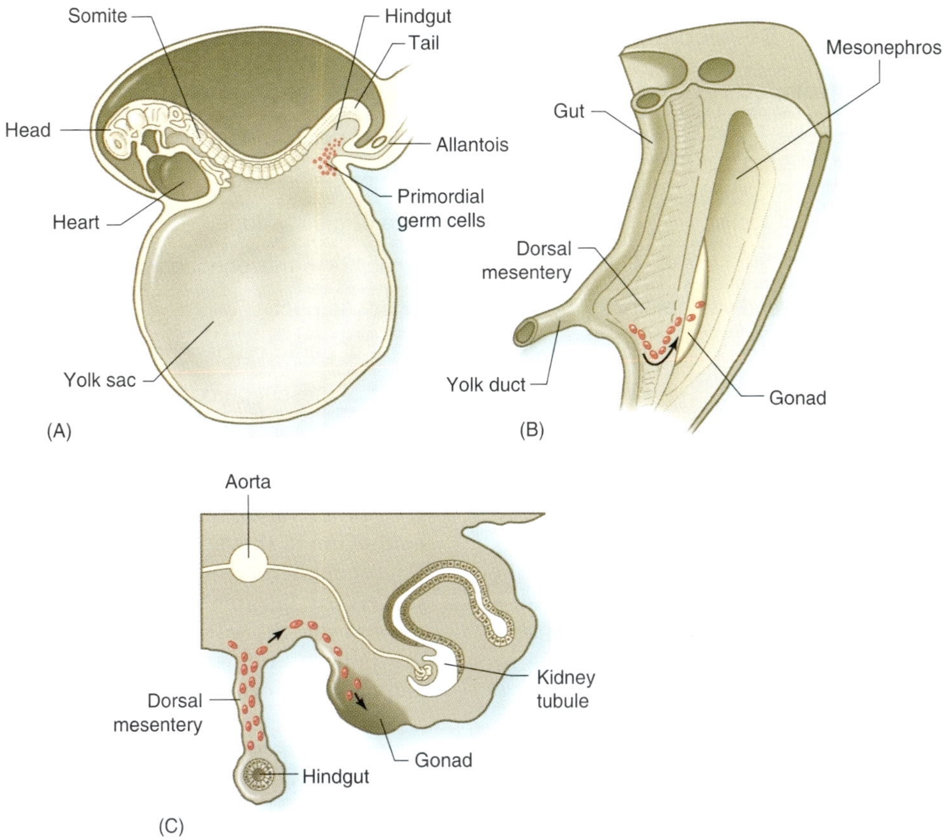

Fig. 18.10 Origin and migration of primordial germ cells in the human embryo. (A) Location of primordial germ cells in the 16-somite human embryo (midsagittal view). (B) Pathway of migration *(arrow)* through the dorsal mesentery. (C) Cross-section showing the pathway of migration *(arrows)* through the dorsal mesentery and into the gonad. (Source: *Human Embryology and Developmental Biology*, 6th ed. 2019.)

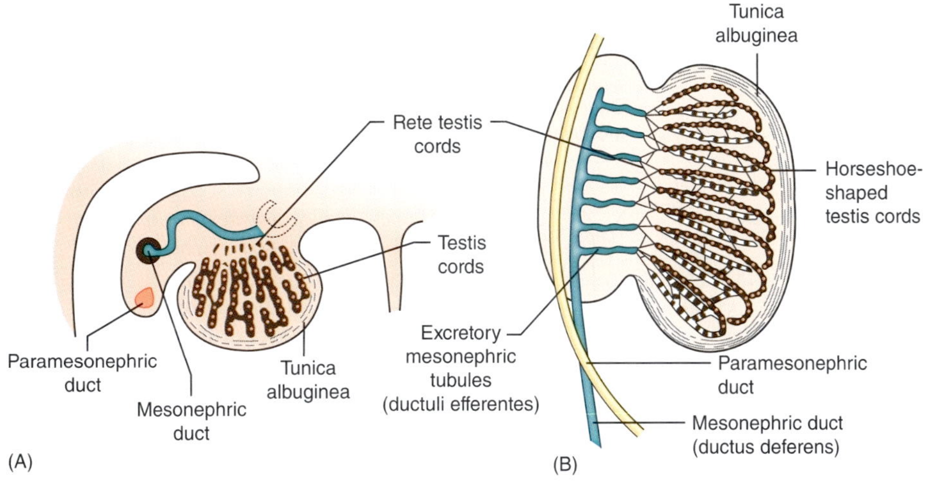

Fig. 18.11 Development of testis.

Table 18.1 Developmental Sources of Structures in Males

Structures Developed	Developmental Sources
Seminiferous tubules	Medulla of genital ridge
Fibrous septa	Medulla of genital ridge
Intrinsic coverings of testis	Medulla of genital ridge
Efferent ductules	Proximal 12–15 mesonephric tubules
Canal of epididymis and vas deferens	Mesonephric duct
Appendix of testis	Remnant of paramesonephric duct
Appendix of epididymis	Remnant of mesonephros

OVARY

- Ovaries are developed from the **cortex** of the genital ridge.
- **Primitive sex cords** form irregular cell clusters containing primitive germ cells.
- The surface epithelium forms **Cortical cords** (Fig. 18.12).
- Cortical cords penetrate mesenchyme and the mesenchyme breaks the cords into number of fragments. The fragmented mass surround oogonium forming the primary ovarian follicle. At birth around **two million primary follicles** are present in the ovary.
- Tunica albuginea is not formed as in testis and hence the surface epithelium covers the ovary. The surface epithelium is very thick and undergoes proliferation and hence called **Germinal epithelium** of the ovary.
- The cephalic end of the genital ridge forms **suspensory ligament of ovary** and the caudal portion merges with the proximal portion of the gubernaculum. The middle part of the genital ridge forms the **definitive Ovary**.

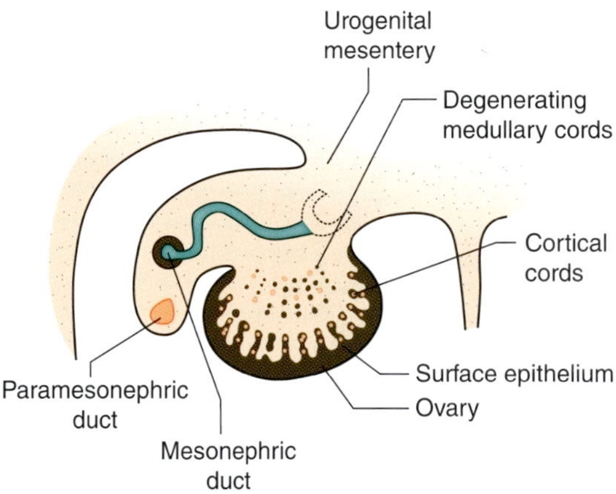

Fig. 18.12 Development of ovary.

DUCTS OF GENITAL SYSTEM

- In the initial stage, both sex have two pairs of genital ducts:
  - **Mesonephric or Wolffian ducts.**
  - **Paramesonephric or Müllerian ducts.**
- The genital ducts in **females** are fallopian tubes, uterus and vagina.
- **Paramesonephric duct** arises on the surface of the urogenital ridge by the invagination of coelomic epithelium.
- **Cranially** it opens into the abdominal cavity as a funnel-like structure.
- **Caudally** the two paramesonephric ducts join in the midline to form the **Uterovaginal canal**. The fusion at first is incomplete due to the presence of a fenestrated septum.
- The caudal part projects into the posterior wall of urogenital sinus as **Müllerian (paramesonephric) tubercle** by around third month.
- The three parts of **Paramesonephric ducts** are:
  1) **Cephalic vertical part** which opens into the coelomic cavity.
  2) **Intermediate horizontal part.**
  3) **Caudal vertical part** which bulges at the dorsal wall of urogenital sinus.

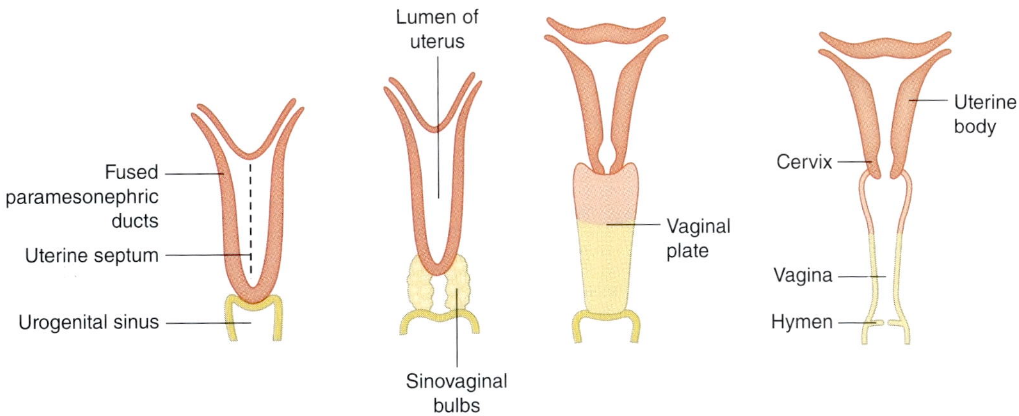

Fig. 18.13 Development of uterus and vagina.

- **Uterine tubes** are developed from the cephalic vertical part and most of the intermediate horizontal parts of the **Paramesonephric ducts** (Fig. 18.13).
- **Uterus** is formed from the cephalic part of **Uterovaginal canal. Fundus** is formed by a segment of horizontal part of paramesonephric duct.
- **Vagina** is developed from three sources (Fig. 18.13):
  - **Upper four-fifths** above the hymen—mucous membrane from the **Sinovaginal bulb** (endodermal outgrowth of urogenital sinus lying between uterovaginal canal and urogenital sinus which later canalize to form a part of vagina) and the **Musculature** from the mesoderm of fused lower vertical part of **Paramesonephric ducts**.
  - **Lower one-fifth** below hymen—endoderm of **Urogenital sinus**.
- **Vaginal orifice—ectoderm** after the rupture of urogenital membrane.
- The mesonephric ducts also open into the urogenital sinus next to the **Müllerian tubercle**.
- The master gene for testes development is **SRY gene**. **SRY** acts along with **SOX9** (autosomal gene) to induce **testicular differentiation**.
- **SOX9** increases the concentration of **AMH (Anti-Müllerian hormone or Müllerian-inhibiting substance)** which results in the regression of **Paramesonephric (Müllerian)** ducts.
- **AMH** is produced by **Sertoli cells**. **Leydig cells** produce testosterone.
- **Testosterone receptor complex** induces the transformation of mesonephric ducts into ejaculatory ducts, vas deferens, seminal vesicles, efferent ductules and epididymis.
- **Dihydrotestosterone complexes** result in the differentiation of male external genitalia.
- Ovary determining gene is **WNT$_4$**. Under the influence of WNT$_4$, **SOX9 is inhibited**.
- **Estrogen** influences the formation of uterine tubes, uterus, cervix and upper part of vagina from paramesonephric duct.
- Estrogen also acts on the **external genitalia** to form labia majora, labia minora, clitoris and lower vagina.

EXTERNAL GENITALIA

- The mesenchyme around the cloacal membrane forms **Cloacal folds** (Fig. 18.14). At the cranial end, the cloacal folds unite to form **Genital tubercle**.
- Caudally it forms two folds:
  - **Anal folds.**
  - **Urethral folds.**
- **Genital swellings** develop on either side of urethral folds to form:
  - **Scrotal swellings** in males.
  - **Labia majora** in females.
- In males the genital tubercle elongates to form the **Phallus (primitive penis)**.
- The urethral folds along the phallus later fuse enclosing the urethral plate from endoderm forming the **Penile urethra**.
- In females the genital tubercles form the **Clitoris**.
- The urethral folds in females instead of fusing forms the **Labia minora**.

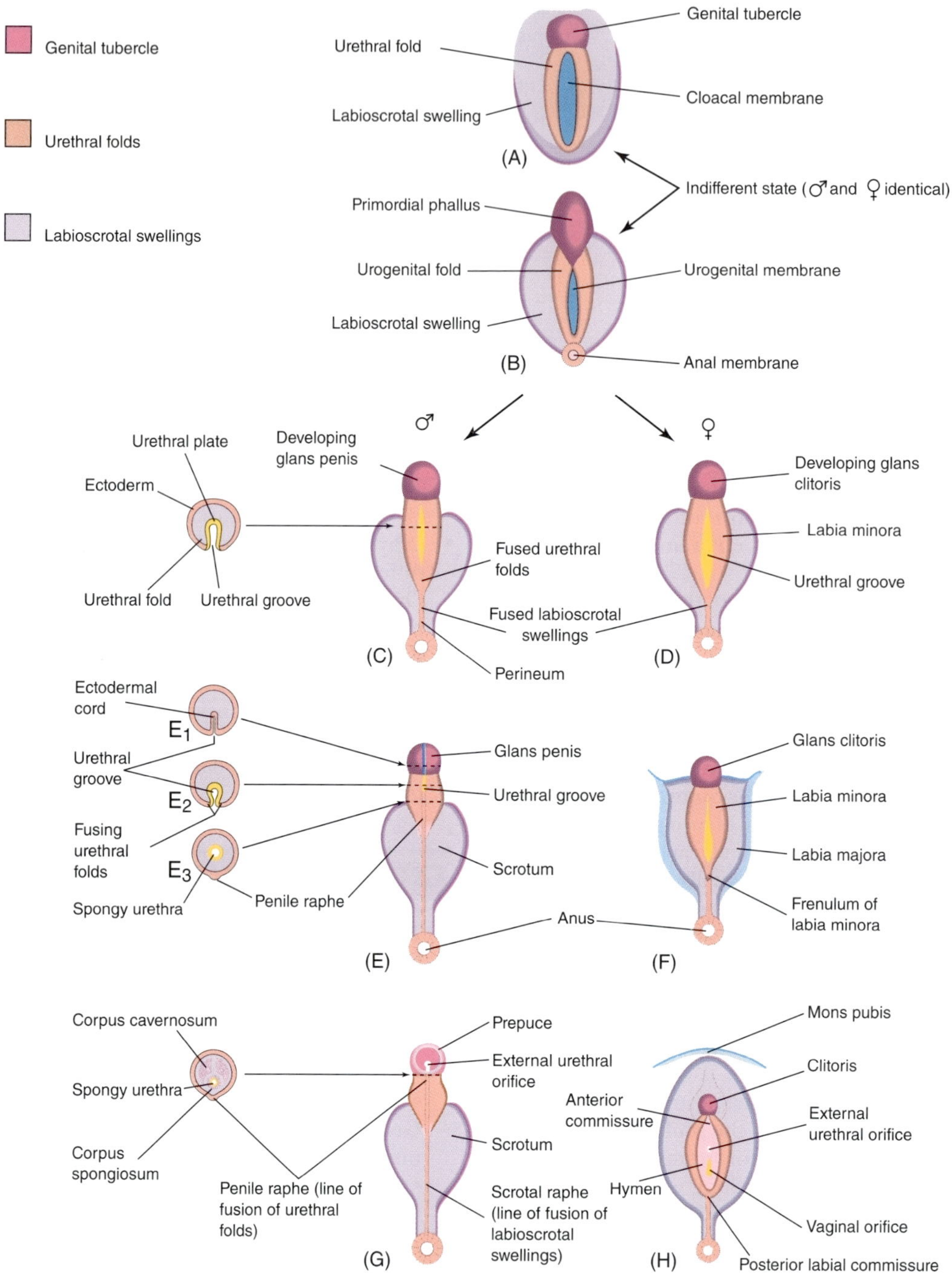

Fig. 18.14 Development of the external genitalia. (A and B) Diagrams illustrating appearance of the genitalia during the indifferent stage (fourth to seventh weeks). (C, E and G) Stages in the development of the male external genitalia at 9, 11, and 12 weeks, respectively. To the left are schematic transverse sections of the developing penis illustrating formation of the spongy urethra and scrotum. (D, F and H) Stages in the development of the female external genitalia at 9, 11 and 12 weeks, respectively. The mons pubis is a pad of fatty tissue over the symphysis pubis. (Source: *Before We Are Born: Essentials of Embryology and Birth Defects*, First South Asia Edition, 2016.)

REMNANTS OF MESONEPHRIC AND PARAMESONEPHRIC DUCTS

- In **males**:
  - **Appendix of epididymis** (cranial end of mesonephric ducts).
  - **Paradidymis** (mesonephric tubules).
  - **Superior aberrant ductules** (mesonephric tubules cranial to vasa efferentia).
  - **Inferior aberrant ductules** (mesonephric tubules caudal to vasa efferentia).
  - **Appendix of testis** (cranial end of paramesonephric duct).
  - **Prostatic utricle** (paramesonephric duct—corresponds to uterus and vagina in females).
- In **females** (mesonephric system) (Fig. 18.15):
  - **Epoophoron** (above the ovary) (remnant of mesonephric tubules).
  - **Paroophoron** (near the ovary) (remnant of mesonephric tubules).
  - **Gartner's duct** (remnant of mesonephric duct).

DESCENT OF THE TESTES

- Testes develop retroperitoneally in the dorsal abdominal wall:
- Urogenital mesentery attaches the testis to the posterior abdominal wall.
- Cephalic end is suspended from the diaphragm by the **suspensory ligament**.
- Caudal part forms caudal genital ligament and **gubernaculum**.
- When the testis reaches the internal inguinal ring, the gubernaculum extends from the inguinal region to the scrotal swellings and finally contacts

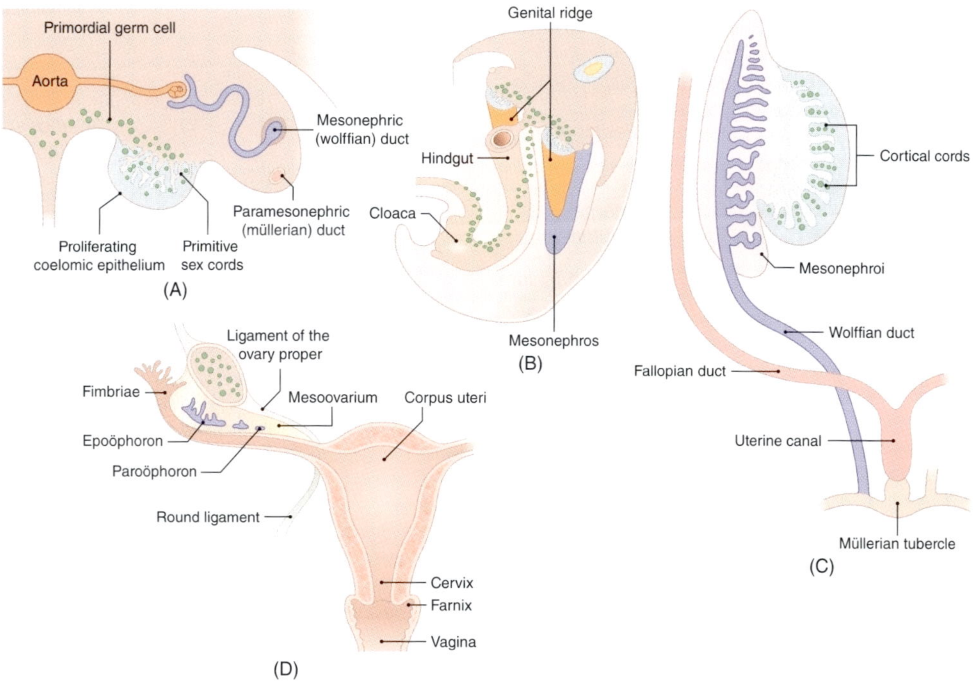

Fig. 18.15 Formation of epoophoron and paroophoron. Female reproductive tract development. (A) Schematic diagram of a transverse section through the genital ridge and mesonephros (*A*, aorta; *MD*, mesonephric (Wolffian) duct; *PCE*, proliferating coelomic epithelium; *PGC*, primordial germ cells; *PMD*, paramesonephric (Müllerian) duct; *PSC*, primitive sex cords). (B) Migrational path of PGCs (*C*, cloaca; *GR*, genital ridge; *HG*, hindgut; *M*, mesonephros). (C) Fusion of lower portions of ducts, with confluence of their cavities (*FD*, fallopian duct; *CCO*, cortical cords of the ovary; *MN*, mesonephroi; *WD*, Wolffian duct; *UC*, uterine canal; *MT*, Müllerian tubercle). (D) Differentiation into uterine corpus, cervix and upper portion of vagina (*F*, fimbriae; *EO*, epoophoron; *PO*, paroophoron; *LoO*, ligament of the ovary proper; *MO*, mesoovarium; *CU*, corpus uteri; *RL*, round ligament; *CX*, cervix; *FX*, fornix; *V*, vagina). (Source: *Potter's Pathology of the Fetus, Infant and Child*. 2nd ed. 2007.)

the scrotal floor. The **gubernacular mesenchyme** forms the coverings of testis and spermatic cord and also gives rise to the cremaster muscle.

- Factors controlling the descent:
  - **Outgrowth of the gubernaculum**—It is the guiding force for the descent of testis. During the last two months of foetal life, the cremasteric muscle developed in the gubernaculum causes rhythmic contraction which accelerates the descent of testes.
  - Increased **Intra-abdominal pressure**.
  - Regression of **gubernaculum**.
  - **Androgens and MIS** (Müllerian-inhibiting substance).
- The evagination of peritoneum as **Processus vaginalis** into the scrotal swelling results in the formation of inguinal canal.
- **Lower scrotal temperature** (4 degree lower than intraabdominal temperature) which is a favourable temperature for spermatogenesis promotes descent of testis into the scrotal sac.
- Straightening of the **foetal curves** accelerates the process of descent.
- Testis reaches (Fig. 18.16) **iliac fossa**—fourth month.
  - **Deep inguinal ring**—seventh month.
  - **Inguinal canal**—seventh to eighth month.
  - **Scrotum**—at birth or shortly after birth.
- **The processus vaginalis** which gets detached from peritoneum forms the parietal and visceral layer of tunica vaginalis covering the testes.
- **The gubernaculum** forms **scrotal ligament** between lower pole of testis and bottom of scrotum. The anomalies of descent of Testes are summarised in Table 18.2.
- Other coverings of testes are derived as follows:
  - Transversalis fascia forms the **Internal spermatic fascia**.

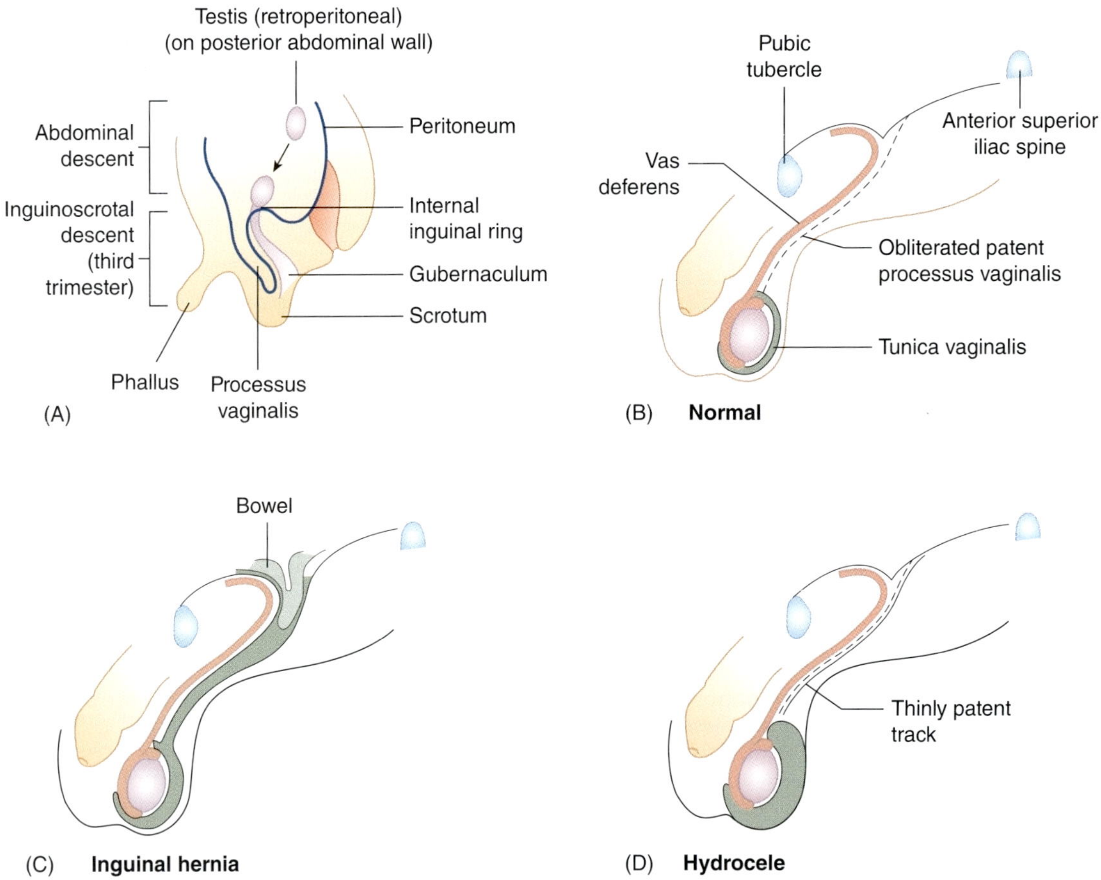

Fig. 18.16 Descent of testis and common anomalies.

Table 18.2 Anomalies of Descent of Testes

Anomaly	Description
Cryptorchidism	Incomplete descent of one or both testes into the scrotum (Fig. 18.17).
Ectopic testis	Testis located in an abnormal position outside the normal descent path, for example perineum, above penis, in front of pubic symphysis, saphenous opening (Fig. 18.17).
Vanishing testis	Testis fails to develop or atrophies after descent, leaving an empty scrotum.
Anorchism	Both testes retained in the abdomen and can go malignant transformation.
Monorchism	Only one testis descends into the scrotum, and the other is absent.
Encysted hydrocele of spermatic cord	Processus vaginalis closed at the upper end of testis and at deep inguinal ring.

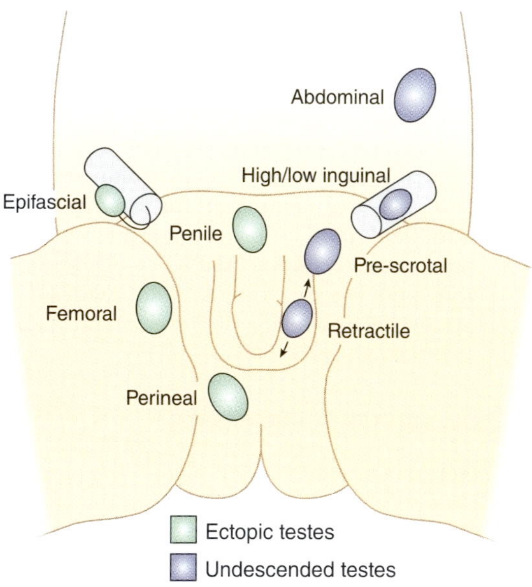

Fig. 18.17 Undescended and ectopic testis.

- Internal oblique abdominis forms **Cremastric fascia and muscle**.
- External oblique abdominis forms **External spermatic fascia**.

DESCENT OF THE OVARIES

Ovaries lie retroperitoneally in the dorsal abdominal wall:

- **Mesovarium** which suspends the ovary first lies at the lumbar region.
- The caudal end is connected to the genital swelling by **gubernaculum of ovary**. The middle portion of gubernaculum is attached to the angle of the developing uterus and this attachment divides the gubernaculum into a proximal portion and distal portion.
- By fifth to sixth week, they descent and lie behind the genital cord.
- In the adult female, they lie on the posterior aspect of the broad ligament.
- The final position of the ovaries is just below the rim of **true pelvis**.
- The reasons for the arrest of further descent are:
  - The **Infundibulopelvic ligament**.
  - Well-developed **Uterus** and **Broad ligament** lying in the front.
- If the ovaries descend up to the inguinal canal or into the labium, it is called **Hernia of the ovary.** This happens when the **Canal of Nuck** (tubular peritoneal pouch) fails to regress after the descent of ovary. This peritoneal pouch extends into the inguinal canal along with gubernaculum just like the processus vaginalis and results in congenital inguinal hernia in females.
- The cranial genital ligaments form **Suspensory ligament of ovary**.
- The caudal genital ligaments form the **ligament of Ovary** (proximal part of gubernaculum) and the **round ligament of Uterus** (distal part of gubernaculum) (Fig. 18.18).

KLINISCHE PERLEN

BARDET-BIEDL SYNDROME

- Bardet-Biedl syndrome (BBS) is a rare genetic disorder that affects **multiple organ systems** in the body.

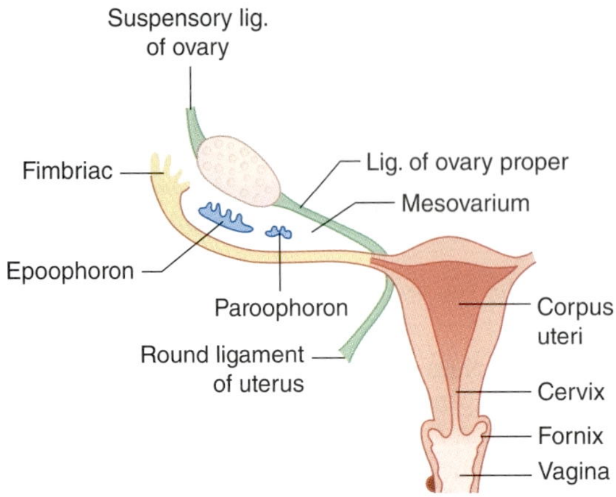

Fig. 18.18 Ligaments of ovary.

- It is a genetically **heterogeneous** disorder, meaning that mutations in several different genes can lead to the development of the syndrome.
- Common features include obesity, retinal degeneration leading to vision problems, extra fingers or toes (polydactyly), kidney abnormalities, intellectual disability and genital anomalies.

MECKEL-GRUBER SYNDROME

- Meckel-Gruber syndrome (MKS) is a rare and severe genetic disorder that primarily affects the development of the **Central nervous system** and the **Kidneys**.
- Several genes have been associated with MKS, including **MKS1, TMEM67, CC2D2A** and others.
- Common features include **occipital encephalocele** (a sac-like protrusion of the brain and its membranes through an opening in the skull), **polydactyly** (extra fingers or toes), **cystic kidneys** and **hepatic ductal proliferation** (liver abnormalities).

POTTER SEQUENCE

- Potter sequence, also known as **Potter syndrome or Oligohydramnios sequence**, refers to a constellation of physical and developmental abnormalities that result from a lack of amniotic fluid (oligohydramnios) during foetal development.
- The condition is typically associated with kidney or urinary tract abnormalities that lead to a reduced production of urine, resulting in decreased amniotic fluid.
- The most common underlying causes of Potter sequence are congenital anomalies affecting the **Kidneys or Urinary tract**.
- Conditions such as bilateral renal agenesis (absence of both kidneys), severe polycystic kidney disease or other urinary tract obstructions can lead to a reduced ability to produce urine.
- The physical features associated with Potter sequence are a consequence of the oligohydramnios and may include **flattened facial features, limb contractures** and **Pulmonary hypoplasia** (underdeveloped lungs).
- The compression of the foetus against the uterine wall due to the lack of amniotic fluid can result in characteristic facial appearances.
- Infants with Potter sequence often exhibit a characteristic facial appearance known as **'Potter facies'**. This includes a flat nose, recessed chin and widely spaced eyes. These features are a result of the facial compression caused by the oligohydramnios.

CONGENITAL POLYCYSTIC KIDNEY DISEASE (CPKD)

- In this condition, the renal tubules become structurally abnormal forming **Cysts**.
- The cysts may also occur in the **Liver, Seminal vesicles** and **Pancreas**.
- The two forms of polycystic kidneys are:
  - **Autosomal dominant (ADPKD)**—adult type and is more common. Mutant genes are located on the short arm of **chromosome 16 or 4**. Classical manifestations are hypertension, flank pain and chronic renal failure.
  - **Autosomal recessive (ARPKD)—Childhood type** and is rare compared to ADPKD. It occurs below the age of 20 years and die at a very early age.

ECTOPIC URETERAL OPENINGS

- The ureters instead of opening into the bladder might open in to the following regions:
  - **Vagina.**
  - **Urethra.**
  - **Vestibule.**
- Usually seen in **duplicated ureters.**

DIFFERENT POSITIONS OF KIDNEY

- **Pelvic kidney**—close to common iliac artery.
- **Horse-shoe kidney.**
  - The inferior poles of both kidneys will be fused.
  - Root of **Inferior mesenteric artery** prevents its ascend (Fig. 18.19).

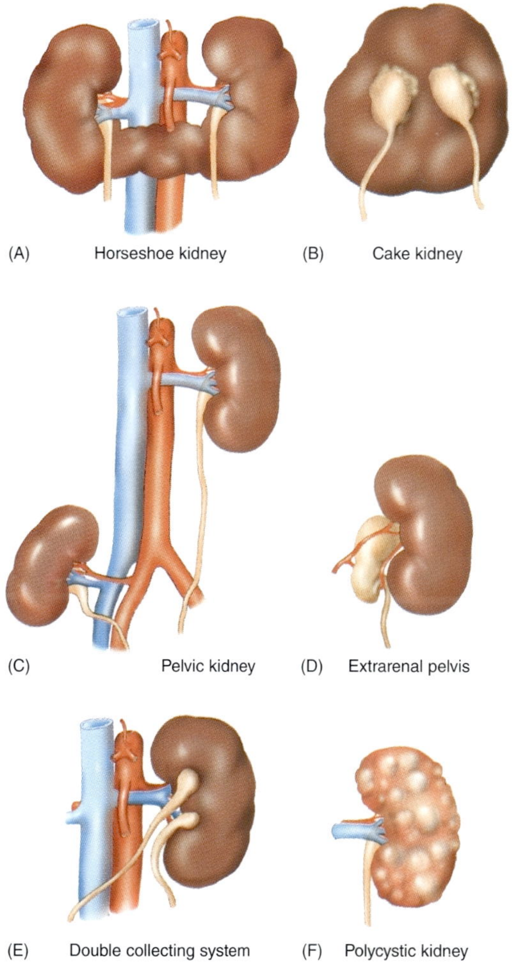

Fig. 18.19 Variations of renal anatomy, position within the retroperitoneal cavity and pathology. (A) Horse-shoe kidney shown as two kidneys connected by an isthmus anterior to the great vessels and inferior to the inferior mesenteric artery. (B) Cake kidney with a double collecting system. (C) Pelvic kidney with one kidney in the normal retroperitoneal position. (D) Extrarenal pelvis. (E) Double collecting system in a single kidney. (F) Polycystic kidney. (Source: *Textbook of Diagnostic Ultrasonography*, 6th ed. 2006.)

ALLANTOIS

- If allantois persists it can present as:
  - **Urachal fistula**—bladder communicates with exterior (Fig. 18.20).
  - **Urachal cyst**—cystic dilatation between umbilicus and bladder.
  - **Urachal sinus**—opens to the exterior, may communicate with the bladder.

EXSTROPHY OF THE BLADDER

- This condition occurs during fetal development when the tissues that form the abdominal wall and the bladder fail to fuse together properly.
- As a result, the bladder mucosa is exposed due to a defect in the ventral body wall often appearing as a red, bladder-shaped protrusion (Fig. 18. 21).

UTERINE ANOMALIES (FIG. 18.22)

- **Uterus didelphys:**
  - Double uterus usually seen along with double vagina.
  - Failure of fusion of **Paramesonephric ducts**.
- **Uterus bicornis:**
  - Two horns of uterus entering a common vagina.
- **Uterus arcuatus:**
  - The fundus is slightly indented in the middle.

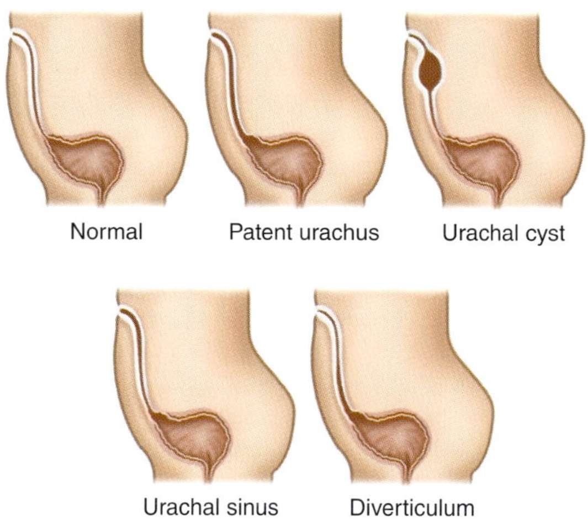

Fig. 18.20 Developmental anomalies of the urachus. (Source: *Surgery for Medical Graduates*, 2018.)

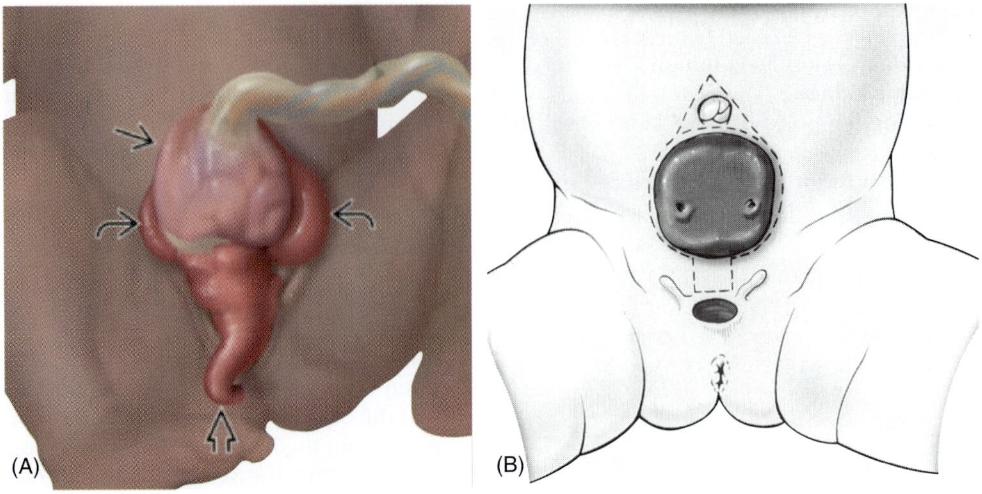

Fig. 18.21 Bladder exstrophy. (A) Graphic of cloacal exstrophy shows an omphalocele, with terminal ileum prolapsed between the two halves of the exstrophic bladder. The appearance of the prolapsed bowel has been likened to an elephant trunk. Note that an omphalocele is not essential for this diagnosis. (B) Typical findings of classic bladder exstrophy in a female and the incision used for repair. (Source: part A, *Diagnostic Imaging: Obstetrics*. 3rd ed. 2016; part B, *Pediatric Surgery*, 6th ed. 2006.)

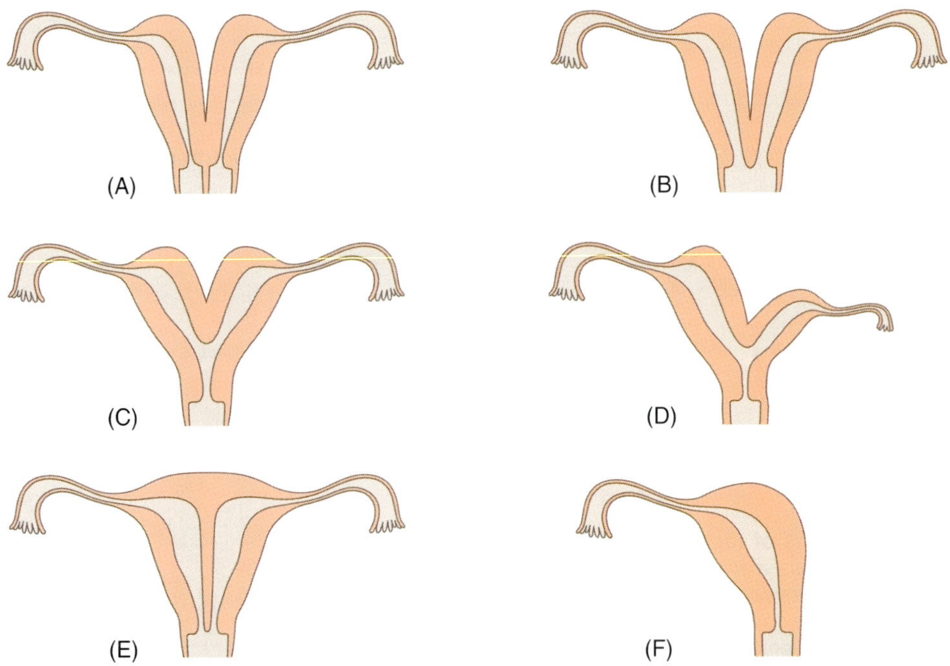

Fig. 18.22 Illustrations of various types of congenital uterine abnormalities. (A) Double uterus and double vagina, (B) double uterus with single vagina, (C) branched (bicornuate) uterus, (D) bicornuate uterus with a small left branch, (E) septate uterus (divided in the middle) and (F) uterus formed from Müllerian duct on one side only. (Source: *Human Reproductive Biology*. 3rd ed. 2006.)

- **Uterus bicornis unicollis:**
  - Partial or complete absence of one of the Paramesonephric ducts.
  - It is seen as a **rudimentary horn** and uterus is developed from the other normal paramesonephric duct.

ANOMALIES OF PENIS

- **Hypospadias** (Fig. 18. 23):
  - Abnormal openings of urethra along the inferior aspect of the penis.
- **Epispadias:**
  - Urethral meatus is seen on the dorsum of penis.
  - Associated with the exstrophy of the bladder.
- **Micropenis:**
  - Caused by primary hypogonadism or hypothalamic or pituitary dysfunction.
- **Double (bifid) penis:**
  - As a result of splitting of genital tubercle.
- **Buried/hidden Penis** (Fig. 18.24):
  - The penis which is normal in length and function is hidden by the excess skin covering it.

AMBIGUOUS GENITALIA (FIG. 18.25)

- Ambiguous genitalia is a medical condition in which an individual's external genitalia do not have the typical appearance of **either a male or a female**. This condition arises due to atypical development of the reproductive system during foetal growth.

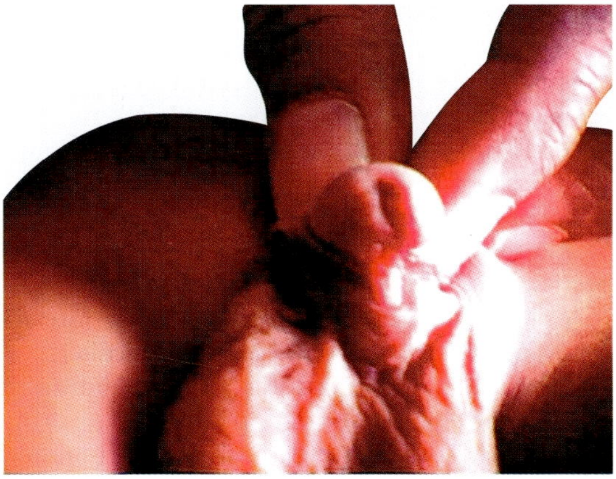

Fig. 18.23 Penis with hypospadias. (Photo courtesy: Dr Aswin.)

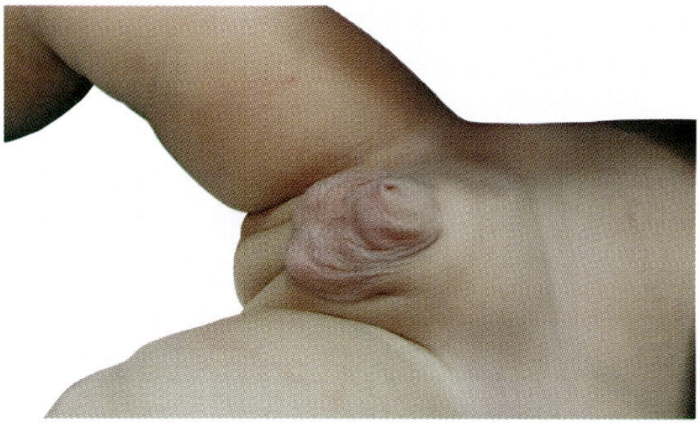

Fig. 18.24 A child with buried or hidden penis. (Photo courtesy: Dr Aswin.)

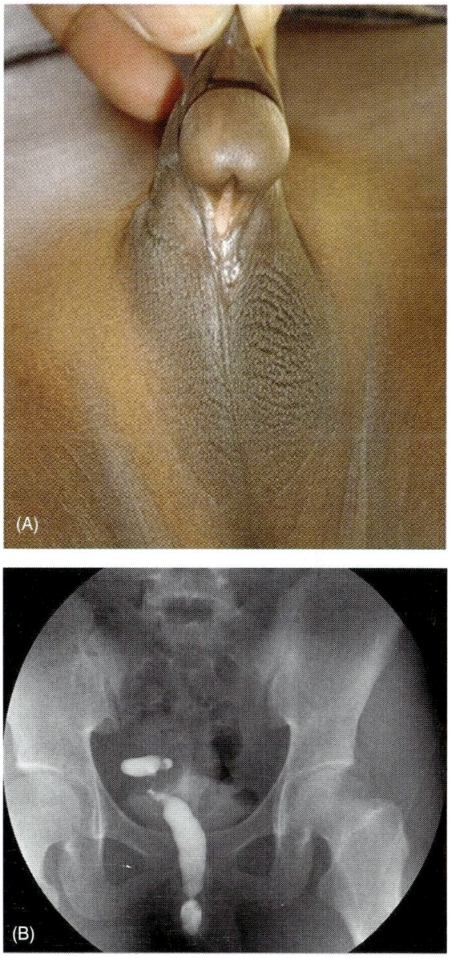

Fig. 18.25 (A) A case of Ambiguous genitalia; (B) Genitogram showing dye in hemiuterus and fallopian tube on right with spillage. (Photo courtesy: Dr Suja.)

- Ambiguous genitalia can result from various genetic, hormonal or environmental factors that influence the development of the reproductive organs during early foetal life. Conditions such as **Congenital adrenal hyperplasia (CAH), Disorders of sexual development (DSD)** and certain genetic syndromes can lead to ambiguous genitalia.
- Hormonal imbalances during foetal development can affect the differentiation of the gonads (testes or ovaries) and the production of sex hormones. An excess of male hormones (androgens) or a deficiency in female hormones (estrogens) can contribute to the development of ambiguous genitalia.

HERMAPHRODITE

- The individuals with characteristics of **both sex**.
- External genitalia and karyotype mostly belong to females **(46,XX)**.
- May have both testicular and ovarian tissue **(ovotestes)**.

CONGENITAL ADRENAL HYPERPLASIA

- Increased **ACTH (Adrenocorticotropic hormone)**
- **21-hydroxylation** is inhibited which results in **masculinization**.
- **17-alpha hydroxylase deficiency** results in female appearance and absence of secondary sexual characteristics.

ANDROGEN INSENSITIVITY SYNDROME (AIS)

- Males with **ineffective Androgens** produced by testes.
- Male genitalia not developed.
- Paramesonephric system is suppressed due to the presence of MIS (Mullerian Inhibiting Substance).

5-ALPHA REDUCTASE DEFICIENCY

- Testosterone not converted into dihydrotestosterone.
- Males with ambiguous genitalia.

KLINEFELTER SYNDROME

- **47, XXY** (nondisjunction of XX homologues).
- 1 in 1000 males.
- Decreased testosterone levels and small testes.
- Gynaecomastia.

GONADAL DYSGENESIS

- Mostly female (phenotypically).
- Oocytes absent and ovaries appear as gonadal streaks.
- For example,
  (a) **Swyer syndrome** (**XY** female gonadal dysgenesis):
    - Point mutation or deletion of **SRY** gene.
  (b) **Turner syndrome:**
    - **45 XO**
    - Short stature, high-arched palate, webbed neck, shield-like chest, inverted nipples, cardiac anomalies and renal anomalies.

CRYPTORCHIDISM

- Cryptorchidism is a condition characterized by the incomplete descent of one or both testes into the scrotum. During normal development, the testes form within the abdomen and gradually descend into the scrotum before birth. Cryptorchidism occurs when this descent process is incomplete, resulting in one or both testes remaining undescended or partially descended in the **inguinal canal or abdomen**.
- It is a relatively common condition in newborns, especially in premature infants. In full-term infants, the incidence is around 3%, and in premature infants, it can be higher.
- In some cases, the undescended testes may descend on their own during the first few months of life. However, if this does not occur, intervention may be needed.
- Premature birth, low birth weight and family history of cryptorchidism are considered risk factors. There may also be a hormonal component involved in the descent process.
- Cryptorchidism can lead to potential complications, including an increased risk of **infertility, testicular cancer and inguinal hernia**.
- The main treatment for cryptorchidism is **Orchidopexy**, a surgical procedure to bring the undescended testis into the scrotum and secure it in place. This procedure is often recommended before the child reaches the **age of 1**.

CONGENITAL INGUINAL HERNIA

- Due to persistent **processus vaginalis**.
- Intestinal loops herniate into scrotum.

POINTS TO PONDER

- The **Intermediate mesoderm** (nephrotome) forms:
  - **Pronephros** in the cervical region.
  - **Mesonephros** in the thoracic and lumbar regions which are drained by mesonephric/Wolffian ducts into the primitive urogenital sinus.
  - **Metanephros**/or definitive kidneys in the sacral region.
- The **Urogenital sinus** expands in the upper part to become the bladder.
- The inferior portion of urogenital sinus forms:
  - The **Pelvic urethra** (membranous and prostatic) and **Penile urethra** in males.
  - The **Pelvic urethra** (membranous) and **Vestibule** of the vagina in females.
- The sexual differentiation of genetic males commences at the end of the sixth week by the expression of **SRY** gene on Y chromosome.
- Embryos in which this gene is not expressed develop as **females**.
- The **SRY protein** leads to the formation of the testes, the male genital ducts, the male external genitalia and male secondary sex characteristics.

BRAIN TEASERS

1. Which part of the developing kidney gives rise to the ureter, renal pelvis, major and minor calyces and collecting tubules?
   A. Pronephros
   B. Mesonephros
   C. Metanephros
   D. Mesoderm
2. What structures make up the collecting system in the developing kidney?
   A. Glomerulus and Bowman's capsule
   B. Ureter, pelvis, major and minor calyces, and collecting tubules
   C. Proximal convoluted tubule, loop of Henle, distal convoluted tubule
   D. Nephrons
3. When does the kidney become functional during development?
   A. 8th week
   B. 10th week
   C. 12th week
   D. 14th week
4. What clinical condition can result from the incomplete division of the ureteric bud?
   A. Polycystic kidneys
   B. Supernumerary kidneys
   C. Wilms tumour
   D. Denys–Drash syndrome
5. Which part of the developing urinary system is obliterated to form the median umbilical ligament in adults?
   A. Allantois
   B. Urachus
   C. Mesonephric duct
   D. Metanephric tissue
6. What does the trigone of the bladder derive its mesodermal origin from?
   A. Mesonephric ducts
   B. Metanephric tissue
   C. Urogenital sinus
   D. Cloaca
7. Which gene mutation is associated with Wilms tumour?
   A. WT1
   B. SOX9
   C. SRY
   D. WNT4
8. Which syndrome is characterized by Wilms tumor, aniridia and gonadoblastoma?
   A. WAGR syndrome
   B. Denys–Drash syndrome
   C. Turner syndrome
   D. Klinefelter syndrome
9. Which chromosome carries the SRY gene, the testis-determining factor?
   A. X chromosome
   B. Y chromosome
   C. Z chromosome
   D. Autosome
10. What is the role of the SRY protein in sex differentiation?
    A. Induces female development
    B. Induces male development
    C. Inhibits testosterone production
    D. Promotes estrogen synthesis
11. Which cells produce anti-Müllerian hormone (AMH)?
    A. Leydig cells
    B. Sertoli cells
    C. Primordial germ cells
    D. Follicular cells
12. What does AMH (anti-Müllerian hormone) lead to in male development?
    A. Regression of paramesonephric ducts
    B. Differentiation of female external genitalia
    C. Formation of uterine tubes
    D. Development of labia majora
13. Which gene is responsible for ovarian development?
    A. SRY
    B. WT1
    C. SOX9
    D. WNT4

14. In males, what does the mesonephric duct transform into after linking with rete testis?
    A. Vas deferens
    B. Uterine tubes
    C. Epididymis
    D. Urethra
15. What is formed by the fusion of genital tubercles in males during external genitalia development?
    A. Labia minora
    B. Scrotal swellings
    C. Clitoris
    D. Phallus
16. What do the genital tubercles form in females during external genitalia development?
    A. Clitoris
    B. Prostate gland
    C. Labia minora
    D. Scrotal swellings

Answers

1. (B); 2. (B); 3. (C); 4. (B); 5. (B); 6. (A); 7. (A); 8. (A); 9. (B); 10. (B); 11. (B); 12. (A); 13. (D); 14. (A); 15. (D); 16. (A).

FURTHER READINGS

Acién P, Acién M. Renal agenesis, associated genital malformations, and responsible genes. *Fertil Steril.* 2021;116(5):1370-1371. https://doi.org/10.1016/j.fertnstert.2021.08.042.

Cornec-Le Gall E, Alam A, Perrone RD. Autosomal dominant polycystic kidney disease. *Lancet.* 2019;393(10174):919-935. https://doi.org/10.1016/S0140-6736(18)32782-X.

Garratt J, Siegelman ES. MR imaging of Müllerian anomalies. *Magn Reson Imaging Clin N Am.* 2023;31(1):11-28. https://doi.org/10.1016/j.mric.2022.06.002.

Grinspon RP, Bergadá I, Rey RA. Male hypogonadism and disorders of sex development. *Front Endocrinol.* 2020;11:211. https://doi.org/10.3389/fendo.2020.00211.

Hill MS, Phelan MW. Polycystic horseshoe kidney. *Kidney Int.* 2022;101(4):835. https://doi.org/10.1016/j.kint.2021.08.010.

Kalfa N, Gaspari L, Ollivier M, et al. Molecular genetics of hypospadias and cryptorchidism recent developments. *Clin Genet.* 2019;95(1):122-131. https://doi.org/10.1111/cge.13432.

Lee BR, Strobel KM, Chu A. The neonate with ambiguous genitalia. *Neoreviews.* 2021;22(4):e241-e249. https://doi.org/10.1542/neo.22-4-e241.

Nguyen V, Ngo L, Jaqua EE. Cryptorchidism (undescended testicle). *Am Fam Physician.* 2023;108(4):378-385.

Sugi MD, Penna R, Jha P, et al. Müllerian duct anomalies: role in fertility and pregnancy. *Radiographics.* 2021;41(6):1857-1875. https://doi.org/10.1148/rg.2021210022.

Xiang H, Han J, Ridley WE, Ridley LJ. Uterus didelphys: anatomic variant. *J Med Imaging Radiat Oncol.* 2018;62(suppl 1):115. https://doi.org/10.1111/1754-9485.58_12784.

Development of Face 19

AN 43.4 Describe the development of face.
AN 43.4 Describe the development of palate.
AN 43.4 Describe the developmental basis of congenital anomalies of face and palate.

ANAMNESE

A child was brought to the paediatric clinic with a diagnosed **Oblique facial cleft**, a rare congenital condition characterized by a noticeable separation in the facial tissues extending from the upper lip to the lower eyelid along a diagonal axis. The parents reported a healthy pregnancy with routine prenatal care, and there were no known genetic predispositions. The medical team conducted a thorough evaluation to identify aetiological factors. While the precise cause remained unclear, the team considered a range of factors, including environmental influences and genetic variations (Fig. 19.1).

Recognizing a person upon initial contact holds significance for humans. The ability to decide whether to confront, evade or seek shelter depends on this swift recognition. While some species rely on olfaction or audition for individual recognition, humans predominantly use their visual system, with a primary focus on faces. When observing a face, two rapid and involuntary processes are initiated: the categorization of the face as part of our own group or species and the identification of the individual face.

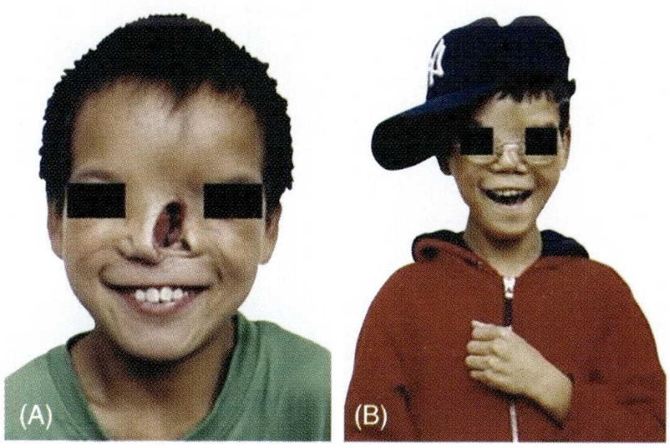

Fig. 19.1 Oblique facial cleft. (Courtesy Dr. J. A. Ascherman, Department of Surgery, Division of Plastic Surgery, Columbia University Medical Center, New York, NY. *The Developing Human: Clinically Oriented Embryology*, 11th ed., Fig. 9.44, Elsevier Inc., 2020.)

DEVELOPMENT OF FACE

- The developmental journey of the face begins in the **fourth week** of gestation.
- By the **sixth week**, the external features of the face also take shape.
- The development of face occurs around stomodeum and the following processes contribute to the formation of face: (AN 43.4)
  - The **Frontonasal process**.
  - A pair of **Maxillary processes**.
  - A pair of **Mandibular processes**.
- Each process consists of mesenchymal core covered by surface ectoderm.

STOMODEUM

- The stomodeum is a surface depression lined with ectoderm that emerges during the head fold of the embryo by fourth week of development.
- It acts as a separator between the developing brain and the pericardium.
- Bounded above by the bulging **forebrain vesicle** and below by the **pericardial swelling**, its lateral wall is formed by the **first pharyngeal arch**, and the floor is composed of the **bucco-pharyngeal membrane**.

FRONTONASAL PROCESS

- The mesenchyme, originating from the caudal part of the forebrain vesicle along with the surface ectoderm, extends downward during the fifth week, forming the frontonasal process.
- It overlaps the upper part of **stomodeum** (Fig. 19.2).

MAXILLARY AND MANDIBULAR PROCESS

- **Maxillary processes** develop as triangular projections from the dorsal part of mandibular arch/first pharyngeal arch.
- **Mandibular processes** are formed from the ventral part of **first pharyngeal arch**.

NASAL PLACODE

- The ectoderm overlying frontonasal process shows localized bilateral thickenings called **Nasal placodes/Olfactory placodes**.
- Nasal placode invaginates and form depressions due to the outgrowth of surrounding mesenchyme, known as **Nasal/Olfactory pits**.
- It becomes continuous with the roof of stomodeum below.

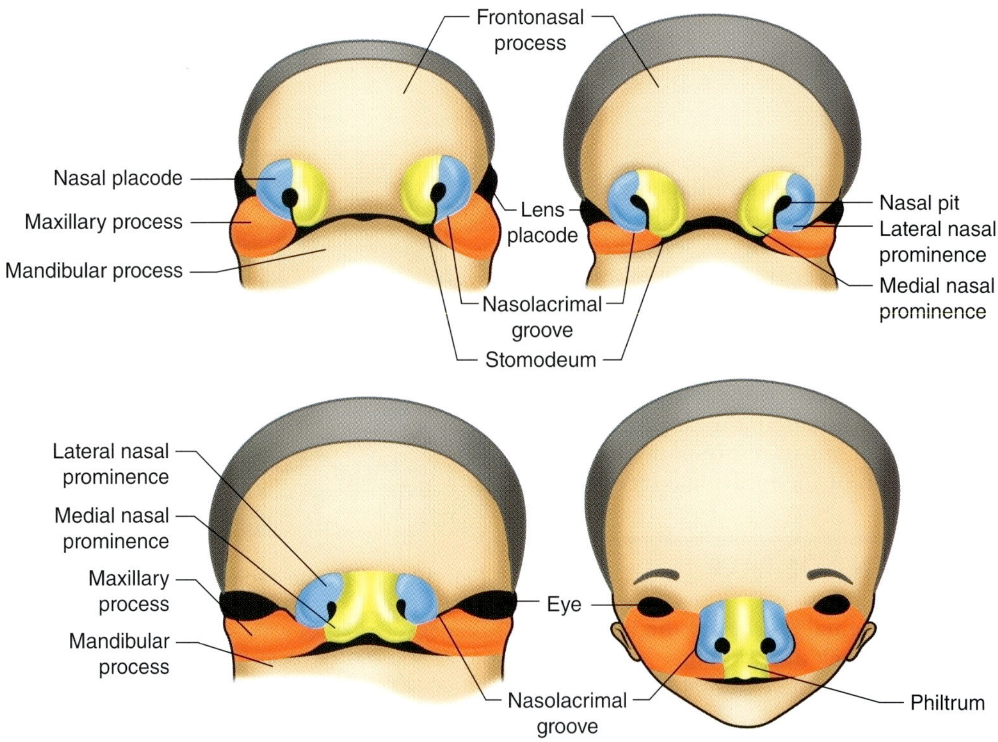

Fig. 19.2 Development of face. (See the text for description)

Continued

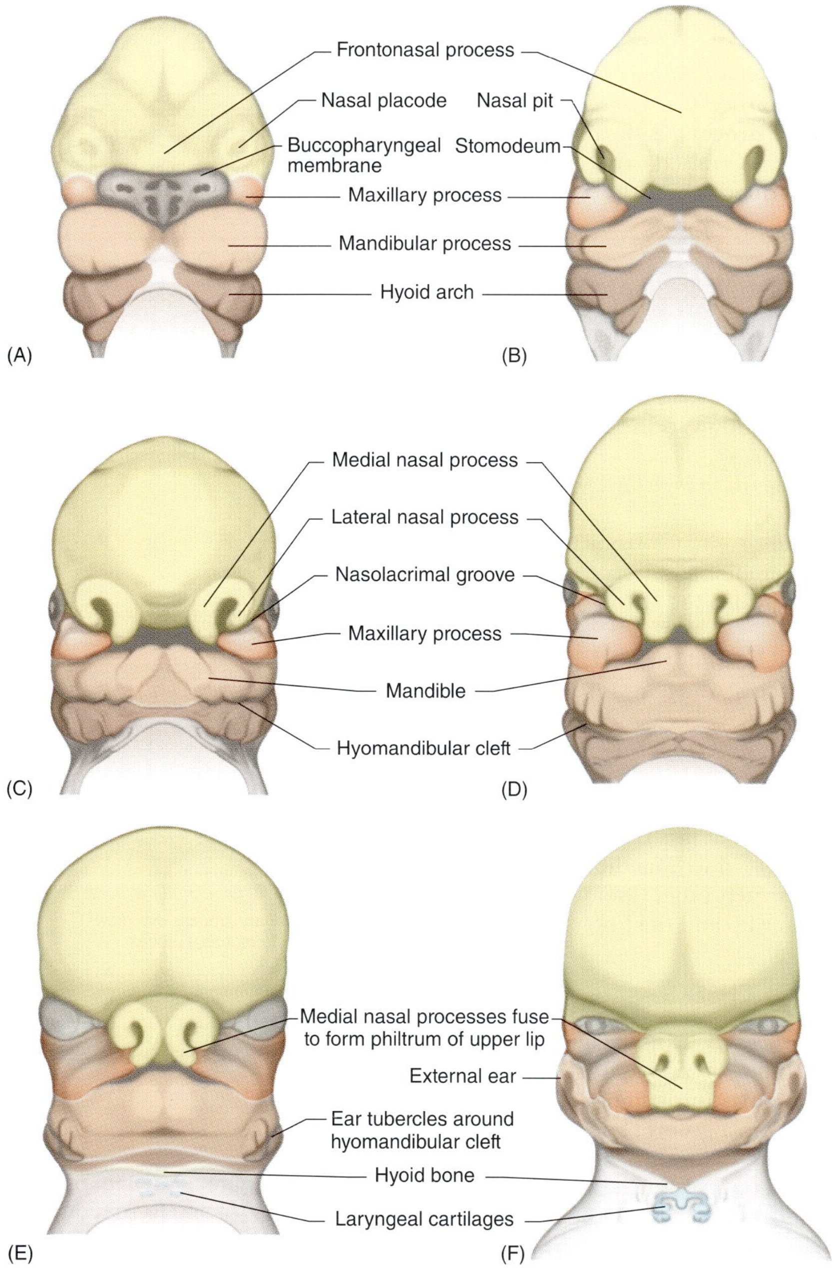

Fig. 19.2, cont'd (A), 5 weeks (B), 5.5 weeks (C), 6 weeks (D), 7 weeks (E) and 8 weeks (F). The frontonasal prominences (processes) are gradually separated from the maxillary prominence by deep furrows. The maxillary prominences (processes) fuse with the medial nasal prominences (processes). The single frontonasal prominence contributes to the forehead, bridge of the nose, and the medial and lateral nasal prominences. The maxillary prominences contribute to the cheeks and the lateral portion of the upper lip. The medial nasal prominences contribute to the philtrum of the upper lip and the crest and tip of the nose. The lateral nasal prominences contribute to the alae of the nose. The mandibular prominences contribute to the lower lip. (Source: *Head and Neck Imaging*. 5th ed. 2011; Credit line: Modified from Strandring, S ed. Gray's Anatomy: *The Anatomical Basis of Clinical Practice*. 40th ed. Madrid: Churchill Livingstone Elsevier, 2008.)

NASAL PIT

- Edges of nasal pit are raised above the surfaces to form **Nasal processes.**
- **Medial nasal process** is formed when the medial edge is raised and **lateral nasal process** is formed when the lateral edge is raised.

FORMATION OF UPPER LIP AND LOWER LIP

- The maxillary process undergoes an increase in size and grows medially.
- Subsequently, it fuses with the medial nasal process, contributing to the formation of the upper lip.
- The upper lip derives from two sources, as shown in Fig. 19.3.
- The **Philtrum** originates from the **Frontonasal process** (medial nasal process), while the lateral part is derived from the **Maxillary process**.
- The **skin** over the philtrum is derived from the **Maxillary process**, which overgrows the frontonasal process.
- Consequently, the ectoderm covering the entire upper lip originates from the maxillary process, and the upper lip is supplied by the maxillary division of the **Trigeminal nerve**.
- Simultaneously, the **Mandibular processes** grow towards each other, eventually fusing to form the lower lip and the lower jaw.

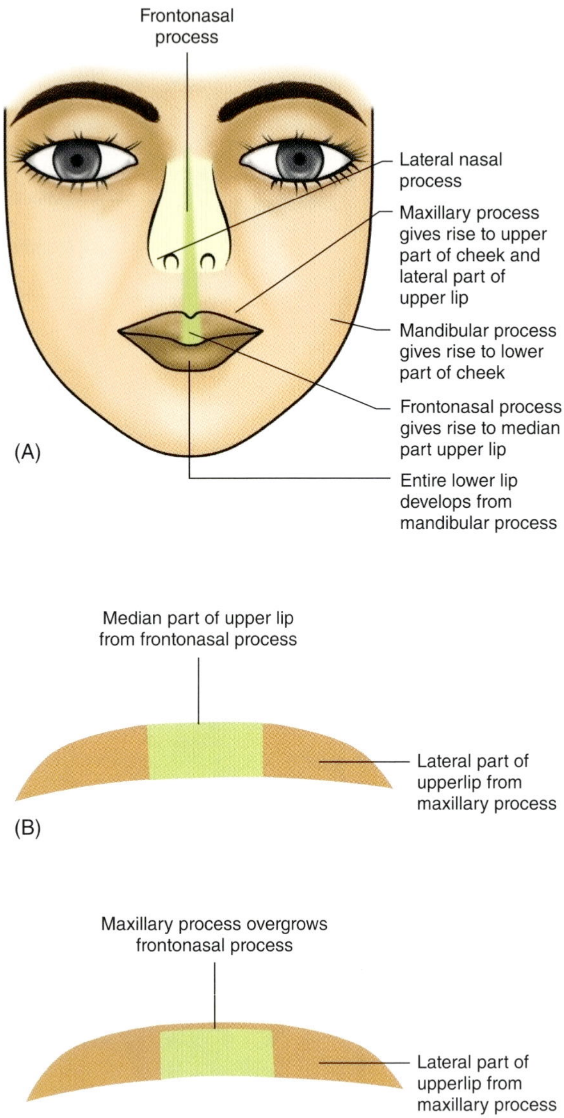

Fig. 19.3 Figure showing derivatives of facial prominences (A) and formation of upper lip (B, C).

FORMATION OF CHEEKS

- Maxillary processes exhibit medial growth, merging with the lateral nasal process.

Nasolacrimal Groove Formation:

- Before fusion, a groove, known as the nasolacrimal groove or furrow, is established between them.
- The surface ectoderm fills the nasolacrimal groove, forming a **solid ectodermal cord**.

Canalization and Duct Formation:

- Subsequent to the fusion of the maxillary and nasal processes, the cord detaches from the surface and undergoes canalization, giving rise to the **Nasolacrimal duct**.
- The nasolacrimal duct extends from the medial angle of the eye to the inferior meatus of the nasal cavity. The upper end of the duct undergoes dilation, forming the **Lacrimal sac**.
- The maxillary process then enlarges, contributing to the development of the **cheeks**.

Table 19.1 Parts of Face and its Embryological Precursor

Frontonasal process	Forehead, bridge of nose
Maxillary process	Upper lip, cheeks
Mandibular process	Lower lip, lower jaw
Medial nasal process	Tip and crest of the nose, philtrum of upper lip
Lateral nasal process	Alae of the nose
Olfactory pits	Anterior nares

FORMATION OF NOSE

- **Bridge formation:** The frontonasal process contributes to the development of the nasal bridge.
- **Tip and crest of the nose:** The medial nasal process is responsible for the formation of the nasal tip and crest.
- **Alae development:** Lateral nasal processes gives rise to the alae of the nose.
- **Primitive anterior nares:** During this process, olfactory pits become detached from the stomodeum roof, persisting as primitive anterior nares.
- The embryological precursors in development of face is given in Table 19.1.

Nerve Supply

- Frontonasal process—**Ophthalmic division** (V_1) of the Trigeminal nerve.
- Maxillary process—**Maxillary division** (V_2) of the Trigeminal nerve.
- Mandibular process—**Mandibular division** (V_3) of the Trigeminal nerve.

DEVELOPMENT OF PALATE (AN 43.4)

- Development of palate begins by 6th week and is completed by 12th week. **Primary palate** is first formed from the frontonasal process.
- Then the **Secondary palate** develops from maxillary process and finally both fuse to form the **Definitive palate** (Fig. 19.4).

PRIMARY PALATE

- **Fusion of Medial Nasal Processes:** The primary palate is a result of the fusion between two medial nasal processes derived from the frontonasal process.
- **Wedge-Shaped Mesenchyme Mass:** Taking on a wedge-shaped form, this mass of mesenchyme encapsulates the upper four incisor teeth.
- **Premaxilla:** The primary palate undergoes ossification, eventually forming the premaxilla.

SECONDARY PALATE

- **Medial Extensions:** Around the sixth week of development, the medial walls of the maxillary process form thin, shelf-like extensions known as **palatal processes** on either side of the tongue as shown in Fig. 19.4.
- **Horizontal Fusion:** Towards the end of the eighth week, these palatal processes undergo horizontal fusion, uniting above the tongue and contributing to the formation of the secondary palate.

DEFINITIVE PALATE

- **Fusion and definite palate formation:** The primary palate and the secondary palate fuse together, creating a **Y-shaped suture** forming the definitive palate.
- **Incisive fossa and foramina:** At the junction of the primary and secondary palate, the incisive fossa becomes evident. **Two incisive foramina** open into this fossa.
- **Intramembranous ossification:** During the subsequent stages, the mesoderm in the anterior three-fourths of the palate undergoes intramembranous ossification, leading to the development of the hard palate.
- **Soft palate:** However, the ossification process does not extend to the posterior **one-fourth**, resulting in the formation of the soft palate.
- **Primary palate and secondary palate** are fused together by a Y-shaped suture to form definite palate.

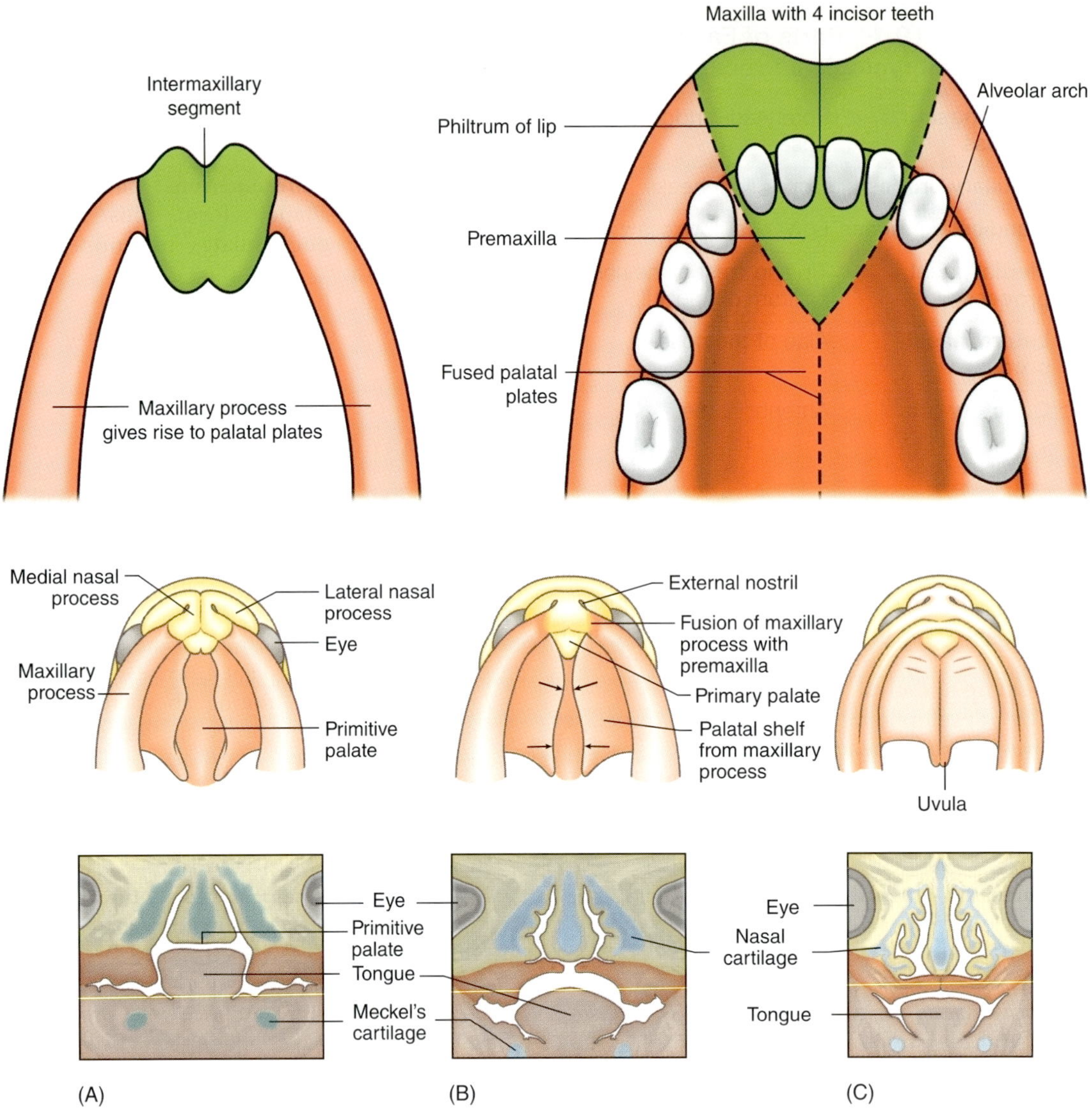

Fig. 19.4 Development of palate. Formation of premaxilla (*first row*). Ventral views (*second row*) and coronal sections (*third row*) of the palatal development during embryonic weeks 7 and 8. (Source: *Head and Neck Imaging*, 5th ed., 2011; Credit Line: Modified from Strandring, S ed. *Gray's Anatomy: The Anatomical Basis of Clinical Practice*. 40th ed. Madrid: Churchill Livingstone Elsevier, 2008.)

CLINICAL NUGGETS

Cleft lip (Cheiloschisis) (AN 43.4)

- Cleft lip, known as **cheiloschisis**, manifests in various forms. It can be categorized as either incomplete, affecting the upper lip exclusively, or complete, extending into the nose.
- **Unilateral and bilateral presentation:** The condition may present unilaterally (affecting one side) or bilaterally (affecting both sides), influencing the severity and visual impact.
- **Underlying cause:** The primary cause of cleft lip lies in the incomplete fusion of the **medial nasal prominence** with the **maxillary process**, disrupting the natural development of the facial structures.
- The **LAHSAL code** was chosen as the preferred classification system.
- LAHSAL is an acronym that indicates the anatomical structures of the palate. It starts from the right side of the patient and goes towards the left. The letters in the acronym are as follows:
  - **L:** Right lip.
  - **A:** Right alveolus.
  - **H:** Hard palate.
  - **S:** Soft palate.
  - **A:** Left alveolus.
  - **L:** Left lip.

  The LAHSAL code indicates whether there is a **complete cleft** (upper case letter), an **incomplete cleft** (lower case letter) or **no cleft**. For example, a complete bilateral cleft lip and palate is represented by all six capital letters—**LAHSAL**.

Cleft palate (Palatoschisis)

- Cleft palate, or palatoschisis, arises from the failure of the **maxillary shelves** to fuse horizontally during embryonic development.
- The severity varies, and in more pronounced cases, the cleft may extend into the upper jaw. The condition can occur as a standalone issue or be associated with a cleft lip.
- Cleft palate can manifest as complete, involving both sides, or incomplete. It may also be **unilateral** (affecting one side) or **bilateral** (affecting both sides).
- Unlike cleft lip, cleft palates are typically diagnosed after birth, often during routine medical examinations. Diagnostic tools, such as the **20-week anomaly scan**, are effective in identifying cleft lip.
- The presence of cleft lip and palate can impact essential functions such as feeding and speech.

DEVELOPMENT OF NASAL CAVITIES

The nasal cavities develop from **Ectodermal nasal placodes**. Nasal placodes undergo invagination to create the nasal pits during early embryonic development (Fig. 19.5).

- **Formation of Nasal Sacs:** Subsequently, the nasal pits deepen, leading to the development of nasal sacs.
- **Primitive Nasal Cavity:** Each nasal sac contributes to the formation of the primitive nasal cavity.
- **Oronasal Membrane:** The oronasal membrane acts as a temporary barrier, separating the primitive nasal cavities from the primitive oral cavity. By the end of the sixth week, the oronasal membrane undergoes rupture, resulting in the creation of **Primitive choanae** situated behind the primary palate. Primitive choanae establish connections between the primitive nasal and oral cavities.
- **Definitive Choanae:** After the development of the secondary palate, definitive choanae

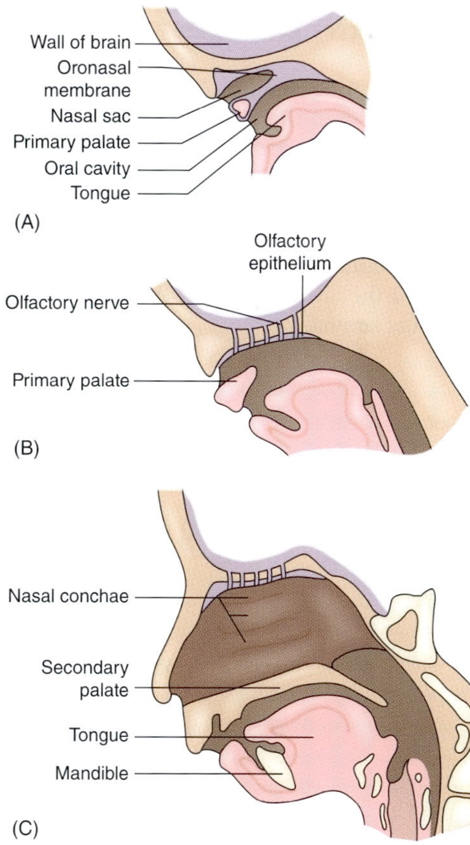

Fig. 19.5 Development of nasal cavity.

form, providing a connection between the **Nasal cavity** and the **Nasopharynx**.

- **External and Dorsal Openings:**
  - **Anterior or External Nares:** The ventral openings of the nasal sacs that emerge on the face.
  - **Posterior Nasal Aperture (Choanae):** The dorsal openings connecting the nasal cavity to the nasopharynx.
- **Frontonasal Process and Nasal Septum:** The frontonasal process, initially wide, undergoes changes as the nasal sacs enlarge. The intervening tissue narrows to form the **Nasal septum**.
- **Lateral Wall of the Nose:** The lateral nasal process contributes to the formation of the lateral wall of the nose, while the **Nasal conchae** (superior, middle and inferior) appear as elevations on the lateral walls of each nasal cavity.
- **Olfactory Epithelium:** The roof of the nasal cavity, lined with ectoderm, gives rise to the olfactory epithelium.

DEVELOPMENT OF TEETH

- **Primary Teeth Formation:** Primary teeth begin forming between the sixth and eighth week of development (Fig. 19.6).
- **Permanent Teeth Development:** Permanent teeth initiation occurs around the **20th week** of development.
- **Dental Lamina:** The epithelium over the convex border of the alveolar process thickens to form the dental lamina.
- **Stages of Tooth Development:**
  - **Bud Stage:** Tooth bud emerges without a clear cellular arrangement, located at the periphery of the dental lamina.
  - **Cap Stage:** Localized proliferation of the lamina results in the formation of the **enamel organ**, a cup-shaped structure housing the dental papilla. Together, they constitute the **tooth germ**.
  - **Bell Stage: Ameloblasts** (columnar cells of the enamel organ) and **odontoblasts** (mesodermal cells in the papilla) are important components separated by a basement membrane. The remaining papilla cells contribute to the tooth's pulp. This stage gives the developing tooth a bell-like appearance.
  - **Maturation (Apposition):**
    - **Ameloblasts:** Responsible for enamel deposition.
    - **Odontoblasts:** Contribute to dentine formation.
    - After enamel formation completion, ameloblasts vanish, forming a thin **dental cuticle**. Odontoblasts persist throughout life, separating dentine from the pulp.
    - **Root establishment** involves continued growth into the underlying mesenchyme, with surrounding mesenchyme forming the periodontal ligament.
    - The **periodontal ligament** connects the tooth's root to the socket.

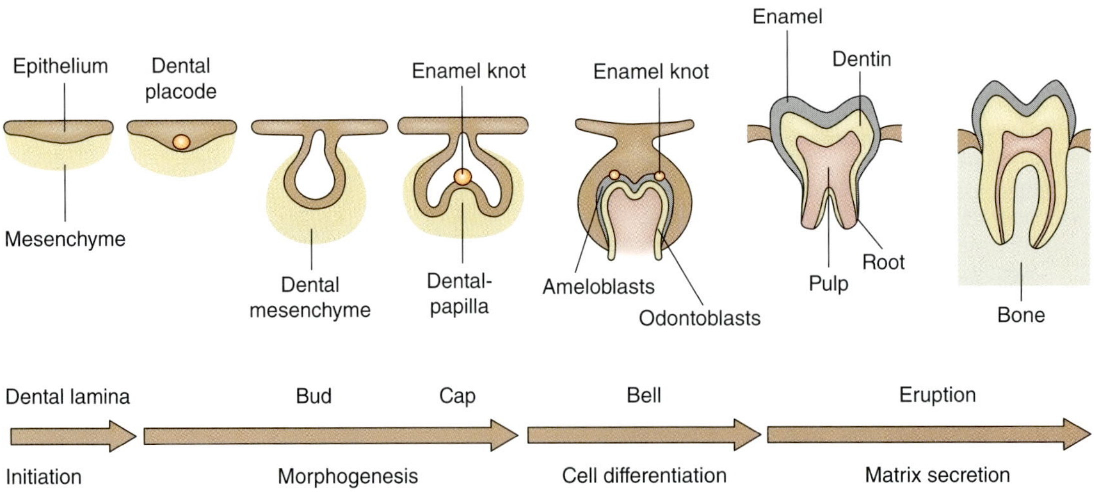

Fig 19.6 Schematic representation of the principal stages of tooth formation.

AVERAGE AGE OF ERUPTION (TABLE 19.2)

Table 19.2 Eruption of Temporary and Permanent Teeth

Temporary or Milk Teeth	
Lower central incisor	6–9 months
Upper incisors	8–10 months
Lower lateral incisor	12–20 months
First molar	12–20 months
Canine	16–20 months
Second molars	20–39 months
Permanent Teeth	
First molar	6–7 years
Central incisor	6–8 years
Lateral incisors	7–9 years
Premolars	10–12 years
Canines	10–12 years
Second molars	11–13 years
Third molars	17–21 years

KLINISCHE PERLEN (AN 43.4)

FACIAL CLEFTS—TYPES AND CHARACTERISTICS: (FIG 19.7)

a) **Anterior Cleft Deformity (Anterior to Incisive Foramen):**
   - Partial or complete failure of fusion between the **Maxillary prominence** and **Medial nasal prominence** (Fig. 19.8).
   - **Examples:**
     - ➢ Lateral cleft lip.
     - ➢ Cleft upper jaw.
     - ➢ Cleft between primary and secondary palates.

b) **Posterior Cleft Deformity (Posterior to Incisive Foramen):**
   - Failure of fusion of **palatine shelves** (Fig. 19.9).
   - **Examples:**
     - ➢ Cleft palate (secondary).
     - ➢ Cleft uvula.

c) **Combination of Both:**
   - Severe form combining anterior and posterior cleft deformities.

d) **Oblique Facial Cleft:**
   - Failure of fusion between the maxillary prominence and lateral nasal prominence (Fig. 19.10). Exposure of the nasolacrimal duct to the surface.

e) **Median Cleft Lip:**
   - Failure of fusion of two medial nasal prominences in the midline. Often associated with brain anomalies.

ANODONTIA

Anodontia refers to the congenital absence of all **primary (deciduous) or permanent teeth**.

- **Causes:**
  - ➢ Genetic factors.
  - ➢ Developmental abnormalities during tooth bud formation.
  - ➢ Environmental factors during prenatal development.
- **Clinical Features:**
  - ➢ Complete absence of teeth in the affected individual.
  - ➢ May occur as an isolated condition or as part of a syndrome.

GERMINATION OF TOOTH

Germination is a dental anomaly where a single tooth germ attempts to divide into two, resulting in a large, often **bifid crown on a single root**.

- **Causes:**
  - ➢ Developmental issues during the formation of the tooth germ.
  - ➢ Genetic factors.
  - ➢ Environmental factors influencing tooth development.
- **Clinical Features:**
  - ➢ Tooth appears larger than normal due to the attempt at division.
  - ➢ The tooth may have a cleft in the crown, resembling two teeth.
  - ➢ Commonly affects **incisors**.

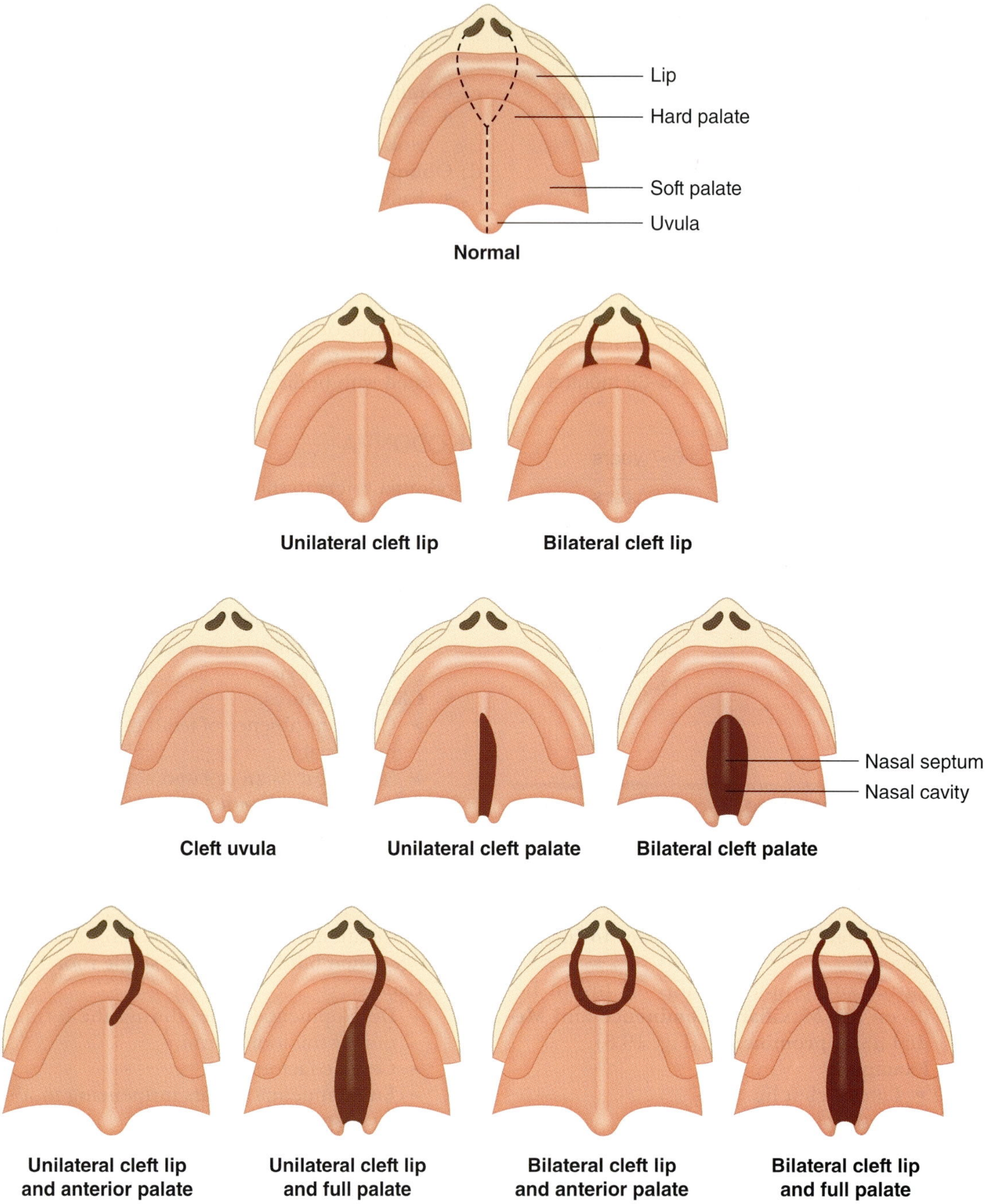

Fig. 19.7 Different types of cleft lip and palate.

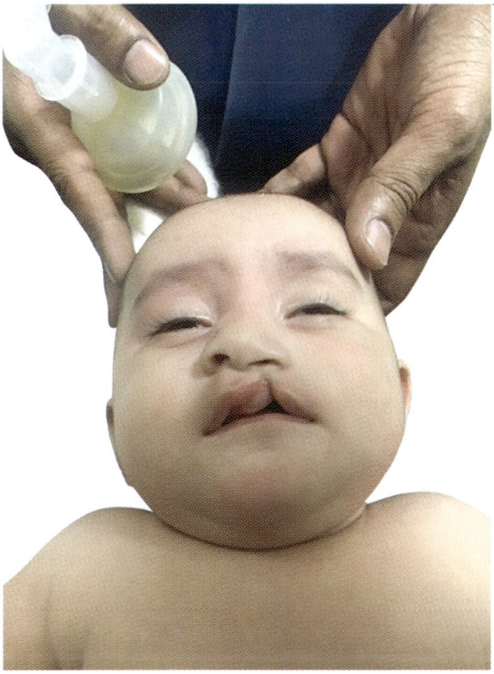

Fig. 19.8 A child with cleft lip. (Photo courtesy: Dr Arjun, Tricity, Institute of plastic surgery, Chandigarh.)

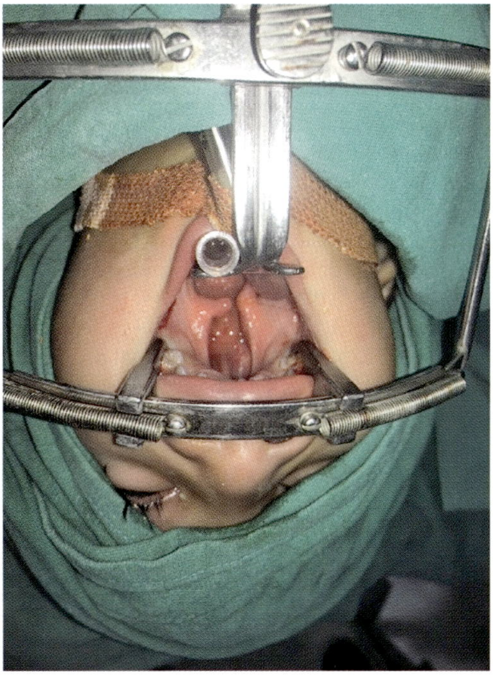

Fig. 19.9 A child with cleft palate. (Photo courtesy: Dr Arjun, Tricity, Institute of Plastic surgery, Chandigarh.)

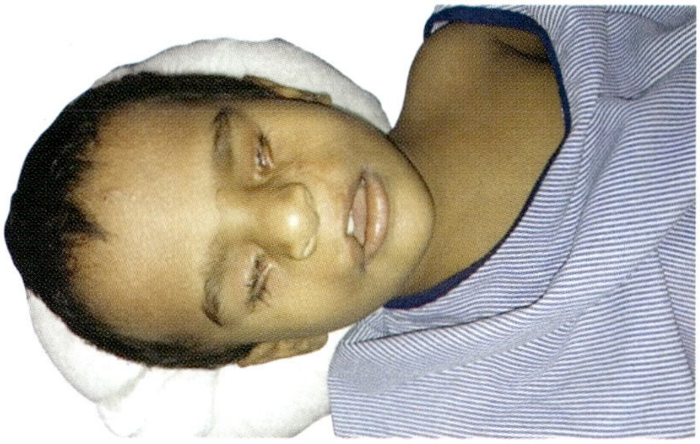

Fig. 19.10 Cleft extending from lips to orbit, associated with ocular defects. (Photo courtesy: Dr Arjun Tricity Institute of plastic surgery, Chandigarh.)

POINTS TO PONDER

The development of the human face occurs between the 4th and 10th weeks of embryonic life, by five facial prominences: the frontonasal, maxillary (pair) and mandibular (pair).

The developmental events are as follows:

Olfactory placodes (fifth week):

- During the fifth week, olfactory placodes emerge on the frontonasal prominence.
- These placodes invaginate to form nasal pits, subsequently dividing the frontonasal prominence into medial and lateral nasal processes.

Facial clefts:

- Defective fusion of facial prominences can result in facial clefts.

Medial nasal processes:

- The medial nasal processes unite, contributing to the formation of essential facial features, including the bridge of the nose, the philtrum (the vertical groove above the upper lip) and the primary palate.

Lateral nasal processes:

- Lateral nasal processes give rise to the lateral aspect of the nose, playing an important role in the overall facial symmetry.

Maxillary processes:

- Maxillary processes play a significant role in cheek development.

Mandibular processes:

- The mandibular processes contribute to the formation of the lower jaw.

Secondary palate formation:

- Shelf-like processes from the maxillary swelling contribute to the formation of the secondary palate.

BRAIN TEASERS

1. What separates the developing brain from the pericardium during embryonic development?
   A. Frontonasal process
   B. Stomodeum
   C. Maxillary process
   D. Nasal placode
2. Which facial prominence gives rise to the bridge of the nose?
   A. Maxillary process
   B. Frontonasal process
   C. Mandibular process
   D. Nasal pit
3. Which nerve supplies the maxillary process during facial development?
   A. Ophthalmic nerve (V1)
   B. Maxillary nerve (V2)
   C. Mandibular nerve (V3)
   D. Facial nerve (VII)
4. How is the upper lip formed during embryonic development?
   A. Fusion of mandibular processes
   B. Fusion of maxillary processes
   C. Fusion of lateral nasal process
   D. Fusion of nasal placode with stomodeum
5. What forms the primitive nasal cavity during development?
   A. Nasal sacs
   B. Nasal placodes
   C. Maxillary process
   D. Nasolacrimal duct
6. What is the clinical term for the condition resulting from the incomplete fusion of the medial nasal prominence with the maxillary process?
   A. Cheiloschisis
   B. Palatoschisis
   C. Cleft lip
   D. Cleft palate
7. When do primary teeth begin to form during embryonic development?
   A. Tenth week
   B. Twentieth week
   C. Sixth week
   D. Fourth week
8. What connects the primitive nasal and oral cavities after the rupture of the oronasal membrane?
   A. Choanae
   B. Nasal septum
   C. Dental lamina
   D. Nasal sacs
9. Which nerve supplies the frontonasal process during facial development?
   A. Ophthalmic nerve (V1)
   B. Maxillary nerve (V2)
   C. Mandibular nerve (V3)
   D. Trigeminal nerve (V)
10. What does the dental Lamina form during tooth development?
   A. Primary teeth
   B. Nasal sacs
   C. Choanae
   D. Secondary palate

Answers

1. (B); 2. (B); 3. (B); 4. (B); 5. (A); 6. (C); 7. (C); 8. (A); 9. (A); 10. (A).

FURTHER READINGS

De Santis D, Sinigaglia S, Faccioni P, et al. Syndromes associated with dental agenesis. *Minerva Stomatol.* 2019;68(1):42-56. https://doi.org/10.23736/S0026-4970.18.04129-8.

Houkes R, Smit J, Mossey P, et al. Classification systems of cleft lip, alveolus and palate: results of an international survey. *Cleft Palate Craniofac J.* 2023;60(2):189-196. doi:10.1177/10556656211057368.

Neagu D, Casal-Beloy I, Luaces Rey R, López-Cedrún JL. Agenesia dental [Tooth agenesis]. *Anales de Pediatria.* 2020;92(6):385-386. https://doi.org/10.1016/j.anpedi.2019.03.002.

Prasad V, Ahmed R, Singh AK, Kumar V. A rare case of bilateral oblique facial cleft and accessory maxilla with repaired unilateral cleft lip and palate. *Natl J Maxillofac Surg.* 2019;10(2):241-244. doi:10.4103/njms.NJMS_67_18.

Song WL, Ma HO, Nan Y, et al. Prenatal diagnosis of isolated lateral facial cleft by ultrasonography and three-dimensional printing: a case report. *World J Clin Cases.* 2021;9(24):7196-7204. https://doi.org/10.12998/wjcc.v9.i24.7196.

Central Nervous System 20

AN 43.4 Describe the development of pituitary gland.

AN 43.4 Describe the developmental basis of congenital anomalies of pituitary gland.

AN 64.2 Describe the development of neural tube, spinal cord, medulla oblongata, pons, midbrain, cerebral hemisphere and cerebellum.

AN 64.3 Describe various types of open neural tube defects with its embryological basis.

ANAMNESE

A newborn was admitted to the Neonatal Intensive Care Unit (NICU) with a diagnosed **Occipital encephalocele**, a rare congenital anomaly characterized by a sac-like protrusion of the brain and meninges through an opening in the skull. Newborn's parents noticed the abnormality shortly after birth when they observed a prominent swelling at the back of her head. Upon examination, the presence of a sizeable encephalocele was confirmed and imaging studies revealed herniation of brain tissue through a defect in the occipital bone. She underwent surgical intervention to repair the defect and protect the exposed brain tissue (Fig. 20.1).

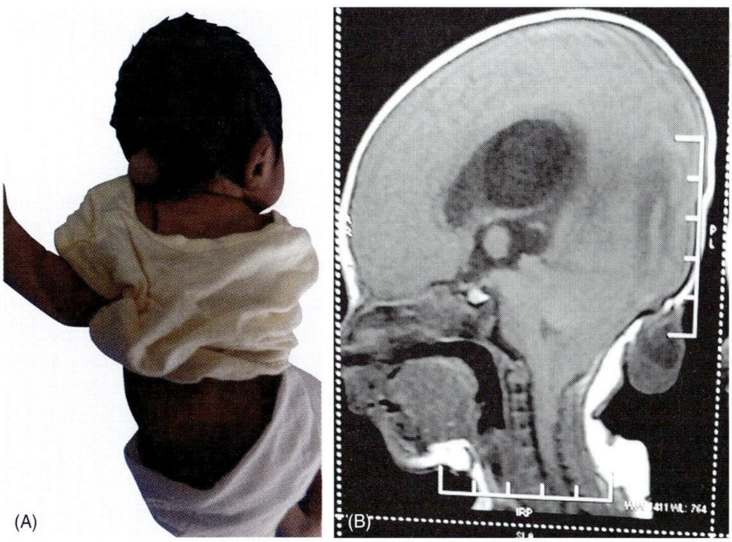

Fig. 20.1 (A) A newborn with occipital encephalocele. (B) MRI showing encephalocele. (Photo courtesy: Dr Nithya.)

Cells that are destined to produce the nervous system begin to form about 3 weeks after fertilization in humans. Most neurogenesis is complete by 5 months, with one important exception being cells in the **Hippocampus**, which continues to form neurons throughout life. **Neural plasticity** or brain plasticity can be defined as the ability of the nervous system to change its activity in response to a stimuli by reorganizing its structures, functions or connections. The human brain is composed of 86 billion neurons. It was believed that **Neurogenesis** or the creation of new neurons stopped shortly after birth. But now it is understood that the brain possesses the remarkable capacity to reorganize pathways, create new connections and, in some cases, even create new neurons.

The central nervous system (CNS) appears in the beginning of the embryonic period (third week to eighth week) from the ectodermal germ layer (Neuroectoderm) that lies over the notochord and in front of the primitive node.

NEURAL PLATE

- The appearance of notochord and prechordal mesoderm induces the development of CNS by the formation of **Neural plate**.
- The thickened ectoderm overlying the notochord is called **Neuroectoderm.** Towards the end of the presomite period, these neuroectodermal cells form an elongated slipper shaped Neural plate.
- The neural plate undergoes neurulation to give rise to **Neural tube**.

NEURULATION

- The neural plate is formed in the beginning of third week following the induction by notochord lying beneath it (Fig. 20.2). By the end of third week (Somite period), the lateral edges of neural plate elevate to form **Neural folds**.
- The longitudinal depression in the middle forms the **Neural groove** which extends from the **Hensen's node** to the **Buccopharyngeal membrane**.
- As the development proceeds, the folds approach each other in the midline and fuse.
- The fusion begins in the cervical region (fourth somite) and continues cranially and caudally, forming the neural tube.

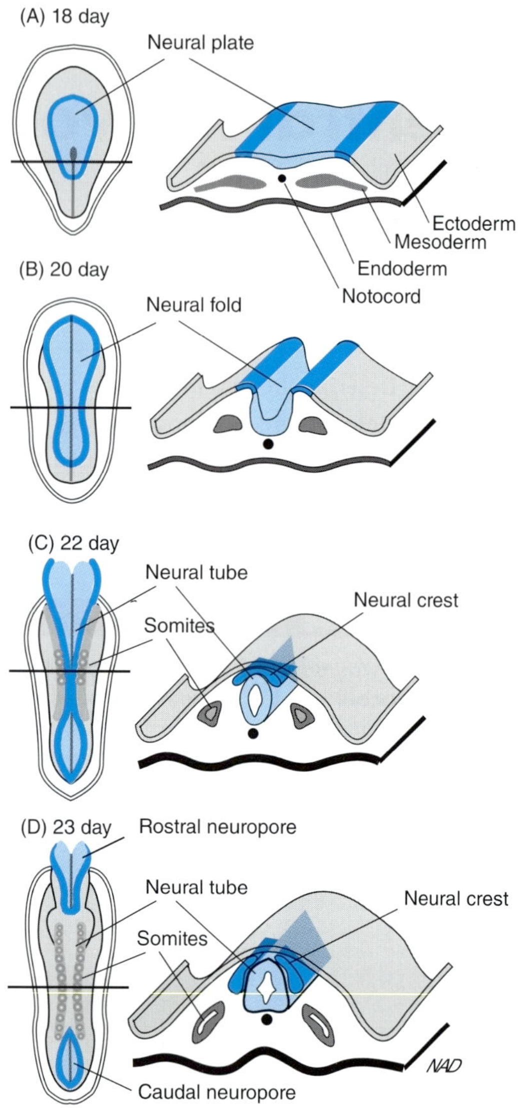

Fig. 20.2 Formation of neural plate, neural crest and neural tube. Human embryos at approximately (A) 18 days, (B) 20 days, (C) 22 days and (D) 23 days. Left side, dorsal view; right side, cross-section at the level indicated on the dorsal view. Note that the neural crest closes into a neural tube in the center first, and this closure moves rostrally and caudally, leaving a neuropore at each end that closes at about 4 weeks. (Source: *Essential Medical Physiology*. 3rd ed. 2003.)

- The neural tube communicates with the amniotic cavity at the cephalic and caudal ends via **Anterior** (cranial) and **Posterior** (caudal) **neuropores,** respectively, till the fusion is complete.

- This communication provides nourishment for the developing neural tube by the **Amniotic fluid** in the amniotic cavity, since vascular nourishment is not established.
- When the neural tube is separated from ectoderm, some cells which were present at the neural folds gets separated to form the **Neural crest cells**.
- Neural crest cells lie just below the ectoderm dorsolateral to neural tube.
- The process of formation of neural tube is known as **Neurulation**.
- The neural crest cells and neural tube formed from the neural plate have different fate and each forms different derivatives.

CLOSURE OF THE NEUROPORES

- Closure of the **Cranial (Anterior) neuropore** occurs at approximately **25th day** (18–20 somite stage) (Fig. 20.2). The anterior neuropore corresponds to the **Lamina terminalis** of the third ventricle in adults.
- The **Caudal (Posterior) neuropore** closes 3 days later **(28th day)** by the end of the fourth week (25 somite stage). This completes neurulation.
- The closed tubular structure represents the CNS of the developing embryo.

NEURAL CREST CELLS

- With the folding of the neural tube, the wedge-shaped mass of cells derived from the neurectoderm lying between the surface ectoderm and the dorsal wall of the neural tube forms the **Neural crest cells**.
- Later this mass splits into two and lies on the dorsolateral aspect of the neural tube as the primitive spinal ganglion (Table 20.1).

Table 20.1 Neural Crest Cell Derivatives

Neural Crest Derivatives	Structures/Formations
Dorsal Mass Derivatives	
Neuroblasts	• Pseudounipolar neurons of dorsal root ganglia for all spinal nerves. • Sensory ganglia of 5th, 7th, 9th and 10th cranial nerves. • Skeletal components of branchial arches. • Parafollicular cells of thyroid gland. • Odontoblasts. • Original bipolar neurons preserved in vestibulocochlear nerves and retina.
Spongioblasts	• Capsular cells around cells of dorsal root ganglia. • Schwann cells.
Pluripotent cells	• Melanoblasts, odontoblasts and cartilage cells of some branchial arches.
Ventral Mass Derivatives	
Small cells/ Sympathoblasts	• Sympathetic ganglion. • Sympathetic trunk. • Sympathetic plexuses. • Cells of parasympathetic ganglion (ciliary, pterygopalatine, submandibular, otic ganglia).
Large cells/Chromaffin Cells/ Phaeochromocytes	• Chromaffin cells of the medulla of suprarenal glands, paraganglia within the ganglia of the sympathetic trunk, para-aortic body around the inferior mesenteric artery, argentaffin and enterochromaffin cells (APUD cells) in the respiratory and gastrointestinal tracts.

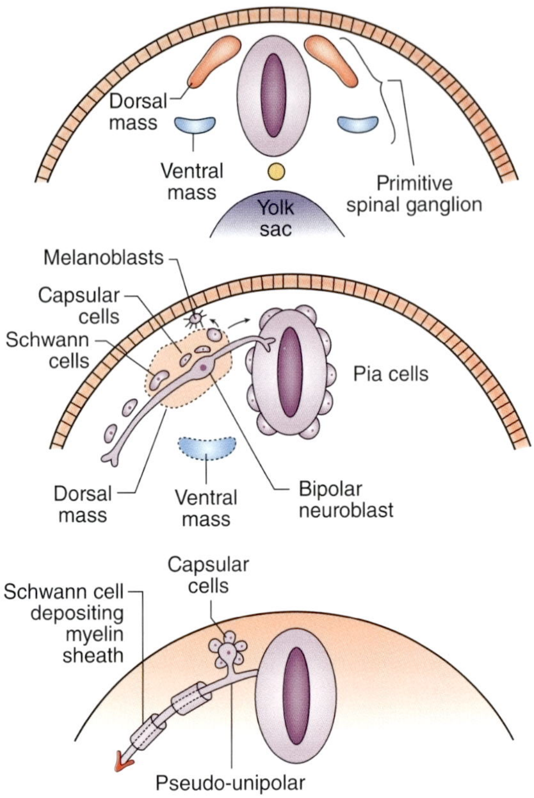

Fig. 20.3 Neural crest cells.

The primitive spinal ganglion then splits into a dorsal and ventral mass (Fig. 20.3).

A) The **Dorsal mass** gives rise to the following structures:
   - **Neuroblasts:** These form the Pseudounipolar neurons of the dorsal root ganglia of all spinal nerves, Sensory ganglia of 5th, 7th, 9th and 10th cranial nerves, Skeletal components of the branchial arches, Parafollicular cells of Thyroid gland and Odontoblasts. **Original bipolar neurons** are preserved in vestibulocochlear nerves and the retina.
   - **Spongioblasts:** These cells differentiate into **Capsular cells** around the cells of Dorsal root ganglia and Schwann cells.
   - **Pluripotent cells:** These cells form Melanoblasts, Odontoblasts and Cartilage cells of some branchial arches.

B) The **Ventral mass** form a syncytium of cells known as **Sympathochromaffin organs.** This later differentiates into small cells and large cells:
   - **Small cells/Sympathoblasts:** These cells form the sympathetic ganglion, sympathetic trunk, sympathetic plexuses, cells of the parasympathetic ganglion (ciliary, pterygopalatine, submandibular, otic ganglia).
   - **Large cells/Chromaffin cells/Phaeochromocytes:** These cells exhibit brownish granules in the cytoplasm when stained with chromium salts. These cells secrete **Noradrenaline**. These cells migrate to various regions and form chromaffin cells of the medulla of suprarenal glands, paraganglia within the ganglia of the sympathetic trunk, para-aortic body around the inferior mesenteric artery, argentaffin and enterochromaffin cells (APUD cells) in the respiratory and gastrointestinal tracts.

CLINICAL NUGGETS

The clavicle

- Arises from neural crest.
- One of the first bones to become ossified (intramembranous).
- Ossification is well advanced by the eighth week.

FATE OF THE NEURAL TUBE (AN 64.2)

- The closed neural tube gives rise to the entire central nervous system. The neural tube which is completely closed has a broader **Cephalic** portion with dilatations called **Vesicles** and a narrow **Caudal** portion, the **Spinal cord**.
- The peripheral nervous system consisting of cranial and spinal nerves and their sensory and sympathetic ganglia are derived partly from neural tube and partly from neural crest cells.
- Further development of the **Cephalic end** of the neural tube is as follows:
- The cephalic end of the neural tube shows three dilatations; the primary brain vesicles (Fig. 20.4):
  1) The **Prosencephalon** or forebrain.
  2) The **Mesencephalon** or midbrain.
  3) The **Rhombencephalon** or hindbrain.

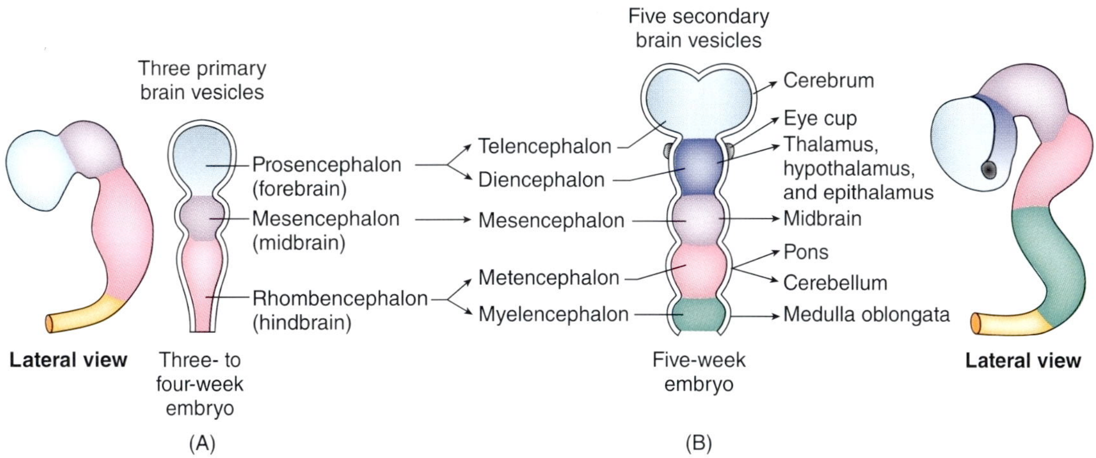

Fig. 20.4 Formation of brain vesicles.

- Simultaneously, it forms a number of flexures (Fig. 20.5):
  - The **Cervical flexure** at the junction of Rhombencephalon (Hindbrain) and Spinal cord. This flexure is concave ventrally and disappears by seventh week with the extension of the embryonic head.
  - The **Cephalic flexure** (mesencephalic flexure) in the Midbrain region develops during head fold of the embryo. This flexure is concave ventrally.
  - The **Pontine flexure** at the middle of Rhombencephalon dividing it into Metencephalon and Myelencephalon. It has a ventral convexity.
  - The **Telencephalic flexure** that occurs late between Telencephalon and Diencephalon.

THE CAVITIES ENCLOSED

- Each subdivision of the developing brain (brain vesicles) encloses a part of the original cavity of the neural tube.
- The cavity of the **Telencephalic** vesicle becomes the **Lateral ventricle** (Fig. 20.6).
- The cavity of the **Diencephalon** (along with central part of telencephalon) becomes **Third ventricle**.
- Each lateral ventricle communicates with the third ventricle through the **Interventricular foramina of Monro**.
- The cavity of the mesencephalon remains narrow and forms **Aqueduct of Sylvius**, which connects the third and fourth ventricles.
- The cavity of **Rhombencephalon** forms **fourth ventricle**. **Central canal** in the Spinal cord is the continuation of the fourth ventricle.

DIFFERENTIATION OF NEURAL TUBE

- The walls of the neural tube gives rise to neurons and neuroglia. The lumen of the tube forms the ventricular system and central canal of spinal cord (Fig. 20.7).
- The neuroepithelial cells lining the neural tube proliferates and form multilayered. They are then organized into three zones: (a) **outer Marginal**, (b) **intermediate Mantle** and (c) **innermost Ependymal**.
  - **Ependymal zone**—Majority of the cells in this germinative zone move outwards into the mantle zone to form Neuroblasts and Spongioblasts. The cells which do not migrate form the **Ependymal lining** of the ventricles and central canal of spinal cord.
  - **Mantle zone**—The neuroblasts of this zone form the **Neurons** and spongioblasts form the **Astrocytes** and **Oligodendrocytes. Microglial cells** are mesodermal in origin and they are seen in both mantle and marginal zone. The grey matter of central nervous system is formed by the mantle zone. Later the cells in the mantle zone migrate to the marginal zone to form the **Cortical grey matter** in cerebrum and cerebellum.
  - **Marginal zone**—The axons of the neuroblasts and neuroglial cells invade this zone. As a result of **Myelination** of nerves in this

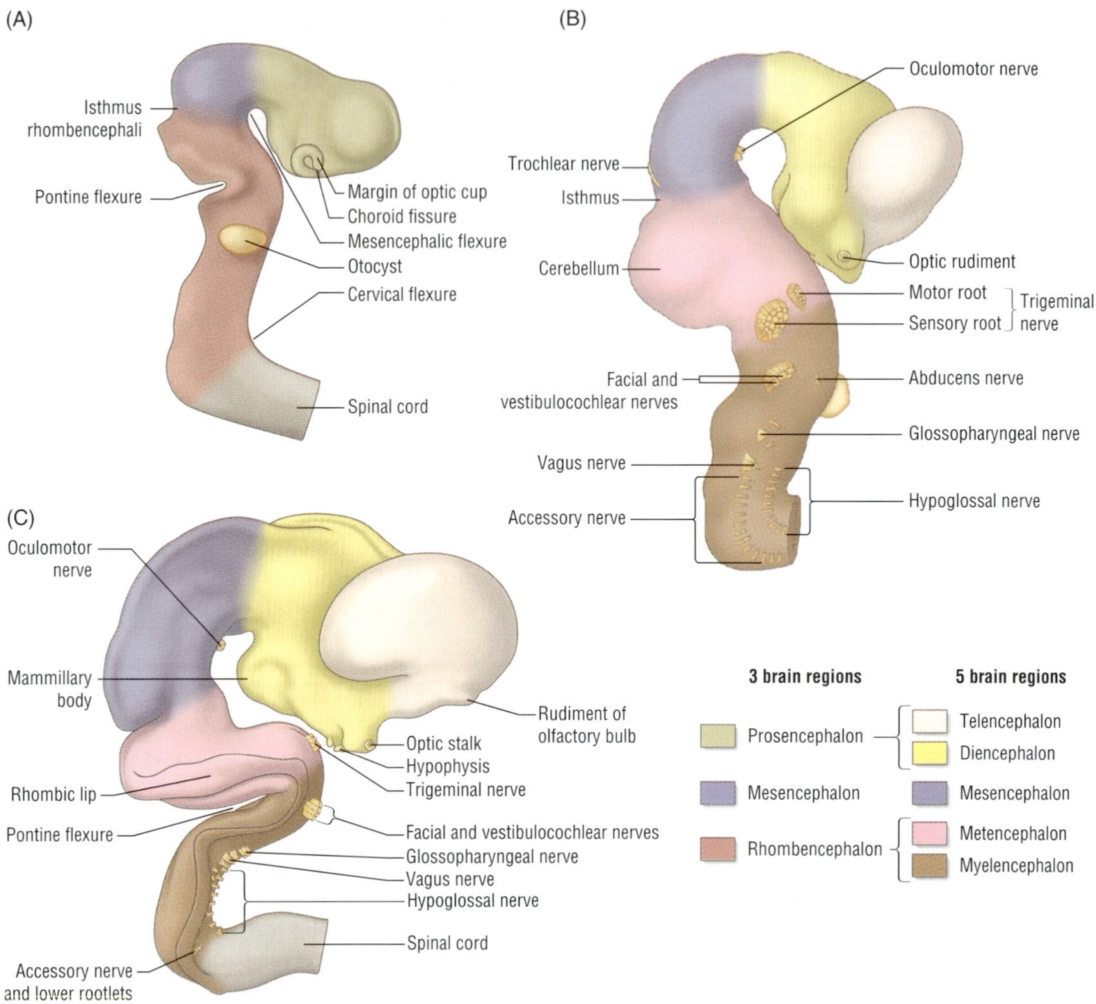

Fig. 20.5 Formation of the mesencephalic, cervical and pontine flexures; human embryos, lateral views. The roof of the rhombencephalon has been removed in each case. (A) 9 mm long. (B) approximately, 10.2 mm long. (C) 13.6 mm long. (Source: *Gray's Anatomy: The Anatomical Basis of Clinical Practice*, 2016.)

layer, this zone appears whitish and forms the white matter of the central nervous system.

DEVELOPMENT OF BRAIN

- The neural tube cranial to the fourth somite forms the brain.
- Brain is often divided into:
  A) **Higher centres** (Cerebral hemispheres and Cerebellum).
  B) **Brain stem** (Myelencephalon, Metencephalon and Mesencephalon).
- The brain is developed from the primary brain vesicles:
  1) **Prosencephalon/Forebrain.**
  2) **Mesencephalon/Midbrain.**
  3) **Rhombencephalon//Hindbrain.**
- The **Prosencephalon** consists of two parts:
  - **Telencephalon**—the primitive Cerebral hemispheres.
  - **Diencephalon**—with an outgrowth of Optic vesicles.
- The **Mesencephalon** which gives rise to **Midbrain** is separated from the rhombencephalon by a deep furrow, the **Rhombencephalic isthmus**.

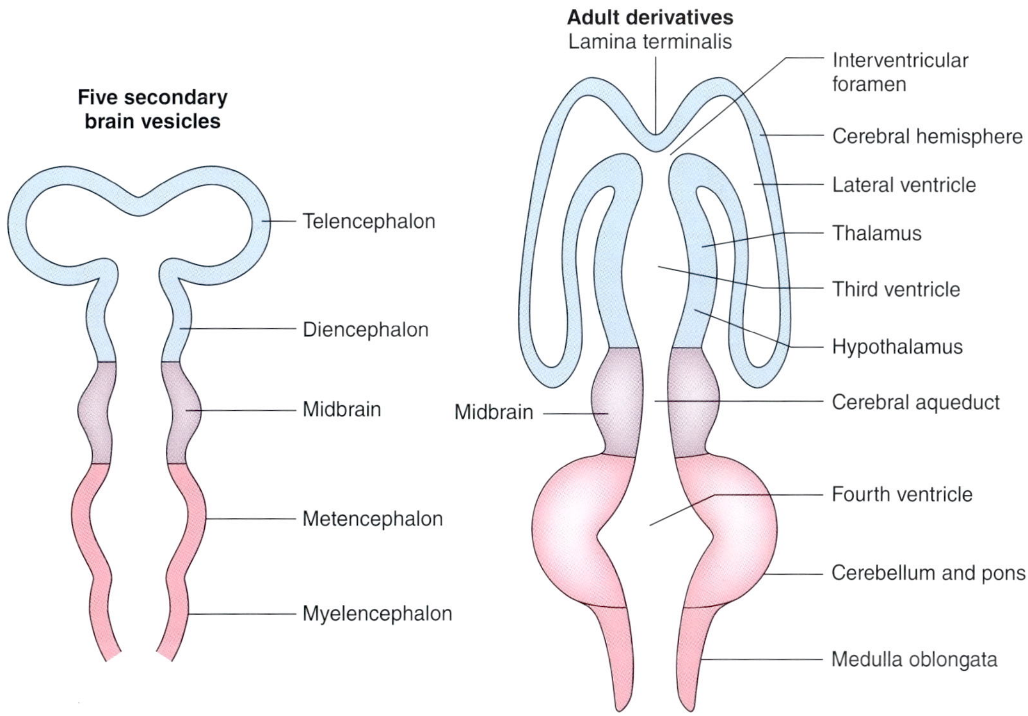

Fig. 20.6 Cavities enclosed in the brain vesicles.

- The **Rhombencephalon** consists of two parts:
  - **Metencephalon** (the pons and cerebellum).
  - **Myelencephalon** (medulla oblongata).
    - These are separated by **Pontine flexure**.
- The **brain stem** is the cranial continuation of spinal cord with a similar structure (**basal** and **alar plates** on each side of the midline).
- The higher centres show prominence of **alar plates** and regression of the basal plates.

RHOMBENCEPHALON (HINDBRAIN)

- It consists of:
  - **Myelencephalon.**
  - **Metencephalon.**
- **Alar** and **basal plates** are clearly distinguished and sulcus limitans separates them.
- The **Basal plate** contains three groups of motor nuclei:
  - **Medial Somatic Efferent (SE) group**, which contains somatic efferent motor column and supplies the striated muscles arising from the myotomes.
  - **Intermediate Special Visceral Efferent (SVE) group**, which contains the visceral efferent motor column and supplies the muscles derived from the branchial arches.
  - **Lateral General Visceral Efferent (GVE) group**, containing motor neurons that supply involuntary musculature of the respiratory tract, intestinal tract and heart (dorsal nucleus of vagus) and secretomotor fibres to various glands.
- The **Alar plate** contains four groups of sensory relay nuclei:
  - **General Visceral Afferent (GVA) group**—interoceptive information from GIT and heart.
  - **Special Visceral Afferent (SVA) group**—taste sensations from the tongue, palate.
  - **General Somatic Afferent (GSA-general sensory) group**—receives exteroceptive sensations from scalp, face and external ear.
  - **Special Somatic Afferent (SSA) group**—impulses from vestibulocochlear nerve for hearing and balancing.

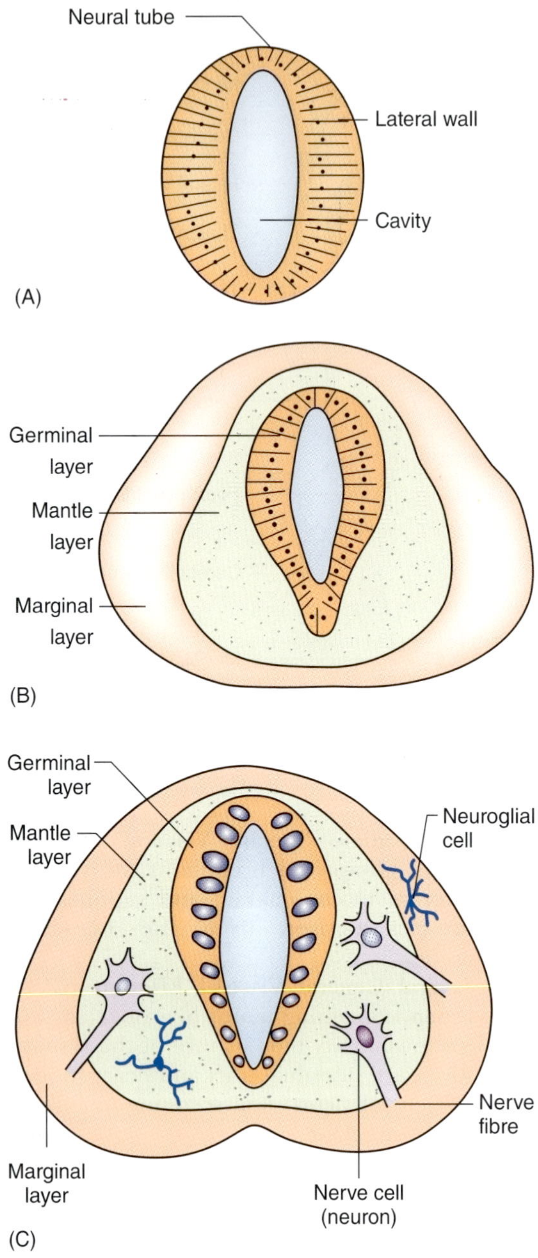

Fig. 20.7 Differentiation of neural tube.

MYELENCEPHALON

- It is the most caudal part of the brain vesicles (Fig. 20.8). It gives rise to **Medulla oblongata**.
- The arrangement of nuclear columns is given in the Table 20.2.
- The roof plate of myelencephalon consists of a single layer of ependymal cells covered by pia mater (tela choroidea). This roof ruptures to form foramina of **Luschka** on lateral side through which CSF flows from the fourth ventricle to the subarachnoid cisternae.
- Tela choroidea with blood vessels form **Choroid plexus** (CSF production).

METENCEPHALON

- It extends from the pontine flexure to rhombencephalic isthmus.
- It has the alar and basal plates. Derivatives are:
  - **Pons**—ventral wall.
  - **Cerebellum**—dorsal wall.

PONS

- The ventral wall of metencephalon gives rise to the pons (Fig. 20.9).
- The arrangement of nuclear columns is given in Table 20.3.
- Axons from pontine nuclei grow transversely to form the middle cerebellar peduncle.
- **Neurobiotaxis** is a phenomenon describing the directional migration of neural structures during development. In the context of brainstem development, the **Nucleus ambiguus** exhibits ventrolateral migration towards the spinal part of the sensory nucleus of the trigeminal nerve.
- Simultaneously, the **Facial nucleus** undergoes caudal migration, positioning itself dorsal to the abducent nucleus before reaching its final ventral location. These migration patterns are explained by the principle of neurobiotaxis, wherein structures move in response to specific **stimulatory cues**, optimizing their positioning during the developmental process.

CEREBELLUM

- It develops from the alar lamina of the **Metencephalon (Rhombic lips)** (Fig. 20.10). Caudally, the lips are separated widely but just below the mesencephalon, the lips fuse in the midline.
- When the pontine flexure becomes deep, the rhombic lips compress to form a dumb bell-shaped **Primitive cerebellum** with vermis in the midline and two cerebellar hemispheres laterally.

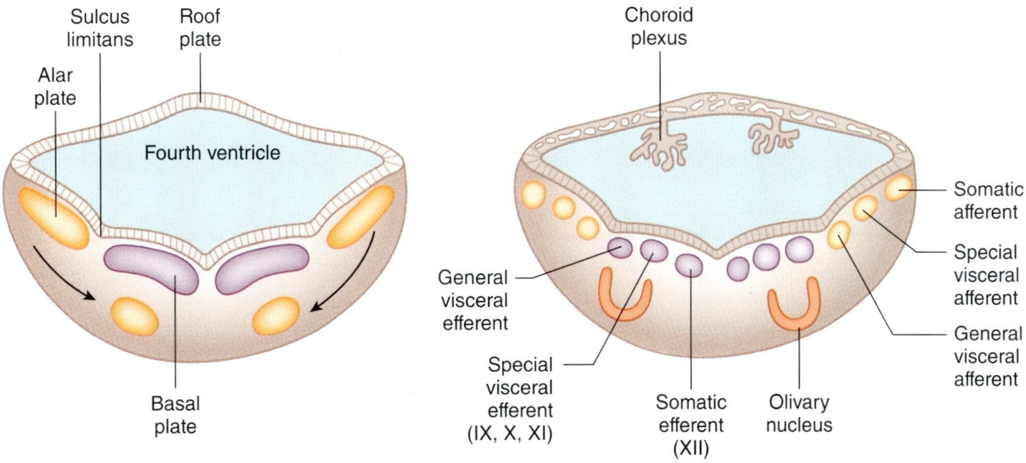

Fig. 20.8 Development of myelencephalon.

Table 20.2 Nuclear Columns in Myelencephalon

Efferent and Afferent Columns of Alar and Basal Lamina	Components
Medial somatic efferent (SE)	Hypoglossal nucleus—tongue.
Intermediate special visceral efferent (SVE)	Nucleus ambiguus (glossopharyngeal, vagus and accessory nerves) for third, fourth and sixth arch muscles.
Lateral general visceral efferent (GVE)	Dorsal nucleus of vagus, inferior salivatory nucleus of glossopharyngeal (parotid).
General visceral afferent (GVA)	Dorsal nucleus of vagus.
Special visceral afferent (SVA)	Nucleus of tractus solitarius (taste).
General somatic afferent (GSA)	Spinal nucleus of trigeminal.
Special somatic afferent (SSA)	Vestibular and cochlear nuclei (nucleus gracilis and cuneatus in the closed part).

- Numerous fissures develop on the dorsal surface and divides the hemispheres into lobes. The first fissure to develop is the **Posterolateral sulcus**. This separates the flocculonodular lobe from the hemispheres.
- The **Flocculonodular lobe (Archicerebellum)** is the most primitive part of the cerebellum, and this lobe is connected to the vestibular nuclei for controlling the posture and equilibrium of the body.
- **Fissura prima**, **fissura secunda** and **postpyramidal fissures** develop during third month on the cephalic slope (fissura prima) and caudal slope (other two) of cerebellum. Fissura prima separates anterior lobe from the remaining part of cerebellum.
- The **Paleocerebellum** consists of anterior lobe, pyramid and uvula. Its connection with the spinal cord controls the tone and posture of the body.
- The remaining part of the cerebellum which make connections with the cerebral cortex forms the **Neocerebellum** and is concerned with voluntary skilful movements.
- The developing cerebellum can be divided into:
  - **Intraventricular part** (into the fourth ventricle).
  - **Extraventricular part** (to the surface)—the major part.

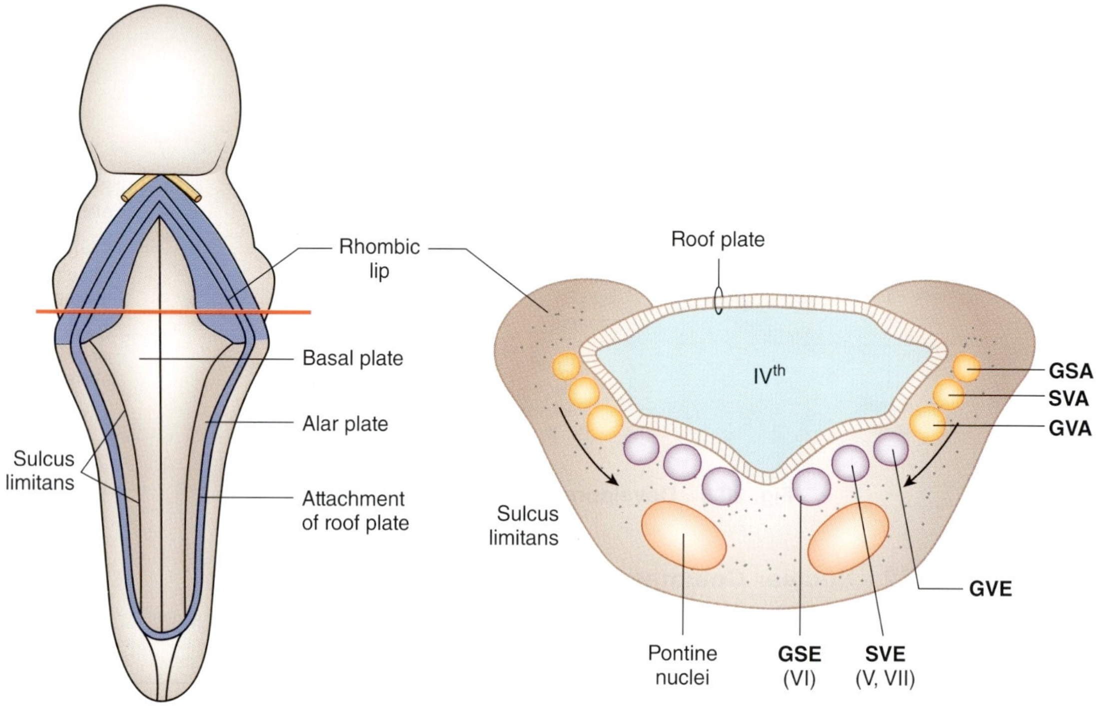

Fig. 20.9 Development of metencephalon—pons.

Table 20.3 Nuclear Columns in Pons

Efferent and Afferent Columns of Alar and Basal Lamina	Components
Medial somatic efferent (SE)	Abducent nucleus.
Intermediate special visceral efferent (SVE)	Motor nucleus of trigeminal and facial for first and second arch muscles.
Lateral general visceral efferent (GVE)	Superior salivatory nucleus of facial nerve (submandibular, sublingual and lacrimal glands).
General visceral afferent (GVA)	Cranial end of dorsal nucleus of vagus.
Special visceral afferent (SVA)	Pontine part of nucleus of tractus solitarius (taste).
General somatic afferent (GSA)	Sensory pontine nucleus of trigeminal.
Special somatic afferent (SSA)	Vestibular and cochlear nuclei.

- The cerebellar rudiment consists of:
  - **Neuroepithelial layer**: External granular layer (Purkinje, Granule cells, Golgi, basket and Stellate cells—differentiation of neuroblasts begin by sixth month of intrauterine life and that of basket and stellate cells continue till 2 years postnatal).
  - **Mantle layer**: dentate, emboliform, globose, fastigii nuclei.
  - **Marginal layer.**

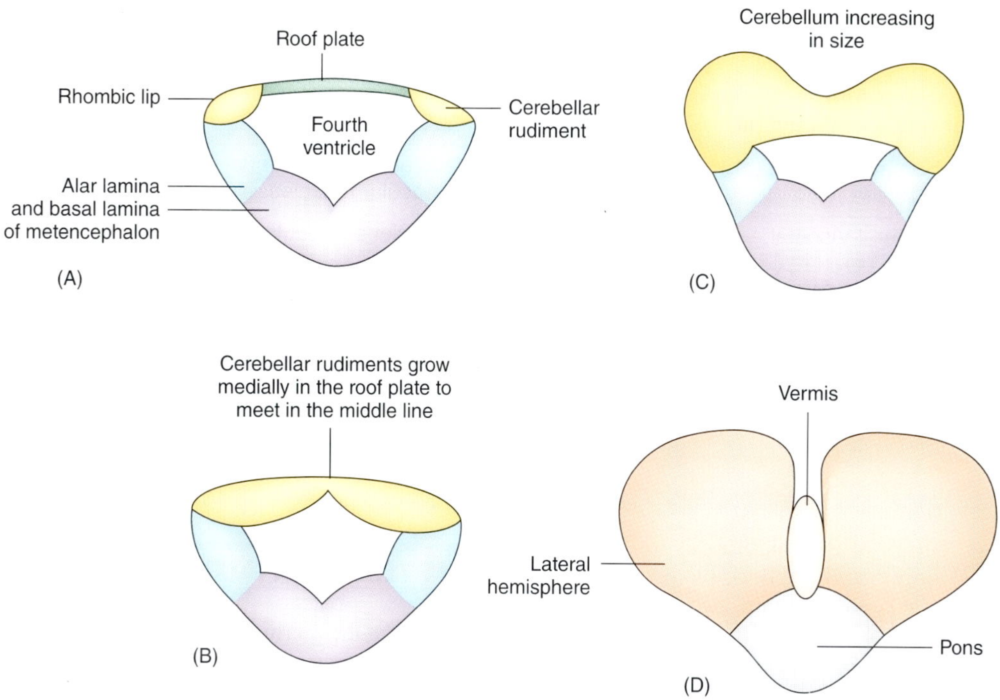

Fig. 20.10 Development of cerebellum.

- The vermis lies at the mesencephalic part of roof of the fourth ventricle, and the part of cerebellar plate anterior to it forms **Anterior medullary velum** and posterior to it forms **Posterior medullary velum**.
- The **Rhombencephalic isthmus** gives rise to trochlear and mesencephalic nucleus of trigeminal which later shifts to its adult position.

MESENCEPHALON (MIDBRAIN)

- The midbrain develops from mesencephalon (Fig. 20.11).
- The cavity within it is **Aqueduct of Sylvius**.
- The mantle is subdivided into **Alar** and **Basal lamina** with the sulcus limitans separating the plates. The tectum of the midbrain is formed by the alar lamina and the roof plate and the

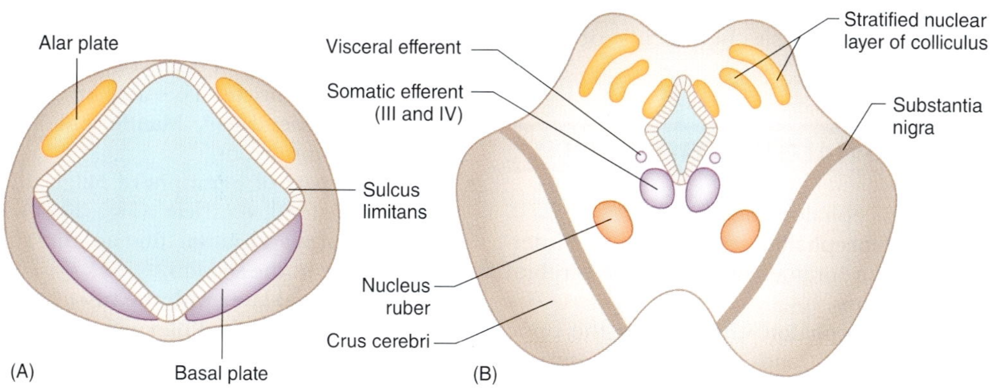

Fig. 20.11 Development of mesencephalon.

Table 20.4 Nuclear Columns in Mesencephalon

Efferent and Afferent Columns of Alar and Basal Lamina	Components
Medial Somatic Efferent (SE)	Oculomotor nucleus and trochlear nucleus (rhombencephalic isthmus)—supplies ocular muscles.
Lateral General Visceral Efferent (GVE)	Edinger–Westphal nucleus of oculomotor nerve—sphincter pupillae and ciliaris.
General Somatic Afferent (GSA)	Mesencephalic nucleus of trigeminal nerve (rhombencephalic isthmus)—proprioceptive stimulus from muscles of mastication, facial and ocular muscles.
Special Somatic Afferent (SSA)	Superior and inferior colliculi—reflex centres for vision and hearing.

tegmentum of the midbrain is formed by the basal lamina and the floor plate.

- The **basal lamina** contains two groups of motor nuclei (Table 20.4):
  - A medial **Somatic Efferent (SE)** group—oculomotor and trochlear nerves.
  - A small **General Visceral Efferent (GVE)** group—the Edinger–Westphal nucleus.
- The alar lamina gives rise to the cells of colliculi.The alar plates initially have two longitudinal elevations. A transverse groove divides each into a superior and inferior colliculus.
- Some cells of the alar lamina move ventrally to form:
  - **Red nucleus.**
  - **Substantia nigra.**
- The expanded region of marginal layer consisting of descending fibres (the corticopontine, corticobulbar and corticospinal) form the basis pedunculi or **Crus cerebri**.

PROSENCEPHALON (FOREBRAIN)

- The Prosencephalon consists of:
  - The **Telencephalon** lies cranial to the interventricular foramen and forms the cerebral hemispheres.
  - The **Diencephalon** which forms the optic cup (retina) and stalk (optic nerve), pituitary, thalamus, hypothalamus and epiphysis.

THE TELENCEPHALON

- It is the most cranial end of the brain vesicles.
- It is seen as two lateral outpouchings on either side of diencephalon.
- The outpouchings form the cerebral hemispheres and the median portion forms the **Lamina terminalis** which corresponds to the cranial end of neural tube (site of closure of anterior neuropore).
- Interventricular foramina of **Monro** connects:
  - The cavities of Telencephalon—the **lateral ventricle**.
  - The cavity of Diencephalon—the **third ventricle**.

CEREBRAL HEMISPHERES

- The cerebral vesicles start appearing by fifth week as bilateral evaginations from **Prosencephalon**, and the cavity of each vesicle is known as the **Lateral ventricle**. The wall of the vesicle consists of **Ependymal, Mantle** and **Marginal zones** from inside out.
- The basal part of hemisphere bulge into the cavity of lateral ventricle (Fig. 20.12). It is named **Corpus striatum** due to the striated appearance in the section.
- The ependymal layer with the vascular mesenchyme form **Choroidal plexus** into the lateral ventricle along the c-shaped choroid fissure.
- Above the choroidal fissure, the hemispheres thicken to form **Hippocampus** (aids in olfaction).

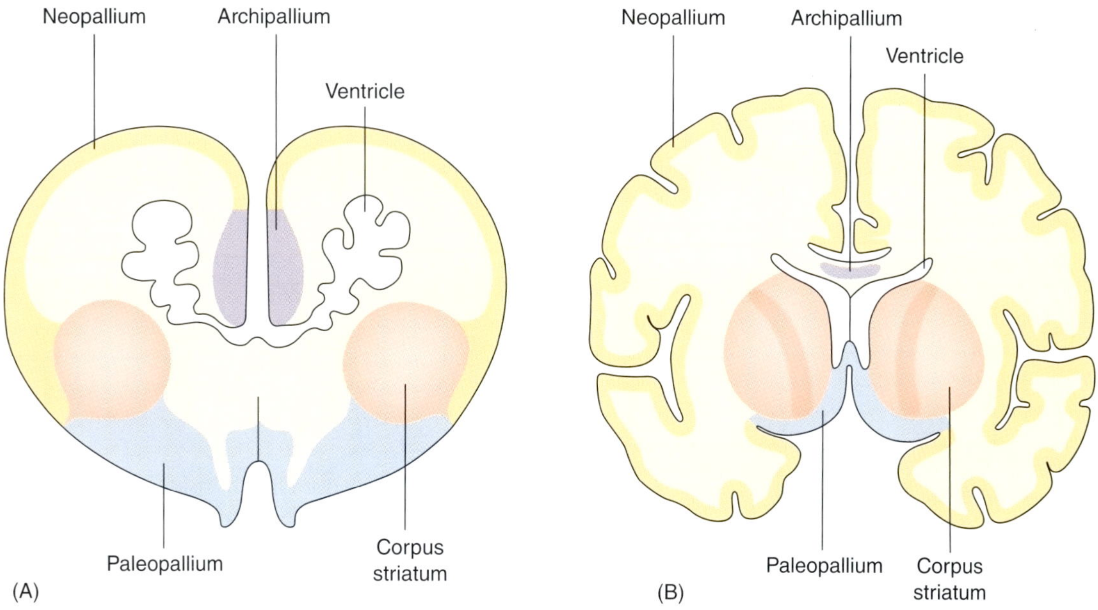

Fig. 20.12 Development of telencephalon.

- **Corpus striatum** bulges posteriorly and forms two parts:
  - A) The **Caudate** nucleus (dorsomedial)—head, body and tail and terminal amygdaloid body.
  - B) The **Lentiform** nucleus (ventrolateral)—putamen and globus pallidus.
- The nerve fibres passing through the corpus striatum from cerebral cortex is called the **Internal capsule**.
- The cerebral hemispheres bulge in different directions forming frontal, temporal and occipital poles.
- The floor of the longitudinal cleft between the medial surfaces of both vesicles are formed by the roof plate of **diencephalon** and **corpus callosum**. The **Falx cerebri** is formed as a result of the differentiation of the mesodermal tissue lying in this cleft.
- Due to the restricted space in the cranial cavity, the primitive posterior pole bends downward and forward as the **Temporal pole** and the **Lateral ventricle** which extends into it forms the **Inferior horn**. The **Frontal** and **Occipital poles** contain the **Anterior** and **Posterior horns** of the lateral ventricle.
- A depression is formed between the frontal and temporal lobes known as **Insula** covered by the adjacent lobes (opercula) which grow over it.
- The hemispheres grow rapidly resulting in convolutions called the **sulci** and **gyri**.
- The differentiation of Neocortex occurs by the migration of cells from the mantle zone to the marginal zone by around eighth month, and it consists of the following layers (outer to inner):
  - ➢ **Molecular layer.**
  - ➢ **Outer granular layer.**
  - ➢ **Pyramidal layer.**
  - ➢ **Inner granular layer.**
  - ➢ **Ganglionic layer.**
  - ➢ **Polymorphous layer.**
- **Fifth** and **sixth** layers are first to differentiate followed by **third** and **fourth** and last to develop are the **first** and **second** layers.
- The migration of cells occur according to the function and the cells of motor cortex are predominantly **pyramidal** and cells of the sensory cortex are predominantly **granular**.
- The **newborn** brain is about one-fourth of the adult brain and by the end of **1 year**, it attains three-fourth of the adult brain size. Full size is attained by around **18 years**.
- The different parts of Telencephalic cortex based on the developmental evolution is summarised in Table 20.5.

Table 20.5 Parts of Telencephalic Cortex Based on Developmental Evolution

A) Archipallium (Migration of ependymal and mantle zones to marginal zone to form definitive cortex begins in archipallium by seventh week)	• Hippocampus, dentate gyrus, fimbria, fornix.
B) Paleopallium	• Uncus and parahippocampal gyrus (piriform cortex).
C) Neopallium	• Frontal, parietal, occipital, temporal lobes and insula. Lateral sulcus—fourth month. Parieto-occipital, postcalcarine, cingulate and central sulci—sixth month. All sulci completed by seventh month.

CLINICAL NUGGETS

Myelination

- It begins in the **Peripheral nervous system** (2–5 months).
- In this, the **motor roots** get myelinated before sensory roots.
- In the spinal cord (11 weeks), myelination follows a craniocaudal gradient.
- After 6 months, myelination commences in the brain in the cranial nerves and motor nerves are myelinated earlier than sensory nerves.
- **Optic nerve** is myelinated by around full term.
- Among the functional tracts, **medial longitudinal bundle** is myelinated first by around sixth month. Myelination in association pathways in the cerebral cortex occurs after birth.
- In the **Corticospinal** tracts, myelination occurs only to the level of the medulla by 40 weeks.
- After birth, myelination continues and it can be appreciated by the increasing mobility of infants in the first year of life. Myelination continues **2–3 years** after birth.

THE DIENCEPHALON

- It is developed from the median portion of the Prosencephalon. It has two lateral walls, thin roof and floor plates.
- There is no representation of basal lamina in the diencephalon and the **Lateral wall** is mainly formed from the alar lamina.
- The hypothalamic sulcus divides the lateral wall into dorsal and ventral areas.
  A) **Dorsal area**—thalamus, medial and lateral geniculate bodies.
  B) **Ventral area**—hypothalamic nuclei.
- The **Roof** has the choroid plexus of the third ventricle. Pineal body and habenular nucleus takes its origin at the roof plate.
- The cells of the **Floor plate** differentiates to form the mamillary bodies, tuber cinereum and hypophysis cerebri. Optic chiasma is formed at the rostral end of floor plate.

PINEAL BODY (EPIPHYSIS)

- It is formed from the caudal part of the **roof plate** as a thickening in the midline (Fig. 20.13).
- Later it evaginates to form the pineal body.
- It is seen on the roof of the **mesencephalon**.
- It is mainly concerned with the diurnal variations.

THALAMUS AND HYPOTHALAMUS

- The alar plates of diencephalon is divided into three parts by two sulci (Fig. 20.13):
  - **The Hypothalamic sulcus.**
  - **The Epithalamic sulcus.**
- The three regions from ventral to dorsal are:
  A) **Hypothalamus.**
  B) **Thalamus.**
  C) **Epithalamus** (Habenular nuclei and Pineal body).
- The thalamic regions fuse in the midline forming **Interthalamic connexus**.
- Mamillary body develops as a protuberance on the ventral surface of hypothalamus.

HYPOPHYSIS OR PITUITARY GLAND (AN 43.4)

- It is formed from two sources (Fig. 20.14):

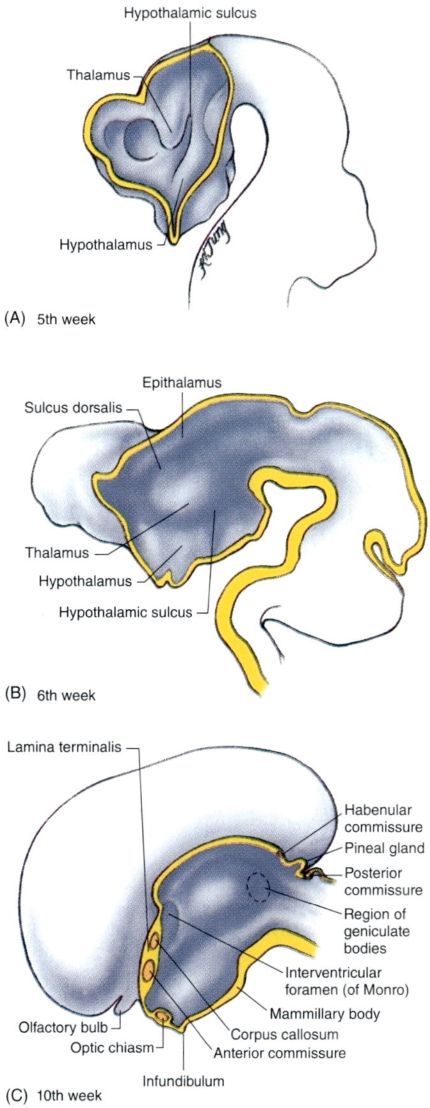

Fig. 20.13 Development of thalamus and pineal gland. Development of the diencephalon. (A) The thalamus and hypothalamus become demarcated by a hypothalamic sulcus during the fifth week. (B) By the end of the sixth week, the thalamus is clearly differentiated from the more dorsal epithalamus by a shallow groove called the sulcus dorsalis. (C) By 10 weeks, additional specializations of the diencephalon are apparent, including the mamillary body, the pineal gland and the posterior lobe of the pituitary. The optic sulci, the posterior and habenular commissures, and the geniculate bodies are also specializations of the diencephalon. (Source: *Larsen's Human Embryology*, 4th ed. 2008.)

  - **Rathke's pouch**—an ectodermal outpouching of the stomodeum in front of buccopharyngeal membrane.
  - **Infundibulum**—downward growth from the diencephalon dorsal to the Rathke's pouch.
- Rathke's pouch detaches from the oral cavity and fuses with the infundibulum (8 weeks) to form the **Hypophysis cerebri**.
- Rathke's pouch proliferates to form:
  A) **Anterior wall**—Pars anterior of the hypophysis (the adenohypophysis).
  B) **Posterior wall**—Pars intermedia.
  C) **Pars tuberalis**—Extension of anterior lobe along the stalk of infundibulum.
- The **Infundibulum** forms:
  - **The stalk.**
  - **Pars nervosa or posterior lobe** (neurohypophysis).
- The posterior lobe contains no nerve cells. **Pituicytes** are neuroglial in nature.
- Pituitary secretes **growth hormone** which can be detected from 10 weeks onward.

CLINICAL NUGGETS

Congenital hypopituitarism (AN 43.4)

- In this condition, there is a decrease in the amount of one or more of the hormones secreted by the **Pituitary gland**.
- Symptoms depend on the type of hormones affected.
- Hypoplasia of the gland or complications with delivery are the usual causes for hypopituitarism.
- Treatment is by replacement of the insufficient hormones (oral/injection).

Secondary hypogonadism

- It can be due to a defect in **Hypothalamus or Anterior pituitary gland**.
- Individuals have depressed levels of **gonadotropins** and **sex steroids**.
- Insufficient secretion of GnRH by the hypothalamus **(Kallmann syndrome)** and the **Fertile Eunuch syndrome** in males are the usual causes.

Craniopharyngioma

- This is a hormone-secreting tumour arising from the remnants of **Rathke's pouch.**
- It results in hydrocephalus and pituitary dysfunction.

DEVELOPMENT OF SPINAL CORD

- The caudal part of the neural tube forms the spinal cord (Fig. 20.15). The cavity of the spinal

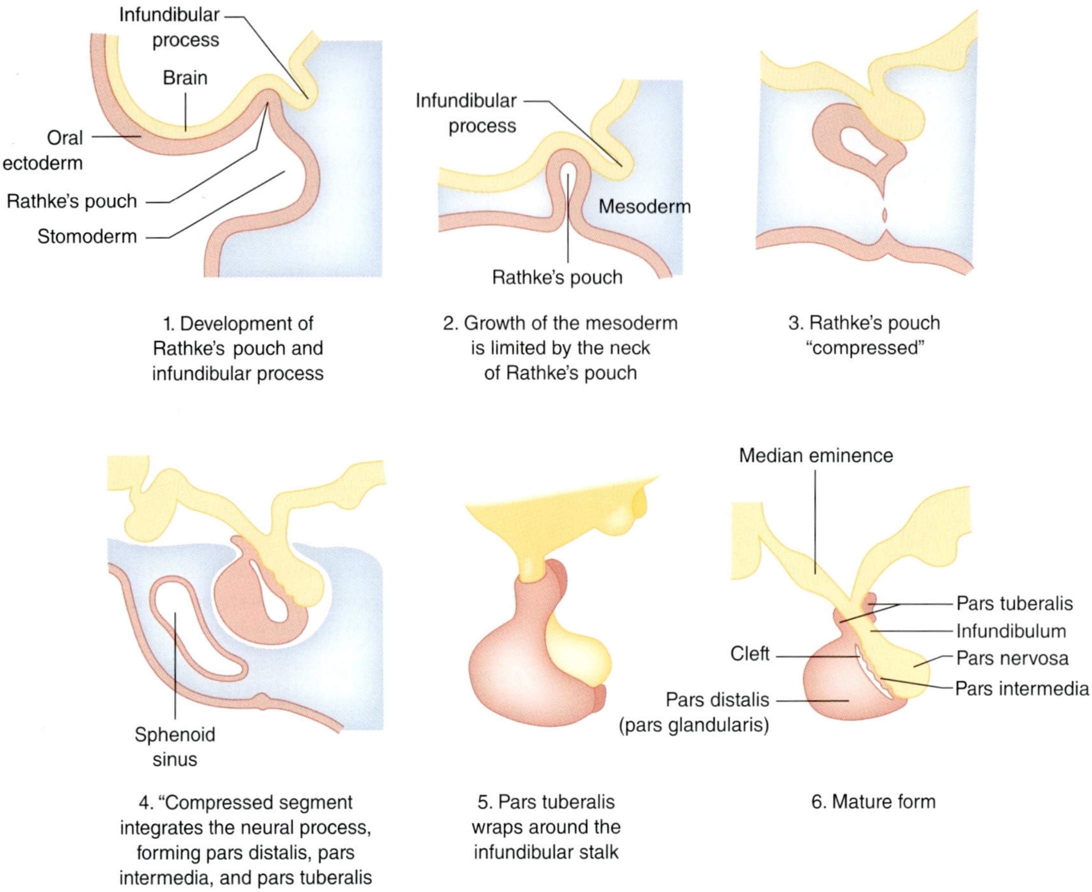

Fig. 20.14 Development of pituitary gland.

cord is called the **Central canal** and its dilated caudal end is known as the **terminal ventricle**.

- The neural tube is lined by pseudostratified epithelium **(Neuroepithelium)**.
- After the closure of neuropores, the neuroepithelial cells form **Neuroblasts**.
- Neuroblasts form the **mantle layer** and the nerve fibres arising from the mantle layer form **marginal layer**.
- Mantle layer forms the **grey matter** and the marginal layer forms the **white matter** of spinal cord.
- **Mantle layer** forms two thickenings:
  - **Dorsal (alar plate)**—Sensory area (posterior horn).
  - **Ventral (basal plate)**—Motor area (nerve cells of the anterior and lateral horns). Motor neurons differentiate earlier than the sensory neurons.
- The **Sulcus limitans** separates the alar and basal lamina.
- The dorsal part of the central canal is obliterated by the fusion of alar lamina and the fusion persists as **posteromedian septum** (ependymal in origin) in the adults.
- A group of neurons between the two lamina forms a small intermediate horn in the thoracolumbar region which later forms the **lateral horn** (the sympathetic outflow).
- The **cervical** and **lumbar enlargements** develop with the appearance of limb buds by around 5–6 weeks.
- The **myelination** occurs when the nerve fibres start functioning. By fourth month, the intersegmental tracts are myelinated first followed by ventral and dorsal roots of spinal nerve by fifth month. **Spinothalamic tracts** are myelinated

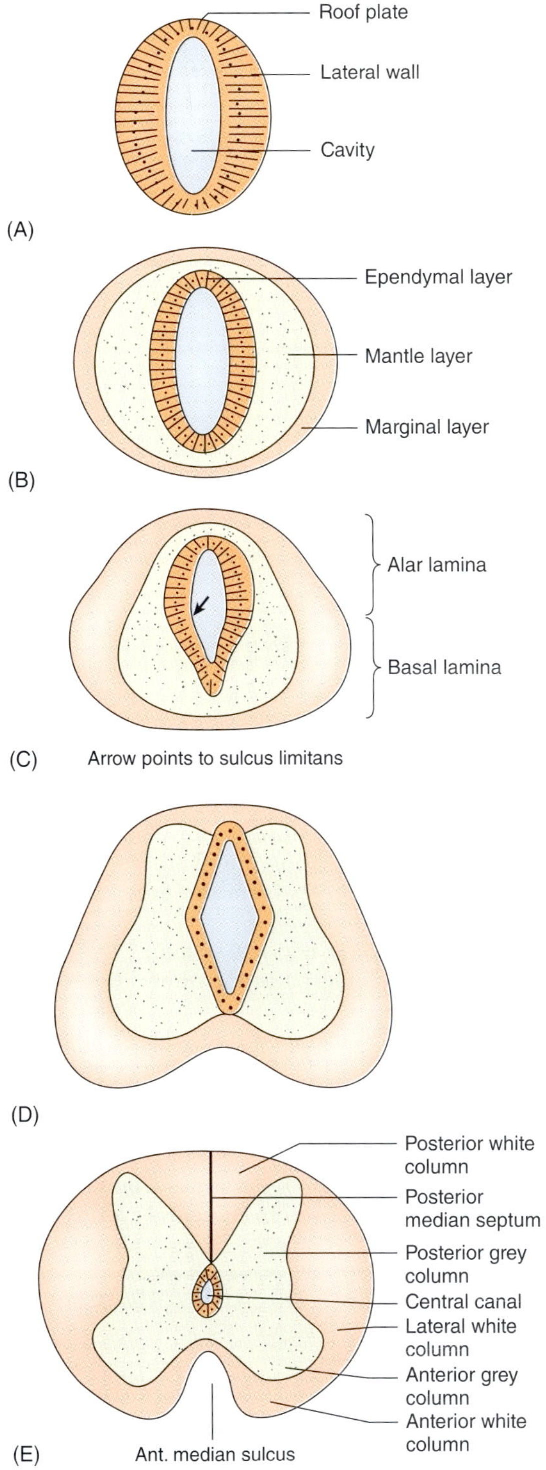

Fig. 20.15 Development of spinal cord.

by seventh month and **Corticospinal tracts** by around ninth month (completed by 3 years after birth).

- Changes in the **position** of the spinal cord (Fig. 20.16):
  - **Third month**—along the entire length of the embryo.
  - **At birth**—it ends at the level of **L3**.
  - **In adults**—it ends at the level of **L1**.
- The dura mater and arachnoid mater ends at the level of **S2**, whereas pia mater remains attached to the **coccyx**. The caudal end of the terminal ventricle obliterates before birth.

DEVELOPMENT OF CRANIAL NERVES

Twelve pairs of cranial nerves are formed by around sixth week of intrauterine life. They are arranged into three groups as follows:

1) **Somatic efferent cranial nerves**—The nerves homologous to the ventral roots of spinal nerves and located in the somatic efferent column of the brainstem belong to this group. They are the greater part of **Oculomotor nerve, Trochlear nerve, Abducens nerve** and **Hypoglossal nerve**. They supply the muscles derived from the preotic and occipital myotomes.
2) **Nerves of pharyngeal arches**—The cranial nerves namely the **Trigeminal nerve, Facial nerve, Glossopharyngeal nerve** and **Vagus nerve** supply the pharyngeal arches and belong to this group. The **Spinal accessory nerve** emerge from the cervical segments of the spinal cord and supply the sternocleidomastoid and trapezius muscles.
3) **Special sensory nerves**—The **Olfactory nerve, Optic nerve** and **Vestibulocochlear nerve** belong to this group.
   - All cranial nerves (except **olfactory and optic**) arise from the brain stem.
   - The **oculomotor** nerve develops outside the hindbrain.
   - The neuroepithelium proliferates to form eight segments of rhombomeres in hindbrain.
   - The **rhombomeres** give rise to motor nuclei of IV, V, VI, VII, IX, X, XI and XII cranial nerves.
   - The **sensory ganglia** which lie outside the brain arises from:
     - **Ectodermal placodes.**
     - **Neural crest cells.**

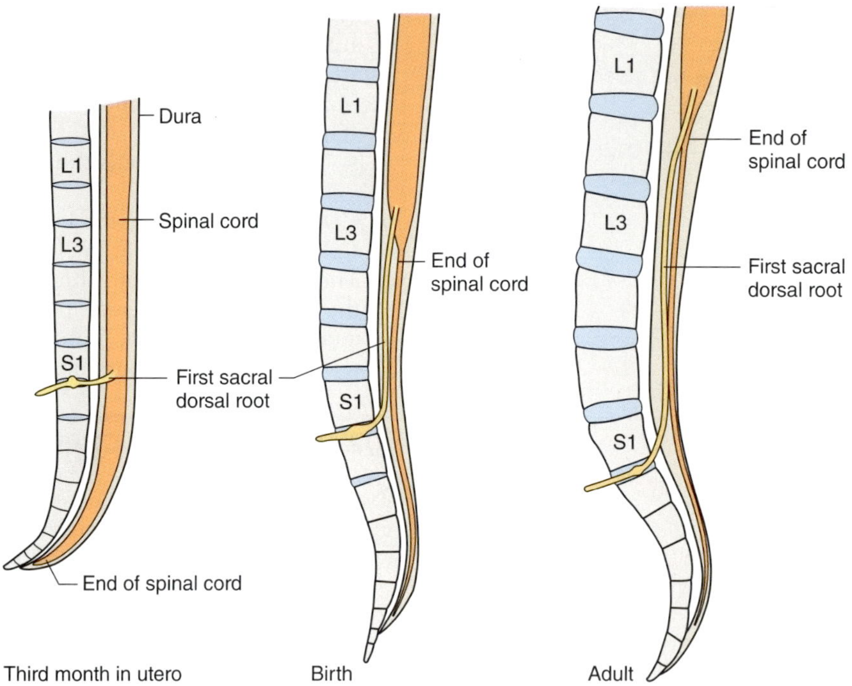

Fig. 20.16 Changes in position of spinal cord.

- The cranial nerves (III–XII) are located in the brainstem and their functional components are commonly organized in longitudinal columns as depicted in the Fig. 20.17.

DEVELOPMENT OF AUTONOMIC NERVOUS SYSTEM

- It consists of:
  - **Sympathetic nervous system.**
  - **Parasympathetic nervous system.**
- **Sympathetic nervous system:**
  - Cells from the **Neural crest** of the thoracic region form the sympathetic ganglia.
  - Sympathetic trunks are formed by the ganglia and interconnecting fibres.
  - The **Neuroblasts** migrate to the cervical and lumbosacral regions, hence the sympathetic trunk extends from the cervical region to sacral region.
  - The nerve fibres from the lateral horn of thoracolumbar segments of spinal cord form the **Preganglionic fibres** (**myelinated**—the white rami communicans).
  - Axons of the sympathetic ganglia form the **Postganglionic fibres (unmyelinated)**.
  - The nerves from the sympathetic trunk to spinal nerves form the **grey rami communicans**.
- **Parasympathetic nervous system:**
  - **Preganglionic** parasympathetic fibres arise from:
    - ➢ The **Brain stem** (via the oculomotor (III), facial (VII), glossopharyngeal (IX), and vagus (X)).
    - ➢ **Sacral region** (S2–S4) of the spinal cord.
  - **Postganglionic** fibres arise from neurons (ganglia) derived from **neural crest cells**.

DEVELOPMENT OF SUPRARENAL GLAND

- The suprarenal gland has two parts (Fig. 20.18):
  - **Cortex** develops from the mesoderm.
  - **Medulla** develops from neurectoderm.
- Mesothelial cells lining the coelomic cavity between root of mesentery and the developing

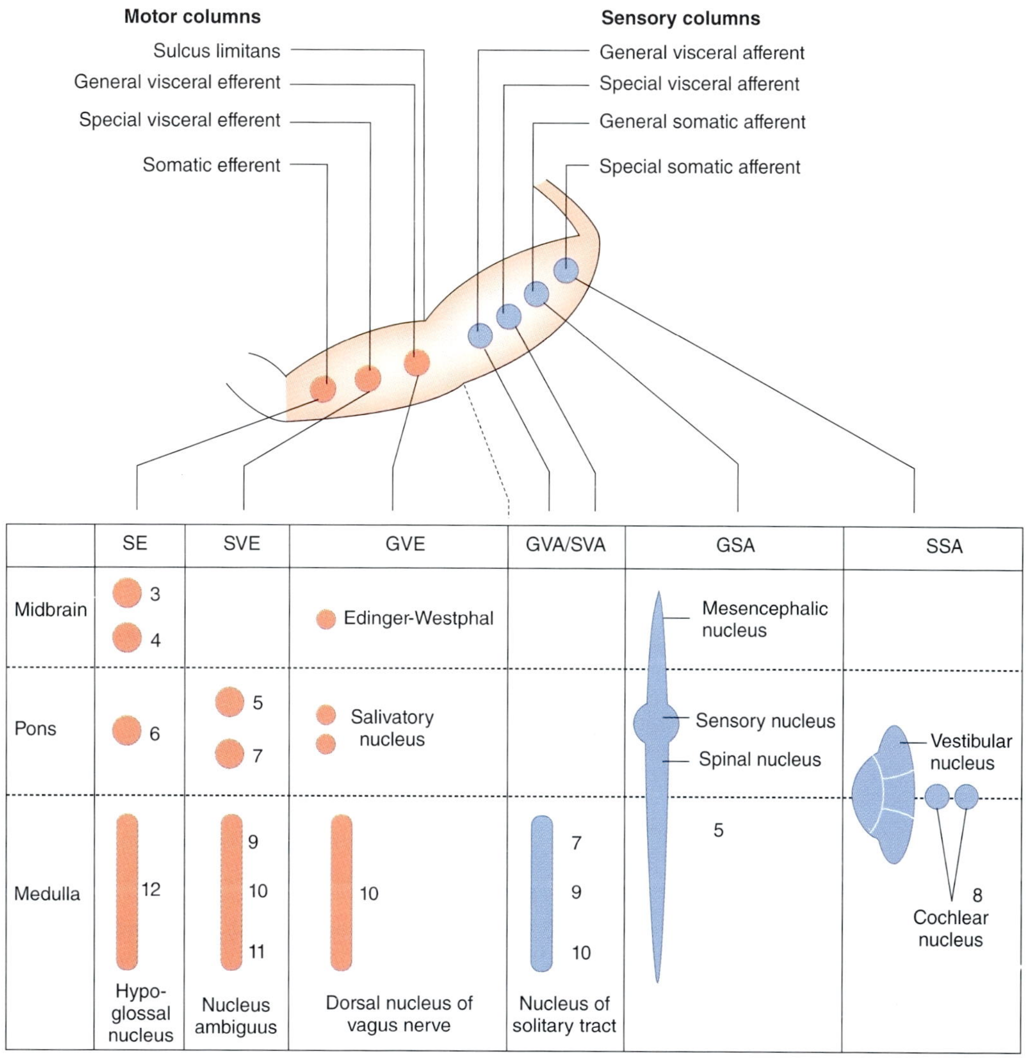

Fig. 20.17 Functional columns of cranial nerve nuclei.

gonads forms an elongated **suprarenal ridge** extending from the 6th thoracic to the 12th thoracic segments. The cells of the suprarenal ridge penetrate the underlying mesenchyme to form the **Primitive cortex** (acidophilic).

- Capillaries from mesonephric arteries invade the ridge and join with the venous sinuses. A fibrous capsule surrounds the cells of the ridge and the neurectodermal cells.
- Cellular cords which proliferate from the ridge cells lie between the radiating capillaries and they later degenerate to form the **Foetal cortex**.
- The cells which lie beneath the capsule form the **Zona glomerulosa** of the definitive cortex. Two weeks after birth the foetal cortex degenerates.
- Zona glomerulosa differentiates to form **Zona fasciculata** and **Zona reticularis** and, as a result, the size of the gland increases and reach the adult size (1/30th of kidney).
- The **Neural crest cells** (the sympathochromaffin masses of primitive spinal ganglia) invade the inner aspect of the cortex to form the medulla.
- Medulla stains **brown** with chromic salts (**chromaffin cells**).

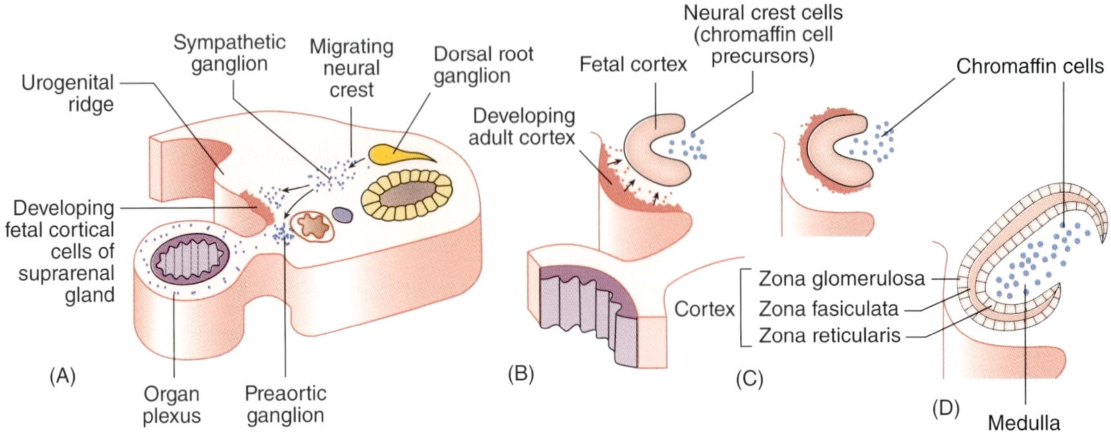

Fig. 20.18 Development of suprarenal gland.

CLINICAL NUGGETS

Neural tube defects (NTDs) (AN 64.3)

- This occur when neurulation fails to occur normally (during **3–4 weeks**). It can be either **open** to the surface or **closed** where it is covered with skin (Fig. 20.19).
- Open NTDs are the most severe, and in **Craniorachischisis**, the entire length of the neural tube opens onto the surface of the head and back **(total dysraphism)**.
- In **localized dysraphism (lumbosacral myeloschisis),** only the lowermost region of the spinal cord is open.
- **Myeloschisis (spina bifida aperta)** means the spinal cord is open to the body surface with bifid vertebral spines.
- **Cranioschisis (anencephaly)** is total dysraphism of the brain with normal spinal cord. In this, there is no functional forebrain (cerebrum) and will not survive more than a few hours after birth.
- **Skin-covered NTDs**:
  - In the spinal cord, it is known as **Spina bifida occulta** (defect is hidden). The location is marked externally on the back by:
    - ➢ **A tuft of hair.**
    - ➢ **Pigmented nevus** (mole).
    - ➢ **Angioma** (port-wine coloured birth mark of the skin).
    - ➢ **Lipoma** (a skin doming caused by an underlying mass of fatty tissue).
    - ➢ **Dimple.**
  - In the brain, it is known as **Encephalocele:** The brain tissue will be protruding through the skull.
- **Myelomeningocele:**
  - The **most** common open NTD.
  - It is a type of spina bifida with **neural tube** and **membranes** (dura mater and arachnoid) protruding from the vertebral canal.
  - It forms a fluid-filled sac or cele. In **meningocele,** only the membranes protrude into the sac without the spinal cord.
- Maternal Serum Alpha-fetoprotein (**MSAFP** screening after 12 weeks of gestation), if elevated can be followed by two other tests: **Ultrasound examination** of the foetal spine and head, and **Amniocentesis** (to measure levels of alpha-fetoprotein contained in amniotic fluid) for confirmation of NTDs since **MSAFP levels** are **elevated** in pregnancies affected by NTDs.
- **Complication** of NTDs: tethered spinal cord resulting in neurological deficit and hydrocephalous.
- NTDs are **multifactorial,** that is it is due to genetic and environmental factors.
- The role of **Retinoic acid, Insulin and high-plasma glucose** in the formation of NTDs have been already proved. **Folic acid (vitamin B9)** supplementation can reduce the incidence of NTDs by up to 75%.

KLINISCHE PERLEN

HOLOPROSENCEPHALY (HPE)

- Mutation of **SHH gene**.
- Loss of midline structures.
- **Single telencephalic vesicle** (lateral ventricles fused).
- Eyes fused.
- Single nasal chamber.
- Single central incisor.

SCHIZENCEPHALY

- Cerebral hemispheres have **large cleft**.
- Brain tissue may be absent.

CRANIORACHISCHISIS (FIG. 20.19)

- Extensive failure of fusion of neural tube cranially and caudally.
- Anencephaly with spinal cord defects.

ARNOLD-CHIARI MALFORMATION

- **Cerebellum herniating** into foramen magnum.
- **Hydrocephalus** (obstruction of CSF flow).
- Associated with abnormal development of spinal cord.

SPINA BIFIDA

Failure of closure of neural tube anywhere from cervical region to caudal region (Chapter 9) (Fig. 20.19).

MICROCEPHALY

- Small cranial vault (Figs 20.14 and 20.20).
- Defective brain development.
- Causes-Toxoplasmosis, Radiation and Teratogens.

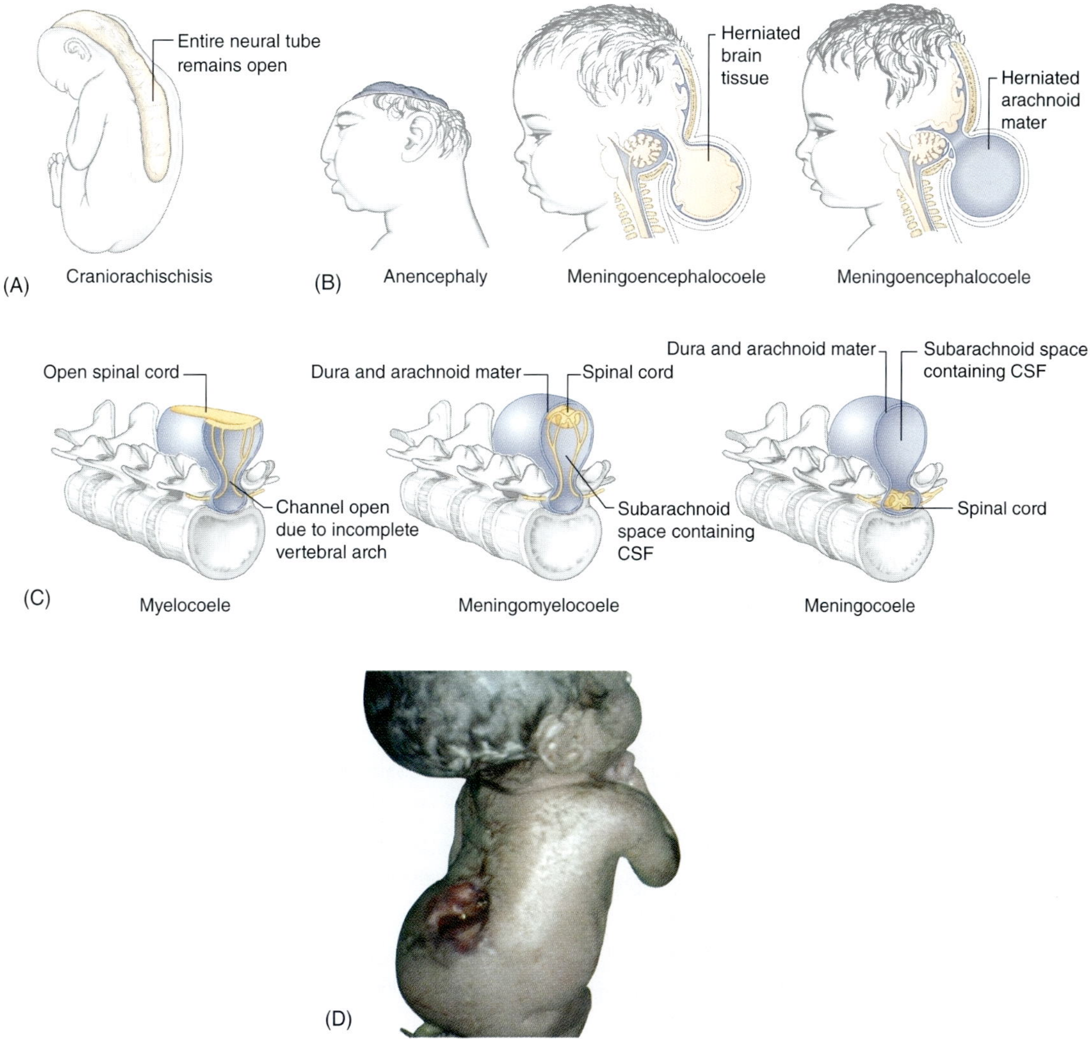

Fig. 20.19 Neural tube defects. (A) Total failure of neurulation. (B) Failure of rostral neurulation. (C) Failure of caudal neurulation. (D) A newborn with spina bifida. *CSF*, Cerebrospinal fluid. (Source: (A, B, C) *Gray's Anatomy: The Anatomical Basis of Clinical Practice*, 2016; part (D) Photo courtesy: Dr Rema.)

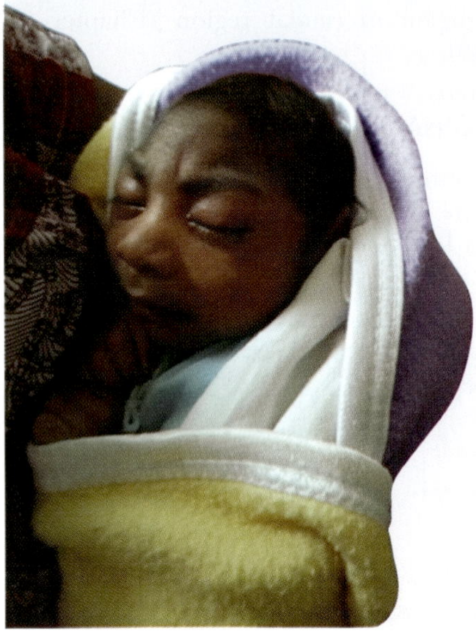

Fig. 20.20 A newborn with microcephaly. (Photo courtesy: Dr Nithya, GMC, Thrissur.)

ENCEPHALOCELE

- It is a **Neural tube defect** (Fig. 20.1).
- Brain along with its membranes protrude like a sac through openings in the skull.
- The defects are caused due to the failure of the neural tubes to close.

POINTS TO PONDER

- The **primordia** of the three brain vesicles—the prosencephalon, mesencephalon, and rhombencephalon—are visible in the neural plate even before neurulation.
- The **secondary brain vesicles** are formed by the subdivision of primary vesicles as follows:
- The Prosencephalon divides into the telencephalon and diencephalon.
- The Rhombencephalon divides into the metencephalon and myelencephalon.
- The Mesencephalon remains undivided.
- The hindbrain divides into **rhombomeres**. The neural tube caudal to the rhombomeres forms the spinal cord.
- **Three flexures** are formed—the mesencephalic (cranial) flexure and cervical flexure which are ventrally directed and pontine flexure which is dorsally directed.
- The **Neuroepithelium** proliferates to form the neurons, glia and ependymal cells.
- The neurons in the ventricular zone form the **Mantle zone**—the precursor of the grey matter. Axons from mantle layer form the **Marginal zone**—the precursor of white matter.
- The mantle zone of the spinal cord and brain stem form alar and basal plates.
- The cranial nerve nuclei **(3–12)** are located in the brain stem.

BRAIN TEASERS

1. What induces the formation of the neural plate?
   A. Notochord
   B. Amniotic fluid
   C. Spinal cord
   D. Neural crest cells
2. When do the lateral edges of the neural plate elevate to form neural folds?
   A. Beginning of second week
   B. End of first week
   C. Beginning of third week
   D. End of third week
3. What is the communication route that provides nourishment to the developing neural tube during fusion?
   A. Primitive pit
   B. Anterior neuropore
   C. Vitelline duct
   D. Posterior intestinal portal
4. What cells are formed when the neural tube separates from the ectoderm?
   A. Neural folds
   B. Neural crest cells
   C. Notochord cells
   D. Amniotic cells
5. When does closure of the cranial neuropore occur?
   A. 18–20 somite stage
   B. 25th day
   C. 30th day
   D. 35th day
6. Where do neural crest cells lie during development?
   A. Beneath the neural tube
   B. Ventral to the neural tube
   C. Dorsolateral to the neural tube
   D. Within the neural tube
7. What is the term for the closure of the caudal neuropore?
   A. 20 somite stage
   B. 23rd day
   C. 25th day
   D. 28th day
8. Which of the following is not a derivative of neural crest cells?
   A. Schwann cells

B. Chromaffin cells
C. Neurons of dorsal root ganglia
D. Neurons of the optic nerve

9. What does the closed tubular structure represent in the developing embryo?
A. Neural crest
B. Notochord
C. Central nervous system (CNS)
D. Amniotic cavity

10. Which part of the brain gives rise to the cerebellum?
A. Metencephalon
B. Myelencephalon
C. Mesencephalon
D. Prosencephalon

11. What structure connects the lateral ventricle with the third ventricle?
A. Interventricular foramina of Monro
B. Choroid plexus
C. Aqueduct of Sylvius
D. Fourth ventricle

12. Which part of the brain develops from the prosencephalon?
A. Midbrain
B. Hindbrain
C. Cerebral hemispheres
D. Spinal cord

13. What is the function of the pineal body (epiphysis)?
A. Olfaction
B. Diurnal variations
C. Motor control
D. Vision

14. From which sources does the pituitary gland (hypophysis) develop?
A. Rathke's pouch and infundibulum
B. Choroid plexus and thalamus
C. Pineal body and hypothalamus
D. Corpus striatum and habenular nuclei

15. What cells form the grey matter of the spinal cord?
A. Neuroblasts
B. Marginal layer
C. Ependymal cells
D. Mantle layer

16. When does myelination in the visual system occur during development?
A. 2–5 months
B. 6 months
C. 11 weeks
D. After birth

Answers

1. (A); 2. (D); 3. (B); 4. (B); 5. (B); 6. (C); 7. (D); 8. (D); 9. (C); 10. (A); 11. (A); 12. (C); 13. (B); 14. (A); 15. (D); 16. (B).

FURTHER READINGS

AlKandery M, AlSaidan L, Owayed F, AlQunaee M, Al-Sihan M, Alterki A. Management of a pediatric patient with spontaneous cerebrospinal fluid leak in the lateral recess of sphenoid sinus and meningoencephalocele: a case report and literature review. *Int J Surg Case Rep.* 2023;110:108727. doi:10.1016/j.ijscr.2023.108727.

Asif M, Abdullah U, Nürnberg P, Tinschert S, Hussain MS. Congenital microcephaly: a debate on diagnostic challenges and etiological paradigm of the shift from isolated/non-syndromic to syndromic microcephaly. *Cells.* 2023;12(4):642. doi:10.3390/cells12040642.

Bosch I Ara L, Katugampola H, Dattani MT. Congenital hypopituitarism during the neonatal period: epidemiology, pathogenesis, therapeutic options, and outcome. *Front Pediatr.* 2021;8:600962. doi:10.3389/fped.2020.600962.

Mateos-Aparicio P, Rodríguez-Moreno A. The impact of studying brain plasticity. *Front Cell Neurosci.* 2019;13:66. doi:10.3389/fncel.2019.00066.

Yu Q, Guan T, Guo Y, Kong J. The initial myelination in the central nervous system. *ASN Neuro.* 2023;15:17590914231163039. doi:10.1177/17590914231163039.

21 Development of Eye

AN 43.4 Describe the development of eye.
AN 43.4 Describe the developmental basis of congenital anomalies of eye.

ANAMNESE

A 5-month-old infant was brought to the ophthalmology clinic with concerns of visual impairment noticed by the parents. The child was born to a mother who had a confirmed case of rubella during the first trimester of pregnancy. Clinical examination revealed bilateral congenital cataracts, significantly affecting the infant's vision. The ophthalmologist diagnosed the condition as congenital cataracts attributed to Rubella infection during foetal development. The case shows the importance of early detection and intervention in congenital cataracts, especially in infants born to mothers with a history of Rubella infection during pregnancy (Fig. 21.1).

DISCOVERY OF EYE FIELD (1920S)

Developmental biologists in the 1920s made a crucial observation that both eyes originate from a singular eye field, subsequently dividing into bilateral hemispheres. The complex structure of the eyeball consists of three layers—sclera, choroid and retina. The sclera, being the toughest, surrounds the outer layer, while the retina, the softest layer, is confined to the distal part of the eyeball, constituting only 72% of the orbit. The unequal thickness of these layers is a characteristic feature. Presently, cellular replacement therapy stands as the sole viable option for treating the loss of retinal cells in the adult eye.

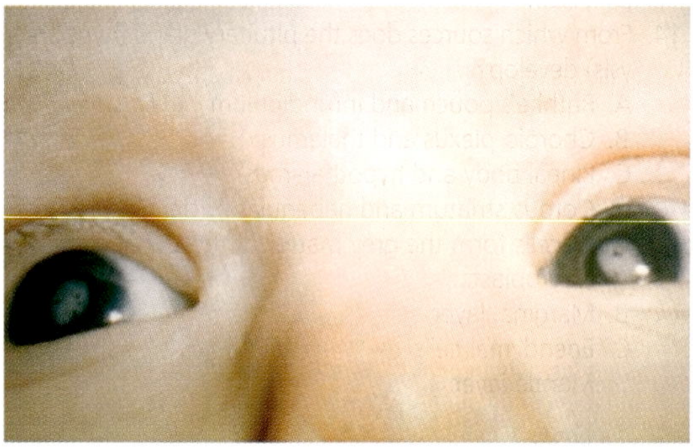

Fig. 21.1 Congenital cataract. (Source: Centers for Disease Control and Prevention [PHIL Photo ID# 4284]. https://www.cdc.gov/rubella/about/photos.html.)

DEVELOPMENT OF EYE

The embryonic journey of eye development initiates around the **22nd day** of gestation. Emerging as a pair of sulci, also known as optic grooves or sulcus, on the sides of the forebrain, the developing eye undergoes complicated processes involving several primordia. Two essential contributors to eye formation are the **Optic vesicle** and the **Lens placode**. The optic sulcus extends into the surrounding mesenchyme, eventually forming the optic vesicle. Simultaneously, the lens placode, a specialized region of the surface ectoderm, transforms to give rise to the lens.

OPTIC VESICLE (AN 43.4)

- The optic sulci, originating from the Prosencephalon, project into the surrounding mesenchyme, setting the surrounding for the formation of optic vesicles. This process marks the beginning of eye development.
- Upon reaching a critical stage, the optic vesicles come into contact with the surface ectoderm. This interaction triggers a series of events leading to the induction of the **Lens placode**—an essential precursor in the development of the eye.
- The proximal segment of the optic vesicle undergoes a transformative phase, becoming constricted and elongated. This results in the formation of the **Optic stalk**.
- Simultaneously, the distal end of the vesicle undergoes dilation and remain as the optic vesicle (Fig. 21.2).

LENS PLACODE

Ectodermal Thickening:

- Overlying the optic vesicle, a specific area of the ectoderm undergoes thickening, initiating the formation of the **Lens placode** (Fig. 21.3).

Lens Vesicle Formation:

- Subsequently, the lens placode descends from the surface ectoderm, transforming into the **Lens vesicle**. Complete separation of lens vesicle from surface ectoderm occurs during **fifth** week.

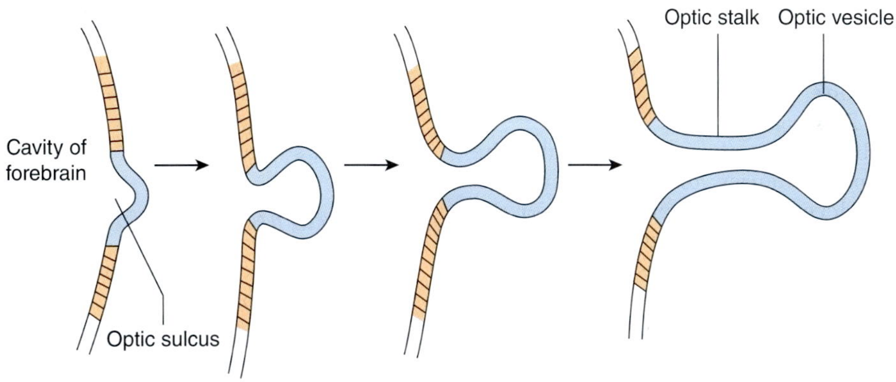

Fig. 21.2 Formation of the optic stalk.

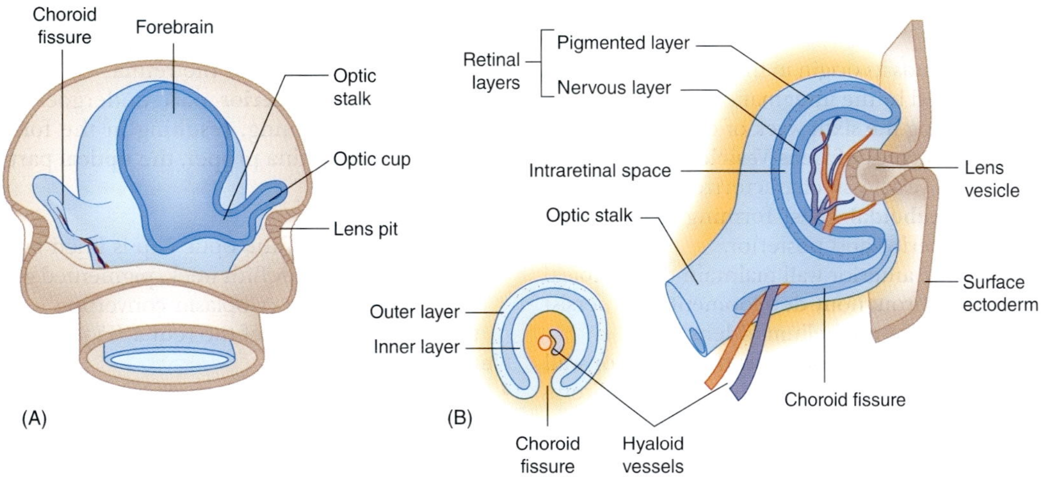

Fig. 21.3 Development of the lens vesicle.

Optic Cup Formation:
- Around the fifth week, the optic vesicle undergoes invagination to accommodate the lens vesicle, resulting in the formation of a double-walled optic cup. The continuous growth of the upper and lateral sides of the cup plays a vital role in enclosing the lens within this evolving structure.

Intraretinal Space:
- The space between the outer and inner layers of the **optic cup** is known as the intraretinal space. Over time, this space disappears, and the layers closely approach each other, contributing to the layering of the developing eye.

Choroid Fissure and Hyaloid Vessels:
- In the inferior part of the vesicle and optic stalk, a **Choroid fissure** develops. Through this fissure, **Hyaloid vessels** extend into the inner chamber of the eye.
- The proximal hyaloid vessels form **Central retinal vessels**, while the distal part undergoes degeneration.

Mesodermal Differentiation:
- Surrounding the developing neural tube, the mesoderm condenses to form meninges. This mesodermal layer extends to cover the optic vesicle, differentiating into **two layers**: a superficial fibrous layer corresponding to the **dura mater** and a deep vascular layer corresponding to the **pia-arachnoid**.

THE COMPONENTS OF EYEBALL

LENS

- The lens finds its origin in the **lens vesicle** which is developed by the invagination of surface ectoderm during the sixth week of development.

Structural Features of Lens Vesicle:
- The lens vesicle is characterized by a single layer of **cuboidal cells**, forming two distinct walls—anterior and posterior.
- Cells in the anterior wall maintain their cubical structure throughout development and persist as the anterior epithelium of lens.
- Significant changes occur as the posterior wall undergoes elongation, leading to the obliteration of the vesicle's lumen (Fig. 21.4).

Transformation Into Lens Fibres:
- Cells in the elongated posterior wall undergo a transformative process, losing their nuclei and becoming the **Primary fibres** that constitute the lens.
- By the conclusion of the seventh week, primary lens fibres reach the anterior wall, while continuous growth involves the addition of **Secondary (new) lens fibres** by equatorial zone cells. The growth of the lens continues till 20th year of life.

Vascular Supply During Development:
- During the developmental phase, the posterior part of the capsule covering the lens is supplied by **Hyaloid artery** and anterior part of the capsule which forms the pupillary membrane by **Anterior choroid arteries**.
- By seventh month, the anterior choroid arteries degenerates and as a result the **pupillary membrane** disappears.
- By eighth month, the distal part of hyaloid artery degenerates and proximal part persists as the **Central artery of retina**.
- Thus, due to lack of blood supply, the lens capsule disappears completely. As the lens undergoes degeneration, it transitions into an avascular structure.

RETINA, IRIS AND CILIARY BODY

- The retina emerges from the outer and inner layers of the optic cup.
- Within the inner layer of the optic cup, two distinct portions are formed—a smaller anterior part and a more extensive posterior part.
  - The **Small anterior part** (single layer of nonnervous cells) contributes to the formation of the epithelial covering for both the ciliary body and iris, representing the **ciliary** and **iridial** aspects of the retina.
  - The **Large posterior part** undergoes substantial thickening, resulting in the formation of the retina proper, the **optical** part of the retina.

Pigmented Layer:
- The outer layer of the optic cup is lined by columnar cells, and by fifth week, pigmented granules appear in the cytoplasm converting it into the pigmented layer of the retina (Fig. 21.5).

Neural Layer:
- Simultaneously, the inner thick layer transforms into the neural layer of the retina with three layers, namely ependymal, mantle and marginal.
  - The **Ependymal layer** lying close to the pigmented layer forms **rods** and **cones**.

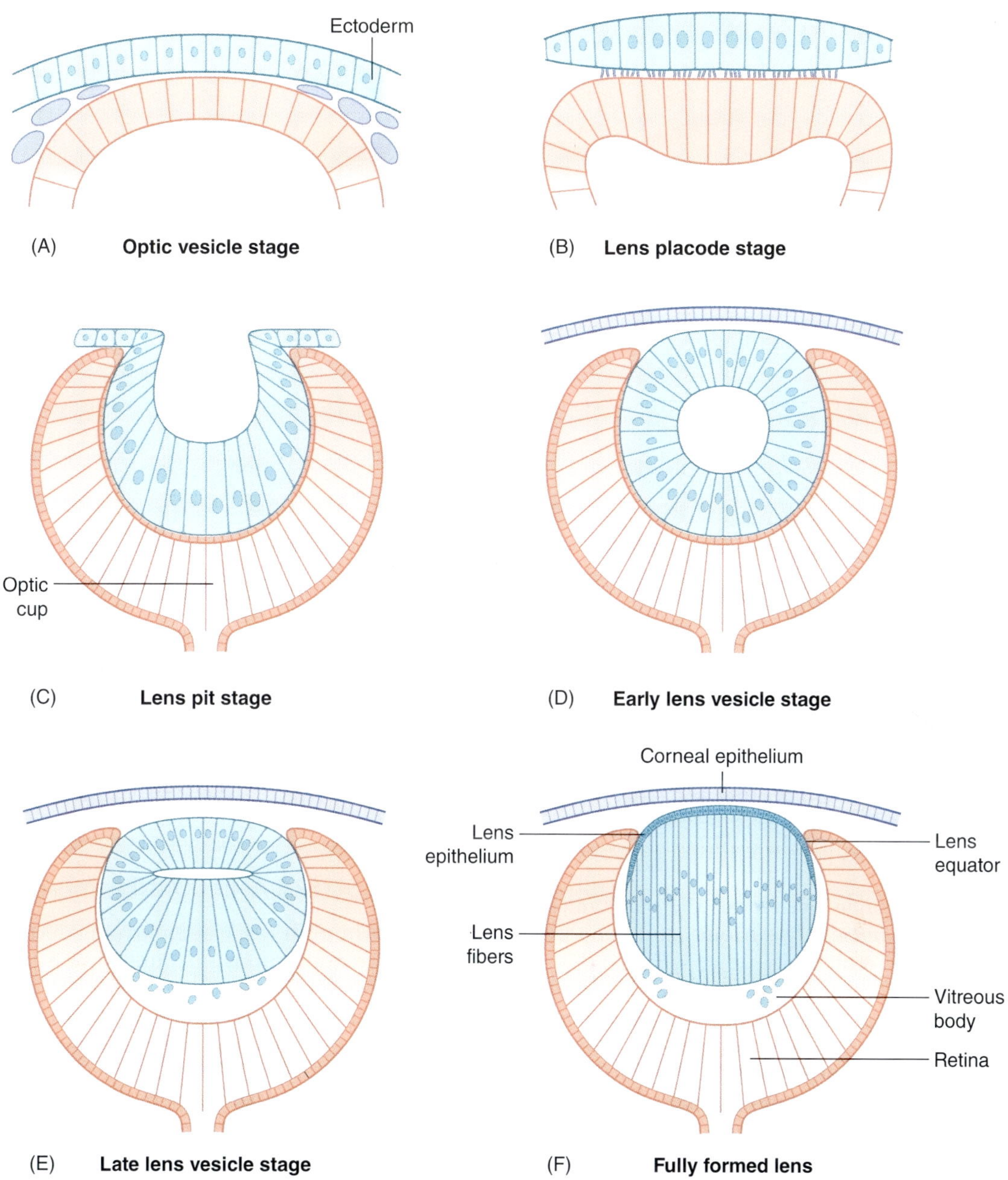

Fig. 21.4 The early stages of lens formation. (A) The lens vesicle contacts the surface ectoderm. (B) The optic vesicle adheres to the surface ectoderm and the prospective lens cells elongate to form the lens placode. (C) The lens placode and the outer surface of the optic vesicle invaginate to form the lens pit and the optic cup, respectively. (D) The lens vesicle separates from the surface ectoderm. (E) The primary lens fibres elongate and begin to occlude the lumen of the vesicle. The posterior of the lens vesicle separates from the inner surface of the optic cup. Capillaries from the hyaloid artery invade the primary vitreous body. (F) The configuration of the lens as it begins to grow. Secondary fibre cells have not yet developed and organelles are still present in all fibre cells. (Source: *Adler's Physiology of the Eye*, 11th ed. 2011; Credit Line modified from McAvoy J. Developmental biology of the lens. In Duncan G (Ed), *Mechanism of Cataract Formation*. Academic Press, pp. 7–46. Copyright Elsevier 1981480.)

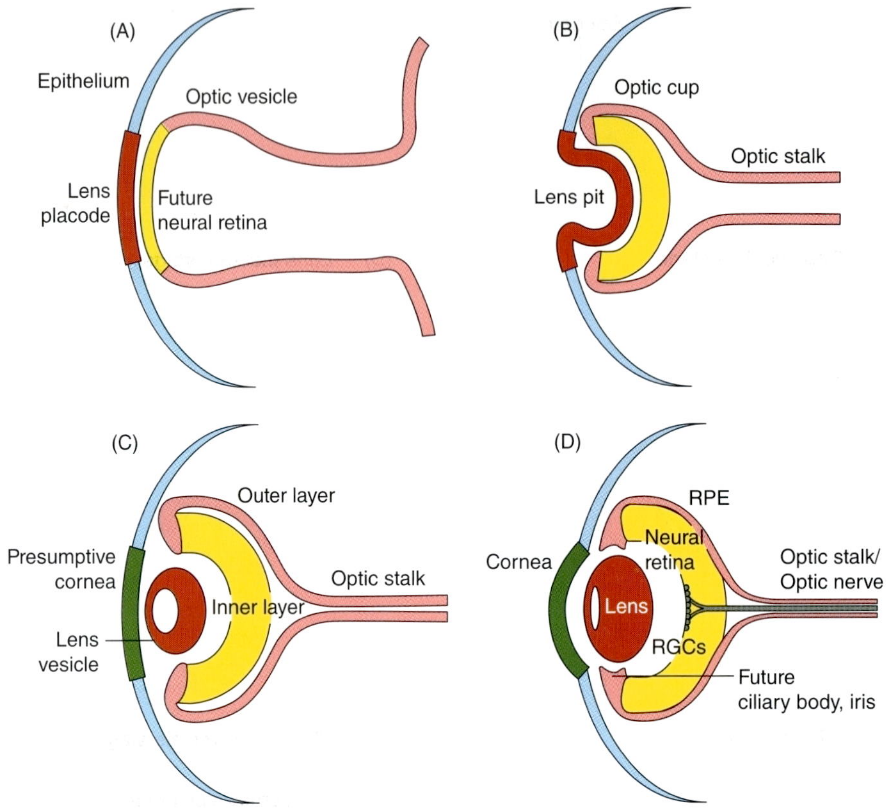

Fig. 21.5 Formation of outer and inner layer of retina. (*RPE*, Retinal pigmented epithelium; *RGC*, retinal ganglionic cells.)

- The **Mantle layer** forms the outer nuclear, inner nuclear, ganglionic and supporting cells of retina.
- The **Marginal layer** forms the stratum opticum with the axons of ganglion cells and the fibres finally form the **optic nerve**.

Fate of Intraretinal Space:

- Over time, the intraretinal space between the outer and inner layers undergoes obliteration during the eighth month of intrauterine life (retinal layers complete differentiation), leading to the fusion of the pigmented layer with the neural layer.
- The plane of cleavage in **Retinal detachment** occurs through this intraretinal space between the pigmented and nervous layer of retina.

Muscle Development:

- The ectoderm contributes to the formation of the **sphincter and dilator pupillae**, while the **ciliaris** muscle traces its origin to mesenchymal sources.

CHOROID, SCLERA AND CORNEA

- Around the fifth week of embryonic development, the optic cup is surrounded by a loose congregation of mesenchymal tissue.
- The initially undifferentiated mesenchyme undergoes a transformative process, giving rise to two layers as follows:
  - **Inner Layer (Analogous to Pia-Arachnoid Mater):** This stratum evolves into the **Choroid**, a richly vascularized pigment layer.
  - **Outer Layer (Resembling Dura Mater):** The outer layer which is fibrous in nature develops into **Sclera**.

Development of Cornea:

- The corneal formation is induced by the lens vesicle and the different sources are as follows:
  - **Epithelial Layer:** Originating from surface ectoderm.
  - **Substantia Propria:** Emerging from the mesoderm and maintaining continuity with the sclera.

- **Endothelial Layer:** Origination from neural crest cells.

Chamber Formation:

- Mesoderm lying between the iris and cornea develops a space within it called the **Anterior chamber**.
- The mesodermal zone bridging the iris and lens results in the formation of the **Posterior chamber**.
- A transient **Pupillary membrane** acts as a temporary separator between the anterior and posterior chambers.
- After the degeneration of the pupillary membrane, a connection is established between the anterior and posterior chambers through the **Pupil**.
- **Persistent pupillary membranes** is a congenital condition with remnants of the blood vessels to the foetal lens (tunica vasculosa lentis). In most patients, it does not affect vision, although it may lead to earlier development of cataract (Fig. 21.6).
- Both the anterior and posterior chambers become reservoirs for **aqueous humour**, produced by the ciliary process of the ciliary body, contributing to ocular fluid balance.

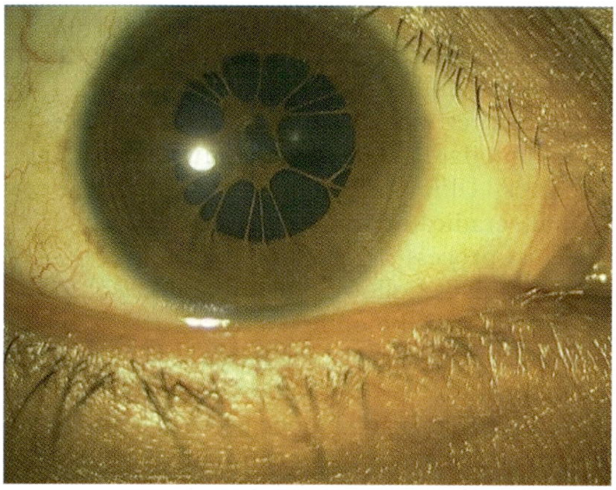

Fig. 21.6 Persistent pupillary membrane covering the pupil (it failed to degenerate). (Photo courtesy: Dr Sanitha.)

VITREOUS BODY

- The vitreous body emerges as a combination of ectodermal (primitive vitreous body) and mesodermal (definitive vitreous body) contributions (Fig. 21.7).

Primitive Vitreous Body:

- The **Primitive vitreous body** takes shape through the processes of ectodermal cells situated between the optic cup and lens vesicle.

Definitive Vitreous Body:

- Mesenchymal cells nestled within the concavity of the optic cup and choroid fissure actively participate in filling the interstices of the primitive vitreous body, transforming it into the **Definitive vitreous body**.
- The processes from the vitreous body forms the following ocular structures:
    - **Suspensory Ligament of Lens:** Encircling the equator of the lens, this structure maintains lens positioning.
    - **Hyaloid Membrane:** Formed at the periphery.
    - **Hyaloid/Cloquet's Canal/Stilling's Canal:** Encircling the hyaloid artery, providing a conduit for vascular elements.

OPTIC NERVE

- The optic stalk, containing the choroid fissure connects the optic cup to the developing brain.
- Retinal nerve fibres traverse through the inner wall of the optic stalk towards the brain.

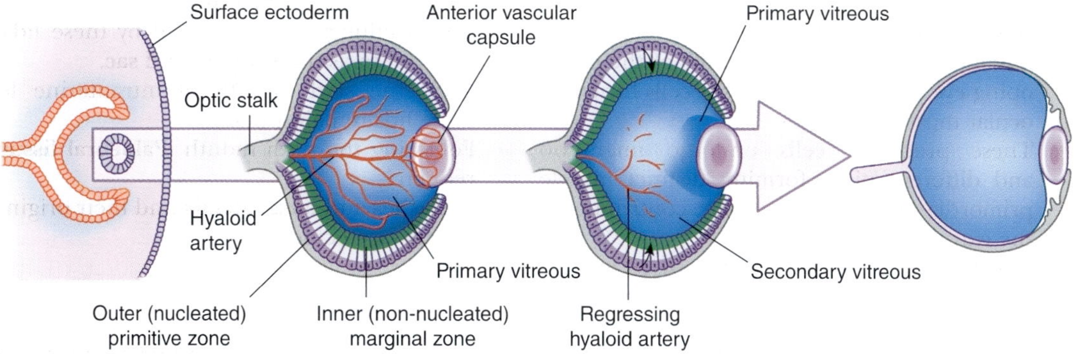

Fig. 21.7 Formation of vitreous body.

- By the seventh week, the **Choroid fissure** undergoes closure, initiating the formation of a slender tunnel within the optic stalk.
- The inner wall of the optic stalk thickens, accommodating the growing number of nerve fibres. Ultimately, it merges with the outer wall, eradicating the intraretinal space.
- This process results in the conversion of the initially hollow optic stalk into a solid cord constituting the optic nerve.
- The **Central artery of the retina** in adulthood is a remnant of the proximal part of the **Hyaloid artery**, persisting at the optic nerve's central core.
- The optic nerve is encapsulated by the pia-arachnoid and dura layers, providing protective coverings for the developing neural tissue.

BLOOD VESSELS

- Blood vessels are of mesodermal origin as a direct extension of the pia-arachnoid.
- A segment of this mesoderm undergoes invagination into the optic cup, initiating the formation of retinal vessels.
- As development progresses, the **central artery** and **vein** of the retina integrate by burying themselves within the optic nerve's central region.
- In the initial stages, the lens finds itself enveloped by a vascular capsule, ensuring a supportive environment for its early growth.

Vascular Supply to Lens:

- The **Hyaloid artery** contributes to the posterior portion of the capsule, while the **Anterior choroid artery** supplies the anterior segment.
- Later, the vascular capsule and hyaloid artery disappear but hyaloid canal in vitreous persists into adulthood.

EXTRAOCULAR MUSCLES

- In the early stages of embryonic development, mesenchymal cells in the vicinity of the developing eye give rise to precursor cells for extraocular muscles.
- These precursor cells undergo migration and differentiation, forming distinct muscle primordia that will eventually contribute to the extraocular muscles.
- The majority of extraocular muscles are derived from the three **Preotic myotomes**.
- They receive innervation from cranial nerves, primarily the **Oculomotor nerve (CN III), Trochlear nerve (CN IV) and Abducens nerve (CN VI)**.
- As the eye structures develop, the extraocular muscles align precisely to ensure coordinated movement and alignment of both eyes.

DERIVATIVES OF EYE AT A GLANCE

Germ Layers	Ocular Structure
Surface ectoderm	• Anterior epithelium of cornea • Lens
Neuroectoderm	• Optic cup (retina) • Sphincter and dilator pupillae • Iris and ciliary body (epithelium) • Optic stalk (optic nerve)
Mesoderm	• Substantia propria of cornea • Sclera • Choroid, ciliary body and iris (stroma) • Vitreous body • Central retinal artery and vein • Extraocular muscles

ACCESSORY STRUCTURES OF EYEBALL

EYELIDS

- Derived from the **surface ectoderm** through reduplication above and below the cornea.
- The mesodermal portion of ectodermal folds contributes to the formation of **muscles** and **tarsal plates**.
- Subsequently, these folds undergo growth and fusion along their margins.
- The resulting space enclosed by these lids is referred to as the **Conjunctival sac**.
- Until the sixth month of intrauterine life, these lids remain united.
- Following the sixth month, **Palpebral fissures** reopen.
- **Eyelashes** and **tarsal glands** find their origin in the surface ectoderm.

LACRIMAL GLAND

It is derived from the **Ectodermal outgrowths** that arise from superior conjunctival fornix.

LACRIMAL SAC AND NASOLACRIMAL DUCT

- Derives from the ectoderm of the **Naso-optic furrow**, located at the junction of the maxillary process and lateral nasal process.
- The naso-optic furrow undergoes modification from a furrow to a solid cord, eventually canalizing.
- The upper part of this canalized structure gives rise to the **Lacrimal sac**, while the lower part forms the **Nasolacrimal duct**.
- **Lacrimal canaliculi** form through the canalization of ectodermal buds originating from the margin of each eyelid near the medial end, extending into the lacrimal sac.
- The regulatory gene **PAX6** governs the regulation of eye development.

CLINICAL NUGGETS

Microphthalmia

- Condition where the eye is abnormally **small**.
- Results from intrauterine infections, such as **Cytomegalovirus** and **Toxoplasmosis**.

Anophthalmia

- Complete absence of the **eye**.
- Occurs when the **Optic vesicle** fails to develop.

Congenital aphakia

- Absence of the **Lens** in the eye.
- Results from the failure of the **Lens placode** to develop.

Aniridia

- Characterized by the absence of the **iris** (refer to Fig. 21.8).
- Caused by a mutation in the **PAX6 gene**.

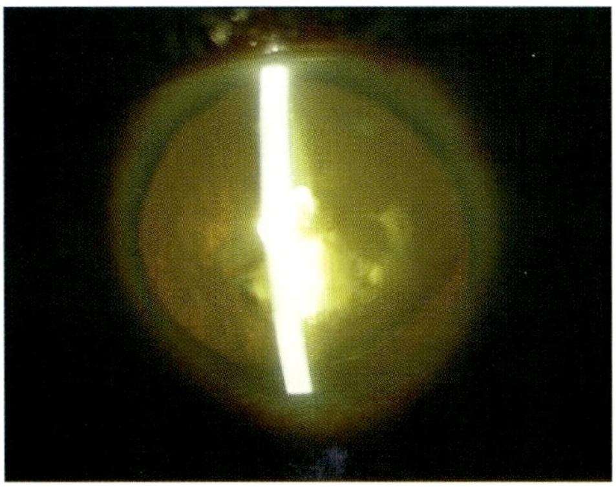

Fig. 21.8 Aniridia (the lens margin can be seen in the nondilated eye due to the absence of iris). (Photo courtesy: Dr Sanitha.)

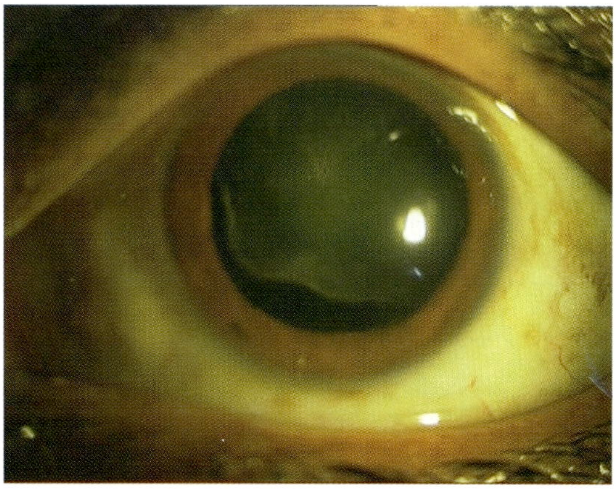

Fig. 21.9 Lens coloboma (the eye is dilated and coloboma of lens is seen as wavy margin on the inferior aspect). (Photo courtesy: Dr Sanitha.)

KLINISCHE PERLEN (AN 43.4)

COLOBOMA

- Anomaly where the **Choroid fissure** fails to close (typically closes by the seventh week of development).
- **Lens coloboma** (Fig. 21.9) results in a cleft in the lens, usually located inferiorly, sometimes associated with uveal colobomas.
- **Coloboma iridis** manifests as a cleft in the iris.
- **Coloboma of Eyelids** involves the absence of a part of the eyelid.
- Linked with a mutation in the **PAX2 gene**.

CONGENITAL CATARACT

- Opacification of the lens during intrauterine life.
- Often associated with **maternal Rubella** infection, particularly if the infection occurs before the seventh week of gestation.
- **Cerulean/blue dot cataract** is a hereditary congenital cataract characterized by bluish and white opacifications in the superficial layers of the foetal and adult **lens nucleus** (refer to Fig. 21.10).

CYCLOPIA AND SYNOPHTHALMIA

- Result from the loss of midline tissue.
- **Cyclopia** is characterized by a **single eye**.
- **Synophthalmia** involves the **fusion of the eyes**.
- Associated with **Proboscis** where nose is represented as a tubular appendage and holoprosencephaly.

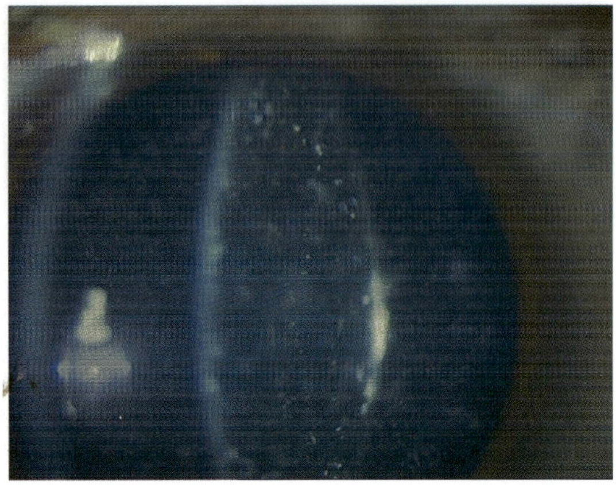

Fig. 21.10 Blue dot cataract (congenital cataract). (Photo courtesy: Dr Sanitha.)

CRYPTOPHTHALMOS

- Congenital absence of **eyelids**.
- The eyeball is defective and covered with **skin**.

RETINAL DETACHMENT

- Can be **congenital or acquired**.
- Involves fluid accumulation between the pigment and neural layers of the retina, which were once separated by the **Intraretinal space**.

LIMBAL DERMOID

- Benign congenital tumours containing **Choristomatous tissue** (tissue not normally found at that site, Fig. 21.11).

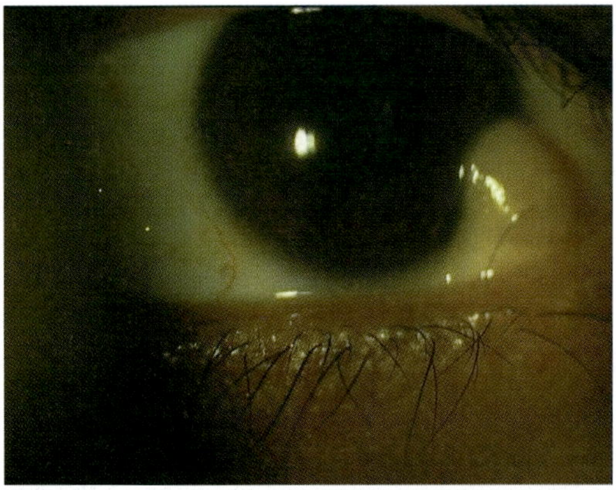

Fig. 21.11 Limbal dermoid. (Photo courtesy: Dr Sanitha.)

- Often found at the inferior temporal quadrant of the **Corneal limbus**.
- May contain various histologically **aberrant tissues**, such as epidermal appendages, connective tissue, skin, fat, sweat glands, lacrimal glands, muscles, teeth, cartilage, bone, vascular structures and neural tissue, including the brain.
- Associated with syndromes like **Goldenhar syndrome**.

POINTS TO PONDER

Developmental Stage	Key Events and Structures Formed
Optic vesicle formation (fourth week)	• The optic sulci, evaginating from the forebrain, form the optic vesicles.
Optic cup formation	• The optic vesicle invaginates, forming an optic cup attached to the forebrain by an optic stalk.
Lens development	• The adjacent surface ectoderm forms the lens placode. Lens placode pinches off to become a lens vesicle (future lens).
Neural retina and pigmented epithelium formation	• Inner wall of the optic cup forms the neural retina. Outer wall gives rise to pigmented epithelium.
Optic nerve formation	• Axons from the neural retina transform the optic stalk into the optic nerve.
Blood supply to lens and retina	• Hyaloid artery supplies the lens and retina through the choroidal fissure groove.
Maturation of lens	• The lens matures, and the artery to the lens degenerates. The remaining artery forms the central artery of the retina.
Extraocular muscles formation	• Mesoderm adjacent to the optic cup differentiates to form the extraocular muscles.
Eyelid formation	• Eyelids arise as folds of surface ectoderm.

BRAIN TEASERS

1. What do optic sulci from the prosencephalon form?
   A. Lens vesicles
   B. Optic vesicles
   C. Neural tube
   D. Retinal vessels
2. When does the complete separation of the lens vesicle from surface ectoderm occur?
   A. Third week
   B. Fifth week
   C. Seventh week
   D. Ninth week
3. What is formed by the invagination of the optic vesicle to accommodate the lens vesicle?
   A. Optic stalk
   B. Lens placode
   C. Optic cup
   D. Intraretinal space
4. Which layer becomes a highly vascularized pigment layer known as choroid?
   A. Outer fibrous layer
   B. Inner fibrous layer
   C. Superficial fibrous layer
   D. Deep vascular layer
5. What is the source of the epithelial layer of the cornea?
   A. Mesoderm
   B. Ectoderm
   C. Endoderm
   D. Neural crest cells
6. Which chamber is formed by the mesoderm between iris and cornea?
   A. Anterior chamber
   B. Posterior chamber
   C. Vitreous chamber
   D. Aqueous chamber
7. What does the primitive vitreous body derive from?
   A. Ectoderm
   B. Mesoderm
   C. Endoderm
   D. Lens vesicle
8. Which structure forms around the hyaloid artery in the vitreous body?
   A. Suspensory ligament of lens
   B. Cloquet's canal
   C. Vitreous body
   D. Optic stalk
9. At what week does the choroid fissure close to form a solid cord of the optic nerve?
   A. 5th week
   B. 7th week
   C. 9th week
   D. 12th week
10. What is the function of the hyaloid artery in the early stage of lens development?
    A. Supply the anterior chamber
    B. Supply the vitreous body
    C. Supply the lens capsule
    D. Supply the posterior chamber
11. From which layers does the retina proper (optical part of retina) originate?
    A. Inner and outer layers of optic cup
    B. Outer and inner layers of meninges
    C. Neural and fibrous layers of optic cup
    D. Superficial and deep layers of optic cup
12. What is mesenchymal in origin in the eye?
    A. Sphincter and dilator papillae
    B. Ciliaris muscle
    C. Iris
    D. Retina
13. Which layer corresponds to the dura mater in the optic cup?
    A. Inner fibrous layer
    B. Outer fibrous layer
    C. Inner vascular layer
    D. Pigmented layer
14. What differentiates into retinal vessels in the optic cup?
    A. Mesodermal layer
    B. Ectodermal layer
    C. Neural crest cells
    D. Optic vesicle

Answers

1. (B); 2. (B); 3. (C;) 4. (D); 5. (B); 6. (A); 7. (A); 8. (B); 9. (B); 10. (C); 11. (A); 12. (B); 13. (B); 14. (A).

FURTHER READINGS

Abdolkarimi D, Cunha DL, Lahne M, Moosajee M. PAX6 disease models for aniridia. *Ind J Ophthalmol.* 2022;70(12):4119-4129. https://doi.org/10.4103/ijo.IJO_316_22.

Kanukollu VM, Blair K, Ahmad SS. Eyelid coloboma. In: StatPearls. *StatPearls* Publishing; 2022.

Kristianslund O, Cholidis S. Persistent pupillary membranes and cataract. *Am J Ophthalmol.* 2021;229:e1. https://doi.org/10.1016/j.ajo.2021.05.030.

Parakh S, Das S, Maheshwari S, Luthra G, Luthra S. Atypical superior iris and chorioretinal coloboma. *Ind J Ophthalmol.* 2022;70(7):2665-2666. https://doi.org/10.4103/ijo.IJO_164_22.

Tripathy K, Salini B. Aniridia. In: *StatPearls.* StatPearls Publishing; 2023.

Vegunta S, Patel BC. Optic nerve coloboma. In: *StatPearls.* StatPearls Publishing; 2023.

22 Development of Ear

ANAMNESE

A 5-year-old male presented with a developmental anomaly of the ear, characterized by a malformed pinna and external auditory canal on the right side. The child's parents reported noticing the abnormality shortly after birth, and subsequent evaluations confirmed the presence of a congenital anomaly affecting the outer ear structures. Audiological assessments revealed no significant hearing impairment in the affected ear, and the child displayed age-appropriate speech and language development. Radiological imaging, including computed tomography scans, provided detailed visualization of the malformed ear anatomy, highlighting a deviation from the typical structure. The case signifies the importance of early identification and assessment of developmental anomalies of the ear and appropriate interventions for better patient outcome.

The distinctive ability of mammals to hear high-frequency sounds can be attributed to evolutionary changes in the middle ear. Notably, the evolution of three distinct middle-ear bones and the development of specific radial and circumferential collagen fibre layers in the eardrum contribute to this unique auditory capacity. Permanent hearing loss, a prevalent congenital disorder affecting **1–3/1000** live births, poses a significant challenge. Fortunately, more than 50% of cases involving permanent childhood hearing impairment can be identified shortly after birth through neonatal hearing screening programmes. It is crucial to note that such screening primarily addresses congenital cases, and progressive or late-onset hearing impairments related to conditions like congenital CMV (Cytomegalovirus) infection or certain genetic disorders often go undetected. Understanding the detailed structure of the ear reveals its three main components:

- **External ear**—Auricle and external auditory meatus.
- **Middle ear**—Tympanic cavity, mastoid antrum, auditory tube, ear ossicles.
- **Inner ear**—Bony and membranous labyrinth (cochlear duct, utricle, saccule, semicircular ducts).

DEVELOPMENT OF EAR

- **Internal Ear:** The **otocyst**, derived from the **ectodermal vesicle**, forms the structural framework for the internal ear.
- **Middle Ear:** The **tubotympanic recess**, originating from the **endoderm** forms the middle ear.
- **External Ear:** The **ectoderm** contributes to the formation of the external ear through the first branchial cleft.
- **Tympanic Membrane:** Serving as the convergence point for all three germ layers, the tympanic membrane *represents* a unique meeting place for ectoderm, mesoderm, and endoderm.
  - **Cuticular Layer:** Derived from the ectoderm.
  - **Fibrous Layer:** Developed from the mesoderm.
  - **Mucous Layer:** Formed from the endoderm of the tubotympanic recess.
- **Structures Assuming Full Size at Birth:**
  - **Internal Ear:** Reaches its complete size during foetal development and assumes its final form at birth.

- **Tympanic Cavity:** Attains full size by birth, contributing to the middle ear's functional development.
- **Mastoid Antrum:** Achieves mature dimensions by birth, constituting an integral part of the temporal bone's anatomy.
- **Ear Ossicles:** The auditory ossicles, including the malleus, incus and stapes, reach their full size at birth, playing a significant role in auditory function.

EXTERNAL EAR

AURICLE

- During the sixth week of development, six distinct mesodermal hillocks become apparent at the external opening of the first branchial cleft, marking a critical stage in the formation of external ear structures (see Fig. 22.1).

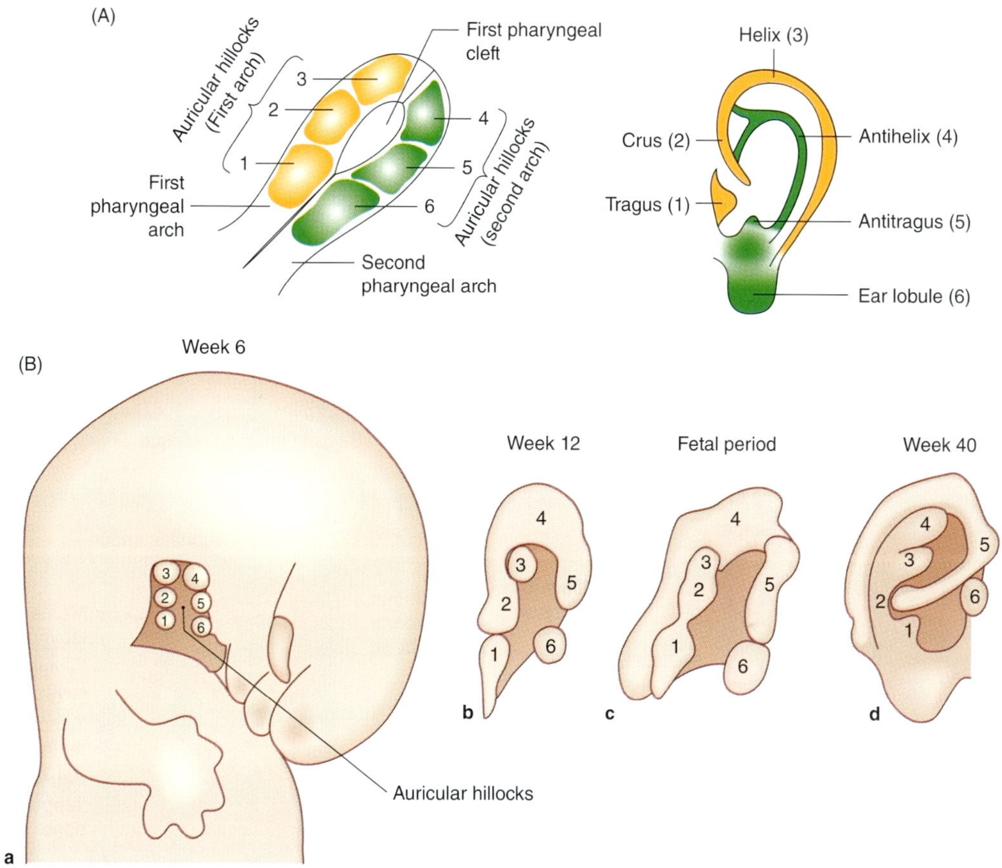

Fig. 22.1 Development of the auricle from the six auricular hillocks, right side. The merger of the auricular hillocks (1-6) is a complex process and, thus, developmental abnormalities are not infrequent. The primordial auricles start to develop at the base of the neck. As the mandible develops, the auricles move cranially to reach their normal position on both sides of the head at the level of the eyes. Ears positioned deeper in the head frequently are associated with (often chromosomal) developmental abnormalities. The external acoustic canal derives from the posterior part of the first pharyngeal groove which extends inwards as a cone-shaped tube to reach the ectodermal epithelial lining of the tympanic cavity (Recessus tubotympanicus). At the beginning of week 9, epithelial cells located at the floor of the external acoustic meatus proliferate to generate a cellular plate, the meatal plug, which normally degenerates by 7 months of foetal development. A persistent plate in the external acoustic meatus is a cause of congenital deafness. (Source: *Sobotta: Atlas of Human Anatomy: Head, Neck, and Neuroanatomy*. 15th ed. 2011.)

- Three hillocks, recognized as **hyoid tubercles** are aligned along the cephalic border, associated with the hyoid arch. Simultaneously, an additional three hillocks, identified as **mandibular tubercles**, arrange themselves along the caudal border, corresponding to the mandibular arch.
- **Formation of External Ear:**
  - **Hyoid Tubercles:** These tubercles contribute to the development of the antihelix, antitragus and lobule.
  - **Mandibular Tubercles:** These tubercles result in the formation of the tragus, helix and crus of helix.

EXTERNAL AUDITORY MEATUS

- Commencing from the dorsal region of the first branchial cleft, ectoderm undergoes invagination, assuming a funnel-like structure in the process of external ear development (Fig. 22.2).
- The invaginated structure transforms into a tube referred to as the **Primary meatus**.
- Ectodermal cells proliferate, forming a solid cord known as the **Meatal plate**, extending towards the developing tympanic cavity.
- In the seventh month of gestation, the cells constituting the meatal plate undergo disinte-

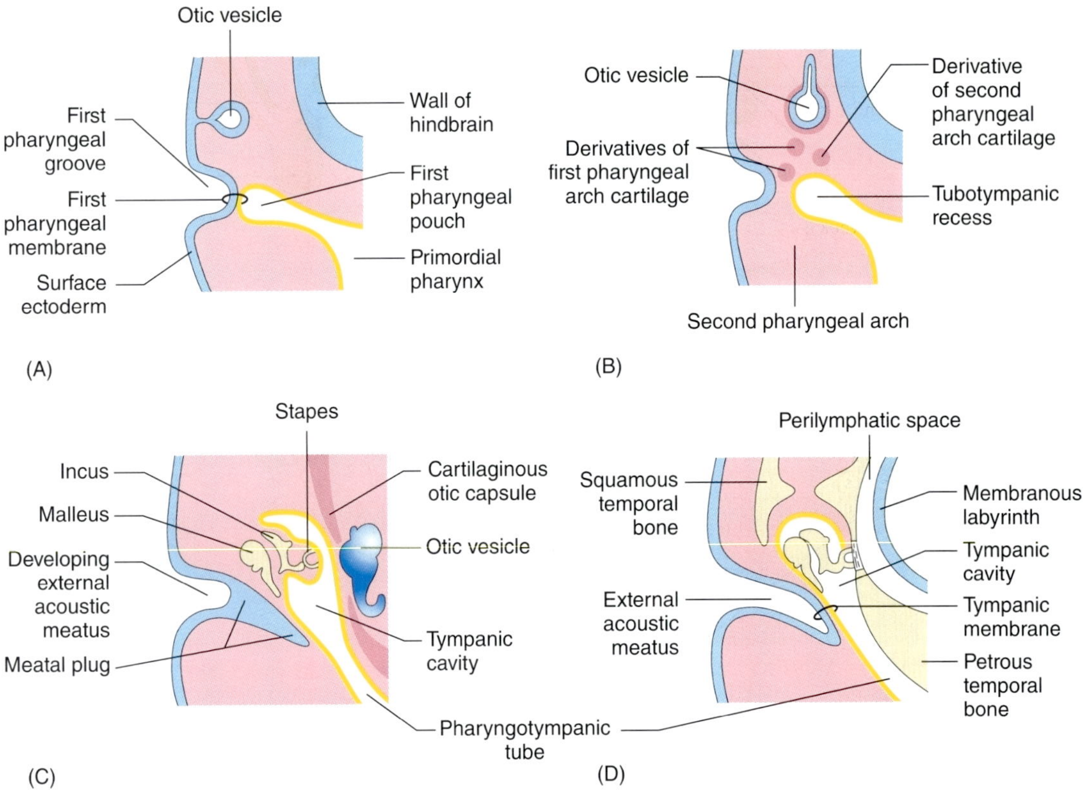

Fig. 22.2 Formation of external acoustic meatus. Schematic drawings illustrating development of the external and middle parts of the ear. Observe the relationship of these parts of the ear to the otic vesicle, the primordium of the internal ear. (A) At 4 weeks, illustrating the relation of the otic vesicle to the pharyngeal apparatus. (B) At 5 weeks, showing the tubotympanic recess and pharyngeal arch cartilages. (C) Later stage, showing the tubotympanic recess (future tympanic cavity and mastoid antrum) beginning to envelop the ossicles. (D) Final stage of ear development showing the relationship of the middle ear to the perilymphatic space and external acoustic meatus. Note that the tympanic membrane develops from three germ layers, surface ectoderm, mesenchyme and endoderm of the tubotympanic recess. (Source: *Before We Are Born: Essentials of Embryology and Birth Defects*. 1st South Asia ed. 2016.)

gration, resulting in the formation of the **Secondary meatus**.

TYMPANIC MEMBRANE

- The cells positioned between the base of the meatal plate and the tympanic cavity contribute to the formation of the tympanic membrane.
- **Definitive Tympanic Membrane:**
  - **Outer Cuticular Layer:** Derived from the ectoderm of the meatal plate, the outermost layer of the definitive tympanic membrane is the cuticular layer.
  - **Middle Fibrous Layer:** Adjoining mesoderm contributes to the middle fibrous layer
  - **Inner Mucous Layer:** Formed from the endoderm of the tubotympanic recess, the innermost mucous layer completes the formation of the definitive tympanic membrane.

MIDDLE EAR

- First pharyngeal pouch (also a part from the second pouch) forms an endodermal diverticulum known as the **tubotympanic recess** during the fifth week.
- The tubotympanic recess extends to the base of the primary external auditory meatus.
- The medial part of the recess which is narrow is positioned between the first and third arches, and it later evolves into the **auditory tube**.
- The dilated lateral part of the recess gives rise to the **primitive tympanic cavity**.
- By the seventh week, three mesodermal thickenings develop in the roof of the tympanic cavity.
- These thickenings undergo chondrification and ossification, resulting in the formation of the **malleus, incus** and **stapes** (Fig. 22.3).
- Malleus and incus originate from the **first arch (Meckel's cartilage)**, while stapes originates from the **second arch (Reichert's cartilage)**.
- **Muscles and Nerves Associated With Ossicles:**
  - **Tensor tympani**, the muscle of the malleus, belongs to the first arch and is supplied by the **mandibular nerve**.
  - **Stapedius**, the muscle of the stapes, belongs to the second arch and is supplied by the **facial nerve**.
- **Formation of Definitive Tympanic Cavity:**
  - Mesenchymal cells surrounding the ossicles disintegrate, forming an extensive cavity known as the **definitive tympanic cavity** by the eighth month.
  - A backward extension of the tympanic cavity contributes to the formation of the **tympanic antrum**.
  - Mastoid air cells mature and are formed by the second year after birth.

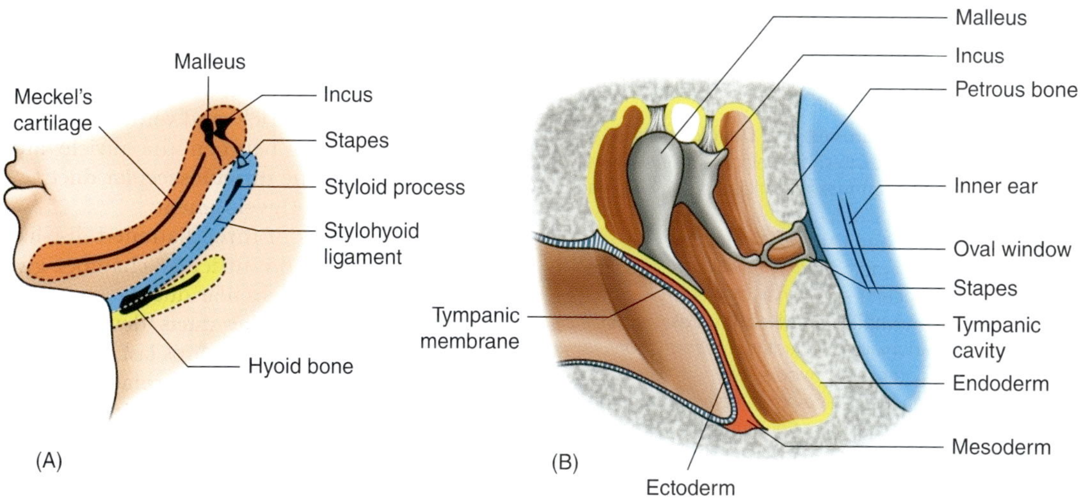

Fig. 22.3 Formation of ear ossicles.

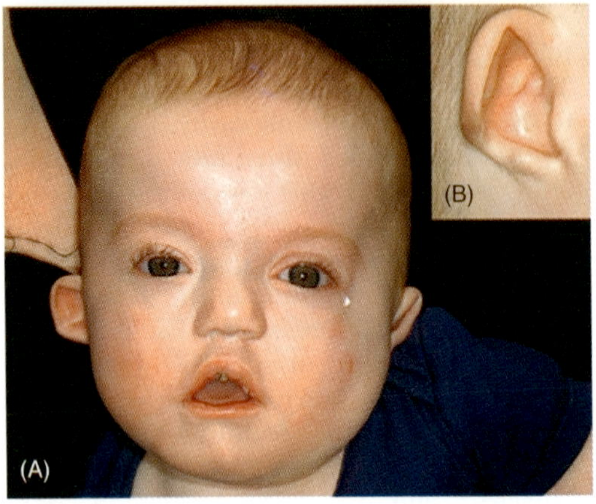

Fig. 22.4 CHARGE syndrome. (Source: *Avery's Diseases of the Newborn*, 11th ed.: Taylor Sawyer, Christine A. Gleason, Fig. 88.12, Elsevier Inc., 2024.)

CLINICAL NUGGETS

Charge syndrome (Fig. 22.4)

- Charge syndrome is a rare genetic disorder characterized by a constellation of congenital anomalies and medical conditions. The acronym '**CHARGE**' represents the key features associated with this syndrome:
  - **C—Coloboma of the Eye:**
    - Coloboma refers to a gap or hole in one of the structures of the eye, such as the iris, retina or optic disc.
  - **H—Heart Defects:**
    - Individuals with charge syndrome may exhibit congenital heart anomalies, which can vary in severity.
  - **A—Atresia of the Choanae:**
    - Choanal atresia is a narrowing or blockage of the back of the nasal passage, leading to breathing difficulties.
  - **R—Retarded Growth and Development:**
    - Delayed growth and developmental milestones are common features, impacting physical and cognitive development.
  - **G—Genital and Urinary Anomalies:**
    - Charge syndrome may involve abnormalities in the genital and urinary systems.
  - **E—Ear Anomalies and Hearing Loss:**
    - Ear anomalies, including malformations of the outer and middle ear, are prevalent. Hearing loss is a common associated feature.
- The syndrome is often caused by mutations in the **CHD7 gene**, which plays a crucial role in embryonic development. The severity and combination of symptoms can vary widely among individuals with charge syndrome.

INTERNAL EAR

The internal ear consists of an outer bony labyrinth and an inner membranous labyrinth. The **bony labyrinth** contains perilymph and connects with the cerebrospinal fluid (CSF) in the subarachnoid space through the cochlear aqueduct. The **membranous labyrinth** forms a closed system, including the cochlear duct, the saccule and utricle, and the three semicircular ducts, and it is filled with endolymph.

MEMBRANOUS LABYRINTH

- **Otic placode** develops as a thickening in the surface ectoderm on each side of the rhombencephalon during the fourth week.
- Otic placode invaginates into underlying mesenchyme, forming the **Otic pit**.
- Otic pit detaches from the surface ectoderm, resulting in the formation of the **Otic vesicle or Otocyst**. Otocyst serves as the structural basis for the membranous labyrinth.
- Neuroepithelial cells separated from the otocyst wall form **bipolar neurons** of the **vestibulocochlear ganglion**.
  - **Peripheral processes** of bipolar neurons form vestibular and auditory nerves, terminating in various structures.
  - **Central processes** terminate in vestibular and cochlear nuclei as the vestibulocochlear nerve.
- A diverticulum from the medial wall of the otocyst forms the **endolymphatic duct** and **sac**.
- **Division Into Utricle and Saccule:**
  - A fold from the lateral wall divides the otocyst into dorsal utricle and ventral saccule.
  - Communication between the utricle and saccule forms the **utriculosaccular duct**.
- **Semicircular Duct Development:**
  - Peripheral rims of three flattened disc-like evaginations in the utricular chamber give rise to three semicircular ducts.
  - **Superior semicircular ducts** develop first, while the **posterior** develops last.
- **Maculae and Cochlear Duct Formation:**
  - Maculae develop from **neuroepithelial cells** of utricle and medial wall of saccule.
  - Cochlear duct forms as an elongation from the caudal end of the **saccular chamber** (Fig. 22.5).

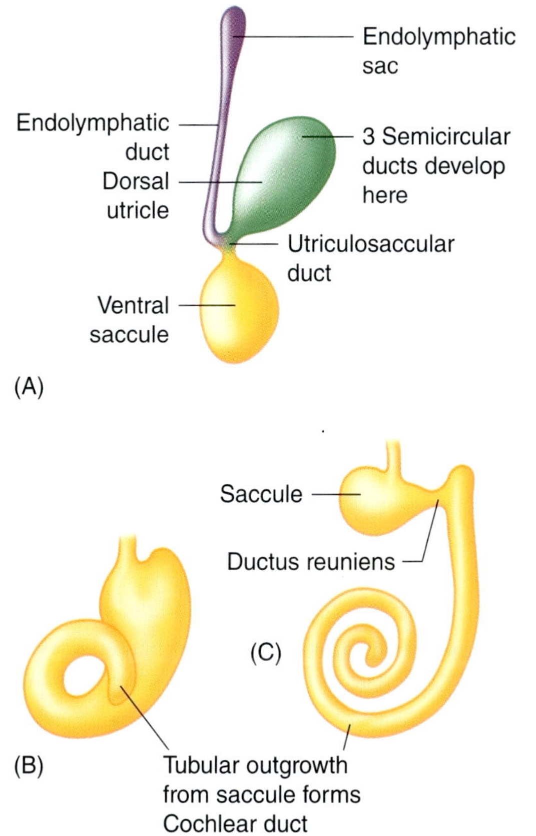

Fig. 22.5 Formation of membranous labyrinth.

BONY LABYRINTH

- Otic capsule forms from the mesenchyme around the otocyst.
- Otic capsule differentiates into cartilage cells, further differentiating into perilymphatic space and bony labyrinth.
- **Modiolus** of cochlea is ossified mesenchyme.
- **Semicircular canals** develop from the bony labyrinth around the semicircular ducts.
- **Vestibule** develops from the bony labyrinth around the utricle and saccule.
- **Scala Tympani and Scala Vestibuli:**
  - Scala tympani and scala vestibuli are derived from **perilymphatic spaces** along the cochlear duct.
  - Scala tympani is separated from the cochlear duct by the **basilar membrane** and scala vestibuli is separated from the cochlear duct by **vestibular or Resissner's membrane**.
  - At the apex of the cochlear duct both scala vestibuli and scala tympani communicate with each other through an aperture called **helicotrema**.
- **Spiral Organ of Corti:**
  - Cells at the **basilar membrane** of the cochlear duct form outer and inner ridges.
  - Spiral organ of corti is derived from outer and inner ridges (Fig. 22.6).

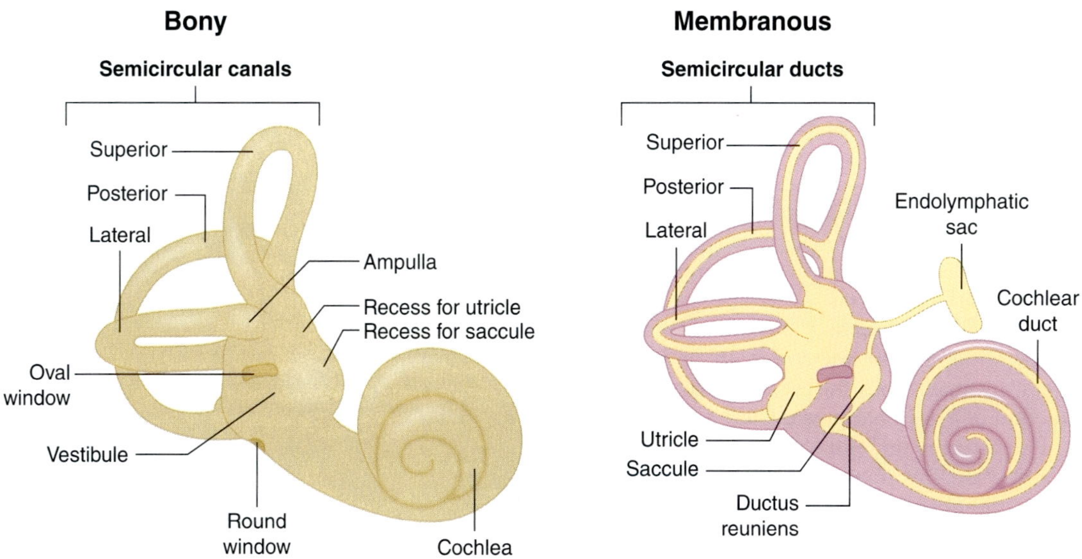

Fig. 22.6 Bony and membranous labyrinths.

CLINICAL NUGGETS

Congenital hearing loss

- Congenital hearing loss, which manifests from birth, occurs when the ear's ability to convert sound's vibratory mechanical energy into electrical impulses is impaired.
- Hearing loss is categorized according to the site of the lesion. In **conductive hearing loss**, the outer or middle ear is affected, while in **sensorineural hearing loss**, the inner ear, auditory nerve or central auditory pathway are impacted.
- **Mixed hearing loss** is characterized by a combination of conductive and sensorineural components.
- In **conductive hearing loss**, sound waves face obstacles in propagating through the ear. This can result from maldevelopment of the middle or external ear or transient obstruction, such as effusion (as seen in otitis media).
- **Sensorineural hearing loss** can be further subdivided into sensory hearing loss (impacting hair cells), central hearing loss (located along the central auditory pathway), or auditory neuropathy spectrum disorder.
- **Auditory Neuropathy Spectrum Disorder:** This disorder may stem from primary lesions in the inner hair cells, auditory nerve, intervening synapses and may involve damage to neuronal populations in the auditory pathway.
- Common causes for congenital hearing loss include genetic factors, rubella, cytomegalovirus and isotretinoin (accutane).

DERIVATIVES OF EAR AT A GLANCE

First Pharyngeal Cleft:
- The external auditory meatus originates from the first pharyngeal cleft.

Auricular Hillocks (First and Second Arch):
- The pinna or auricle is derived from the auricular hillocks associated with the first and second pharyngeal arches.

First Pharyngeal Arch:
- The malleus and incus are derived from the first pharyngeal arch.

First Pharyngeal Pouch:
- The auditory tube and structures of the middle ear originate from the first pharyngeal pouch.

Junction of First Pharyngeal Cleft and Pouch:
- The tympanic membrane is formed at the junction of the first pharyngeal cleft and pouch, with contributions from three sources.

Second Pharyngeal Arch:
- The stapes and stapedius muscle are derivatives of the second pharyngeal arch.

Utricular Part:
- The utricular part gives rise to the utricle, endolymphatic duct and sac, and the semicircular ducts.

Saccular Part:
- The saccular part contributes to the development of the saccule and the cochlear duct.

KLINISCHE PERLEN

PREAURICULAR PITS

- Preauricular pits are small holes in front of the ear, towards the face, present since birth.
- These pits are connected to a sinus tract beneath the skin.
- The presence of preauricular pits results from the abnormal development of auricular hillocks.

PREAURICULAR APPENDAGES (FIG. 22.7)

- Preauricular appendages refer to abnormal protrusions or skin tags located near the external ear.
- These appendages result from the presence of **accessory auricular hillocks** during embryonic development.
- While generally benign, preauricular appendages may prompt further examination, especially

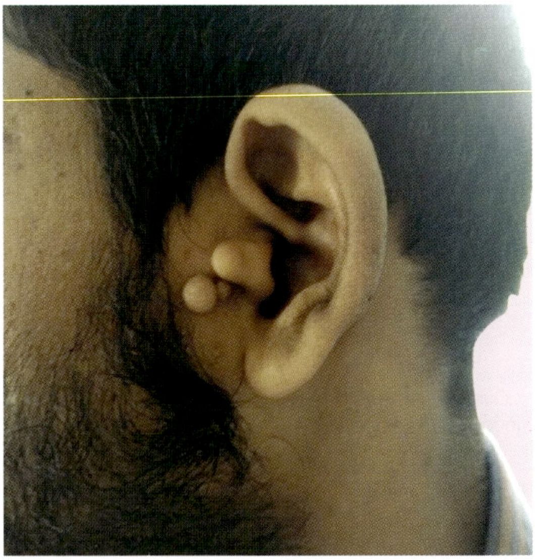

Fig. 22.7 Preauricular appendages. (Photo courtesy: Dr Jeena.)

in the context of other ear anomalies, to ensure a complete understanding of any associated conditions or developmental variations.

CONGENITAL DEFORMITY OF THE PINNA

- **Microtia** is a congenital deformity characterized by underdeveloped pinna (Fig. 22.8). It can occur unilaterally (affecting one side) or bilaterally (affecting both sides).
- **Aural atresia**, the underdevelopment of the middle ear and canal, is often seen in association with microtia.
- In cases where the pinna is completely undeveloped, it is termed **Anotia**.

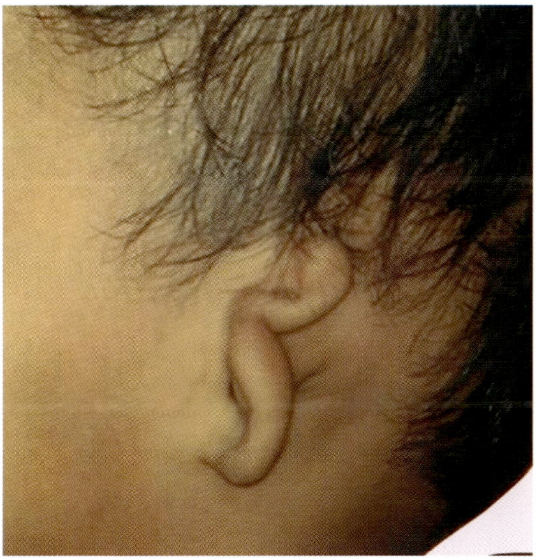

Fig. 22.8 A child with microtia. (Photo courtesy: Dr Jeena.)

OTOCEPHALY

- Otocephaly is a rare and severe congenital malformation characterized by the fusion or absence of structures in the head and neck region, particularly those related to the ear and face.
- The condition often involves abnormalities in the development of the **mandible, maxilla** and **facial bones**.
- Severe cases may exhibit the absence of the lower jaw or the fusion of the lower jaw with the upper jaw.

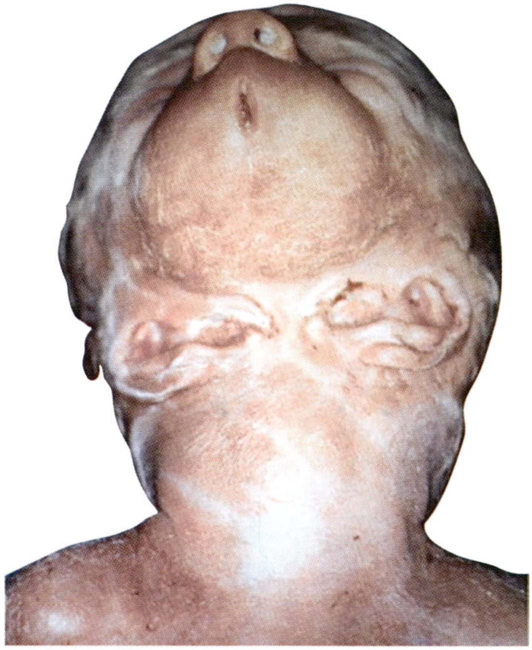

Fig. 22.9 Otocephaly. (Source: *Potter's Pathology of the Fetus, Infant and Child*, 2nd ed.: Enid Gilbert-Barness, Fig. 3.7, Elsevier Inc., 2007.)

- Otocephaly is commonly associated with abnormalities in the formation of the external ears and may involve the absence or fusion of ear structures (Fig. 22.9).

POINTS TO PONDER

External Ear

- The external ear originates from six mesenchymal masses surrounding the first pharyngeal cleft.

Middle Ear

- The middle ear develops from the first pharyngeal cleft and the associated arches, with the formation of ossicles and muscles within its cavity.

Inner Ear

- The inner ear takes shape from the surface ectoderm by the induction of hindbrain through a sequential process.
  - Ectodermal thickening (placode).
  - Invagination to form an otic vesicle.
  - Division into auditory (cochlea) and vestibular (semicircular canals) portions.

BRAIN TEASERS

1. What contributes to the unique capacity for high-frequency hearing in mammals?
   A. Evolution of the external ear
   B. Changes in the inner ear
   C. Evolution of three distinct middle-ear bones
   D. Development of the tympanic membrane
2. Permanent hearing loss is a common congenital disorder with an incidence of:
   A. 1–20/1000 live births
   B. 2–10/1000 live births
   C. 1–3/1000 live births
   D. 3–15/1000 live births
3. What structure is the meeting point of the three germ layers in the ear?
   A. Tympanic cavity
   B. Mastoid antrum
   C. Tympanic membrane
   D. Auditory tube
4. What ectodermal structure forms the outer cuticular layer of the definitive tympanic membrane?
   A. Meatal plate
   B. Tubotympanic recess
   C. Ectoderm of the second branchial cleft
   D. Otic vesicle
5. What forms the antihelix, antitragus and lobule of the external ear?
   A. Hyoid tubercles
   B. Mandibular tubercles
   C. Meatal plate
   D. Tubotympanic recess
6. When does the secondary meatus form in the development of the external auditory meatus?
   A. Fifth week
   B. Sixth week
   C. Seventh month
   D. Eighth month
7. The auditory tube forms from the narrow medial part of which structure?
   A. Tubotympanic recess
   B. External auditory meatus
   C. First pharyngeal pouch
   D. Mastoid antrum
8. Which nerve supplies the tensor tympani muscle, a muscle of the ear ossicles?
   A. Facial nerve
   B. Trigeminal nerve
   C. Vagus nerve
   D. Mandibular nerve
9. What structure forms the structural basis of the membranous labyrinth in the internal ear?
   A. Otic vesicle
   B. Vestibulocochlear nerve
   C. Endolymphatic duct
   D. Otic pit
10. The communication between the utricle and saccule forms which structure?
    A. Vestibulocochlear nerve
    B. Utriculosaccular duct
    C. Endolymphatic duct
    D. Semicircular ducts
11. Which semicircular duct develops first in the inner ear?
    A. Superior semicircular duct
    B. Posterior semicircular duct
    C. Lateral semicircular duct
    D. Anterior semicircular duct
12. The cochlear duct is formed as an elongation from the caudal end of which chamber?
    A. Vestibular chamber
    B. Saccular chamber
    C. Utricular chamber
    D. Endolymphatic duct
13. Which syndrome is often associated with ear anomalies and hearing loss?
    A. Down syndrome
    B. Turner syndrome
    C. Charge syndrome
    D. Klinefelter syndrome
14. What is the function of the stapedius muscle, a muscle of the stapes (ear ossicle)?
    A. Regulating pressure in the middle ear
    B. Controlling balance and equilibrium
    C. Contraction during loud sounds
    D. Facilitating taste perception
15. At what week does the otic placode form as a thickening in the surface ectoderm?
    A. Second week
    B. Third week
    C. Fourth week
    D. Fifth week

Answers

1. (C); 2. (C); 3. (C); 4. (A); 5. (A); 6. (C); 7. (A); 8. (D); 9. (A); 10. (B); 11. (A); 12. (B); 13. (C); 14. (C); 15. (C).

FURTHER READINGS

Korver AM, Smith RJ, Van Camp G, et al. Congenital hearing loss. *Nat Rev Dis Primers.* 2017;3:16094. doi:10.1038/nrdp.2016.94.

Usman N, Sur M. CHARGE Syndrome. In: *StatPearls.* StatPearls Publishing; 2023.

Wernheden E, Krogerus C, Andersen PS, Hesselfeldt-Nielsen J. Congenital anomalies of the external ear. *Ugeskr Laeger.* 2019;181(48):V05190300.

Wu W, Kamat D. A review of benign congenital anomalies. *Pediatr Ann.* 2020;49(2):e66-e70. https://doi.org/10.3928/19382359-20200121-03.

Zhang Y, Wang C, Yang M, Pan B. Inheritance analysis and family history for microtia: a hospital-based study in China. *In J Pediatr Otorhinolaryngol.* 2023;171:111613. https://doi.org/10.1016/j.ijporl.2023.111613.

The Integumentary System

23

AN 9.3 Describe the development of breast.

ANAMNESE

A newborn presented with severe skin abnormalities, prompting a thorough examination to determine the underlying cause. The characteristic symptoms, including thick and diamond-shaped plates of skin, suggested a diagnosis of **Harlequin ichthyosis**. The medical team conducted genetic testing to confirm the presence of specific mutations associated with this rare and severe genetic skin disorder. The diagnosis was further supported by the distinct cracked and armour-like appearance of the skin. Following confirmation, the infant received specialized care from a team of dermatologists and paediatric specialists (Fig. 23.1).

The remarkable phenomenon of scarless healing in early-gestation foetal wounds is attributed to the inherent regenerative capacity of foetal skin. This unique ability is particularly evident in certain mammals, including humans, where the tips of digits can fully regenerate after injury. The presence of the overlaying nail organ and the proliferative blastemal contributes to this regenerative process, guided by a mechanism dependent on **Wnt signalling**. Examining the molecular complexities of digit tip regeneration offers understanding in the development of translational therapies aimed at regrowing more extensive portions of limbs and other traditionally nonregenerative tissues.

Integumentary system constitutes of skin and its appendages (sebaceous glands, sweat glands, hair and nails).

DEVELOPMENT OF SKIN

- Skin consists of two layers:
  - The superficial layer, known as the **Epidermis** (see Fig. 23.2).
    - Characterized by keratinized stratified squamous epithelium (avascular).
    - The strata, arranged from superficial to deep, include the stratum corneum, stratum lucidum, stratum granulosum, stratum spinosum and stratum basale.
  - The deep layer, identified as the **Dermis or corium**:
    - It is highly vascularized.
    - It consists of the outer **papillary** layer and the inner **reticular** layer.
    - It also contains the **pilosebaceous unit (thin skin)**, including the arrectores

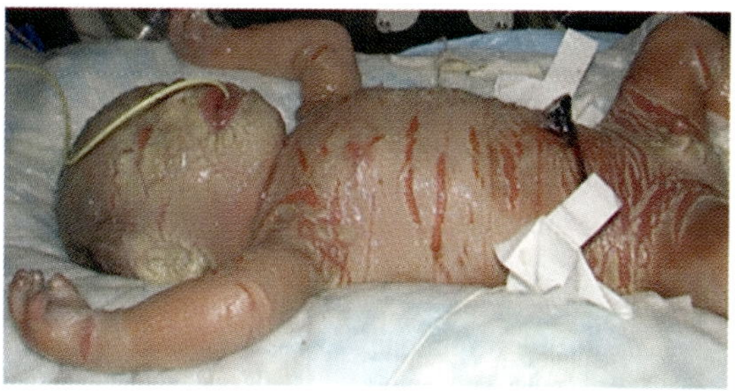

Fig. 23.1 Harlequin ichthyosis. (Source: *Andrews' Diseases of the Skin Clinical Atlas*, 2nd ed.: Robert G. Micheletti, Dirk M. Elston, William D. James, et al., Fig. 27.63, Elsevier Inc., 2023.)

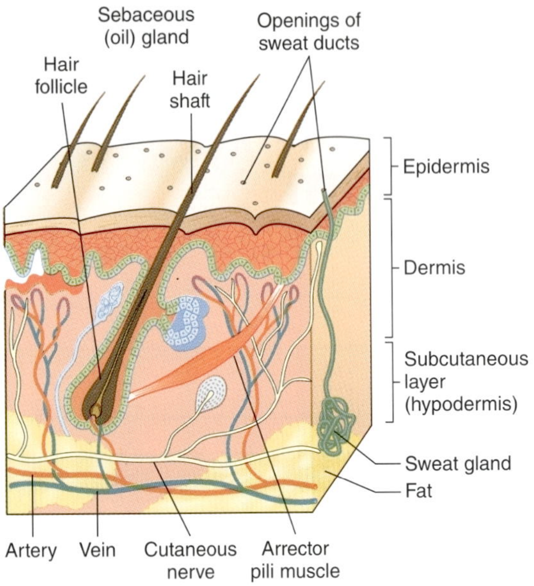

Fig. 23.2 Structure of skin.

pilorum muscle, sebaceous gland and hair follicle.

- The two sources of development of skin are:
  - **Surface ectoderm** (epidermis).
  - **Mesoderm** (dermis and hypodermis).

SURFACE ECTODERM

- Initially, the surface ectoderm consists of a single layer of cubical cells, that is **Stratum germinativum**.
- In the second month, these cells proliferate and form a second layer of flattened cells called **Periderm/epitrichium**.
- Proliferation of the germinative stratum results in the formation of the remaining layers by the end of third month.
  - **Basal layer (Stratum basale):**
    - ➢ Columnar cells that constantly divide **mitotically** and move superficially to renew epidermis.
    - ➢ **Melanoblasts** (dendritic cells) which appear in the basal layer during the third month are derived from **neural crest cells**.
  - **Spinous layer (Stratum spinosum):**
    - ➢ Irregular prickle cells **(keratinocytes)** with spine-like process.
  - **Granular layer (Stratum granulosum):**
    - ➢ Contains **keratohyalin granules** due to process of keratinization.
  - **Stratum lucidum:**
    - ➢ A layer of cells with scanty nuclei forming a **homogenous** layer superficial to granular.
  - **Horny layer (Stratum corneum):**
    - ➢ Several layers of flattened scale-like cells that are continuously shed off.
    - ➢ Cytoplasm of these cells are filled with keratin granules and these are **devoid of nucleus**.
    - ➢ By third month, the differentiation is complete and the shed-off cells get mixed with the secretions of sebaceous gland to form a paste-like substance: **Vernix caseosa**.
    - ➢ Vernix caseosa protects the foetus from the macerating effects of amniotic fluid.

MESODERM

- Lateral plate mesoderm and paraxial mesoderm differentiates into **superficial dermis** and **deep hypodermis/subcorium**.
- **Dermis** consists of two layers:
  - **Papillary layer.**
  - **Reticular layer.**
- Dermal papillae projects into epidermis from dermis.
- Subcutaneous tissue is derived from hypodermis.

EPIDERMAL RIDGES AND DERMAL PAPILLAE

- The epidermis exhibits thickenings that extend into the dermis, forming distinctive **epidermal ridges**.
- The portions of the dermis extending between these ridges are termed **dermal papillae**.
- Epidermal thickenings result in surface ectodermal ridges on the palm, sole and ventral surface of fingers and toes, contributing to the formation of **fingerprints**.
- The development of these epidermal thickenings is not solely governed by **genetics**; it is also influenced by the **uterine environment**. Consequently, these patterns are unique to each individual, even among **identical twins**.
- This uniqueness forms the foundation for personal identification through **fingerprint analysis**, particularly in medicolegal contexts.

- In children with chromosomal abnormalities, the ectodermal patterns on the hands and fingers serve as a diagnostic tool.

DEVELOPMENT OF HAIR

- Hair develops as solid epidermal proliferations from the germinative layer that penetrates the underlying dermis obliquely forming hair bud.
- The terminal part of the hair bud becomes **club**-shaped and forms the hair bulb invaginated by the mesenchyme of the dermis, and the hair bulb now becomes **inverted cup**-shaped structure.
- The dermis within the cup-shaped hair bulb is called **dermal papilla**.
- The cells of the hair bulb at the summit of dermal papilla form the **'germinal matrix'** or the growth zone of hair that later produces the hair.
- The peripheral cells of developing hair follicle form **epithelial root sheath**. The dermis condenses around this sheath to form **dermal root sheath**.
- The cells of the germinal matrix proliferate to form **root** of the hair.
- As it grows, it is pushed outside the hair follicle on the surface of skin as a **shaft** of hair follicle by the third month of intrauterine period.
- The melanoblasts migrate into the hair bulbs and differentiate into the **melanocytes**.
- **Melanin** responsible for colour of hair is formed by these melanocytes which are transferred to proliferating cells of the germinal matrix.
- First hairs that appear are fine, soft, lightly pigmented and silky called **lanugo hairs** which are cast off at birth.
- Lanugos **(downy hairs)** are replaced by fine hairs **(vellus hair)** during the postnatal period.
- In the scalp and eyebrows, **coarser terminal hairs** replace vellus hairs.
- In axillary and pubic regions, they are replaced at puberty by even coarser terminal hair.
- The **Arrectores pilorum** muscles are derived from surface ectoderm and they extend between the hair follicles and the epidermis at an obtuse angle.
- The hair growth cycle consists of three main stages (Fig. 23.3):
  - **Anagen Phase (Growth Phase):** This is the **active phase** of hair growth. During anagen, cells in the hair follicle divide rapidly, and the hair shaft is formed. The duration of the anagen phase varies depending on the location of the hair on the body. Scalp hair, for example, has a longer anagen phase compared to eyebrows or body hair. The **majority of hair** (about 85%–90%) is in the anagen phase at any given time.
  - **Catagen Phase (Transition Phase):** The catagen phase is a **transitional phase** that marks

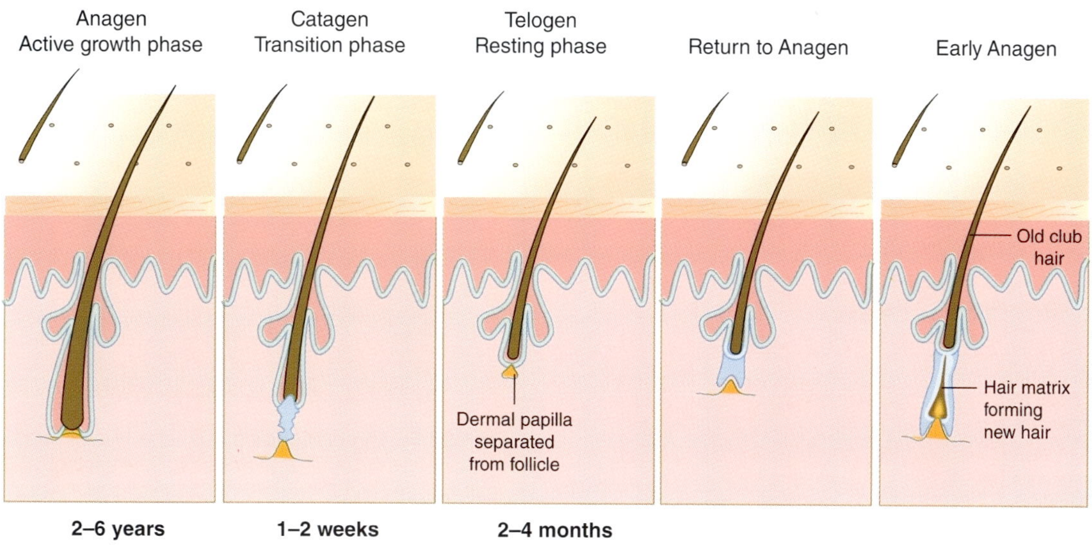

Fig. 23.3 Stages of hair growth.

the end of the active growth of a hair. It is a relatively **short phase** that lasts a few weeks. During catagen, the hair follicle shrinks, and the lower part is destroyed. This phase prepares the hair for the next stage.

- **Telogen Phase (Resting Phase):** The telogen phase is a resting phase, during which the hair is no longer actively growing. It lasts for a few months. At the end of the telogen phase, the hair follicle re-enters the anagen phase, and a new hair begins to form. About **10%–15% of hair** is in the telogen phase at any given time. After the telogen phase, the cycle repeats, and a new hair begins to grow.

DEVELOPMENT OF NAILS

- Nails develop from **Surface ectoderm** approximately at 10th week.
- At the tip of each digit, the ectoderm becomes thickened and form **primary nail field**.
- The cells in the most proximal part of nail field proliferate to form **germinal matrix** which corresponds to the **stratum lucidum** of skin (Fig. 23.4).
- Stratum corneum which first covers the surface of the nails disappears and persist as **eponychium**.
- **Hyponychium**—epidermal thickening of under surface of free border of nail.
- The developing nails shift from the tip of the digits to the dorsal surface.

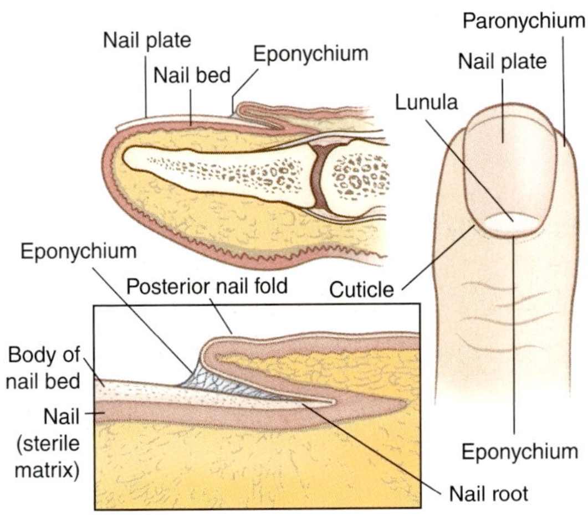

Fig. 23.4 Structure of a nail.

CLINICAL NUGGETS

Hypertrichosis

- It is a medical condition characterized by excessive hair growth on areas of the body where **terminal hair** does not normally grow. Terminal hair is the thick, long and pigmented hair that grows on the scalp, face (for men), armpits and pubic area (Fig. 23.5).
- There are two main types of hypertrichosis:
  1. **Generalized Hypertrichosis:** Excessive hair growth occurs all over the body.
  2. **Localized Hypertrichosis:** Excessive hair growth is limited to a specific area of the body.

Atrichia or atrichosis

- It refers to the absence or loss of hair, where individuals are born without hair or gradually lose their hair over time. There are different forms of atrichia, and the condition can be congenital (present at birth) or acquired (developed later in life).
  - **Congenital Atrichia:** This is a rare genetic condition in which a person is born without hair. It is often associated with other features, and different genetic mutations can lead to congenital atrichia.
  - **Acquired Atrichia:** This form of atrichia occurs when a person loses their hair later in life due to various factors such as autoimmune diseases, certain medications, infections or other underlying medical conditions.

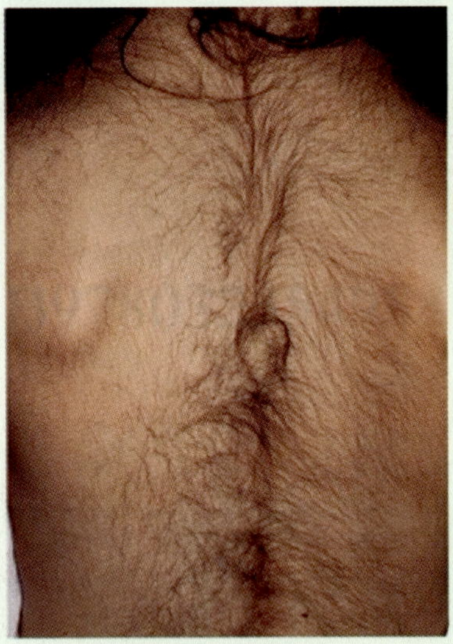

Fig. 23.5 Hypertrichosis. (Source: Paller and Mancini – Hurwitz Clinical Pediatric Dermatology: A Textbook of Skin Disorders of Childhood and Adolescence, 6th ed.: Anthony J. Mancini, Amy S. Paller, Anthony J. Mancini, Fig. 7.56, Elsevier Inc., 2022.)

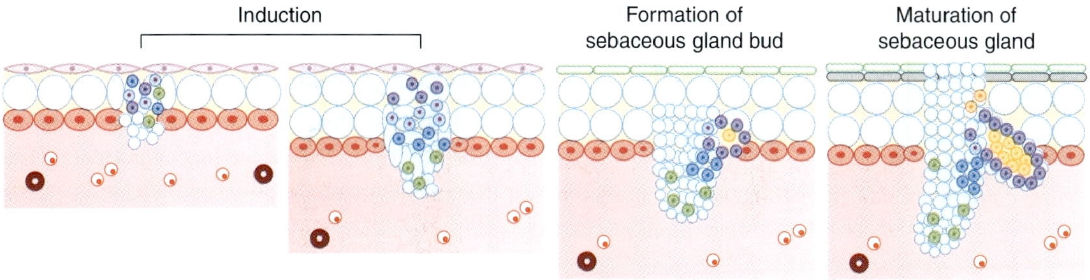

Fig. 23.6 Development of sebaceous glands.

DEVELOPMENT OF GLANDS

SEBACEOUS GLANDS

- The sebaceous gland initiates its development as a bud emerging from the epithelial root sheath of the hair follicle (Fig. 23.6).
- This bud extends into the surrounding dermis, branching into primordia that give rise to several alveoli and their associated ducts.
- Cells positioned at the centre of the alveoli undergo degeneration, producing an oily secretion known as **sebum**.
- Sebum is released into the hair follicle, creating a cavity and subsequently flows to the skin's surface.
- The sebaceous glands are classified as **holocrine glands (disintegration of the entire glandular cell in releasing its product)**, as new cells formed from the gland walls fill the cavity during the secretion process. Palms and soles lack sebaceous glands.
- Sebaceous glands are not directly supplied by nerves. Instead, the regulation of their secretions is influenced by sex hormones, underscoring their hormonal sensitivity.

SWEAT GLANDS

- There are two type of sweat (sudoriferous) glands (Fig. 23.7):
  1) **Eccrine sweat gland:**
     - ➢ Arises from a downward growth of the epidermis into the underlying dermis.
     - ➢ The downgrowth elongates, and its terminal segment coils. This solid downgrowth subsequently canalizes to form a lumen.
     - ➢ The terminal coiled part serves as the secretory section, while the proximal straight part forms the duct.
     - ➢ Eccrine sweat glands are found in the skin of most parts of the body.
     - ➢ Primarily acts as a **thermoregulator** by inducing cooling effects through the evaporation of surface secretions.
     - ➢ Innervated by **cholinergic nerves**.
  2) **Apocrine sweat glands:**
     - ➢ Develop from the same epidermal buds that form the hair follicles and hence open into the **hair follicles** (above sebaceous gland opening) instead of opening on the skin surface.

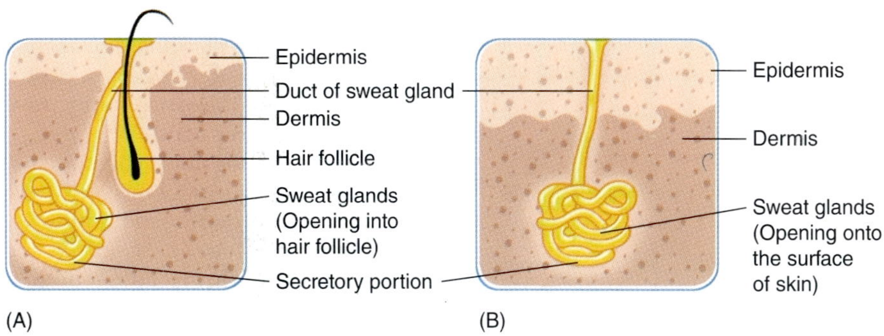

Fig. 23.7 Structure of sweat glands. (A) Apocrine. (B) Eccrine.

- Found in the axilla, pubic, perineal regions, and areolae of nipples (develop during puberty).
- Innervated by **adrenergic nerves**.
- Specialized Types: Include **Ceruminous glands** (earwax-producing) and **Mammary glands** (milk-producing).

CLINICAL NUGGETS

Waardenburg syndrome

- This syndrome is named after **P.J. Waardenburg**, a distinguished Dutch ophthalmologist.
- The primary manifestations of Waardenburg syndrome include congenital sensorineural hearing loss and pigmentary disturbances affecting the eyes, hair and skin (Fig. 23.8).
- Depending on the presence of additional symptoms, Waardenburg syndrome (WS) is categorized into four types:
  - **WS I (Type 1):**
    - Mode of Inheritance: **Autosomal dominant**.
    - Associated with facial deformities, such as dystopia canthorum (lateral displacement of the inner canthi).
  - **WS II (Type 2):**
    - Mode of Inheritance: **Autosomal dominant**.
    - Typically characterized by sensorineural hearing loss and pigmentary changes without further associated symptoms.
  - **WS III (Type 3)—Klein-Waardenburg Syndrome:**
    - Mode of Inheritance: **Autosomal dominant**.
    - Shares similarities with WS I, accompanied by musculoskeletal abnormalities, primarily affecting the upper limbs.
  - **WS IV (Type 4)—Shah-Waardenburg Syndrome:**
    - Mode of Inheritance: **Autosomal recessive**.
    - Linked with Hirschsprung disease, a condition affecting the large intestine and causing difficulties with bowel movements.

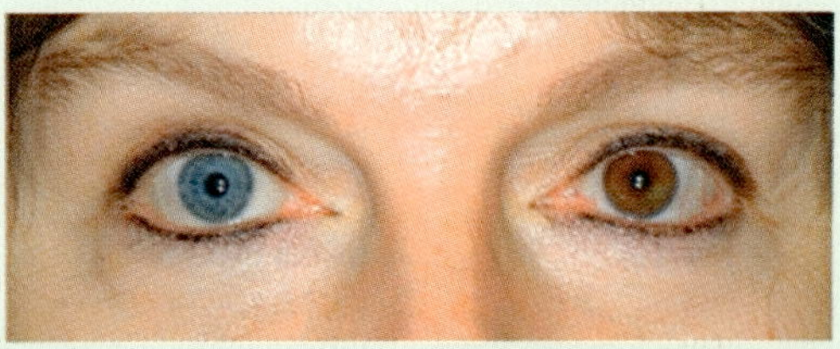

Fig. 23.8 Waardenburg syndrome. (Source: Paller and Mancini—*Hurwitz Clinical Pediatric Dermatology: A Textbook of Skin Disorders of Childhood and Adolescence*, 6th ed.: Anthony J. Mancini, Amy S. Paller, Fig. 11.22, Elsevier Inc., 2022.)

DEVELOPMENT OF MAMMARY GLANDS (AN 9.3)

- Mammary glands are modified sweat glands which develop from **Surface ectoderm** (the parenchyma—alveoli and ductules) and **underlying Mesoderm** (fibrofatty stroma).
- It appears as bilateral band of thickened epidermis called **Mammary (Schulz) lines/Mammary ridges** (Fig. 23.9A).
- Normally, mammary ridge and associated mammary buds disappear, except in the pectoral region.
- About **15–20 mammary buds** develop as solid downgrowths of the epidermis into the underlying mesenchyme along the mammary ridge on each side.
- In the pectoral region, the mammary bud presents a surface depression called **Mammary pit**.
- By the end of prenatal period, epithelial sprouts which grow inward from the pits are canalized to form **lactiferous duct** (Fig. 23.9B). Initially, lactiferous duct opens into small epithelial pit.
- The pits later evaginates due to the mesodermal growth and gets transformed as **nipples**.
- The mammary epithelium is rudimentary at birth. It consists of a few small ducts until puberty.
- With the onset of puberty, the ducts undergo morphogenesis which is influenced by **Growth hormone (GH), Oestrogen and Insulin-like growth factor-1 (IGF1)**.
- Later, short tertiary branches form under the influence of progesterone.
- **Alveologenesis** occurs during pregnancy with the induction of **Prolactin (PRL)** and **Progesterone**.
- PRL stimulation results in the stage of **lactogenesis** and milk production.
- **Human placental lactogen** (somatomammotropin) which is a placental hormone also stimulates breast to the effects of oestrogens and progesterone, thereby resulting in the synthesis of milk constituents.
- Secretion of the **milk** components (**proteins** and **fats**) occurs as follows:
  - **Apocrine**—caseins and lactose.
  - **Merocrine**—fat.
- During **weaning** involution occurs, and the mammary gland is remodelled back to its original adult state.
- **Witch's milk**—the milk expressed after birth in **newborns** (both sex) due to the action of maternal hormones.

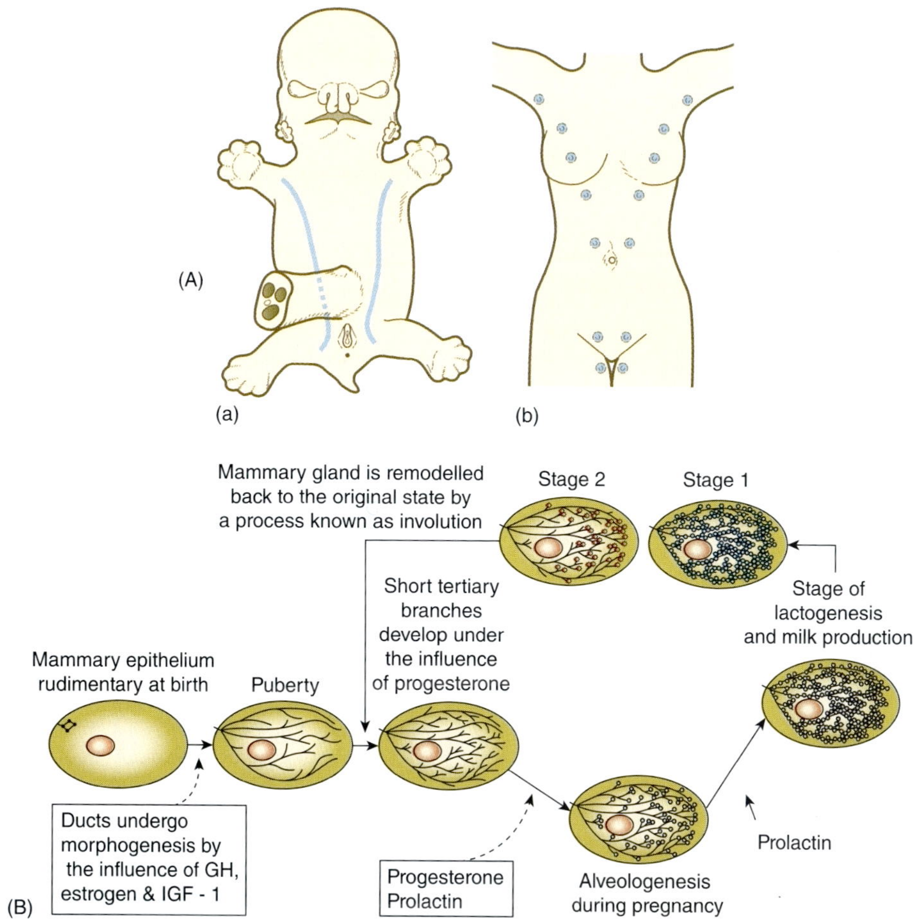

Fig. 23.9 (A) Mammary lines. (a) Milk lines *(blue)* in a generalized mammalian embryo. Mammary glands form along these lines. (b) Common formation sites for supernumerary nipples or mammary glands along the course of the milk lines in the human. (B) The stages of postnatal mammary gland development. (Source: *Human Embryology and Developmental Biology*. 4th ed. 2009.)

CLINICAL NUGGETS

Amastia

- Bilateral absence of the mammary glands.
- *Characterized by* complete absence of mammary tissue.

Polymastia

- Presence of accessory breasts.
- Manifests as the development of additional breast tissue beyond the typical mammary glands.

Gynaecomastia

- In this condition, mammary glands in adult males undergo an increase in size.
- Enlargement of breast tissue, often associated with hormonal imbalances as in **Klinefelter syndrome** or medication side effects.

KLINISCHE PERLEN

HARLEQUIN ICTHYOSIS

- Excessive keratinization of skin:
  Harlequin ichthyosis represents the most severe form of congenital ichthyosis (Fig. 23.1).
- Remarkably rare, occurring at a frequency of 1 in 300,000 births.
- Typically inherited as an **Autosomal recessive** trait.
- Abnormalities in skin function are closely tied to the malfunction of **lamellar granules** responsible for secreting lipids crucial for maintaining the skin barrier.
- As a result, massive water loss occurs between skin layers due to compromised lipid secretion.

- Neonates exhibit a distinctive hyperkeratotic '**coat of armor**' covering the entire body, marked by red fissures and skin patterning reminiscent of a **harlequin's costume**. Movement is notably restricted due to the rigid skin.
- **Complications:**
  - Respiratory insufficiency: Limited chest expansion leads to respiratory challenges.
  - Possible skeletal deformities: In some cases, skeletal abnormalities may coexist.

POLYTHELIA

- Polythelia refers to the presence of supernumerary nipples along the milk ridges (Fig. 23.10).
- The incidence varies between 0.2% and 5.6%. More frequently observed in the axilla.
- Generally, it is more commonly seen in males than females.
- Polythelia may be linked to other congenital disorders. It has been associated with urologic malformations and, in some cases, **urogenital malignancies**.

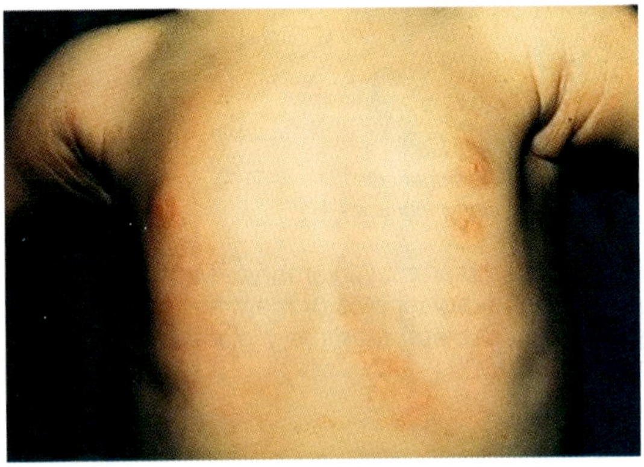

Fig. 23.10 Polythelia. (Courtesy: Dr. A.E. Chudley, Section of Genetics and Metabolism, Department of Pediatrics and Child Health, Children's Hospital and University of Manitoba, Winnipeg, Manitoba, Canada.)

POINTS TO PONDER

- **Structural Layers**
  The skin is composed of two primary layers, namely the epidermis and the dermis.
- **Epidermis Origins**
  The epidermis is derived from the surface ectoderm during embryonic development.
- **Cellular Derivatives**
  Neural crest cells contribute to the development of **Melanocytes** and **Merkel** cells, while Langerhans cells originate from bone.
- **Dermis Composition**
  The dermis is primarily a mesodermal tissue, although in the head region, it is predominantly derived from neural crest cells.
- **Epidermal Glands**
  - **Sebaceous Glands:** Responsible for secreting sebum, a lubricating substance for the skin and hair.
  - **Apocrine Glands:** Found in regions such as the axilla and pubic area, secreting odorous substances.
  - **Sweat Glands:** Contribute to temperature regulation through sweat secretion.
  - **Mammary Glands:** Specialized glands associated with lactation.
- **Nail Development**
  - **Nail Primordia:** The initial stages of nail formation occur at the distal tips of the digits. The nail plate extends from the stratum germinativum in the nail fold of the epidermis.

BRAIN TEASERS

1. What is the initial structure formed by the surface ectoderm during embryonic development?
   A. Stratum basale
   B. Stratum spinosum
   C. Stratum germinativum
   D. Stratum granulosum
2. During the second month of development, what is the name of the second layer formed by the proliferation of cells?
   A. Stratum corneum
   B. Stratum spinosum

C. Vernix caseosa
D. Periderm/epitrichium

3. Which layer of the epidermis contains irregular prickle cells (keratinocytes) with spine-like processes?
A. Stratum basale
B. Stratum spinosum
C. Stratum granulosum
D. Stratum lucidum

4. What is the function of the Vernix caseosa in foetal development?
A. Provides nutrients to the foetus.
B. Protects against UV radiation.
C. Acts as a thermal insulator.
D. Protects against the macerating effects of amniotic fluid.

5. Which cells in the basal layer of the epidermis are derived from neural crest cells?
A. Melanoblasts
B. Keratinocytes
C. Merkel cells
D. Langerhans cells

6. What are the two layers of the dermis?
A. Papillary layer and reticular layer
B. Stratum basale and stratum spinosum
C. Stratum granulosum and stratum lucidum
D. Epidermis and dermis

7. What influences the development of epidermal ridges and dermal papillae, contributing to unique fingerprint patterns in individuals?
A. Genetic factors only
B. Uterine environment
C. Hormonal factors
D. Both A and B

8. What medical application uses the uniqueness of epidermal ridge patterns for personal identification?
A. DNA analysis
B. Fingerprint analysis
C. Blood typing
D. X-ray imaging

9. What is the name of the homogenous layer superficial to the granular layer in the epidermis?
A. Stratum lucidum
B. Stratum corneum
C. Stratum granulosum
D. Stratum spinosum

10. Which cells in the basal layer constantly divide mitotically and move superficially to renew the epidermis?
A. Melanoblasts
B. Langerhans cells
C. Merkel cells
D. Basal columnar cells

Answers

1. (C); 2. (D); 3. (B); 4. (D); 5. (A); 6. (A); 7. (D); 8. (B); 9. (A); 10. (D).

FURTHER READINGS

Farrer LA, Grundfast KM, Amos J, et al. Waardenburg syndrome (WS) type I is caused by defects at multiple loci, one of which is near ALPP on chromosome 2: first report of the WS consortium. *Am J Hum Genet.* 1992;50(5):902-913.

Fonseca GM, Cantín M. Familial polythelia associated with dental anomalies: a case report. *Colomb Med.* 2014;45(1):45-47.

Halleland HH, Balling E, Tei T, Arcieri S, Mertz H, Mele M. Polythelia in a 13-year old girl. *G Chir.* 2017;38(3):143-146.doi:10.11138/gchir/2017.38.3.143.

Kim MR, Oji V, Valentin F, et al. Vitamin D status in distinct types of ichthyosis: importance of genetic type and severity of scaling. *Acta Derm Venereol.* 2021;101(9):adv00546.doi:10.2340/00015555-3887.

Prasad P, Bennett A, Speirs V, Shaaban AM. Morphological features and immunohistochemical profiling of male breast gynaecomastia; a large tissue microarray study. *Front Oncol.* 2022;12:875839. doi:10.3389/fonc.2022.875839.

24 Skeletal System

AN 13.8 Describe the development of upper limb.
AN 20.10 Describe the basic concept of development of lower limb.

ANAMNESE

A 14-year-old boy was referred to the paediatric clinic when his parents noticed that he was unusually tall and lanky for his age, with disproportionately long limbs and fingers. Physical examination revealed classic features of **Marfan syndrome**, including a tall stature, arachnodactyly (long, slender fingers) and a high-arched palate. Further evaluation, including echocardiography, confirmed the presence of Aortic root dilation, a common cardiovascular manifestation of Marfan syndrome. Genetic testing subsequently confirmed a mutation in the **FBN1 gene**, confirming the diagnosis.

The skeletal system originates from the mesodermal germ layer and neural crest during embryonic development. Bone formation occurs through two distinct processes. In the axial skeleton, which includes the vertebral column and ribs, as well as the appendicular skeleton comprising the limbs, a cartilage model serves as the initial framework, which is eventually replaced by bone through a process known as **endochondral ossification**. In contrast, the bones of the skull form directly from mesenchymal cells through **intramembranous ossification**. The skeletal system is a dynamic structure where the ongoing processes of bone deposition and resorption continuously reshape and maintain bone size, shape and integrity. Imbalances in this dynamic equilibrium can lead to conditions such as osteoporosis, arthritis and various hereditary skeletal disorders.

- The skeletal system is categorized into two parts:
  - **Axial skeleton**—vertebral column, ribs, sternum and skull.
  - **Appendicular skeleton**—pectoral and pelvic girdles and limb bones.

AXIAL SKELETON

VERTEBRAL COLUMN

- The vertebral column consists of 33 vertebrae categorized into 5 regions: 7 cervical, 12 thoracic, 5 lumbar, 5 sacral and 4 coccygeal.
- The different stages of vertebral development are:
  - **Blastemal or membranous.**
  - **Cartilaginous.**
  - **Bony.**
- The **Somites** developed from the paraxial mesoderm is composed of sclerotome and dermomyotome.
- By the fourth week of embryonic development, cells from the sclerotome migrate medially around the notochord and contribute to the formation of the **centrum** of the blastemal vertebra (Fig. 24.1).
- Sclerotome cells extend dorsally, forming **neural arches** that converge at the midline to shape rudimentary spines.
- Each neural arch generates **costal elements** near the centrum and extends laterally through the myotomes.

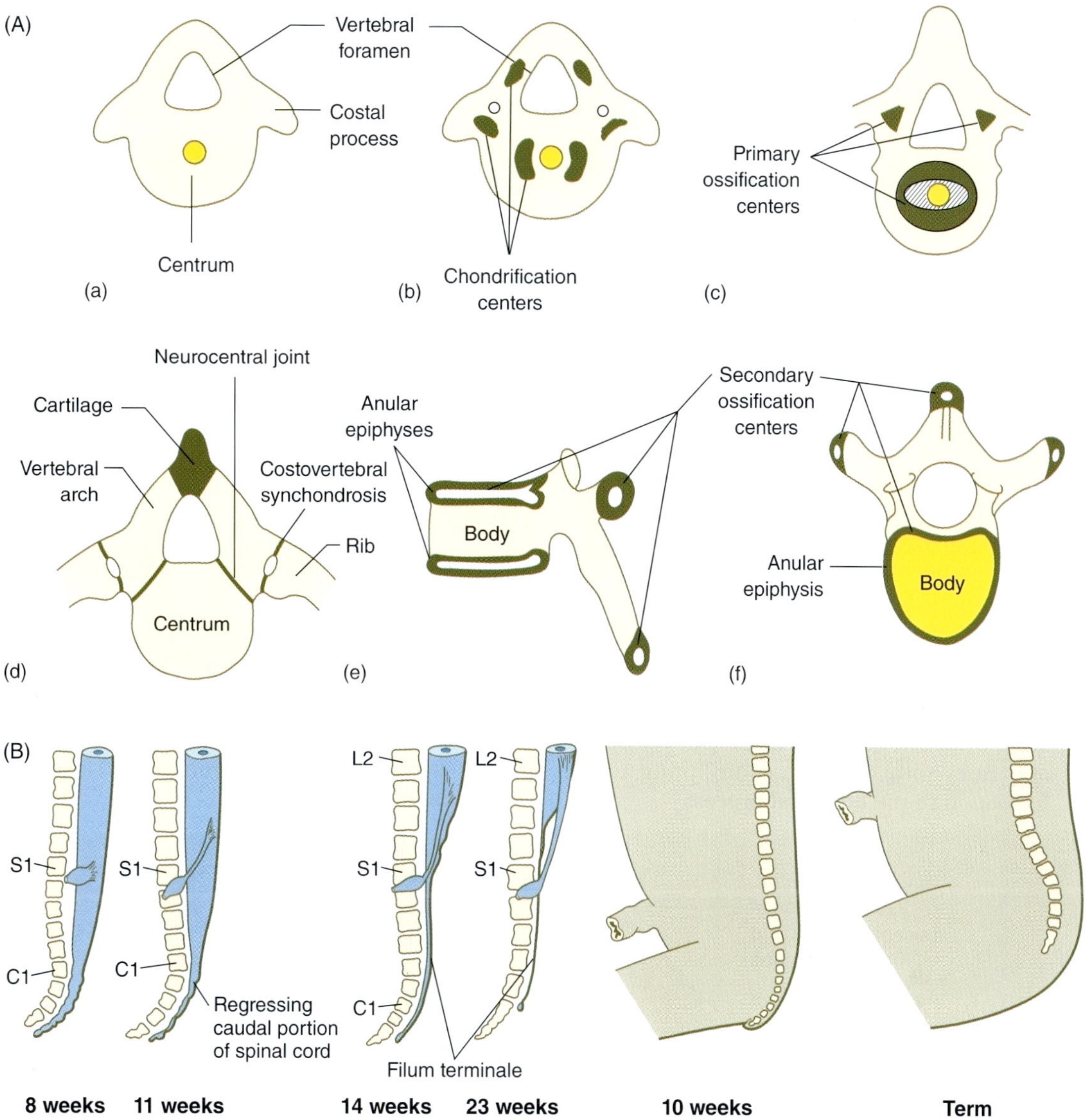

Fig. 24.1 Development of vertebra. (A) Drawings illustrating the stages of vertebral development. (a) Mesenchymal vertebra at 5 weeks. (b) Chondrification centres in a mesenchymal vertebra at 6 weeks. (c) Primary ossification centres in a cartilaginous vertebra at 7 weeks. (d) A thoracic vertebra at birth consisting of three bony parts. Note the cartilage between the halves of the vertebral arch and between the arch and the centrum (the neurocentral joint). (e and f) Two views of a typical thoracic vertebra at puberty, showing the location of the secondary centres of ossification. (B) Changes in the level of the end of the spinal cord in relation to bony landmarks in the vertebral column during foetal development and development of the curvature of the spine. (Source: (A) From Moore KL. *The Developing Human: Clinically Oriented Embryology*. 4th ed. Philadelphia: Saunders, 1988:339; *Caffey's Pediatric Diagnostic Imaging*. 11th ed. 2008; (B) *Human Embryology and Developmental Biology.* 4th ed. 2009.)

- Segments of the sclerotome are divided into cranial and caudal parts by a horizontal **sclerotomic fissure**.
- The definitive centrum forms through the fusion of the caudal part of one segment with the cranial part of the succeeding segment (**intersegmental development**) (Fig. 24.2).
- The sclerotomic fissure and surrounding mesoderm give rise to the **perichordal disc**, which persists into adulthood as the **intervertebral disc**.
- Notochordal cells in the disc centre become the **Nucleus pulposus**, while the surrounding perichordal mesenchyme forms the **Annulus fibrosus**.
- **Chondrification** commences in the blastemal vertebra around the sixth week, with centres appearing in the centrum and neural arch.
- **Ossification** starts in the cartilaginous vertebrae around the seventh week, involving three primary centres and five secondary centres (Fig. 24.1).
- In the upper three cervical vertebrae, the costal elements initially fuse but subsequently degenerate, except in the first cervical vertebra, where they persist as the **hypochordal bow**.
- The hypochordal bow eventually undergoes ossification to form the **anterior arch** of the atlas, while the centrum of the atlas separates and fuses with the axis, contributing to the formation of the **odontoid process**.

CERVICAL VERTEBRAE

- In cervical vertebra, the costal element and transverse element fuse to form **Foramen Transversarium**.
- The components of **costal element** are:
  - **Anterior root.**
  - **Anterior tubercle.**
  - **Costotransverse bar.**
  - **Posterior tubercle.**
- **True transverse element**—posterior root.
- **Cervical rib**—bony spicule from the anterior root of **seventh cervical transverse process** (1%). Effects of compression on brachial plexus and subclavian artery are usually seen associated with this condition.

LUMBAR VERTEBRAE

- Transverse process are derived from costal elements.
- True transverse elements form **Mammillary** and **Accessory tubercles**.

SACRAL VERTEBRAE

- Costal and transverse elements fuse to form the **lateral mass**.

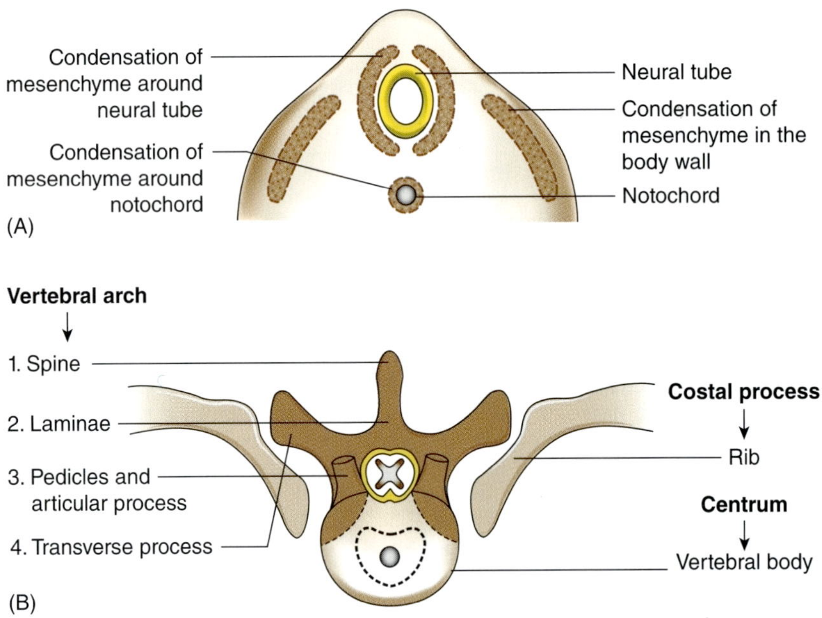

Fig. 24.2 Development of thoracic vertebra.

- Anterior two-thirds of lateral mass is from **costal element**.
- Posterior one-third of lateral mass is from **transverse element**.

THORACIC VERTEBRAE

- Costal elements independently grow to form **ribs** (Fig. 24.2).

DEVELOPMENT OF RIBS

- **Costal elements** of thoracic vertebra independently grow to form ribs.
- As they grow through myotomes of the body wall, they form **costal arches** which are completely chondrified.
- Ventral end of upper seven arches unite on each side to form a **cartilaginous sternal plate** which fuses in the midline to form rudiment of the sternum.
- A typical rib has a **primary centre** at the **posterior angle** (seventh week) and three **secondary centres** (head—1, tubercles—2).
- At **birth**, the ventral part of costal arch remains cartilaginous and persist throughout life.
- After **second year**, the vertebral end of upper ribs migrates cranially crossing the boundary of vertebra above and hence the rib articulates with the corresponding vertebra and vertebra above it.

THE STERNUM

- Two longitudinal cartilaginous plates fuse to form sternum (Fig. 24.3).
- It occurs in craniocaudal direction (**manubrium** (one ossification centre), **body** (four ossification centres) and **xiphoid process** (one ossification centre)).

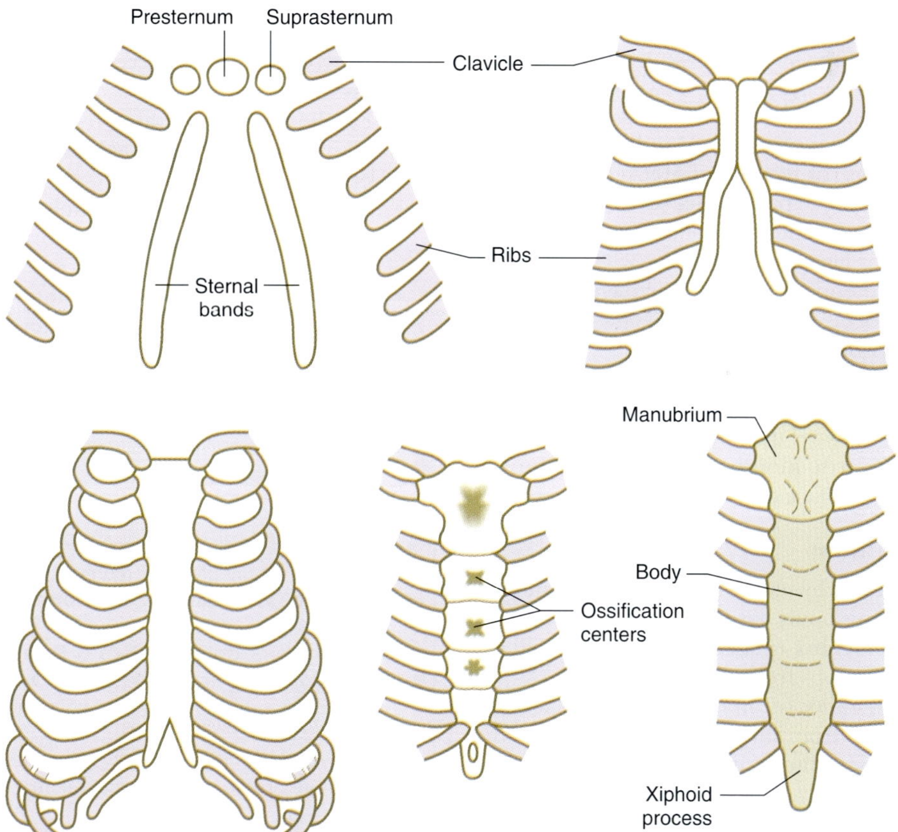

Fig. 24.3 Successive stages in the development of the sternum. (Source: *Human Embryology and Developmental Biology*. 6th ed. 2019.)

- Fusion is completed by **ninth week** and ossification completed by **ninth month** except for xiphoid process.
- Xiphoid process is ossified during second or third year after birth.
- The segments forming the body of sternum are known as **Sternebrae** (four in number).
- **Sternal foramen:** This anatomical variation occurs between the third and fourth sternebrae and results from the incomplete fusion of sternal plates.

THE SKULL

- It has two parts:
  - **Viscerocranium** (skeleton of face).
  - **Neurocranium** (case around brain).

Viscerocranium

Facial skeleton is derived from the cartilaginous plates of first arch and dorsal part of second arch.

- **First arch (Meckel's cartilage):**
  - **Maxillary process**—Maxilla, zygomatic bone and part of temporal bone.
  - **Mandibular process**—Mandible (intramembranous ossification of Meckel's cartilage).
  - Intermediate part of **Meckel's cartilage** forms anterior ligament of Malleus and sphenomandibular ligament.
  - Dorsal end of **Meckel's cartilage** (mandibular) forms malleus and dorsal end of maxillary process forms **Incus**.
- **Second arch (Reichert's cartilage):**
  - Dorsal end of the second arch forms **Stapes**.
- Ear ossicles are the **first** bones to completely ossify (fourth month). Mesenchyme for the bones of the face comes from **neural crest cells**.

Neurocranium

- The mesenchymal condensation around the developing brain has two parts:
  - **Endomeninx** (pia mater and arachnoid mater develops from this part).
  - **Ectomeninx** (dura mater and cranial bones develop from this layer).
- According to the ossification they are classified as follows:
  - Bones forming **base of the Skull** (cartilaginous part/chondrocranium).
  - Bones forming **Cranial vault** (membranous part/flat/dermal bones).
  - Some are formed partly in cartilage and partly in membrane.
- **Chondrocranium:**
  - **Prechordal**—which lies in front of notochord is derived from **Neural crest cells**.
  - **Chordal**—which lies posterior to prechordal is derived from **Occipital myotomes** (paraxial mesoderm).
  - These cartilages undergo **endochondral ossification** and fuse to form base of the skull.
  - Ossification of chondrocranium starts in foetal life and is completed after puberty.
  - The cartilaginous plate remaining between basiocciput and sphenoid bone disappears by **25th year** by bony fusion.
- **Membranous neurocranium:**
  - The bones covering the vault and side wall of skull are ossified in membrane (frontal bone with orbital plates, parietal bone, squamous part of temporal and part of occipital bone lying between parietal bones).
  - Derived from **neural crest cells** and **paraxial mesoderm**.
  - Flat bones are separated by **coronal** (paraxial mesoderm) and **sagittal** (neural crest cells) sutures.
  - Sutures are wide at fontanelles which are nothing but unossified membranes (more than two bones meet).
  - There are **six fontanelles**—anterior, posterior, 2 anterolateral and 2 posterolateral.
  - Anterior fontanelle closes by **18 months**.
  - Posterior fontanelle closes by **1–2 months**.

CLINICAL NUGGETS

Craniosynostosis

- Craniosynostosis is a condition characterized by the premature closure of one or more cranial sutures.
- This process is regulated by **Transforming Growth Factor beta**.
- An example of craniosynostosis is **Scaphocephaly** (Fig. 24.4), which involves the premature closure of the sagittal suture, resulting in an elongated and narrow skull.
- **Brachycephaly** is another type, caused by the premature closure of the coronal sutures, leading to a short skull.
- **Plagiocephaly** is characterized by the premature closure of the coronal suture on one side, causing the skull to appear flattened and asymmetric.

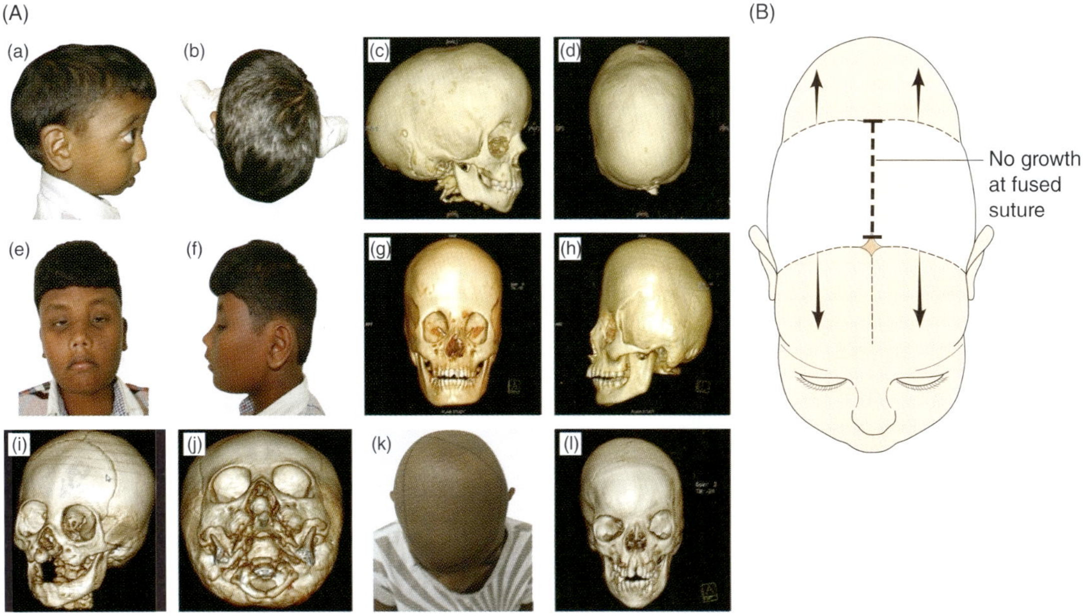

Fig. 24.4 Craniosynostosis. (A) (a-d) Scaphocephaly-premature sagittal synostosis. (e-h) Turricephaly-tower head deformity-premature synostosis of bicoronal with other sutures. (i, j) Trigonocephaly-premature metopic suture synostosis. (k) Plagiocephaly showing flattened left forehead. (l) Premature fusion of left coronal suture. (B) Sagittal suture craniosynostosis. The sagittal suture is prematurely fused (*broken line*). Growth normally occurs perpendicular to the suture line. In this case, the skull cannot widen, as there is no growth at the fused suture, which may be palpable as a ridge in the midline. There is compensatory growth at the coronal and lambdoid sutures, leading to an elongated head shape (scaphocephaly), with bulging of the forehead (frontal bossing) in severe cases. (Source: Part A, *Textbook of Oral and Maxillofacial Surgery*. 3rd ed. 2017; Part B, *Principles and Practice of Surgery*, 5th ed. 2007.)

APPENDICULAR SKELETON

(AN 13.8; AN 20.10)

- It consists of pectoral girdle, pelvic girdle and the limbs.
- By the fourth week, limb buds will be visible (Fig. 24.5).
- Upper limb appears (at **24 days** opposite to fourth cervical to second thoracic somites) first followed by lower limb (at **28 days** opposite to lumbo sacral somites).
- Each limb bud consists of:
  - Core of **Mesenchyme** from parietal layer of lateral plate mesoderm (bones and connective tissue).
  - **Ectoderm** (cuboidal layer).
- As the limb grows, three axes will be established:
  - **Anteroposterior:**
    - Runs from thumb to little finger.
    - A small area known as **Zone of Polarizing Activity (ZPA)** located at the base of posterior limb is responsible for polarization along the anteroposterior axis.
  - **Dorsoventral:**
    - Runs from dorsum to palm of the hand.
    - It is regulated by **non-Apical ectodermal ridge** (AER) ectoderm.
  - **Proximodistal:**
    - Extends from trunk to the tip of the digits.
- The bones of the limb develop in the following sequence:
  - **Pectoral/pelvic girdle.**
  - **Upper arm/thigh bones.**
  - **Forearm/leg bones.**
  - **Bones of hand and foot.**
- It is controlled by the **AER**-thickening of ectoderm at the distal end of the limb (Fig. 24.6). AER induce the proliferation of mesenchyme.
- The proliferating cells as they move away from AER differentiates to form muscle and cartilage.
- Distal end broadens to form:
  - **Hand plate.**
  - **Foot plate.**

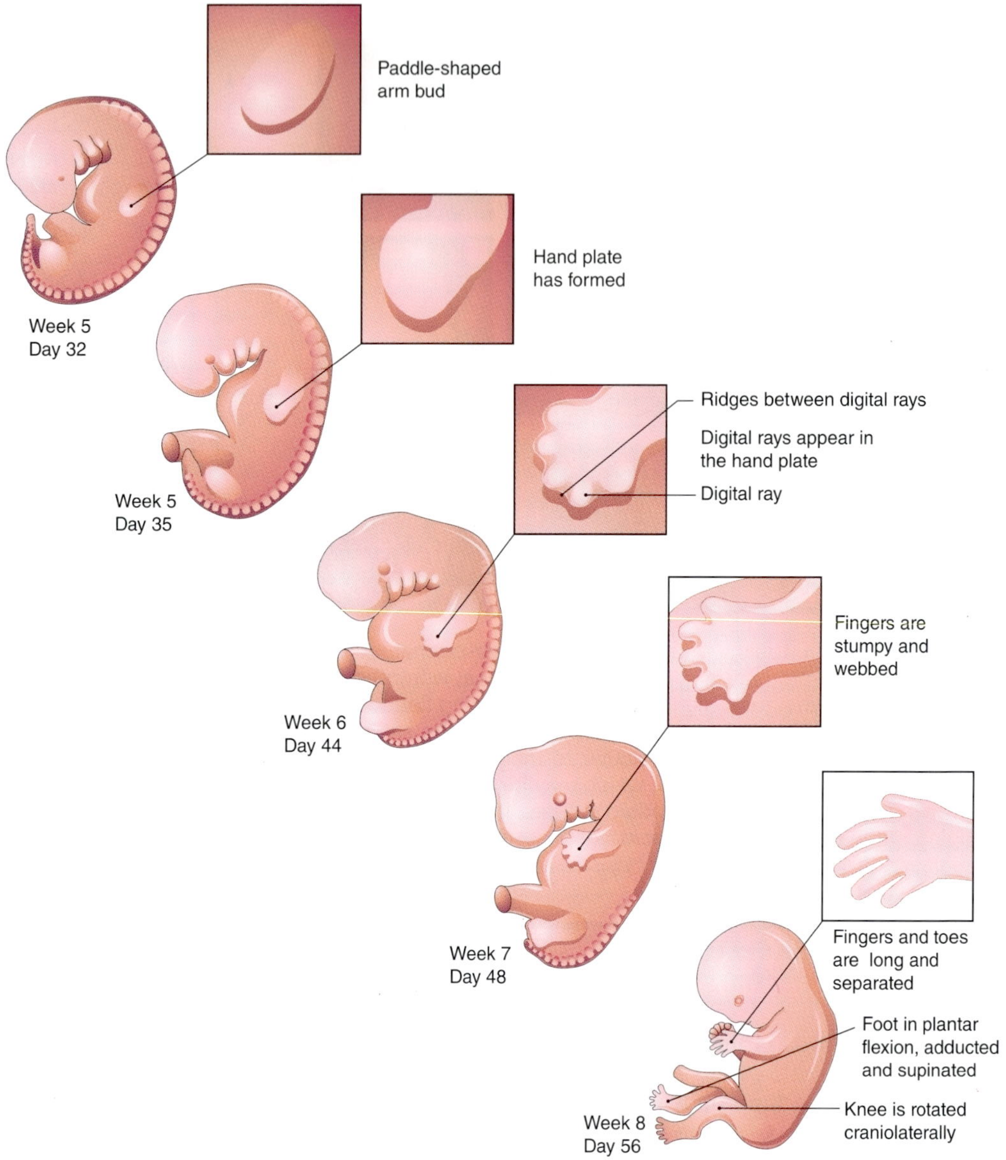

Fig. 24.5 Formation of limb buds. Development of the extremities in week 5-8; schematic illustration. The extremities begin to develop in week 4. The fin-like arm bud develops on day 26-27, thus two days prior to the development of the leg bud. At this point in time, the primordial extremities consist of a mesenchymal core of connective tissue deriving from the mesodermal somatopleura and of an encasing surface ectoderm which later forms the epidermal layer of the skin. Ectoderm of the distal edge of the limb bud (ectodermal ridge) expresses growth factors which attract muscle cell precursors from somites of the mesoderm of the trunk area. In week 5-6, the limb buds display a spatial pattern formation in the primordial arms and legs. Beginning in week 6, digital rays are forming through programmed cell death (apoptosis) in the interpositioned tissue. The fingers and toes are completely separated by the end of week 8. In contrast to the arm anlage, the primordial legs rotate laterally during week 8 resulting in the knee to be oriented in a craniolateral position. As a consequence of this rotation, the extensor muscles of the leg are in a ventral position, in contrast to the dorsal position of the extensor muscles in the arm. Furthermore, at week 8 the foot is positioned in plantar flexion, adduction, and supination. This position is reversed until week 11. (Source: Moore: *The Developing Human*, 11th ed. 2020.)

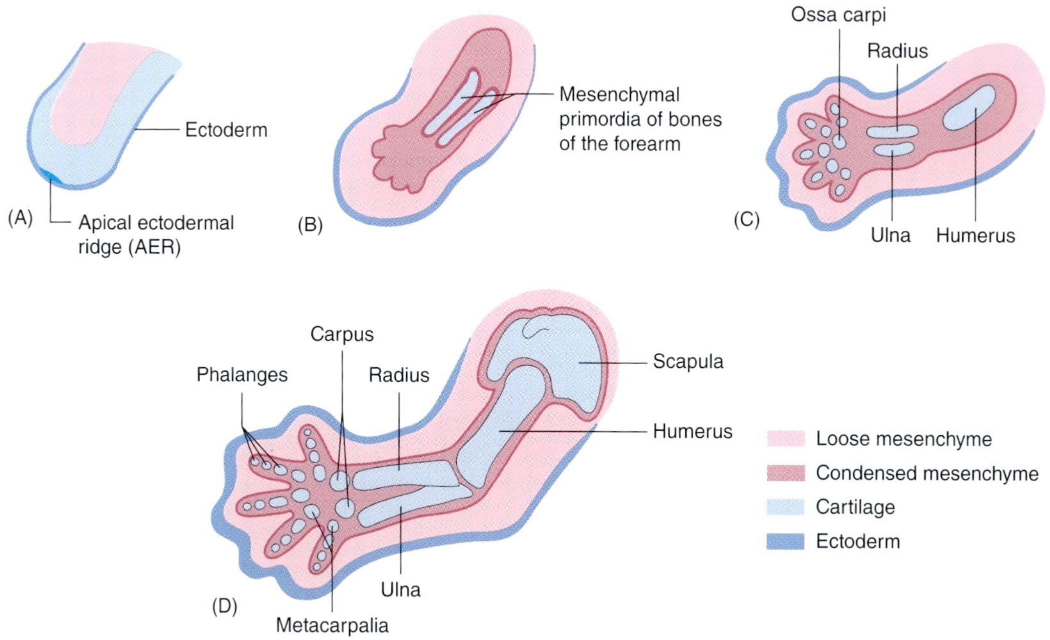

Fig. 24.6 Formation of bones in the extremities. Development of the cartilaginous precursors of the bones of the upper extremities in weeks 4-8; schematic longitudinal sections. In week 4 the primordial limbs consist of a connective tissue (mesenchymal) core and a sheath of surface ectoderm which later forms the epidermis of the skin. Condensation of the mesenchyme results in formation of a cartilaginous skeleton during weeks 4-6 in the arm and weeks 6-8 in the leg. The cartilaginous skeleton serves as precursor for the formation of bones at a later point in time. This process advances from proximal to distal. Within this cartilaginous skeleton primary ossification centres begin to establish in week 7 which initiates the restructuring of the cartilage into bones (endochondral ossification). Ossification progresses according to a specific pattern. At week 12, ossification centres are present in all bones of the upper limb except for the carpus. Ossification centres of the carpus only form postnatally between 1 and 8 years of age. As an exception, ossification of the clavicle proceeds directly from the mesenchyme (desmal ossification). Ossification in the lower extremity occurs with delay. Ossification centres in the femur are present already at the 6th month, but ossification of the phalanges occurs only between the 5th and 9th month. Ossification of the tarsus and the pelvic girdle occurs during the first to fourth year of age and up to the 20th year of age, respectively. Closure of the epiphyseal plates with resulting cessation of the longitudinal growth of the extremities takes place between years 14 and 25, for most of the bones before year 21. (Source: Moore: *The Developing Human*, 11th ed. 2020.)

- These plates are separated from the main bud by a constriction.
- The main bud is further divided into two segments by a second constriction.
- AER is divided into **five segments** by the programmed cell death of certain regions of the ridge.
- Cartilaginous **digital rays** in each segment form the digits.
- Each limb bud projects laterally at right angles from the trunk with a **preaxial** and **postaxial border**.
- **Rotation of limbs** (seventh week):
  - Upper limb rotates **laterally** (90 degrees).
  - Lower limb rotates **medially** (90 degrees).
- As a result of rotation, thumb lies laterally and big toe lies medially.
- At first mesenchymal condensation occurs, then a cartilaginous model is laid down by sixth week followed by ossification.
- **Endochondral ossification** of hyaline cartilaginous models starts by eighth week.
- All long bones of the body will have **primary** ossification centre by the end of **3 months**.

Primary centres for **carpal bones, navicular** and **cuneiform** develop **after birth**.
- Epiphysis remains cartilaginous even after birth. The **epiphyseal plate** lying between the epiphysis and diaphysis determines the length of the bone.
- Long bones have **two** epiphyseal plates and short bones (phalanges) have **one** epiphyseal plate.
- **Secondary ossification** centres appear after birth except lower epiphysis of femur and upper epiphysis of tibia (appear by ninth month of foetal life).
- All limb bones develop in cartilage except **clavicle** which is ossified in membrane during fifth and sixth week, and it is the first bone to ossify in the body.
- **Interzone** is the region lying between the ends of two cartilaginous models and they develop cleft-like spaces, which later coalesce to form **synovial joint** during the third month of intra-uterine life.
- The **mesenchyme** of the interzone differentiates into:
  - **Articular cartilage.**
  - **Synovial membrane.**
  - **Menisci.**
  - **Ligaments.**
  - **Fibrous joints** (Fig. 24.7).
- The mesenchymal cells around the interzone forms the **joint capsule**.
- The muscles of the limb are derived from the somites which migrate into the limb buds during fifth week. The muscle mass is arranged as **ventral** (flexors and pronators of upper limb and flexors and adductors of lower limb) and **dorsal mass** (extensors and supinators of upper limb and extensors and abductors of lower limb).
- The ventral mass is supplied by ventral branches of ventral primary rami and dorsal mass is supplied by dorsal branches of **ventral rami**.
- The **motor axons** form plexus (brachial and lumbar) at the base of the limb buds

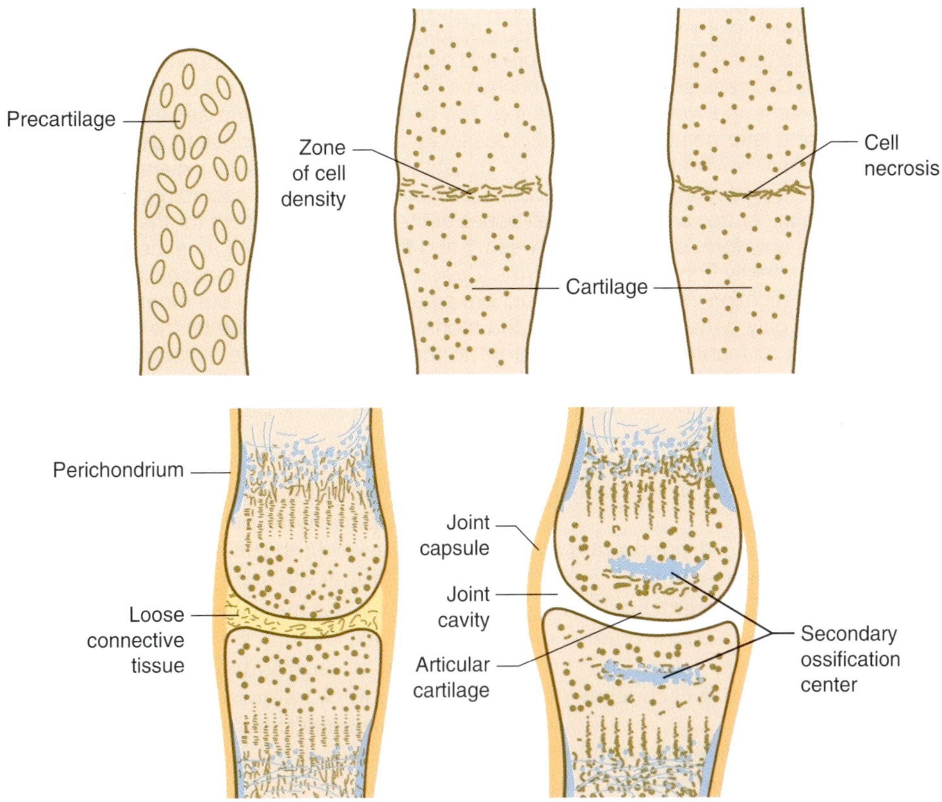

Fig. 24.7 Formation of joints. Sequence of the formation of the joints in the limbs. (Source: *Human Embryology and Developmental Biology*. 4th ed. 2009.)

(decision-making regions for the axons). The axons from these plexus follow the growth pathway of limb bud to reach their target muscle. Later the sensory fibres grow along the motor axons.
- The connective tissue for the muscle is derived from **lateral plate mesoderm**.

CLINICAL NUGGETS

- **HOX genes** play a pivotal role in specifying the segmental origins of limb buds:
  - The upper limb buds originate from segmental levels C5–T2.
  - The lower limb buds have their beginnings at segmental levels L2 to S2 (Fig. 24.8).
- The **Apical Ectodermal Ridge (AER)** secretes Fibroblast Growth Factors (FGFs) to regulate growth in the proximal-distal direction.
- Patterning and growth along the anteroposterior axis are governed by the **Zone of Polarizing Activity (ZPA)**, located at the posterior border of the limb bud, which releases **Sonic Hedgehog (SHH)**.

KLINISCHE PERLEN

CRANIOSCHISIS

- Cranioschisis is a rare congenital condition characterized by the incomplete closure of the cranial bones (cranial vault is not formed due to failure of closure of **cranial neuropore**), resulting in an opening or defect in the skull. Brain degenerates since exposed to amniotic fluid and results in **Anencephaly**.
- Some of the genes associated with cranial development include **HOX** genes, **BMP** genes and **SHH** genes, which play roles in the patterning and growth of cranial structures. Mutations or dysregulation of these genes can disrupt the normal development of the cranial bones and potentially lead to cranioschisis.

ACHONDROPLASIA

- Achondroplasia is the **most common** form of skeletal dysplasia and results in disproportionately short stature and several distinct physical features.
- Individuals with achondroplasia have shorter arms and legs compared to their trunk, resulting in a characteristic dwarfed appearance. They often have a relatively **large head** with a prominent forehead.
- The fingers and toes may be short and stubby, often described as **'trident hands'** due to the spacing between the middle and ring fingers.
- It can lead to spinal abnormalities, including a narrowed spinal canal and compression of the spinal cord.
- The genetic basis of achondroplasia involves mutations in the **FGFR3** (fibroblast growth factor receptor) gene. This **autosomal dominant** genetic mutation is typically sporadic, meaning it occurs as a new mutation rather than being inherited from parents.

THANATOPHORIC DYSPLASIA

- Thanatophoric dysplasia is a **lethal** and most common form of neonatal skeletal dysplasia. It primarily involves mutations in the **FGFR3** (fibroblast growth factor receptor) gene. Both **Type 1** and **Type 2** are inherited as **autosomal dominant**.
- Foetuses with thanatophoric dysplasia have extremely short arms and legs, often described as **'micromelia'**. This shortening is a hallmark feature of the condition.
- The chest and thoracic cavity are abnormally narrow, which can lead to respiratory difficulties and may be life-threatening.
- Thanatophoric dysplasia may result in skull abnormalities, including a prominent forehead, a **cloverleaf-shaped skull** (**Kleeblattschaedel deformity**—all sutures closed prematurely and brain grows through fontanelle) and an overall reduction in the size of the skull.

PFEIFFER'S SYNDROME

- Pfeiffer's syndrome is a rare genetic disorder characterized by **craniosynostosis**, resulting in a cloverleaf-shaped skull.
- Individuals with Pfeiffer's syndrome typically exhibit broad great toes and thumbs, as well as an underdeveloped facial appearance.
- This condition is associated with mutations in the **FGFR1 gene**, which plays a crucial role in normal cranial development and bone growth.

APERT'S SYNDROME

- Apert's syndrome is a rare genetic condition characterized by **craniosynostosis**, leading to an underdeveloped facial appearance.
- It is often associated with symmetrical **syndactyly**, where the hands and feet exhibit fused digits.
- This condition is primarily linked to mutations in the **FGFR2** gene.

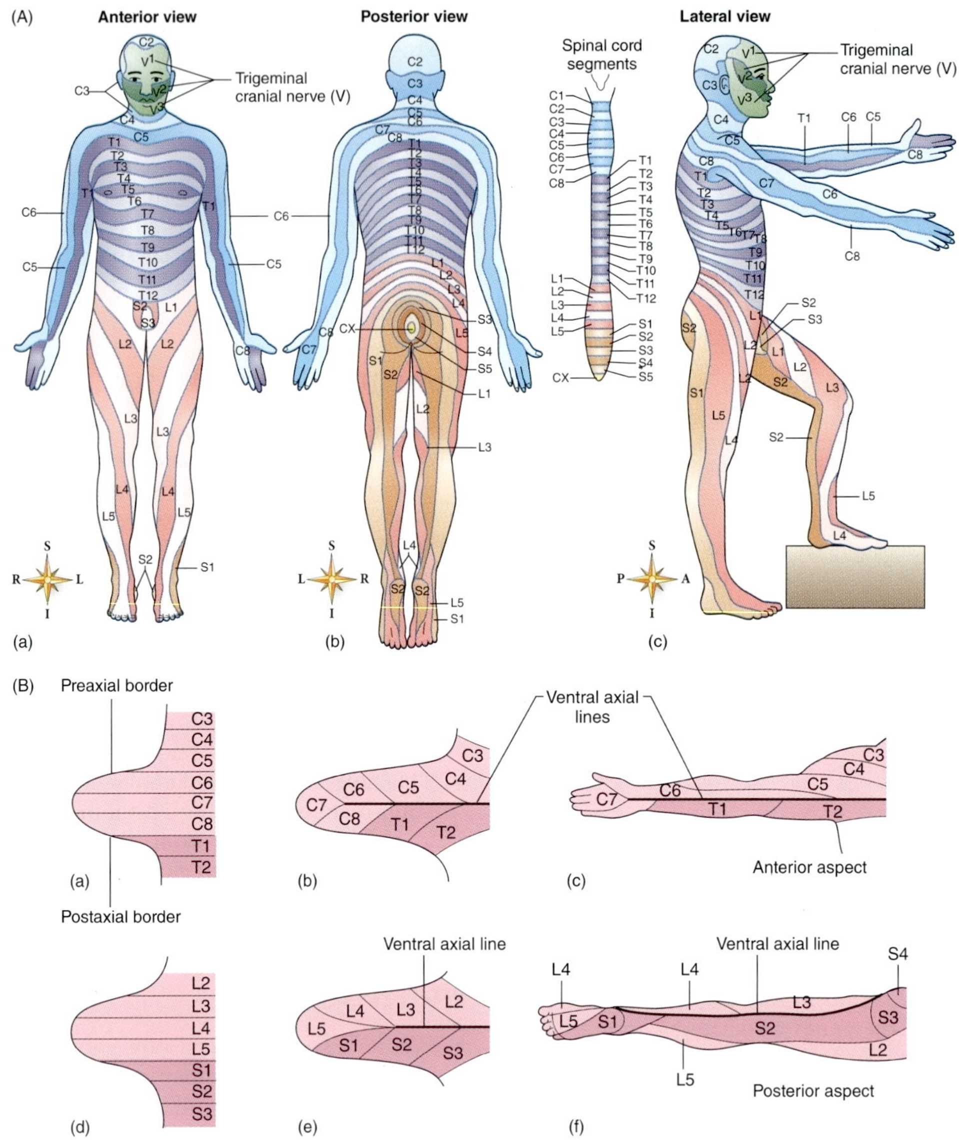

Fig. 24.8 Arrangements of dermatomes in upper limb and lower limb. (A) Dermatome distribution of spinal nerves. (a) The front of the body's surface. (b) The back of the body's surface. (c) The side of the body's surface. The inset shows the segments of the spinal cord connected with each of the spinal nerves associated with the sensory dermatomes shown. *C*, Cervical segments and spinal nerves; *T*, thoracic segments and spinal nerves; *L*, lumbar segments and spinal nerves; *S*, sacral segments and spinal nerves. (B) Development of the dermatomal patterns of the limbs. The *axial lines* indicate where there is no sensory overlap. (a and d) Ventral aspect of the limb buds early in the fifth week. At this stage, the dermatomal patterns show the primordial segmental arrangement. (b and e) Similar views later in the fifth week showing the modified arrangement of dermatomes. (c and f) The dermatomal patterns in the adult upper and lower limbs. The primordial dermatomal pattern has disappeared, but an orderly sequence of dermatomes can still be recognized. In (f) note that most of the original ventral surface of the lower limb lies on the back of the adult limb. This results from the medial rotation of the lower limb that occurs toward the end of the embryonic period. In the upper limb, the ventral axial line extends along the anterior surface of the arm and forearm. In the lower limb, the ventral axial line extends along the medial side of the thigh and knee, to the posteromedial aspect of the leg to the heel. (Source: Part A. *Anatomy & Physiology*, 7th ed. 2010. Part B, *Before We Are Born: Essentials of Embryology and Birth Defects*. 1st South Asia ed. 2016.)

CLEIDOCRANIAL DYSOSTOSIS

- Individuals with cleidocranial dysostosis typically have underdeveloped or **missing clavicles**, late closure of the fontanelle and generalized bone and dental tissue dysplasia.

ACROMEGALY

- Acromegaly is a congenital condition that results from hyperpituitarism, causing increased levels of **Growth hormone**.
- This overproduction of growth hormone leads to the enlargement of facial features, hands and feet, often in a disproportionate manner.

MARFAN SYNDROME

- Marfan syndrome is an autosomal dominant disorder primarily associated with mutations in the **FBN1** gene.
- This condition leads to characteristics such as long limbs and face, high-arched palate, lens dislocation, abnormal joint flexibility, aortic dissection and variations in chest wall shape (**Pectus carinatum/excavatum**).

OSTEOPETROSIS

- Osteopetrosis, also known as '**stone bone**' or '**marble bone**' disease, results in increased bone density and brittleness (Fig. 24.9).
- This condition can cause stunted growth, frequent fractures and a thinning or absence of the medullary cavity, leading to bone marrow failure.

POINTS TO PONDER

- Bone development commences within the mesenchymal regions of the embryo during the fourth week of gestation.
- Two distinct modes of bone formation are observed:
  - **Endochondral Ossification:** This process involves the initial formation of a cartilage model, which is subsequently replaced by bone. It predominantly contributes to the formation of the **axial skeleton** consisting of the vertebral column and ribs, as well as the **appendicular skeleton** (limbs), excluding the clavicle.
  - **Intramembranous Ossification:** In this mode of bone formation, bone directly arises from mesenchymal cells without preceding cartilage formation. It plays a critical role in shaping most **facial** and **cranial** bones.
- Three types of cells are involved in endochondral bone formation:
  - **Chondrocytes**, responsible for secreting cartilage and its matrix.
  - **Osteoblasts**, which secrete osteoid and bone matrix.
  - **Osteoclasts**, tasked with bone resorption.
- The bones forming the central trunk originate from the **somites**, with the sclerotome giving rise to the axial skeleton's bones. Conversely, the lateral plate mesoderm contributes to the formation of **limb bones**, while neural crest cells are responsible for generating the bones of the **head and neck**.
- The vertebral column takes shape through the resegmentation of the **sclerotomes**. This re-segmentation process results in motor axons and dorsal root ganglia residing between vertebrae rather than traversing through them.

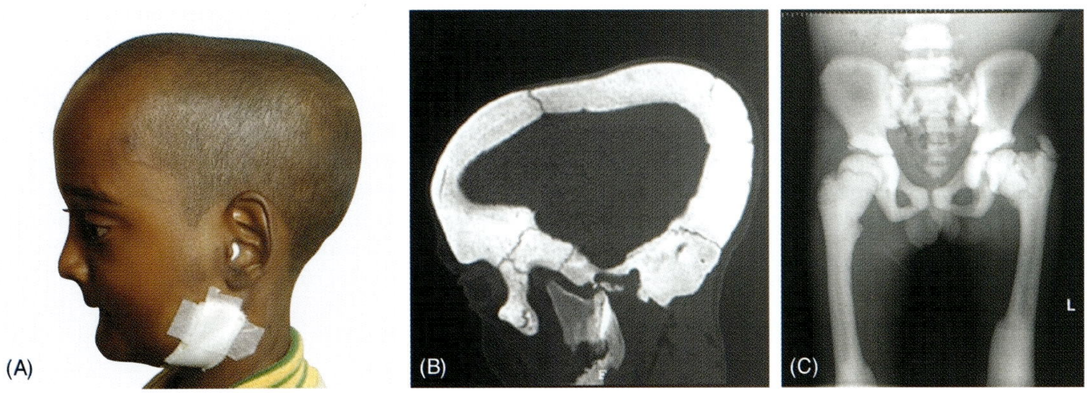

Fig. 24.9 (A) A child with osteopetrosis. (B) X-ray of osteopetrosis skull. (C) X-ray of pelvis with femur, showing increased density of bones and fractures. (Photo courtesy: Dr Suja.)

BRAIN TEASERS

1. What is the final stage in the development of vertebrae?
   A. Blastemal
   B. Membranous
   C. Cartilaginous
   D. Bony
2. Which embryonic structure gives rise to both the sclerotome and dermomyotome?
   A. Notochord
   B. Paraxial mesoderm
   C. Neural crest cells
   D. Lateral plate mesoderm
3. At what week of embryonic development do cells from the sclerotome migrate to form the centrum of the blastemal vertebra?
   A. Second week
   B. Fourth week
   C. Sixth week
   D. Eighth week
4. What is the anatomical variation that occurs due to the incomplete fusion of sternal plates between the third and fourth sternebrae?
   A. Sternum bifurcation
   B. Xiphoid deviation
   C. Sternal foramen
   D. Rib separation
5. How many fontanelles are present in the human skull?
   A. 2
   B. 4
   C. 6
   D. 8
6. At what age does the anterior fontanelle typically close?
   A. At birth
   B. 1–2 months
   C. 18 months
   D. 25 years
7. What type of ossification occurs in the flat bones covering the vault and side wall of the skull?
   A. Endochondral ossification
   B. Intramembranous ossification
   C. Epiphyseal ossification
   D. Cortical ossification
8. What is the most common skeletal dysplasia?
   A. Thanatophoric dysplasia
   B. Achondroplasia
   C. Pfeiffer's syndrome
   D. Cleidocranial dysostosis
9. Which genetic mutation is primarily associated with achondroplasia?
   A. FGFR1
   B. FGFR2
   C. FGFR3
   D. FBN1
10. Which form of skeletal dysplasia is considered the most common neonatal skeletal dysplasia and is lethal?
    A. Pfeiffer's syndrome
    B. Apert's syndrome
    C. Cleidocranial dysostosis
    D. Thanatophoric dysplasia
11. Which gene is involved in both type 1 and type 2 thanatophoric dysplasia?
    A. FGFR1
    B. FGFR2
    C. FGFR3
    D. FBN1
12. What is the typical cranial shape associated with Pfeiffer's syndrome?
    A. Micromelia
    B. Cloverleaf skull
    C. Prominent forehead
    D. Syndactyly of hands and feet

Answers

1. (D); 2. (B); 3. (B); 4. (C); 5. (C); 6. (C); 7. (B); 8. (B); 9. (C); 10. (D); 11. (C); 12. (B).

FURTHER READINGS

Lin GH, Zhang L. Apical ectodermal ridge regulates three principal axes of the developing limb. *J Zhejiang Univ Sci B.* 2020;21(10):757-766. doi:10.1631/jzus.B2000285.

Impellizzeri A, Midulla G, Romeo U, La Monaca C, Barbato E, Galluccio G. Delayed eruption of permanent dentition and maxillary contraction in patients with cleidocranial dysplasia: review and report of a family. *Int J Dent.* 2018;2018:6591414. doi:10.1155/2018/6591414.

Wolters TLC, Netea MG, Riksen NP, Hermus ARMM, Netea-Maier RT. Acromegaly, inflammation and cardiovascular disease: a review. *Rev Endocr Metab Disord.* 2020;21(4):547-568. doi:10.1007/s11154-020-09560-x.

Gülaşı S, Atıcı A, Çelik Y. A case of thanatophoric dysplasia type 2: a novel mutation. *J Clin Res Pediatr Endocrinol.* 2015;7(1):73-76. doi:10.4274/jcrpe.1703.

Muscular System 25

AN 79.4 Describe the development of somites.

ANAMNESE

A 14-year-old adolescent presented with concerns about noticeable physical asymmetry in the chest and upper limb on the left side of their body. The adolescent and their family reported that the right chest wall appeared underdeveloped and lacked the normal muscle bulk, causing a visible concavity. Additionally, the right hand displayed subtle differences, including a smaller size and underdeveloped fingers. The patient expressed feelings of self-consciousness due to these physical disparities and sought medical evaluation for both cosmetic and functional reasons. Upon examination, the diagnosis of **Poland syndrome** was confirmed, which explained the congenital absence of the right pectoral muscles, affecting the chest and the upper limb on the same side.

Musculoskeletal malformations can be identified through prenatal ultrasound, with these anomalies potentially impacting an individual's entire life. Various imaging techniques, including **USG, CT,** and **MRI**, are employed to visualize primary abnormalities. The utilization of **3D-HCT** and **3D-USG** has proven to be more effective in detecting abnormalities than traditional 2D-USG. Diagnoses are typically made between **27** and **36 weeks of gestation**. The advantage of **3D-HCT** over 3D-USG lies in its ability to provide a comprehensive foetal image.

Regarding the development of the muscular system, it is essential to understand that, except for specific smooth muscle tissues like sphincters, dilator pupillae, arrector pili and myoepithelial cells derived from the ectoderm, the majority of the muscular system originates from muscle precursor cells of the **mesodermal germ layer**. Specifically, **Skeletal muscle** derives from the **paraxial mesoderm**, giving rise to somitomeres in the head and somites from the occipital to sacral regions. **Smooth muscle**, on the other hand, differentiates from the **splanchnic mesoderm** surrounding the gut, as well as from the ectoderm. Lastly, **Cardiac muscle** originates from the **splanchnic mesoderm** surrounding the heart tube.

DEVELOPMENT OF STRIATED OR SKELETAL MUSCLE (AN 79.4)

SOMITE DIFFERENTIATION

- During the third week of development, the **paraxial mesoderm** undergoes a remarkable transformation, organizing into structures called **somitomeres**. This process initiates in the cephalic region and proceeds cephalocaudally (as illustrated in Fig. 25.1).
- Each somitomere is composed of mesodermal cells arranged in concentric whorls. Head mesenchyme is formed through the combination of somitomeres and neuromeres (resulting from the segmentation of the neural plate) in the head region.

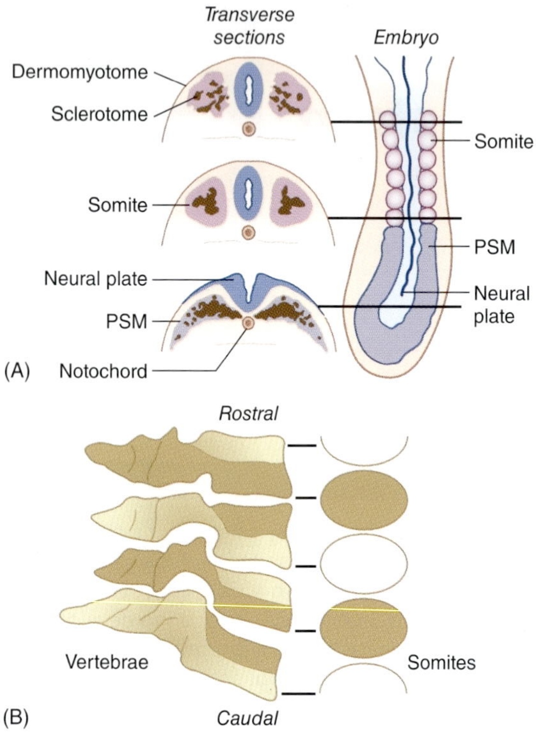

Fig. 25.1 Somite differentiation. (A) Embryologic differentiation of the mesoderm into pairs of somites on either side of the spinal cord. Somites divide further to form the ventral sclerotome and dorsal dermomyotome. (B) Cells from the rostral and caudal half of adjacent somites fuse to form future vertebral bodies and arches. Defects in this process have been theorized in Klippel-Feil syndrome. *PSM*, paraspinal muscles. (Source: Murphy RF, Hedequist DJ, Glotzbecker MP. Congenital anomalies of the cervical spine. In: Garfin SR, Eismont FJ, Bell GR, Fischgrund JS, Bono CM (eds). *Rothman-Simeone and Herkowitz's The Spine*. 7th ed. Elsevier, 2018; Credit line modified from Tracy MR, Dormans JP, Kusumi K. Klippel-Feil syndrome. *Clin Orthop*. 2004;424:183-190.)

- The first pair of somitomeres emerges in the occipital region around the 20th day of development, with a total of **42–44 pairs** present by the conclusion of the fifth week. The age of an embryo can be accurately determined by counting these somites.
- An important role played by these mesenchymal cells of the somites is their migration to envelop the neural tube and notochord, eventually giving rise to the **Sclerotome**, which differentiates into essential structures like vertebrae and ribs.

FATE OF SOMITES

- Each **Somite** is composed of three distinct components: the **sclerotome**, **myotome** and **dermatome**. The sclerotome plays a crucial role in giving rise to the vertebral column and ribs. On the other hand, the dermatome is responsible for forming the dermis of the skin and the subcutaneous tissue. The myotome, in turn, is the origin of striated or skeletal muscle (Fig. 25.2).
- The myotome undergoes a transformation, losing its epithelium to adopt a spindle-shaped structure, which ultimately leads to the formation of **Myoblasts**. These myoblasts fuse together, forming **Myotubes**, which then differentiate into muscle fibres. By the third month of development, the muscle tissue develops a striated appearance due to the presence of myofibrils in the cytoplasm (Fig. 25.3).
- As the vertebral column develops with the outgrowth of transverse processes, the myotome is divided into two distinct parts: a smaller dorsal section known as the **epimere** and a larger ventral portion known as the **hypomere** (Fig. 25.4). The septum observed between these two subdivisions persists as the **thoracolumbar fascia** in adults.

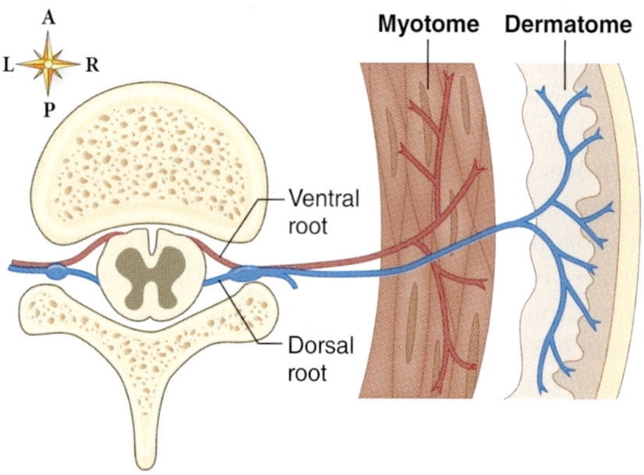

Fig. 25.2 Segmental distribution of spinal nerves. A dermatome is a region of skin supplied by afferent (sensory) fibers of a given spinal nerve. A myotome is a region of skeletal muscle innervated by efferent (motor) fibers of a given spinal nerve. Spinal nerves at different segments of the spinal cord innervate different sets of dermatomes and myotomes. (Source: Patton KT, Thibodeau GA. Peripheral nervous system. In: *Anatomy & Physiology*. 7th ed. 2010.)

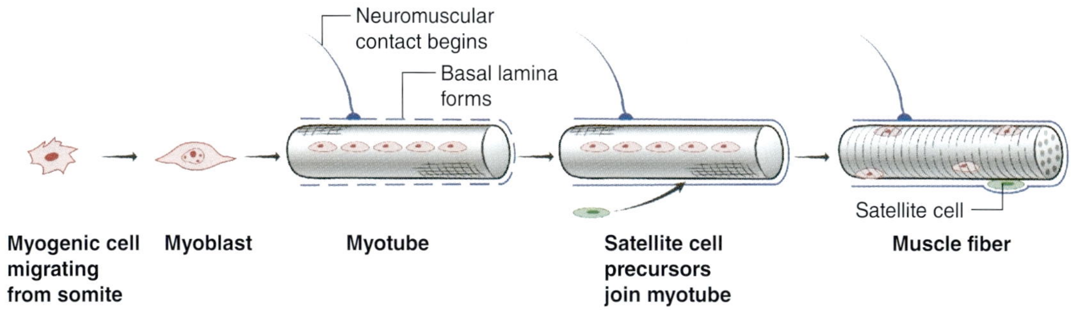

Fig. 25.3 Embryonic development of a skeletal muscle fiber from a myogenic cell. Many myoblasts fuse to form a single myotube, which then matures to become muscle fiber. (Source: Carlson BM. Tissues. In: *The Human Body: Linking Structure and Function*. 2019; Credit line from Carlson (2007), with permission.)

- The epimere eventually gives rise to the **extensor** muscles, including the erector spinae of the vertebral column. Conversely, the hypomere forms the **flexor** muscles of the trunk, contributing to the muscles of the body wall. It is important to note that epimeres, or back muscles, are innervated by **dorsal primary rami**, while hypomeres, which include limb and body wall muscles, are innervated by **ventral primary rami.**
- According to recent theory, **epaxial** (above the axis) muscles are innervated by dorsal primary rami and **hypaxial** (below the axis) muscles by ventral primary rami.
- The musculature of the **axial skeleton**, body wall and limbs is derived from somites that extend from the occipital region to the coccygeal region. **Tendons** are derived from sclerotome cells situated near the myotomes at the anterior and posterior edges of the somites.
- During development, the **occipital/precervical somites** initially number four, but later, the first one disappears. The occipital myotomes, along with the hypoglossal nerve, invade the developing **tongue** through the epipericardial ridge, forming the muscles of the tongue (Fig. 25.5).
- The extrinsic muscles of the **eyes** are developed from three **preotic myotomes** arranged around the developing eyes and are innervated by the third, fourth and sixth cranial nerves (Fig. 25.5).
- Muscles of the branchial arches are discussed in conjunction with the branchial apparatus.
- Muscles of the upper and lower limb buds are derived from mesodermal somites that migrate

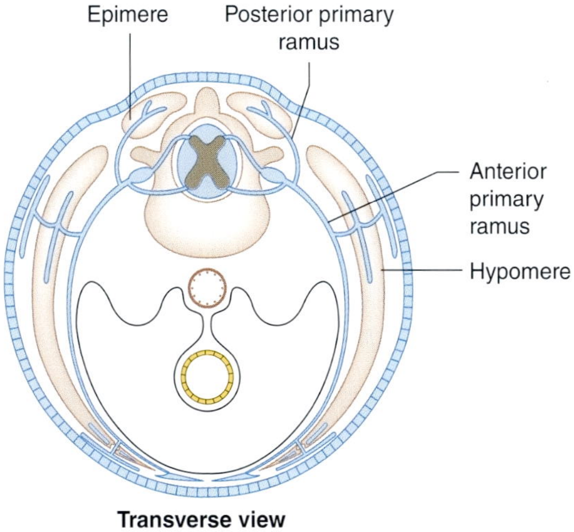

Fig. 25.4 Epimere and hypomere.

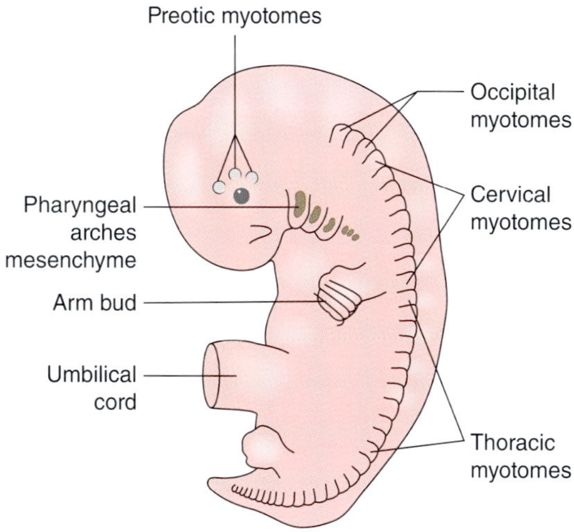

Fig. 25.5 Distribution of somites.

into the developing limb buds during the fifth week of the intrauterine period. Premuscle cells enter the limb buds along the axis of skeletal elements, forming ventral and dorsal muscle masses that occupy the flexor and extensor compartments of the limb buds.
- The ventral primary rami supply all muscle masses of the limb buds, with the **ventral mass** being supplied by ventral branches and the **dorsal mass** being supplied by dorsal branches of the ventral rami. The connective tissue covering and their tendons are formed from the somatopleuric mesenchyme.

DEVELOPMENT OF CARDIAC MUSCLE

- The development of **cardiac muscle** stems from the formation of the **Myoepicardial mantle**, which arises from the thickening of the **splanchnic mesoderm** surrounding both the endothelial heart tube and the pericardium (as depicted in Fig. 25.6).
- During this process, **myoblasts** adhere to each other through attachments that will subsequently evolve into **intercalated discs**. The **myofibrils** develop within cardiac muscle cells in a manner similar to skeletal muscle, but unlike skeletal muscle, myoblasts in cardiac muscle do not fuse.
- The heart's conducting system is composed of specific bundles of muscle cells known as **Purkinje fibres**, which have an irregular distribution of myofibrils. These specialized fibres play a critical role in coordinating and regulating the rhythmic contractions of the heart.

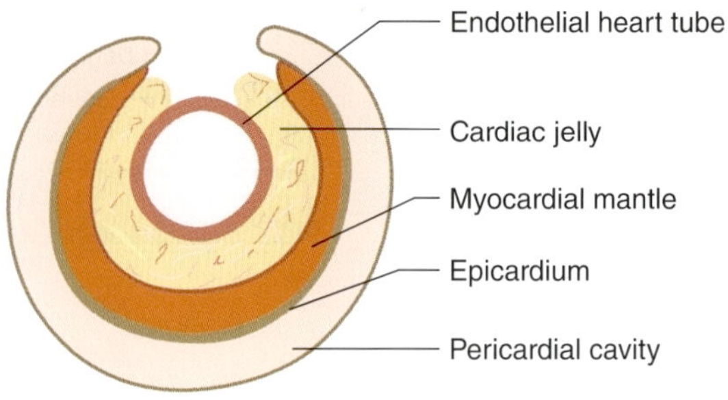

Fig. 25.6 Development of cardiac muscle.

DEVELOPMENT OF SMOOTH MUSCLE

- The development of **smooth muscles** is characterized by the predominance of their derivation from **mesenchyme**. The sources of smooth muscle cells can vary in different anatomical locations.
- The smooth muscle in the **dorsal aorta** and **large arteries** is primarily derived from the **lateral plate mesoderm** and **neural crest cells**, contributing to their formation. The **coronary arteries** rely on the differentiation of smooth muscle from **proepicardial cells** and **neural crest cells** (Fig. 25.7).
- The smooth muscle found in the walls of the **gut** and its derivatives originates from the **lateral plate mesoderm**, enveloping these structures.
- Specific structures like the **dilators** and **sphincters of the pupil, smooth muscle in sweat** and **mammary glands,** and **arrector pili** have a distinct origin and are derived from the **ectoderm**.

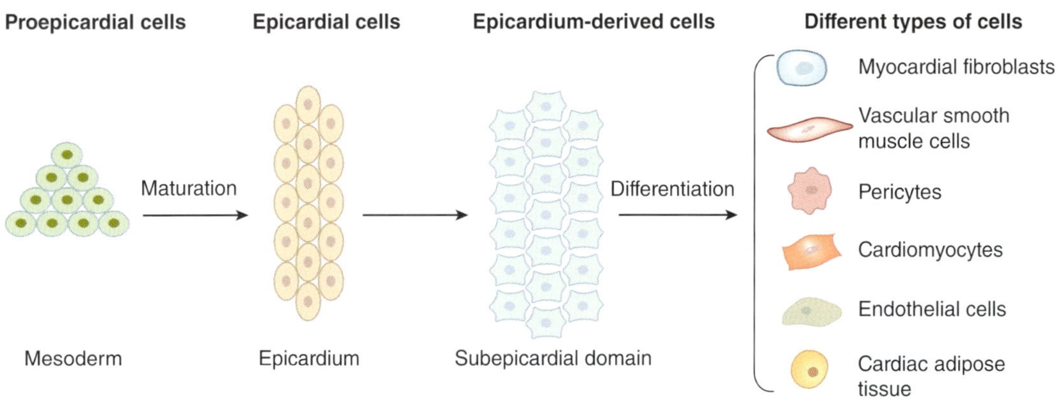

Fig. 25.7 Fate of proepicardial cells.

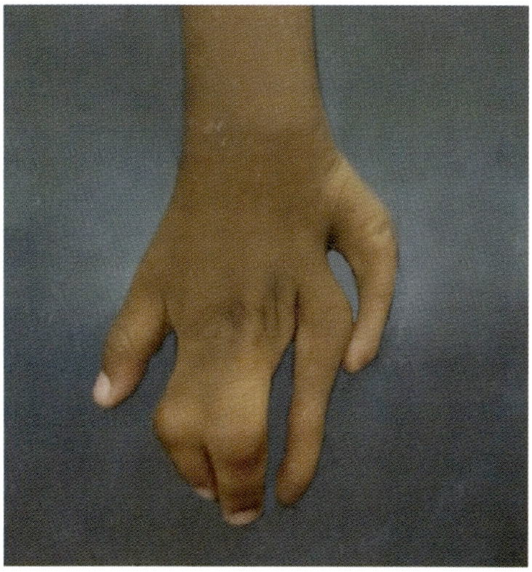

Fig. 25.8 Syndactyly: The Index and middle fingers are fused. (Source: Photo courtesy Dr Nithya.)

CLINICAL NUGGETS

Poland sequence

- Poland syndrome is a rare congenital condition that primarily affects the development of **chest muscles**, typically on one side of the body (see Fig. 26.9A).
- In addition to the chest wall deformity, Poland syndrome can also involve the underdevelopment or absence of the sternal portion of the **Pectoralis major** muscle, and in some cases, it may affect the breast and hand (**syndactyly** (Fig. 25.8), **brachydactyly**) on the same side of the body.
- While Poland syndrome usually does not impact vital organ function, it can pose significant cosmetic and psychological challenges. The severity and specific features of Poland syndrome can vary from one individual to another.

KLINISCHE PERLEN

MUSCLE DEVELOPMENT DOMAINS

1. **Primaxial Domain:**
   - Comprised of cells derived from **somites** (paraxial mesoderm).
   - Located around the **neural tube**.
   - Muscles arising from this region include:
     - Scalene.
     - Geniohyoid.
     - Intercostals.
     - Prevertebral.
     - Latissimus dorsi.
     - Levator scapulae.
     - Rhomboids.
2. **Abaxial Domain**:
   - Formed by **somite cells** and **lateral plate mesoderm** (parietal layer).
   - Muscles originating from this domain include:
     - Infrahyoid muscles.
     - Lower limb muscles.
     - Distal muscles of the upper limb.
     - Pectoralis major and minor.
     - Abdominal wall muscles.
     - Pelvic diaphragm.

DUCHENNE MUSCULAR DYSTROPHY

- Duchenne muscular dystrophy (DMD) is a severe and progressive genetic disorder that primarily affects the muscles. It is one of the most common forms of muscular dystrophy and primarily affects **males**, although females can be carriers of the gene mutation (Fig. 25.9).
- Key characteristics of Duchenne muscular dystrophy include:
  - **Genetic Cause:** DMD is caused by a mutation in the **DMD gene,** which is located on the X chromosome. Because it is an **X-linked recessive** disorder, it primarily affects males. Females can be carriers of the mutated gene.
  - **Muscle Degeneration:** DMD leads to the progressive degeneration and weakening of muscle tissues. This typically begins in early childhood.
  - **Symptoms:** Common symptoms include **muscle weakness**, difficulty with motor skills, frequent falls and an abnormal gait. As the disease progresses, individuals with DMD may experience difficulty in walking, standing and eventually become wheelchair-bound.
  - **Cardiac Involvement:** DMD can also affect the heart muscles, leading to cardiomyopathy and an increased risk of heart problems.
  - **Respiratory Complications:** Weakened respiratory muscles can result in breathing difficulties, and some individuals with DMD may require ventilatory support.
  - Diagnosis is typically made through genetic testing to identify the mutation in the DMD gene. Muscle biopsies and imaging studies may also be used.
  - Ongoing research in the field of genetics and muscle biology is exploring potential treatments, including **gene therapy** and **exon-skipping techniques**.

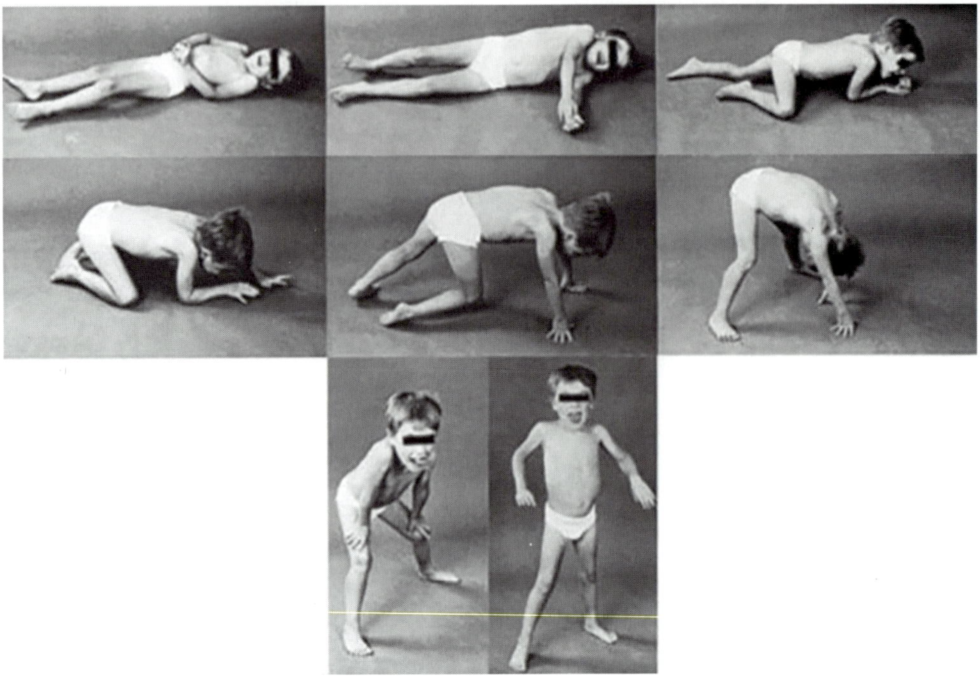

Fig. 25.9 Duchene muscular dystrophy. (Source: Source: Wayne Harris, Practical Paediatrics: Neuromuscular disorders, 4th ed. Churchill Livingstone; 2012.)

PRUNE BELLY SYNDROME

- Prune belly syndrome, also known as **Eagle-Barrett syndrome or triad syndrome**, is a rare congenital disorder that primarily affects male infants. It is characterized by a set of distinctive features (Fig. 25.10).
    1. **Abdominal Muscle Deficiency:** The hallmark feature of prune belly syndrome is the absence or severe underdevelopment of the abdominal muscles, which gives the abdomen a **wrinkled** or 'prune-like' appearance. This muscle deficiency can lead to a thin, translucent abdominal wall.
    2. **Urinary Tract Anomalies:** Individuals with prune belly syndrome often have a range of urinary tract abnormalities. This can include dilation of the urinary tract (**hydronephrosis**), abnormalities in the kidneys and issues with the bladder, such as poor muscle tone or nonobstructive urinary retention.
    3. **Cryptorchidism:** Many males with this syndrome are born with undescended testicles (cryptorchidism).
- Other features and complications of prune belly syndrome may include:
    - Gastrointestinal anomalies.
    - Orthopaedic issues, such as joint contractures.
    - Respiratory problems.
    - Pulmonary hypoplasia (underdeveloped lungs).
    - Risk of vesicoureteral reflux (urine flowing backward from the bladder to the kidneys).

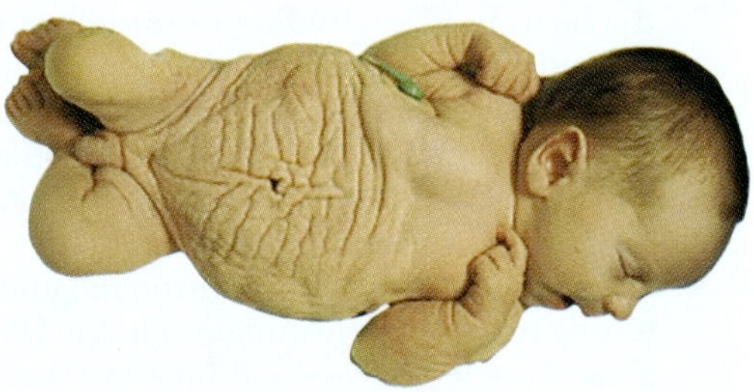

Fig. 25.10 Prune Belly syndrome. (Source: Zitelli and Davis' *Atlas of Pediatric Physical Diagnosis,* 8th ed.: Jessica Garrison, Basil j. Zitelli, Andrew J. Nowalk, et. al. Fig. 14.22, Elsevier Inc., 2023.)

POINTS TO PONDER

- Muscle development in the embryo is a complex process that unfolds during the fourth week of gestation, giving rise to three distinct types of muscles: skeletal, smooth and cardiac. This begins with the formation of **myoblasts**, which subsequently differentiate into myocytes.
- Skeletal muscle development undergoes two key phases: **primary myogenesis** in the embryonic stage and **secondary myogenesis** in the foetal stage. Postnatally, muscle growth and repair are facilitated by satellite cells, which respond to factors like exercise and muscle damage.
- The muscles in the trunk, limbs and tongue find their origins in the **somites**, with the dermomyotome region of the somite contributing to their formation. Facial, masticatory and laryngeal muscles originate from the unsegmented paraxial mesoderm.

BRAIN TEASERS

1. What are the three distinct components that make up each somite during embryonic development?
   A. Dermatome, myotome and hypomere
   B. Dermis, epimere and sclerotome
   C. Myotome, epimeres and thoracolumbar fascia
   D. Sclerotome, myotome and dermatome
2. What happens to the myotome during development?
   A. It becomes a new type of tissue not related to muscle.
   B. It retains its original epithelial structure.
   C. It forms myoblasts, which eventually develop into myotubes.
   D. It remains dormant and does not contribute to muscle development.
3. Which muscles are innervated by dorsal primary rami?
   A. Back muscles, including the erector spinae.
   B. Limb and body wall muscles.
   C. Facial and masticatory muscles.
   D. Muscles of the tongue.
4. What are the muscles of the upper and lower limb buds derived from during development?
   A. Neural crest cells
   B. Somites
   C. Epimeres
   D. Sclerotome cells
5. During cardiac muscle development, what is the role of Purkinje fibres in the heart?
   A. Formation of cardiac muscle myoblasts.
   B. Coordination and regulation of heart contractions.
   C. Intercalated disc formation.
   D. Development of myofibrils in cardiac muscle cells.
6. How do cardiac muscle cells differ from skeletal muscle cells in terms of myoblast fusion?
   A. Cardiac muscle cells fuse to form myoblasts.
   B. Both cardiac and skeletal muscle cells fuse to form myoblasts.
   C. Cardiac muscle cells do not fuse to form myoblasts.
   D. Skeletal muscle cells do not fuse to form myoblasts.
7. Which germ layer primarily contributes to the formation of smooth muscles in the dorsal aorta and large arteries?
   A. Endoderm
   B. Ectoderm
   C. Lateral plate mesoderm and neural crest cells
   D. Mesenchyme
8. Where is the source of smooth muscle cells for the coronary arteries during development?
   A. Neural crest cells
   B. Lateral plate mesoderm
   C. Mesenchyme
   D. Proepicardial cells and neural crest cells
9. Which embryonic layer contributes to the formation of structures like the dilators and sphincters of the pupil, sweat and mammary gland muscles, and arrector pili?
   A. Mesoderm
   B. Endoderm
   C. Lateral plate mesoderm
   D. Ectoderm
10. The smooth muscle in the walls of the gut and its derivatives primarily derives from which embryonic source?
   A. Neural crest cells
   B. Splanchnic mesoderm
   C. Lateral plate mesoderm
   D. Ectoderm

Answers

1. (D); 2. (C); 3. (A); 4. (B); 5. (B); 6. (C); 7. (C); 8. (D); 9. (D); 10. (B).

FURTHER READINGS

Ferizovic N, Summers J, de Zárate IBO, et al. Prognostic indicators of disease progression in Duchenne muscular dystrophy: a literature review and evidence synthesis. *PLoS One*. 2022;17(3):e0265879. doi:10.1371/journal.pone.0265879.

Pradhan BS, Prószyński TJ. A role for caveolin-3 in the pathogenesis of muscular dystrophies. *Int J Mol Sci*. 2020;21(22):8736. doi:10.3390/ijms21228736.

Straub V, Guglieri M. An update on Becker muscular dystrophy. *Curr Opin Neurol*. 2023;36(5):450-454. doi: 10.1097/WCO.0000000000001191.

SECTION 4

SPECIAL TOPICS

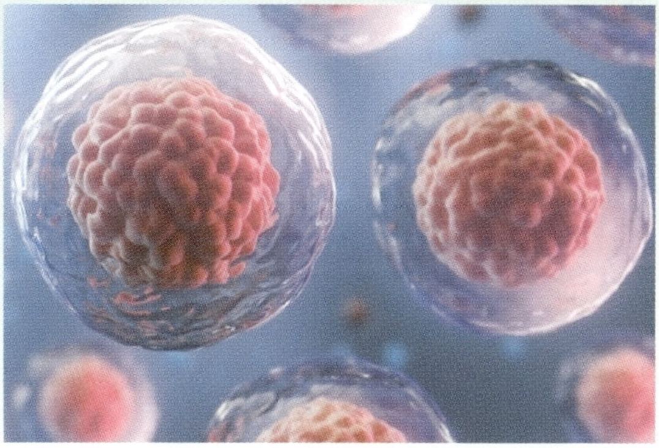

Teratology 26

AN 77.6 Describe teratogenic influences.
AN 79.6 Describe the role of teratogens.

ANAMNESE

A 32-year-old pregnant woman who, during the critical first trimester, was exposed to a specific teratogen—high doses of retinoids commonly found in acne medication. She had been using the medication without realizing the risks during pregnancy. Her newborn, born at full term, exhibited a range of congenital anomalies, including facial malformations, heart defects and developmental delays. This case serves as an example of the harmful impact of retinoid exposure during pregnancy, underlining the importance of educating expectant mothers on the hazards of certain medications and emphasizing the need for caution and informed decision-making during pregnancy to protect the health of the unborn child.

Teratology emerged as a modern scientific discipline in the 1930s, marked by a significant breakthrough when a series of experiments involved feeding pregnant pigs a diet deficient in **Vitamin A**. The resulting piglets displayed a spectrum of malformations, prominently characterized by a lack of eyes. This pioneering work was credited to the physician **Josef Warkany**, often referred to as the **father of experimental teratology**. Warkany's research, conducted in the 1930s and 1940s, was groundbreaking in demonstrating that external factors could induce congenital developmental disorders in mammals. His investigations not only paved the way for understanding genetic and environmentally induced structural defects but also established teratology as the study of prenatal pathology.

- Teratology, also known as **embryopathy**, specifically focuses on the pathological conditions affecting the unborn.
- In cases of severe defects, the consequences may lead to abortions or foetal deaths, essentially illustrating natural selection's role in eliminating such pregnancies.
- Milder forms of defects manifest as abnormal phenotypes, underlining the wide spectrum of outcomes within the realm of teratology.

BIRTH DEFECTS

The causative factors can be classified into four primary categories:

A) **Genetic factors** (gene and chromosome abnormalities).
B) **Environmental factors** (radiations, drugs, maternal infections, hormonal influences and nutritional aspects).
C) **Multifactorial** (genetic and environmental factors).
D) **Uncertain aetiology** (includes more than 50% of congenital anomalies, attributing to this category) (Fig. 26.1).

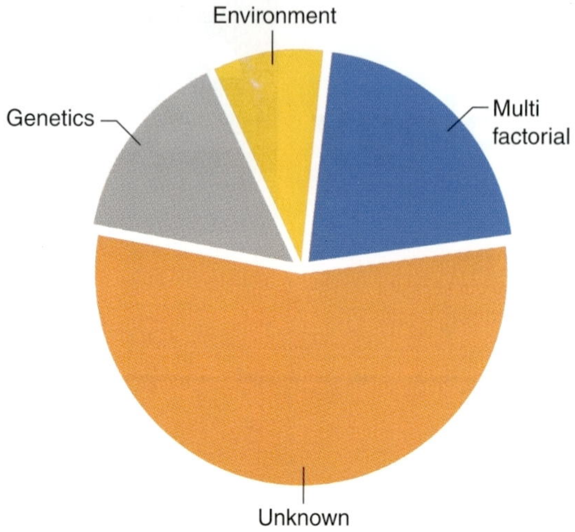

Fig. 26.1 Causes of birth defects.

BIRTH DEFECTS CAUSED BY GENETIC FACTORS

Chromosomal Abnormalities

It includes numerical and structural irregularities within both autosomes and sex chromosomes.

- **Numerical aberrations** stem from the nondisjunction of chromosome pairs during mitosis or meiosis, resulting in two daughter cells, one with a pair of chromosomes and one without any.
- Two main types of numerical aberrations include **Aneuploidy** (characterized by one chromosome more, i.e. trisomy, or one chromosome less, i.e. monosomy) and **Polyploidy** (involving a chromosome number that is a multiple of the haploid number and usually not compatible with survival).
- Examples of numerical aberrations include monosomy of sex chromosomes (e.g. **Turner's** syndrome, 45,X0), trisomy of sex chromosomes (e.g. **Klinefelter's** syndrome, 47,XXY (Fig. 26.2) and **Triple X** syndrome, 47,XXX) and trisomy of autosomes (e.g. Trisomy 21/**Down's** syndrome, Trisomy 18/**Edwards's** syndrome, and Trisomy 13/**Patau** syndrome).
- **Structural abnormalities** result from chromosomal breakage and abnormal rejoining. Translocation and inversion are two common structural abnormalities transmitted from parents to children.
  - **Translocation:** It involves the transfer of a segment of one chromosome to a nonhomologous chromosome, as seen in **Down's syndrome** (**Translocation D/G; 21/22; 21/21**).
  - **Deletion:** A portion of a chromosome breaks and may be lost, as observed in **Cri-du-chat** syndrome (terminal deletion from the short arm of **chromosome 5**).
  - **Microdeletion:** This pertains to the deletion of a specific band on a chromosome, as seen in **Prader-Willi** syndrome and **Angelman** syndrome (involving the deletion of **band q12 on chromosome 15**).
  - **Inversion:** In this anomaly, a segment of a chromosome is reversed, with the most common inversion found in **chromosome 9**, typically without harmful effects.

Anomalies by Mutant Genes

- Mutations denote permanent, heritable changes that lead to loss or alteration in the function of a gene.
- These mutations consist of various types, including autosomal dominant traits like Achondroplasia and Marfan's syndrome, autosomal recessive traits like inborn errors of metabolism such as Albinism and Phenylketonuria, haemoglobinopathies like Sickle-cell anaemia and Thalassaemia, and X-linked recessive traits like Haemophilia and Duchenne muscular dystrophy.

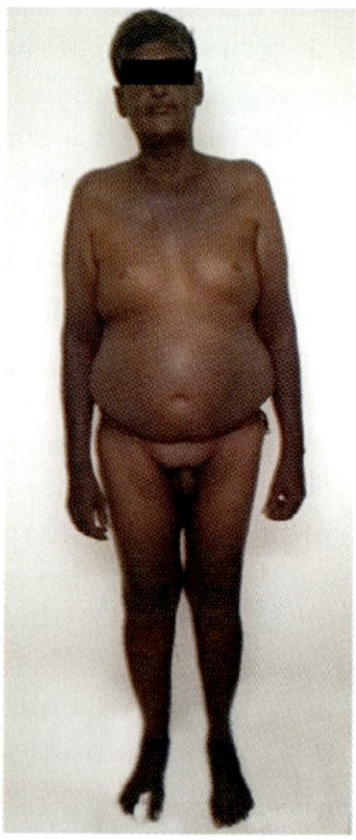

Fig. 26.2 A male with Klinefelter syndrome showing less body hair, gynaecomastia, smaller genitals and is taller than normal. (Photo courtesy: Dr Suja.)

BIRTH DEFECTS CAUSED BY ENVIRONMENTAL FACTORS (AN 77.6)

- **Teratogens** are agents that can be defined as substances capable of causing or increasing the occurrence of congenital anomalies within a population.
- Human embryos exhibit an unusual sensitivity to external teratogenic agents, stressing on the importance of securing prenatal development (Fig. 26.3).
- The occurrence of teratogenesis depends on three primary factors:
  1. **Developmental Stage of the Embryo:** Critical periods for teratogenic susceptibility

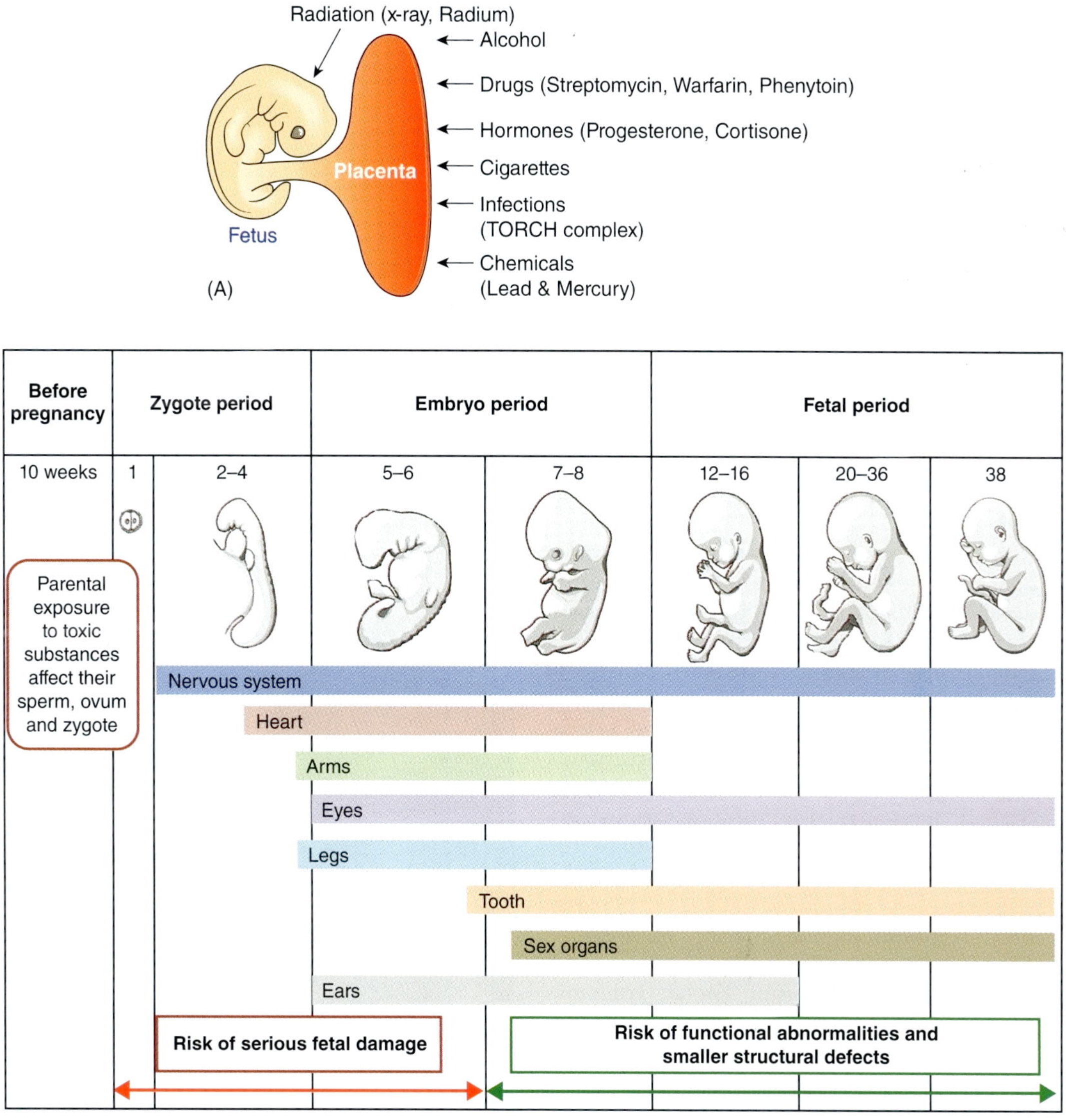

Fig. 26.3 The teratogenic factors affecting foetus. Sensitivity of individual organs to damage during exposure to teratogenic factors depending on the week of pregnancy (pictures present the main changes in the shape of the foetus). (Source: *TRAC*, 2018.)

are most during the germinal period (first 3 weeks) and the embryonic period (4–8 weeks), which marks the organogenesis phase.

2. **Teratogen Dosage:** The degree of exposure plays an important role, with prolonged exposure leading to more severe congenital anomalies.
3. **Genetic Makeup of the Embryo:** It is important to recognize that not all embryos exposed to a teratogenic agent will develop congenital anomalies; the outcome depends on the specific genetic constitution of the embryo. Hence, susceptibility to teratogenic effects may vary according to the embryo's genotype.

TERATOGENIC FACTORS ARE CLASSIFIED AS (FIG. 26.3) (AN 79.6)

- Drugs.
- Chemicals.
- Radiation.
- Hormones.
- Infections.
- Nutritional excess/deficiency.

Drugs

- Numerous drugs administered during pregnancy can exert teratogenic effects on the developing foetus. For instance, high doses of antibiotics like **Streptomycin**, an antitubercular agent, can lead to deafness or damage to the eighth cranial nerve in infants.
- Anticoagulants, such as **Warfarin**, used to treat thromboembolic disorders during pregnancy, can result in nasal cartilage hypoplasia, microcephaly, mental retardation and various central nervous system defects, leading to the condition known as **Foetal Warfarin syndrome** (Fig. 26.4). Alternatively, the use of heparin, which is not teratogenic, may be considered.
- Anticoagulants like **Phenytoin** can also induce teratogenic effects, causing **Foetal Hydantoin syndrome** (Fig. 26.5) characterized by intrauterine growth restriction, microcephaly, mental retardation and digital hypoplasia. Similarly, the use of **Valproic acid** during pregnancy can result in craniofacial and neural tube defects.

Commonly Used Drugs and Associated Anomalies:

- **Thalidomide** (sleeping pill) can affect the development of limb buds, leading to

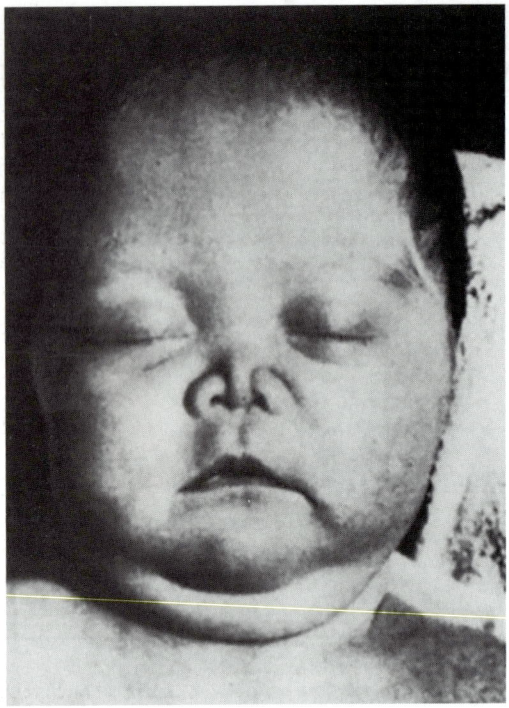

Fig. 26.4 Foetal warfarin syndrome. (From Pauli RM, Madden JD, Kranzler KJ, Culpepper W, Port R. Warfarin Therapy Initiated During Pregnancy and Phenotypic Chondrodysplasia Punctata. J Pediatr 88(3): 506–508, 1976.)

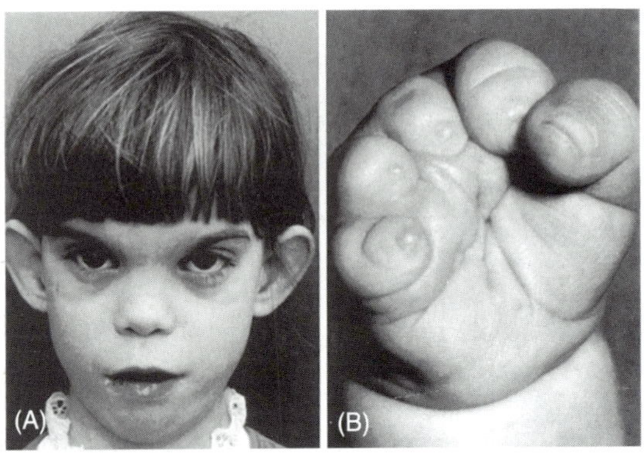

Fig. 26.5 Foetal hydantoin syndrome. (Source: (A), Courtesy Dr. A. E. Chudley, Section of Genetics and Metabolism, Department of Pediatrics and Child Health, Children's Hospital, Winnipeg, Manitoba, Canada. (B), From Chodirker BN, Chudley AE, Reed MH, Persaud TV: Possible prenatal hydantoin effect in a child born to a nonepileptic mother, Am J Med Genet 27:373, 1987.)

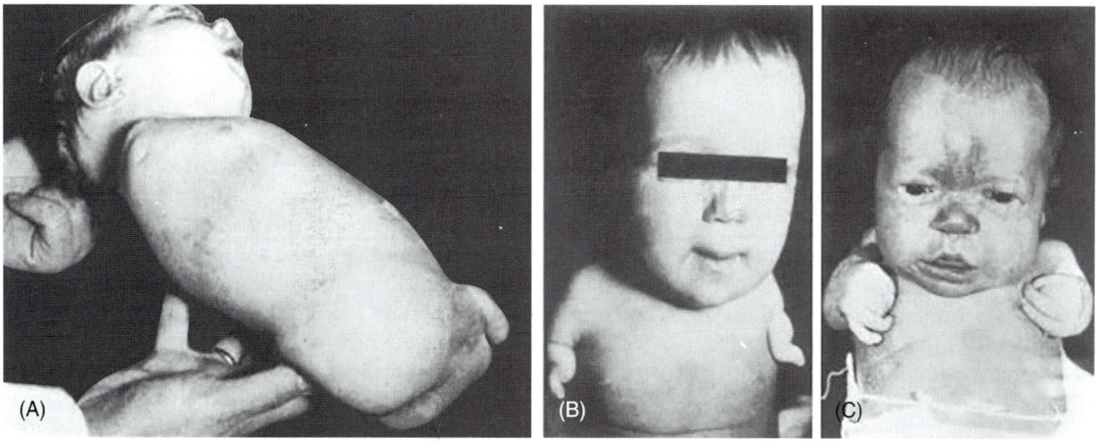

Fig. 26.6 Effects of thalidomide on limb buds. (Source: From Lenz W, Knapp K: Foetal malformation due to thalidomide, Geriatr Med Monthly 7:253, 1962.)

conditions like amelia and meromelia (Fig. 26.6).

- **Diazepam** (tranquilizer) is associated with cleft lip.
- **Tetracycline** (antibiotic) may cause bone and tooth anomalies.
- **Lysergic acid diethylamide (LSD)** exposure can result in limb and central nervous system malformations.

Chemicals

- Environmental pollutants, industrial and agricultural chemicals, and food additives are among the factors contributing to teratogenic effects.
- For instance, elevated levels of **organic mercury** in maternal consumption of fish can lead to **Foetal Minamata** disease, resembling cerebral palsy with neurological and behavioural disturbances.
- The presence of **lead,** a common environmental pollutant, crossing the placental barrier and accumulating in foetal tissues, can result in intrauterine growth restriction (IUGR), abortions, psychomotor disturbances and foetal anomalies.
- Maternal alcohol abuse can lead to **Foetal Alcohol Syndrome (FAS),** characterized by a range of distinctive features, including a thin upper lip, a short nose, joint anomalies and congenital heart defects (Fig. 26.7).

Radiation

Exposure to radiation during pregnancy can have deleterious effects on the developing foetus, depending on several factors, including the type of radiation, the dose and the stage of foetal development. Here are some effects of radiation exposure on the foetus:

- **Growth Retardation:** Radiation exposure can impair the normal growth and development of the

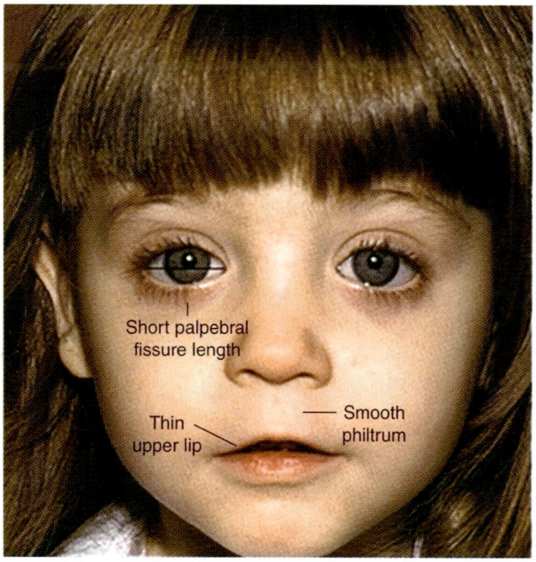

Fig. 26.7 Foetal alcohol syndrome. (Source: From Williams JF, Smith VC. AAP committee on substance abuse. Fetal alcohol spectrum disorders. Pediatrics. 2015;136[5]:e1395–e1406; copyright 2022 Susan (Astley) Hemingway PhD, University of Washington.)

foetus. This may result in low birth weight and a smaller-than-average size for gestational age.

- **Developmental Abnormalities:** High doses of radiation during foetal development can lead to structural abnormalities. For example, exposure during the **embryonic stage (4–8 weeks)** may cause organ malformations and developmental issues.
- **Mental Retardation:** Severe radiation exposure at critical stages can lead to cognitive impairments, intellectual disabilities and learning difficulties in the child.
- **Skeletal Anomalies:** Radiation exposure can affect the development of the skeletal system, leading to bone abnormalities in the foetus.
- **Central Nervous System (CNS) Malformations:** High doses of radiation during pregnancy can result in malformations of the foetal brain and spinal cord.
- **Spina Bifida:** Radiation exposure may increase the risk of neural tube defects such as spina bifida, where the neural tube remains open either completely or in parts.
- **Behavioural and Neurological Issues:** Children exposed to radiation in utero may be at a higher risk of developing behavioural and neurological problems, such as attention deficits and hyperactivity.
- **Cancer Risk:** Prenatal radiation exposure can increase the child's risk of developing cancer later in life, as it may damage the genetic material in cells.

Hormones

Hormonal imbalances or exposure to certain hormones during pregnancy can have a range of effects on the developing foetus. The specific effects can vary depending on the timing and duration of hormonal exposure, as well as the type and quantity of hormones involved. Here are the effects of hormonal imbalances or exposure on the foetus:

- **Masculinization or Feminization:** Hormonal imbalances can lead to atypical sexual development. For example, exposure to excess **androgens** (male sex hormones) during foetal development can result in masculinization of female foetuses, leading to ambiguous genitalia or virilization. Prolonged use of **progesterone** during pregnancy can have masculinizing effects on female children.
- **Foetal Growth:** Hormones like insulin and growth hormone are essential for foetal growth. Abnormal levels of these hormones can result in either excessive or restricted foetal growth, leading to conditions like **Macrosomia** (excessive foetal growth) or **Intrauterine growth restriction** (IUGR) where the foetus does not reach its full growth potential. Maternal diabetes can lead to neonatal deaths, abortions and the birth of large babies.
- **Cleft Palate and Lip:** Certain hormonal imbalances or exposures can contribute to orofacial clefts, such as cleft lip and cleft palate. The use of **cortisone** during early pregnancy may result in deformed children with cleft palates.
- **Development of Endocrine Organs:** Hormonal imbalances can disrupt the development of endocrine organs like the thyroid, pancreas or adrenal glands in the foetus, leading to hormonal deficiencies or overactivity.
- **Metabolic Effects:** Hormonal imbalances during pregnancy can impact the foetal metabolic system, increasing the risk of metabolic disorders in the child, such as obesity, diabetes or metabolic syndrome.
- **Cognitive and Behavioural Effects:** Hormonal imbalances or exposure to stress hormones during foetal development may affect cognitive and behavioural development, contributing to conditions like **Attention deficit hyperactivity disorder (ADHD)** or other behavioural challenges.
- **Immune System Function:** Hormonal imbalances may influence the development of the foetal immune system, affecting the child's susceptibility to infections and autoimmune disorders.
- **Neurological and Brain Development:** Hormones, such as thyroid hormones, are important for proper brain development. Thyroid hormone imbalances during pregnancy can lead to neurological and cognitive deficits in the child.

Infections

- Microorganisms can cross the placental barrier and enter the foetal bloodstream, causing **congenital anomalies**. Bacteria, viruses and other organisms are vertically transmitted from mother to foetus and are collectively known as the **TORCH complex.**
    - **T**—Toxoplasmosis.
    - **O**—Others, for example chicken pox, HIV, syphilis.

  - **R**—Rubella.
  - **C**—Cytomegalovirus.
  - **H**—Herpes simplex virus.
- **Toxoplasmosis,** a parasitic infection, can lead to hydrocephalus and ocular defects. Maternal infection can occur through the consumption of poorly cooked meat (pork/lamb) containing toxoplasma cysts or close contact with infected domestic animals, particularly cats.
- Maternal **Varicella** (chickenpox) infection can result in hypoplasia of limbs, eye issues and brain damage.
- **Retrovirus (HIV)** infection can cause growth failure and specific craniofacial anomalies.
- **Syphilitic** infection can lead to congenital deafness, abnormal teeth (Hutchinson teeth) and bone abnormalities.
- **Rubella** (German measles) virus infection can manifest as Congenital Rubella syndrome, characterized by cataracts, cardiac defects and deafness (Fig. 26.8).
- **Cytomegalovirus (CMV)** infection in the first trimester may lead to spontaneous abortions, while infections occurring later in pregnancy can result in severe anomalies like chorioretinitis, blindness and cerebral palsy.
- **Herpes simplex** virus infection in early pregnancy typically leads to abortion, while infections in the third trimester may cause prematurity.

Nutritional Excess or Deficiency

Nutritional excess or deficiency during pregnancy can have significant effects on the developing foetus. Adequate nutrition is crucial for proper foetal growth and development, and imbalances in nutrient intake can lead to various health issues.

Nutritional Deficiency:

- **Intrauterine Growth Restriction:** Inadequate nutrition can result in IUGR, where the foetus does not reach its full growth potential. This condition is associated with low birth weight and can lead to a range of health problems for the infant.
- **Neurological and Cognitive Impairments:** A lack of essential nutrients, particularly

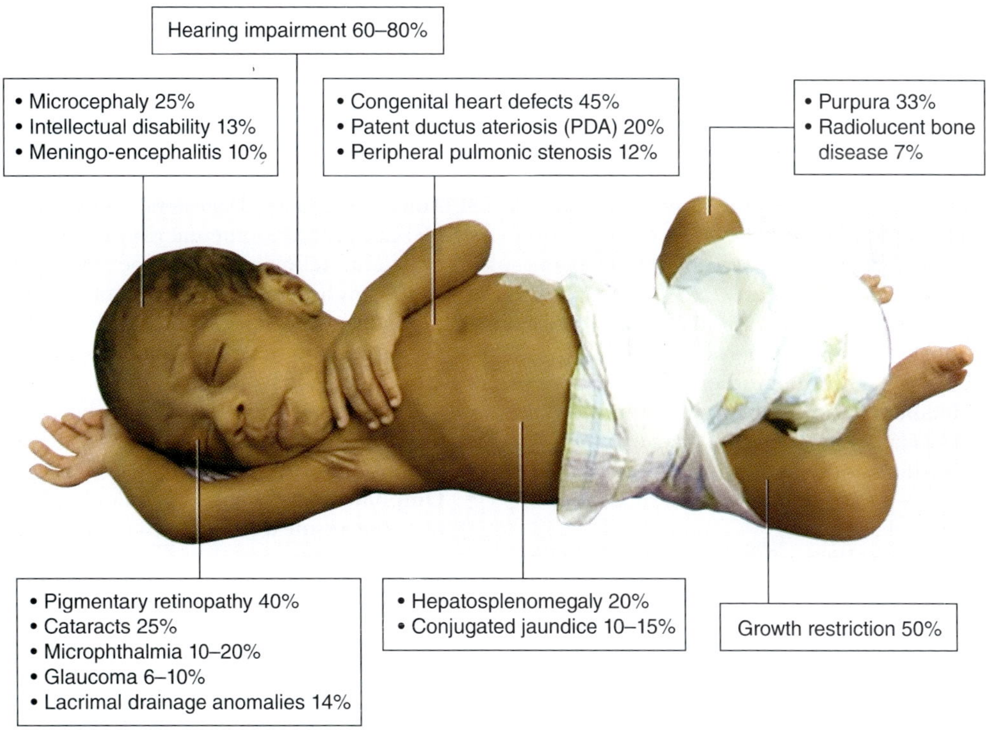

Fig. 26.8 Congenital rubella syndrome. (Source: Taylor & Hoyt's *Pediatric Ophthalmology and Strabismus*, 6th ed.,: Scott R Lambert, Christopher J Lyons, Fig. 11.7, Elsevier Inc., 2023.)

during critical periods of brain development, can lead to neurological and cognitive impairments in the child, causing learning disabilities and developmental delays.

- **Preterm Birth:** Inadequate nutrition can contribute to preterm birth, increasing the risk of neonatal health problems and long-term developmental challenges.
- **Congenital Abnormalities:** Some nutritional deficiencies, such as **folic acid** deficiency, are associated with an increased risk of congenital abnormalities, including neural tube defects like spina bifida.
- **Weakened Immune System:** Inadequate nutrition can compromise the foetal immune system, making the child more susceptible to infections and illnesses.
- **Anaemia: Iron deficiency** during pregnancy can lead to maternal anaemia and increase the risk of anaemia in the infant.
- **Iodine deficiency** in the mother can lead to congenital cretinism, resulting in stillborn or malformed children.

Nutritional Excess:

- **Macrosomia:** Excessive maternal nutrition, particularly excessive calorie intake, can lead to foetal macrosomia, where the baby is born significantly larger than average. Macrosomia increases the risk of complications during delivery and need for a caesarean section.
- **Childhood Obesity:** Babies born to mothers with excessive nutrition during pregnancy may have a higher risk of developing childhood obesity and related health problems.
- **Gestational Diabetes:** Excessive maternal nutrition can increase the risk of gestational diabetes, which can lead to complications for both the mother and the baby.
- **Metabolic Disorders:** High maternal intake of certain nutrients can lead to metabolic disorders in the child, such as glucose intolerance and an increased risk of developing type 2 diabetes.
- **Increased Risk of Allergies and Asthma:** Some studies suggest that excessive maternal nutrient intake, particularly during the later stages of pregnancy, may increase the child's risk of developing allergies and asthma.
- Prolonged exposure to high doses of **Vitamin A** can harm the brain and result in mental retardation.

BIRTH DEFECTS CAUSED BY MULTIFACTORIAL INHERITANCE

Birth defects due to multifactorial inheritance result from the complex interactions of both genetic and environmental factors. These defects are typically influenced by the combination of multiple genetic variants along with various environmental factors. Here are some examples of birth defects that are thought to have a multifactorial basis:

- **Cleft Lip and Palate:** Cleft lip and palate are among the most common congenital anomalies, and their development is influenced by both genetic and environmental factors. While specific genes have been associated with clefts, environmental factors such as maternal smoking, alcohol consumption and nutrient deficiencies also play a role.
- **Congenital Heart Defects:** Many congenital heart defects have a multifactorial basis. Genetic predisposition, including family history and maternal factors, such as viral infections during pregnancy, can contribute to the development of these defects.
- **Neural Tube Defects:** Neural tube defects, such as spina bifida and anencephaly, are influenced by a combination of genetic and environmental factors. Folate deficiency in the mother's diet is a well-known environmental risk factor for these defects.
- **Autism Spectrum Disorders:** Autism is a complex neurodevelopmental disorder with a multifactorial aetiology. While specific genes have been implicated, environmental factors like prenatal exposure to certain medications, infections and maternal stress may also contribute.
- **Hypospadias:** Hypospadias is a birth defect affecting the male urethra. It is believed to have multifactorial causes involving genetic susceptibility and environmental factors.
- **Omphalocele:** This is an abdominal wall defect that result from a combination of genetic and environmental factors, including maternal smoking and certain medications.

BIRTH DEFECTS DUE TO UNKNOWN AETIOLOGY

- Birth defects with an unknown aetiology, also known as idiopathic or unexplained birth defects, are those for which the exact cause remains unclear or unidentified despite extensive research and investigation More than 50% of human congenital anomalies occur due to unknown aetiology. These anomalies occur without a clear genetic, environmental or multifactorial explanation. Some examples of birth defects with an unknown aetiology include:

- **Clubfoot (Talipes Equinovarus):** Clubfoot is a congenital condition in which one or both feet are turned inward and downward. While genetic and environmental factors have been studied, many cases are still classified as idiopathic, with no discernible cause.
- **Amniotic Band Syndrome:** This condition involves the presence of fibrous bands in the amniotic fluid that can wrap around foetal body parts, leading to constriction and deformities. The exact cause of amniotic band syndrome is not well understood.
- **Hirschsprung's Disease:** This condition affects the large intestine and is characterized by a lack of nerve cells in the intestinal wall. While some cases are linked to genetic mutations, others have an unknown aetiology.
- **Microtia and Anotia:** These conditions involve underdeveloped or absent external ear structures. While some cases are attributed to genetic factors, others remain unexplained.
- **Bladder Exstrophy:** Bladder exstrophy is a congenital anomaly in which the bladder and sometimes other pelvic organs are exposed outside the abdominal wall. The cause of this condition is not fully understood.
- **Poland Syndrome:** Poland syndrome is characterized by the underdevelopment or absence of chest muscles and other associated anomalies. The exact cause is not clear, although it is believed to have both genetic and environmental components (Fig. 26.9).
- **Congenital Diaphragmatic Hernia (CDH):** CDH involves a hole or defect in the diaphragm, which allows abdominal organs to move into the chest cavity. While some cases are associated with known genetic syndromes, the cause for many remains unknown.

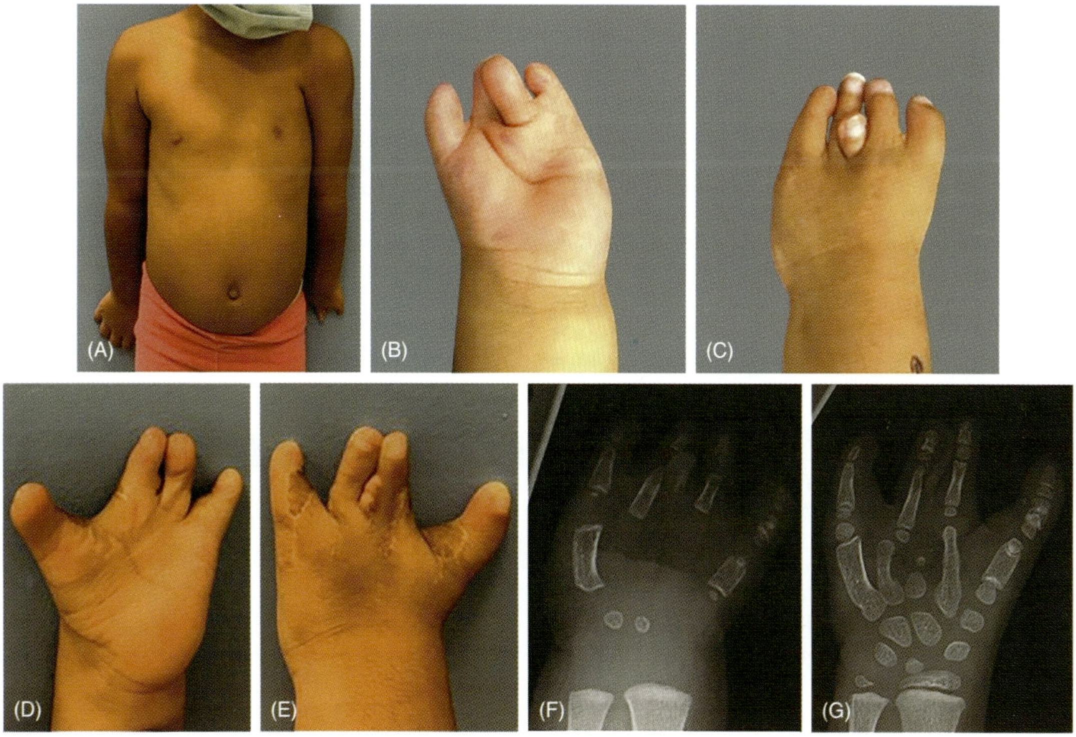

Fig. 26.9 Poland syndrome. (Source: *Plastic Surgery: Volume Six: Hand and Upper Extremity*, 5th ed.: James Chang, Fig. 33.3, Elsevier Inc., 2024.)

- **Prune Belly Syndrome:** Prune belly syndrome is a rare condition characterized by a lack of abdominal muscles, urinary tract anomalies and undescended testicles in males. The aetiology is not fully understood, and it is considered a complex condition with genetic and environmental factors (see Fig. 25.10).
- TeraTox's analysis of altered gene expression patterns may aid in grouping toxicologically similar compounds and potentially uncovering common modes of action.
- This innovative assay and the accompanying dataset serve as valuable resources for the assessment of drug teratogenicity.

KLINISCHE PERLEN

PREPLACENTAL EMBRYONIC TERATOGENICITY

- Here, teratogens act before the formation of the gestational sac and placenta. Placental biomarkers help evaluate direct, time-dependent teratogenic effects.
- Chronic exposure at conception directly affects early embryo development, allowing teratogenicity without placental transfer. This can impact the embryo's cell lineage determination, leading to effects on both embryonic and extraembryonic structures.
- Teratogenic outcomes may include limb wall defects, neural tube defects, gastroschisis and cleft palate.
- The **ADAM syndrome** demonstrates gestational sac pathology associated with environmental exposures. Detecting these effects in the first trimester often relies on circulating biomarkers originating from the embryo or placenta.
- **Alpha-fetoprotein (AFP)** is one such biomarker, capable of predicting spina bifida when elevated early in pregnancy, with malformations in early embryonic and extraembryonic structures influencing its presence.

TERATOX ASSAY

- To enhance sensitivity, researchers have introduced the TeraTox test, a novel multilineage differentiation assay utilizing **3D human-induced pluripotent stem cells**.
- TeraTox assesses primary output parameters like concentration-dependent cytotoxicity and altered gene expression induced by test compounds.
- These data are then processed by an interpretable machine-learning model to make predictions regarding the concentration-dependent human teratogenicity potential of drug candidates.

POINTS TO PONDER

The Principles of Teratology

First Principle:

- An embryonic structure is most susceptible to the effects of teratogens during specific **sensitive periods,** which typically coincide with phases of differentiation and morphogenesis.
- Therefore, a teratogen can influence embryonic development only if it is administered during these critical periods.
- As the major events of organogenesis take place within the first 8 weeks of development, this period is particularly vulnerable to teratogenic influences.

Second Principle:

- The impact of a teratogen on an embryonic structure is dependent on the **dose administered**.
- According to this principle, the lowest dose of a teratogen has no effect, while the highest dose can be lethal to the embryo.

Third Principle:

- The susceptibility to teratogens varies based on the **genetic makeup** of the embryo or foetus.
- When two embryos are exposed to the same dose of a teratogen, only one may be affected, influenced by its genetic constitution.
- This principle highlights the importance of genetic factors in determining susceptibility to teratogenic effects.

BRAIN TEASERS

1. During which stage of embryonic development is the foetus most vulnerable to teratogens?
   A. Third trimester
   B. Second trimester
   C. First trimester
   D. Postnatal stage
2. What is the primary function of the TeraTox test in drug development?
   A. Measuring drug concentration in blood.
   B. Assessing maternal health during pregnancy.
   C. Predicting human teratogenicity potential.
   D. Testing for genetic disorders in foetuses.

3. Which of the following is a birth defect that can result from nutritional excess during pregnancy?
   A. Intrauterine growth restriction (IUGR)
   B. Congenital heart defects
   C. Macrosomia
   D. Neural tube defects
4. What is the role of the first principle of teratology?
   A. Identifying genetic causes of birth defects.
   B. Determining the genetic constitution of the embryo.
   C. Defining the sensitive periods for teratogen exposure.
   D. Predicting the dose of teratogen required for an effect.
5. Maternal infection with rubella virus during pregnancy can lead to which of the following foetal anomalies?
   A. Neural tube defects
   B. Limb defects
   C. Cataracts and heart malformations
   D. Craniofacial abnormalities
6. What birth defect is associated with the exposure to thalidomide during pregnancy?
   A. Cleft palate
   B. Limb defects
   C. Heart malformations
   D. Clitoral hypertrophy
7. Maternal use of androgenic steroids during pregnancy can lead to which specific anomaly in female foetuses?
   A. Heart malformations
   B. Limb defects
   C. Cataracts
   D. Clitoral hypertrophy
8. Foetal exposure to radioiodine therapy is linked to what developmental issue?
   A. Thyroid deficiency
   B. Neural tube defects
   C. Craniofacial anomalies
   D. Limb malformations
9. Exposure to diazepam, a tranquilizer, during pregnancy is associated with which congenital issue in infants?
   A. Bone and tooth anomalies
   B. Limb defects
   C. Cleft lip
   D. Neural tube defects
10. The antibiotic tetracycline may lead to which types of anomalies in newborns?
    A. Limb and central nervous system malformations
    B. Heart defects
    C. Tooth and bone anomalies
    D. Cataracts and deafness

Answers

1. (C); 2. (C); 3. (C); 4. (C); 5. (C); 6. (B); 7. (D); 8. (A); 9. (C); 10. (C).

FURTHER READINGS

Adibi JJ, Layden AJ, Birru RL, et al. First trimester mechanisms of gestational sac placental and foetal teratogenicity: a framework for birth cohort studies. *Hum Reprod Update.* 2021;27(4):747-770. doi:10.1093/humupd/dmaa063.

Challa AP, Beam AL, Shen M, et al. Machine learning on drug-specific data to predict small molecule teratogenicity. *Reprod Toxicol.* 2020;95:148-158. doi:10.1016/j.reprotox.2020.05.004.

Jaklin M, Zhang JD, Schäfer N, et al. Optimization of the TeraTox assay for preclinical teratogenicity assessment. *Toxicol Sci.* 2022;188(1):17-33. doi:10.1093/toxsci/kfac046.

Marikawa Y, Chen HR, Menor M, Deng Y, Alarcon VB. Exposure-based assessment of chemical teratogenicity using morphogenetic aggregates of human embryonic stem cells. *Reprod Toxicol.* 2020;91:74-91. doi:10.1016/j.reprotox.2019.10.004.

27 Recent Advances in Embryology

ANAMNESE

A couple eagerly anticipating the arrival of their first child became apprehensive as complications surfaced during routine check-ups, causing an increased risk of preterm birth, even though the pregnancy had been progressing healthily. In the past, breakthroughs in embryology, including advanced genomic screening, genetic analysis and imaging technologies, played a major role in understanding factors contributing to preterm birth. In a research programme, a couple's embryonic development underwent close monitoring, revealing genetic markers associated with preterm birth risk. Researchers used **CRISPR-Cas9** for targeted intervention and continuous precision monitoring through wearable devices and AI provided real-time observations. Successfully identifying and modifying the genetic anomaly, the pregnancy progressed to full term, resulting in the birth of a healthy baby. This case highlighted the transformative impact of recent embryological advances in preventing preterm birth, the potential of personalized approaches for maternal and foetal health, offering hope to families facing pregnancy challenges (Fig. 27.1).

It is always interesting to go through the research work where the different aspects and clinical implications of embryology are unravelled. In this chapter, some of the handpicked researches are mentioned with the reference links for further reading.

1. On recent advances in **human engineering-provocative trends in embryology**, **genetics and regenerative medicine**.
   - Embryogenic methods are weaving into a new **'in vivitro' (in life in glass) fabric**.

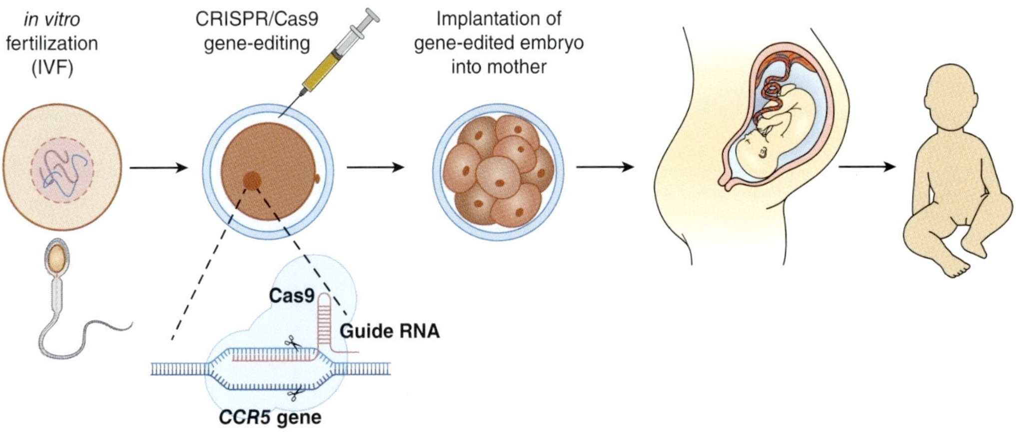

Fig. 27.1 CRISPR/Cas 9 gene editing.

- These methods known to be in use promise to bring society to choices and predicaments, to supply **rejuvenating stem** cells, to prevent, treat, cure or even someday eradicate diseases having genetic or epigenetic mechanisms.
- With humanity's human-engineering era now begun, procedural prohibitions, funding restrictions, institutional controls and transparency rules are proving ineffective.

2. **Horseshoe crab perivitelline fluid (PVF)** triggers the human bone marrow stem cell differentiation into **cardiomyocyte** in vitro.

- Advances in cardiomyocyte regeneration are being made in human embryonic stem cell research due to their ability to differentiate into any cell type in the adult body.
- **Embryonic stem cells** are another possible source for cardiac repair cells.
- Itskovitz-Eldor et al. demonstrated that human embryonic stem cells can reproducibly differentiate in culture into embryoid bodies made up of cell types of three embryonic germ layers.
- In the horseshoe crab embryo, the space between the inner egg membrane and embryo (called **perivitelline space**) is filled with a fluid which is known as the perivitelline fluid.
- The PVF of the fertilized eggs of the Indian horseshoe crab contains peptide(s) capable of positively influencing differentiations of specific organs.
- **PVF-8,** a fraction of PVF obtained from the fertilized eggs of the horseshoe crab helped in increasing the differentiation of CD 34+ stem cells into myocytes.
- It is concluded that PVF8 contains an active component enhancing the differentiation of stem cells in myocytes.
- This can have therapeutic application in ischaemic cardiomyopathy and vascular diseases.

3. Tumour suppressors and endodermal differentiation of **P19 embryonic stem cells**.

- The **P19 embryonic stem (ES)** cells are derivatives of the inner cell mass of a mouse blastoderm.
- They are **multipotent** and can give rise to all three germ layers.
- Depending on the nature of inducers, P19 ES cells differentiate into all three germ layers. This is used extensively to study early developmental events.
- **Dimethyl sulfoxide (DMSO)** treatment of P19 ES cell aggregates results in differentiation into cardiac- and skeletal muscle-like cells.
- **Retinoic acid (RA)** induces differentiation into neurons, glia and fibroblast-like cells.
- Understanding the mechanism by which the tumour suppressors are regulated by the morphogen, RA may prove useful in developing retinoid-based therapies for various diseases, especially cancer.

4. Bridging the gap: understanding **embryonic intervertebral disc (IVD)** development.

- The IVD development is a fundamental aspect of axial skeletogenesis in vertebrates.
- With the advent of technologies such as RNA-sequencing **(RNA-Seq),** chromatin immunoprecipitation sequencing **(ChIP-Seq)** and chromatin interaction analysis with paired-end tag sequencing **(ChIAPET),** it is apparent that innumerable factors (miRNAs, noncoding RNAs and cis-regulatory elements), other than genes, regulate the molecular mechanisms of developmental processes.
- By understanding the mechanisms in detail, we would be able to fine-tune the cell therapy process for Degenerative discs as well as for other diseases.

5. New advances in human embryology: morpho-functional relationship between the **embryo** and the **yolk sac**.

- During organogenesis, normal development depends on two factors: nutrition and a functional transport system for the distribution of nutrients and for waste disposal.
- **The yolk sac (YS),** a highly differentiated adnexal organ, is known to accomplish this fundamental task during early pregnancy.
- The endodermal cells are involved in the synthesis of numerous proteins which are transported by the bloodstream to the embryo.
- The mesothelial surface is provided with cell-surface differentiation that promotes a protective coat to prevent damage of the YS wall against the amnios, umbilical cord and chorionic cavity wall during growth.
- The mesenchyme is the main site for blood vessel formation.
- The **vitelline duct** is not functional after week 5 because of the closure of its lumen and hence its functional period of activity, and its possible role in the physiology of exchange during the embryonic period is assessed.

6. **New advances in human embryology: implications of the preimplantation diagnosis of genetic disease.**
- Embryos might be typed by noninvasive methods, by assessing their uptake of metabolites.
- The methods of diagnosis including enzyme assays and the use of DNA probes and the difficulties related to these techniques are debated in many articles.
- Certain embryological factors such as the high incidence of chromosomal imbalance and the problems of 'imprinting' might obscure certain diagnoses.

7. **Organoids and 3D Culture Systems:**
- The contemporary term 'organoid' describes cells cultivated in a controlled three-dimensional (3D) setting *in vitro*, giving rise to mini-clusters of cells that autonomously organize and differentiate into functional cell types. This process mimics the structure and function of an organ *in vivo*, earning organoids the alternative designation of **'mini-organs'**.
- Organoids can be generated from **embryonic stem cells (ESCs), induced pluripotent stem cells (iPSCs) or neonatal and adult stem cells (ASCs)**, mirroring the organizational process observed during the natural development of an organ (Fig. 27.2).

8. **Single-Cell Sequencing:**
- Advances in **single-cell RNA sequencing** techniques have allowed researchers to analyse gene expression at the single-cell level.
- This technology has provided insights into the heterogeneity of cell populations during embryonic development, allowing for a more detailed understanding of cell fate decisions.

9. **Gene Editing Technologies:**
- The development and refinement of gene editing tools, such as **CRISPR-Cas9**, have revolutionized the study of embryonic development.
- These tools enable precise manipulation of genes, allowing researchers to investigate the function of specific genes and understand their role in development.
- CRISPR holds the potential for direct application in patients, either *in vivo* or *ex vivo*, facilitating therapeutic gene editing.

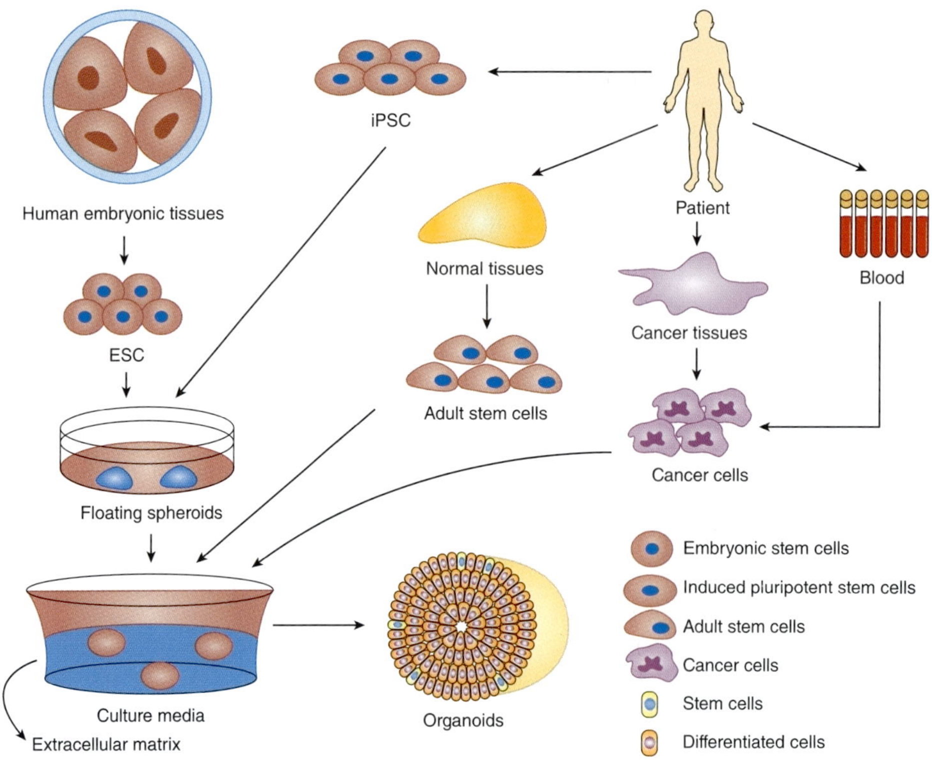

Fig. 27.2 Organoids and 3D culture systems.

- **In vivo** gene editing entails modifying genes directly within the organism, achieved by delivering CRISPR/Cas9 directly to the target cells.

10. Stem Cell Research:
- Stem cells, especially **iPSCs**, continue to be a focus of research in embryology.
- iPSCs can be differentiated into various cell types, providing a valuable resource for studying early embryonic development and potential therapeutic applications.

11. Synthetic Biology:
- The fundamental aspects of synthetic biology includes the creation of genetic material from scratch and an engineering-oriented methodology for designing components, organisms and products.
- This includes efforts to create **artificial embryos** and study the fundamental principles of embryonic development.

12. Epigenetics and Epitranscriptomics:
- Understanding the role of epigenetic modifications and RNA modifications in embryonic development is an active area of research.
- These modifications play crucial roles in regulating gene expression and cell fate determination.
- Neurodevelopment depends on temporal and spatial gene regulation, producing the diverse cellular subtypes observed in the adult mammalian brain.
- Epigenetic mechanisms, involving modifications to DNA, histone proteins and subsequent RNA, play an important role in guiding this gene expression diversity

13. In Utero Imaging:
- Advancements in imaging technologies, such as high-resolution ultrasound and advanced MRI techniques, have improved our ability to study embryonic development in utero.
- This provides a noninvasive way to monitor development and detect abnormalities.

14. Artificial Intelligence (AI) in Data Analysis:
- The increasing complexity of data generated in embryology research has led to the integration of AI and machine learning techniques for data analysis.
- The latest research on employing AI for embryo selection suggests that AI models exhibit superior performance in both embryo morphology assessments and predictions of reproductive outcomes compared to embryologists.
- It is important to note that reported accuracies in current studies vary due to differences in methods, sample sizes and datasets used for AI training and validation, emphasizing the need for standardized evaluation metrics.

FURTHER READINGS

Anton J. On recent advances in human engineering provocative trends in embryology, genetics, and regenerative medicine. *Politics Life Sci.* 2016;35(2): 54-78. doi:10.1017/pls.2016.17.

Alam H, Sumedha C, Pati S, Dash BP, Chatterji A. Horseshoe crab perivitelline fluid triggers the human bone marrow stem cell differentiation into cardiomyocyte in vitro. *Cell Dev Biol.* 2015;4:162. doi:10.4172/2168-9296.1000162.

Kanungo J. Tumor suppressors and endodermal differentiation of P19 embryonic stem cells. *Cell Dev Biol.* 2015;4:e138. doi:10.4172/2168-9296.1000e138.

Corrò C, Novellasdemunt L, Li VSW. A brief history of organoids. *Am J Physiol Cell Physiol.* 2020;319(1): C151-C165. doi:10.1152/ajpcell.00120.2020.

Wen L, Li G, Huang T, et al. Single-cell technologies: from research to application. *Innovation (Camb).* 2022;3(6):100342. doi:10.1016/j.xinn.2022.100342.

Dasgupta I, Flotte TR, Keeler AM. CRISPR/Cas-dependent and nuclease-free in vivo therapeutic gene editing. *Hum Gene Ther.* 2021;32(5-6):275-293. doi:10.1089/hum.2021.013.

Lendahl U. 100 plus years of stem cell research-20 years of ISSCR. *Stem Cell Rep.* 2022;17(6):1248-1267. doi: 10.1016/j.stemcr.2022.04.004.

Shapira P, Kwon S, Youtie J. Tracking the emergence of synthetic biology. *Scientometrics.* 2017;112(3):1439-1469. doi:10.1007/s11192-017-2452-5.

Mao N, Aggarwal N, Poh CL, et al. Future trends in synthetic biology in Asia. *Adv Genet (Hoboken).* 2021; 2(1):e10038. doi:10.1002/ggn2.10038.

Salih M, Austin C, Warty RR, et al. Embryo selection through artificial intelligence versus embryologists: a systematic review. *Hum Reprod Open.* 2023;2023(3): hoad031. doi:10.1093/hropen/hoad031.

Diakiw SM, Hall JMM, VerMilyea MD, et al. Development of an artificial intelligence model for predicting the likelihood of human embryo euploidy based on blastocyst images from multiple imaging systems during IVF. *Hum Reprod.* 2022;37(8):1746-1759. doi: 10.1093/humrep/deac131.

SECTION 5

GENETICS

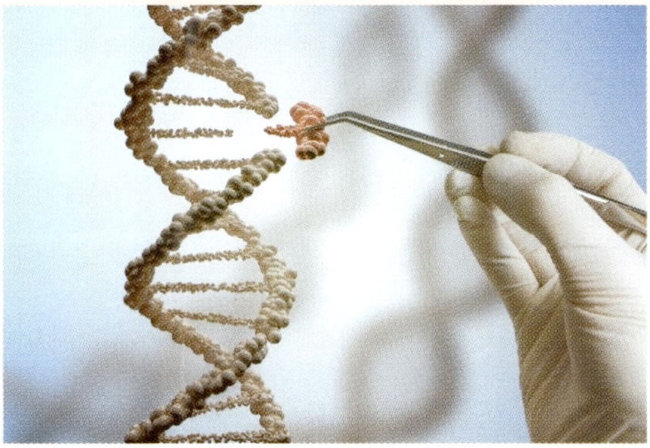

28 Medical Genetics

AN 73.1 Describe the structure of chromosomes with classification.

AN 73.2 Describe technique of karyotyping with its applications.

AN 73.3 Describe the Lyon's hypothesis.

AN 74.1 Describe the various modes of inheritance with examples.

AN 74.2 Draw pedigree charts for the various types of inheritance and give examples of diseases of each mode of inheritance.

AN 74.3 Describe multifactorial inheritance with examples.

AN 74.4 Describe the genetic basis and clinical features of achondroplasia, cystic fibrosis, vitamin D-resistant rickets, haemophilia, Duchenne's muscular dystrophy and sickle cell anaemia.

AN 75.1 Describe the structural and numerical chromosomal aberrations.

AN 75.2 Explain the terms mosaics and chimeras with example.

AN 75.3 Describe the genetic basis and clinical features of Prader-Willi syndrome, Edwards syndrome and Patau syndrome.

AN 75.4 Describe genetic basis of variation-polymorphism and mutation.

AN 75.5 Describe the principles of genetic counselling.

ANAMNESE

A 32-year-old female, gravida 2, para 1, was referred to the genetic counselling clinic due to recurrent pregnancy losses. The couple had experienced two consecutive spontaneous abortions during the first trimester. Given the unexplained nature of these losses, karyotyping was recommended to investigate potential chromosomal abnormalities. The karyotypic analysis revealed a **balanced translocation** involving chromosomes 5 and 14 in the mother. The presence of this translocation increased the risk of chromosomal imbalances in the offspring, contributing to the recurrent pregnancy losses. The couple was provided with genetic counselling, various reproductive options, including preimplantation genetic testing or prenatal diagnosis in future pregnancies to alleviate the risk of chromosomal anomalies.

STRUCTURE OF CHROMOSOME

(AN 73.1)

DNA STRUCTURE

- Deoxyribonucleic acid (DNA) serves as the genetic code passed from one generation to the next.
- DNA molecules consist of two linear chains of nucleotides, forming a double helix (Fig. 28.1).
- **James Watson** and **Francis Crick** introduced the double helix model in 1953.
- Histones wrap around DNA to create chromosomal structures.
- The nucleotide, the structural unit of DNA, consists of sugar, phosphate and a nitrogenous base.

Nitrogenous Bases:

- The nitrogenous bases are **Purines** (adenine (A), guanine (G)) and **Pyrimidines** (thymine (T), cytosine (C) and uracil (U)).
- DNA and RNA share adenine (A), guanine (G) and cytosine (C).
- **Thymine** (T) is unique to DNA, while **uracil** (U) is exclusive to RNA.

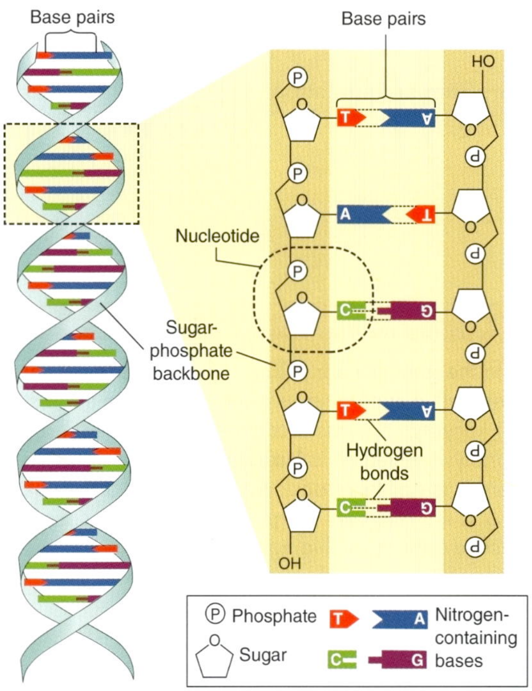

Fig. 28.1 Structure of DNA.

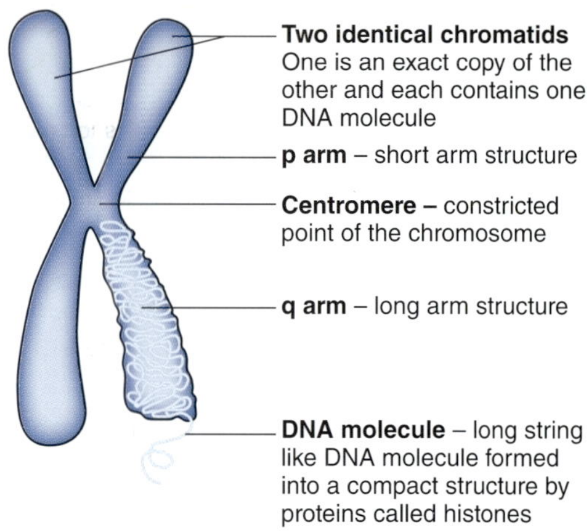

Fig. 28.2 Structure of a chromosome.

- Base pairing involves A with T (two hydrogen bonds) and G with C (three hydrogen bonds).

Nucleotide Chain:

- Phosphodiester bonds connect adjacent sugars, forming the nucleotide chain.
- The 5' end concludes with the 5' carbon of the sugar molecule, and the 3' end concludes with the 3' carbon.
- DNA strands lie antiparallel in the duplex.

Location of DNA and RNA:

- **RNA** is present in the cytoplasm and nucleolus.
- **DNA** primarily resides in chromosomes within the nucleus.
- The nuclear DNA quantity equals the total length of DNA in the chromosomes.

Coiling Levels of DNA:

- **Primary coiling** forms the DNA double helix.
- **Secondary coiling** involves histone-coiled nucleosomes.
- **Tertiary coiling** creates chromatin fibres, tightly coiled to form chromosomes (solenoid structure).

CHROMOSOME STRUCTURE

- Chromosomes consist of sister chromatids formed by DNA replication in the **S (synthesis) phase.**
- Sister chromatids are joined at the centromere, the **primary constriction** (Fig. 28.2).
- Chromosomes are divided into arms: **'p' (petite)** for the short arm and **'q' (grande)** for the long arm.

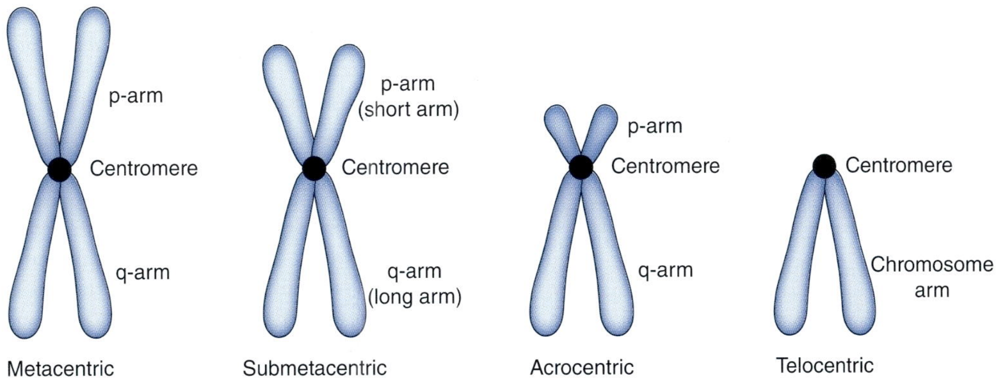

Fig. 28.3 Classification of chromosomes.

- There are **23 pairs** of chromosomes:
  - **22 pairs of autosomes.**
  - **1 pair of sex chromosomes (XX/XY).**

CHROMOSOMAL CLASSIFICATION

- Depending on the position of centromere, chromosomes are classified as follows (Fig. 28.3):
  A) **Metacentric chromosomes** have a central centromere, and both arms are of equal length (e.g. human chromosome 1 and 3).
  B) **Submetacentric** chromosomes have a slightly shifted centromere, resulting in asymmetry (e.g. human chromosomes 4–12 and X chromosome).
  C) **Acrocentric** chromosomes have a centromere away from the centre, with one long and one short arm (e.g. human chromosomes 13, 14, 15, 21 and 22 and Y chromosome). Stalk-like appendages known as **Satellites** that form the nucleolus of resting interphase cell are seen in Acrocentric chromosomes.
  D) **Telocentric** chromosomes have a centromere at the extreme end (not found in humans).

KARYOTYPING (AN 73.2)

- Karyotyping is a method used to examine chromosomes in a cell sample.
- Any living nucleated cell undergoing division is suitable for chromosome analysis.

Cell Selection and Preparation:
- **Circulating lymphocytes** from peripheral blood are frequently chosen for karyotyping.
- Other sources, such as skin cells, bone marrow cells, chorionic villi or amniotic fluid cells, can also be utilized.

Chromosome Arrangement:
- Chromosomes are arranged based on their **size**.
- The classification follows 22 pairs of autosomes, succeeded by the sex chromosomes X and Y at the end (Fig. 28.4).

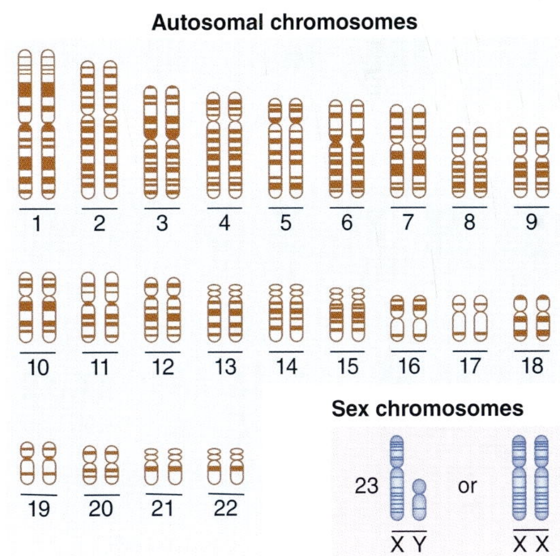

Fig. 28.4 Chromosome arrangement.

DENVER LONDON SYSTEM

- The Denver London system of classification (1960) is employed for organizing chromosomes.
- Chromosomes are categorized into **seven groups** labelled **A–G** (Fig. 28.5).
- The arrangement is according to decreasing length and centromere position. This systematic classification helps in the accurate analysis of chromosomal abnormalities and variations.

Group A: Chromosomes 1–3

- The **largest** pairs of chromosomes are seen in this group.
- The centromeres are located in the middle **(Metacentric)**.
- Chromosomes 1 and 2 have same length, but they differ in positions of centromere.
- Chromosome 1 has its centromere in the middle.
- **Chromosome 2** has its centromere slightly shifted towards the short arm **(Submetacentric)**.
- Chromosome 3 also has its centromere in the middle similar to chromosome 1, but it is shorter than chromosome 1.

Group B: Chromosomes 4 and 5

- They are large chromosomes with centromeres in the subterminal regions **(Submetacentric)**.

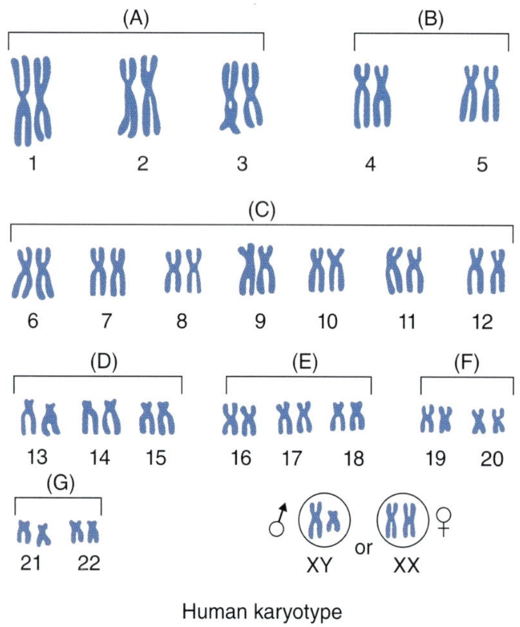

Fig. 28.5 Denver London classification of chromosomes.

- Chromosomes 4 and 5 are very much similar and hard to distinguish from each other.

Group C: Chromosomes 6–12 and X

- This group consists of **middle-sized** chromosomes.
- Since it contains **X chromosome,** males carry **15** group-C chromosomes, and females carry **16.**
- Centromeres are located either in the middle or subterminal regions **(Submetacentric)**.
- **Chromosome 6** is the largest among the group-C chromosomes.
- **Chromosome 12** is the smallest pair of chromosomes.

Group D: Chromosomes 13–15

- In this group, the centromeres are located terminally **(Acrocentric)**.
- The entire length of the chromosome corresponds to the short arm of chromosome 3.
- All the chromosomes bear an **'s' (satellite)** which may not be visible in each cell.

Group E: Chromosomes 16–18

- This group consists of chromosomes that are slightly smaller than group-D chromosomes **(Submetacentric)**.
- Chromosome 16 has the centromere near the middle.
- Chromosomes 17 and 18 have centromeres in more distal regions.

Group F: Chromosomes 19 and 20

- It consists of short chromosomes with their centromeres in the middle **(Metacentric)**.

Group G: Chromosomes 21, 22 and Y

- In this group, two pairs of autosomes are seen with an 's' at the end of every short arm and they are the smallest chromosomes and acrocentric.
- The Y chromosome may also contain an 's' and it is slightly longer than chromosomes 21 and 22.

SAT CHROMOSOMES

- In **acrocentric chromosomes** 13, 14, 15, 21 and 22, apart from centromere, there are secondary constrictions which separate a segment of chromosome from the rest of the chromosome. These segments are known as **satellite bodies** (Fig. 28.6).

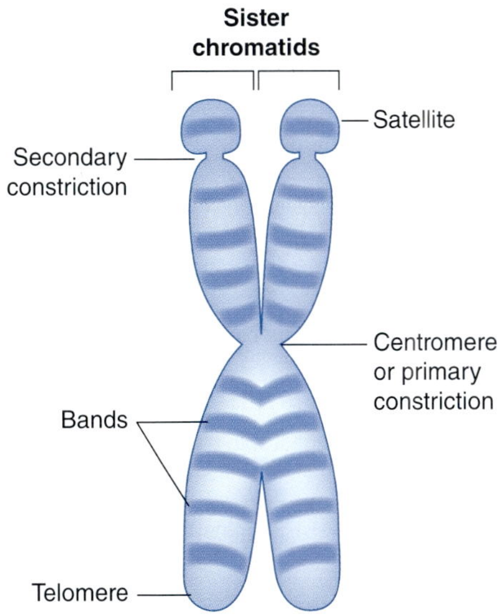

Fig. 28.6 Sat chromosome.

- The chromosomes which possess satellite bodies are known as **sat chromosomes.**
- For example, chromosome 13, 14, 15, 21 and 22.

TECHNIQUE OF CHROMOSOME PREPARATION

Selection of Tissue:

- Tissues commonly used for chromosome preparation include skin, bone marrow and peripheral blood (Fig. 28.7).
- For **foetal analysis**, amniocentesis or chorionic villi sampling is performed.

Chromosome Preparation From Peripheral Blood:

- Peripheral blood is commonly used for chromosome analysis.
- The process begins with the collection of **2 mL** of blood from a vein.
- The blood is heparinized, and **Phytohaemagglutinin (PHA)** is added to induce T-lymphocyte proliferation by mitosis. (Note: PHA is not used in bone marrow specimens because cells are visualized in interphase and there is no need of inducing cell division.)
- Mature erythrocytes are selectively sedimented.

Lymphocyte Incubation:

- Lymphocytes are incubated in culture media for **3 days at 37°C.**
- **RPMI 1640** (Rosewell Park Memorial Institute media) or **TC 199** is commonly used as culture media, with streptomycin and penicillin as preservatives.
- Carbon dioxide formed during incubation is released, and tubes are gently mixed every 24 hours.

Metaphase Chromosomes:

- In metaphase, chromosomes with their chromatids assemble around the centriole.
- **Colchicine** (0.01%) is added to the culture media at the **69th hour** and kept for 2 hours to arrest cell division at metaphase.
- Harvesting is done at the **71st hour**.

Centrifugation

- The culture tube is centrifuged at **1500–2000 RPM** for 10 minutes to collect cells.
- The supernatant is removed, and 5 mL of **KCl** is added, incubating for 4 ½ minutes to induce cell swelling and chromosome release.
- Centrifugation is repeated to remove the supernatant with red blood cells.

Fixation:

- 10 mL of fixative **(methanol and glacial acetic acid)** is added, and overnight fixation in the refrigerator is performed.
- Tubes are centrifuged until a **white pellet** forms.
- Fixative is added to the pellet according to its size to create a cell suspension.

Slide Mounting:

- The cell suspension is mounted on slides as drops and allowed to dry at room temperature.

STAINING

- In order to classify chromosomes, **Giemsa stain** is used conventionally.
- With the new banding technique, different stains are used to identify the different banding patterns in chromosomes.
- **Idiogram/karyogram** is the standard format of arranging photomicrographs of chromosomes.
- The different banding techniques are as follows:
  - **C-banding:**
    - This stains highly repetitive **DNA** sequences when the chromosomes are treated with **acid** and **alkali** before Giemsa staining.
  - **G-banding:**
    - Before Giemsa staining, the chromosomes are treated with **trypsin** which denatures the protein in it.

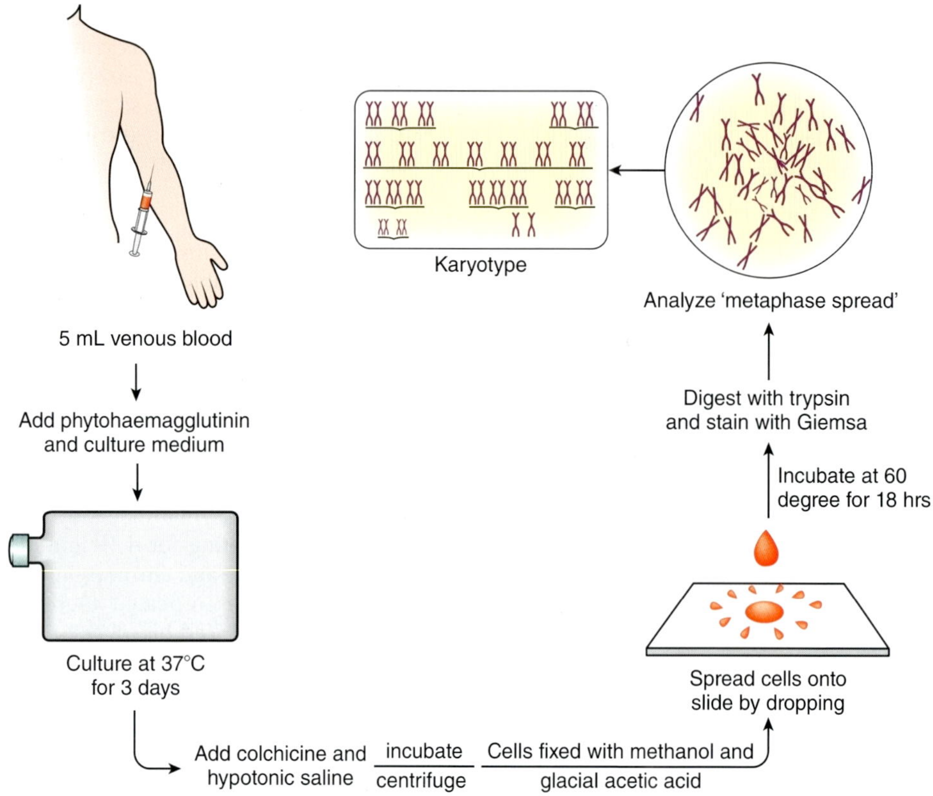

Fig. 28.7 Steps in karyotyping.

- Less protein is associated with A-T rich DNA.

- **R-banding:**
  - Prior to Giemsa staining, the chromosomes are **heated** to 87°C.
  - Here the interband regions are demonstrated which is just the **reverse** of G-banding.
- **Q-banding:**
  - In this, the chromosomes are stained with **quinacrine mustard.**
  - Q bands in A-T bases of DNA are seen as fluorescent regions under **Fluorescent microscopy**.

APPLICATIONS OF KARYOTYPING

Stillbirth and neonatal death:

- Chromosome abnormalities are much higher among stillbirths than live births.
- Chromosome analysis should be performed for all stillbirths and neonatal deaths to rule out a chromosome abnormality. In such cases, karyotyping is essential for **Genetic counselling**. (AN 75.5)
- Karyotyping provide important information for prenatal diagnosis in future pregnancies.

Mosaicism:

- In this condition, two or more different chromosome complements are present in an individual. It can be detected by karyotyping.
- A common cause of mosaicism is nondisjunction.
- For example, mosaic **Down syndrome** or mosaic **Turner syndrome.**

Down syndrome:

- Abnormal karyotype for Down syndrome has little effect on the phenotype of the patient but it is essential for determining the **recurrence risk**.

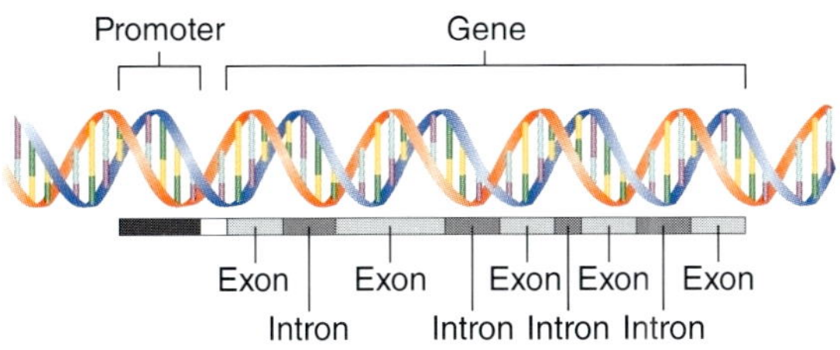

Fig. 28.8 Structure of a gene.

- In **translocation Down syndrome**, there is a high-recurrence risk in families when a parent is a carrier of the translocation.
- Hence, karyotyping of the parents and relatives is essential for providing genetic counselling.

Turner syndrome:

- It is not associated with advanced maternal or paternal age.
- The diagnosis is confirmed by karyotyping of chorionic villi or amniocytes before birth.
- If someone with Turner syndrome becomes pregnant, most of the offspring had congenital anomalies such as **congenital heart disease, Down syndrome** and **spina bifida.**

GENE

- A gene stands as the fundamental unit of DNA, the unit of inheritance.
- Coined by **Johannsen** in 1909, the term 'gene' signifies the core functional component in genetic information.

Gene Components

- Genes consists of coding sequences known as **exons** and noncoding sequences referred to as **introns** (Fig. 28.8).
- Exons contribute to the actualization of genetic instructions, while introns play regulatory roles.
- The nuclear genome harbours approximately **25,000–30,000 genes.**
- Surprisingly, this is just under **2%** of the entire genome devoted to encoding proteins in humans.

Chromosomal Disparities

- Chromosomes exhibit significant variations in gene density.
- Chromosomes 19 and 22 emerge as **gene-rich**, while chromosomes 4 and 18 are comparatively deficient in genes.

THE LYON'S HYPOTHESIS (AN 73.3)

- Formulated by **Dr Mary Lyon**, the Lyon hypothesis explains the process of X chromosome inactivation (Fig. 28.9).

Mosaic Nature of Women

- According to Lyon, normal women show mosaicism with respect to their two X chromosomes.
- Despite microscopic similarities in cells, Lyon presumes that during early embryonic development (day 12), **one X chromosome** in each cell of the female foetus becomes inactive.

Random Inactivation Process

- The inactivation process is random, with each cell independently determining which X chromosome becomes inactive.
- As a consequence, approximately half of the cells exhibit inactivation of the **maternal X** chromosome, while the **paternal X** chromosome is active, and vice versa for the remaining cells.

Singular X Chromosome in Men

- Men, possessing only one X chromosome, necessitate its functionality in every cell.

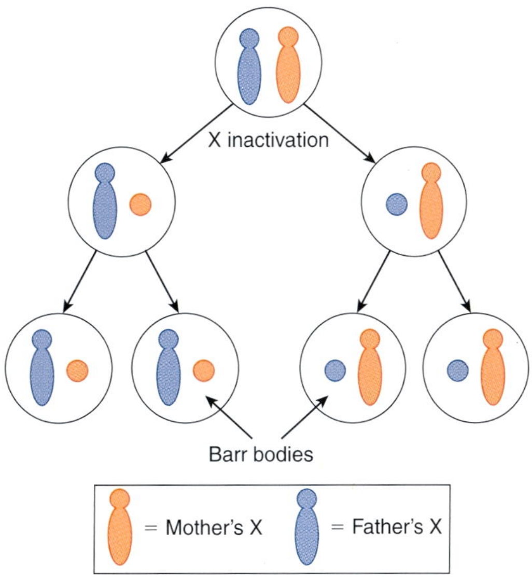

Fig. 28.9 X chromosome inactivation.

Autosomes

- An extra autosome leads to mental deficiency, while the absence of one is lethal.
- The dynamics change with the X chromosome.

X Chromosome Variations

- Contrary to autosomes, **XXX** individuals do not consistently exhibit mental deficiencies.
- The **Barr body**, a dark-staining mass inside the nuclear membrane of normal females, is indicative of X chromosome inactivation. The number of Barr bodies is always **one less than the total X chromosomes** present.

Tetraploid Cells and Barr Bodies

- In females with tetraploid cells (e.g. leukaemia), possessing four complete sets of chromosomes (eight X chromosomes), four Barr bodies can be observed. Each complete set of autosomes has one working X chromosome.

MODES OF INHERITANCE

(AN 74.1, AN 74.2, AN 74.3)

- The external appearance of a human being is called **Phenotype**. Phenotype is determined by his or her genotype.
- The genotype depends on the alleles received from the parents.
- More than **16,000 traits** in humans exhibit single gene or Mendelian inheritance, whereas certain characteristics like height and disorders like diabetes and hypertension do not follow this pattern of inheritance.
- Dominant or recessive traits are decided by the **alleles.**
- If only one copy of the allele is required for a trait to manifest, such traits are known as **Dominant trait**.
- If two copies of an allele are required, they are known as **Recessive**.
- If the allele for a particular trait is carried on the **X chromosome**, they are called **X-linked.**
- **Autosomal traits** are carried by alleles located on any chromosome other than the X or Y.
- **Punnett square** is used to determine the probability of producing a child with a particular trait (Fig. 28.10).
- **Pedigree** is a diagrammatic representation that allow individuals to visualize the modes of inheritance through their **family history** (Fig. 28.11).
- The common symbols used in pedigree are as follows:
  - **Squares**—males.
  - **Circles**—females.
  - **Shading**—a particular individual with the trait that is being studied in the pedigree.

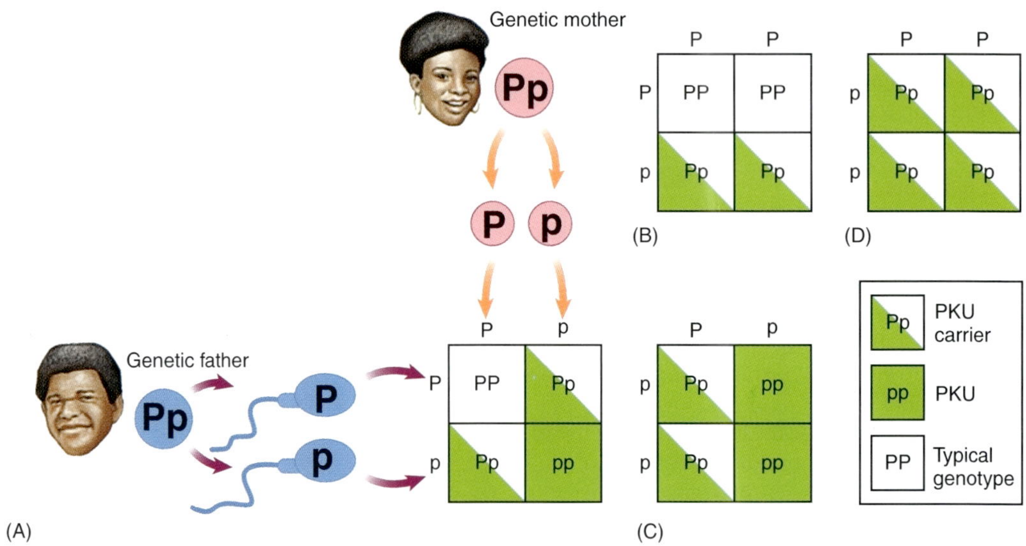

Fig. 28.10 Punnet square. (Source: *The Human Body in Health & Disease*, 8th ed.: Peggie Williamson, Terry Thompson, Frank Bell, et. al., Fig. 25-13, Elsevier Inc., 2024.)

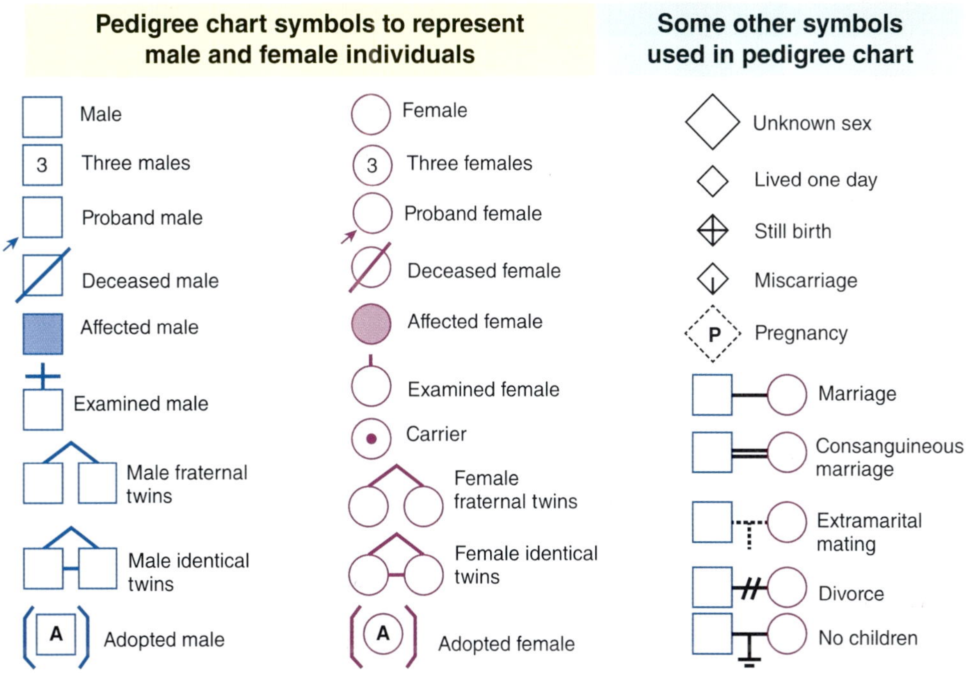

Fig. 28.11 Pedigree chart symbols.

- **A diagonal line** through an individual—family member is deceased.
- **A horizontal line** connecting two individuals—couple.
- **Parallel** branched line below the couple—offspring.

- Knowledge about mode of inheritance helps to predict whether a particular couple will have a child who inherits a particular condition.
- The transmission of a particular trait depends on whether the gene is on an autosome or on a sex chromosome, and whether it is recessive or dominant autosomal inheritance.

AUTOSOMAL DOMINANT INHERITANCE

- A trait can appear in **either sex** since an autosome carries the gene.
- A child receives the trait since at least one parent possess it (Fig. 28.12). Such traits do not skip generations.
- **Huntington** disease is an autosomal dominant condition. Other examples are **Marfan syndrome, Hereditary spherocytosis, Neurofibromatosis, Osteogenesis imperfecta, Achondroplasia** and **Tuberous sclerosis.**
- **Criteria for an autosomal dominant trait:**
  - Males and females can be affected **equally.**
  - **Male-to-male** transmission can occur.
  - Successive generations are affected.
- Transmission stops when no one inherits the mutation in a generation:

AUTOSOMAL RECESSIVE INHERITANCE

- Such traits can appear in **either sex**. Affected individuals have a **homozygous recessive** genotype (Fig. 28.13).
- Heterozygotes will act as **carriers**.
- If a couple has a child with an autosomal recessive illness, each of their next children faces the same **25% risk** of inheriting the condition.
- Autosomal recessive condition is seen in **consanguineous marriages** because the related parents may carry the same alleles from a common ancestor.
- **Sensorineural hearing impairment** is an autosomal recessive trait. Other examples are **Thalassaemia, Sickle cell anaemia, Cystic fibrosis, Albinism, Galactosaemia, Phenylketonuria, Homocystinuria** and **Alkaptonuria.**

Pathophysiology review

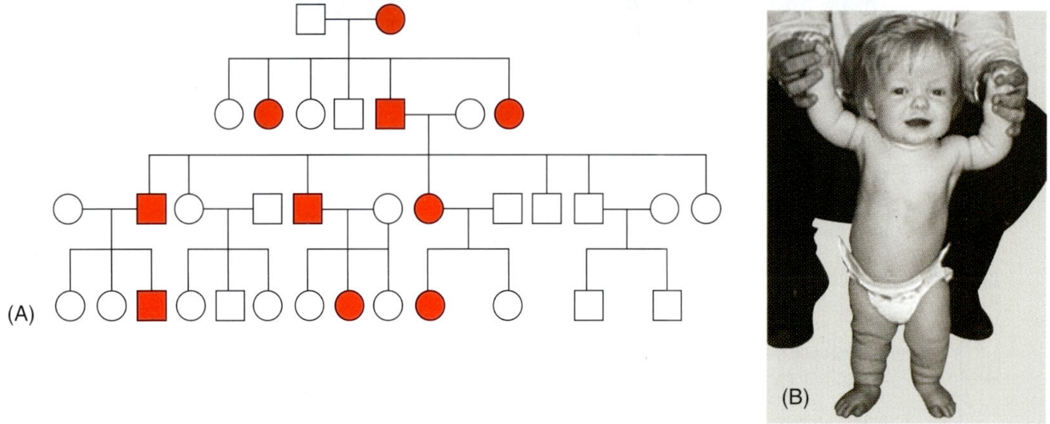

Fig. 28.12 Autosomal dominant inheritance. (Source: From Jorde, L. B., Carey, J. C., Bamshad, M. J., et al. [2003]. *Medical genetics* [3rd ed.]. St. Louis, MO: Mosby.)

- **Criteria for an autosomal recessive trait:**
  - Males and females can be affected in **equal** proportions.
  - Affected males and females **transmit** the gene.
  - The trait can **skip** generations.
  - Parents are heterozygous or have the trait.
  - Parents can be **consanguineous**.

SEX-LINKED INHERITANCE

- The genes for sex linked inheritance are located on the **sex chromosomes**.
- In **X-linked** inheritance genes are carried on the X chromosome and in **Y-linked** inheritance genes are carried on the Y chromosome.

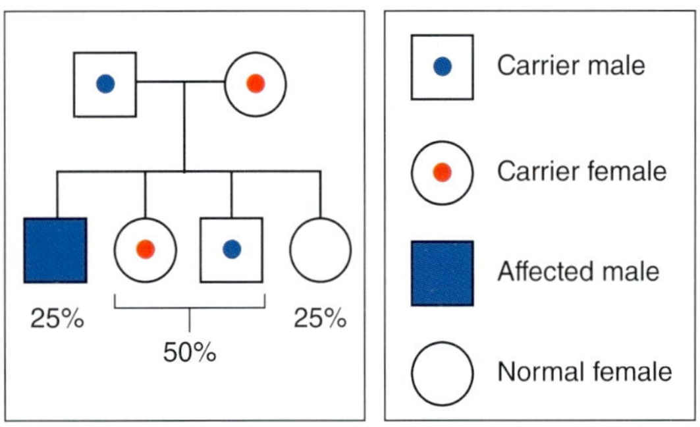

Fig. 28.13 Autosomal recessive inheritance.

X-linked recessive inheritance

- This type of inheritance is determined by a gene carried on the X chromosome (Fig. 28.14).
- It manifests only in **males**.
- Diseases are transmitted by heterozygous female carriers to affected males, and from affected males to their carrier daughters, thereby to male grandchildren through carrier daughters.
- The pedigree might show **'diagonal'** or a **'knight's move'** pattern of transmission.
- **Haemophilia, G-6-PD deficiency, Duchenne muscular dystrophy (DMD)** and **Colour blindness** are examples.
- **Criteria for X-linked recessive inheritance:**
  - **Only males** usually affected.
  - Transmitted through unaffected female carriers.
  - Males cannot transmit the trait to their sons (**no male-to-male** transmission).

X-linked dominant inheritance

- This has got some resemblance with autosomal dominant trait.
- Both the daughters and sons of an affected female have a **50%** chance of getting the disease (Fig. 28.15).
- But an **affected male** transmits the trait to all his daughters but not to his sons.
- Direct male-to-male transmission is also not possible.

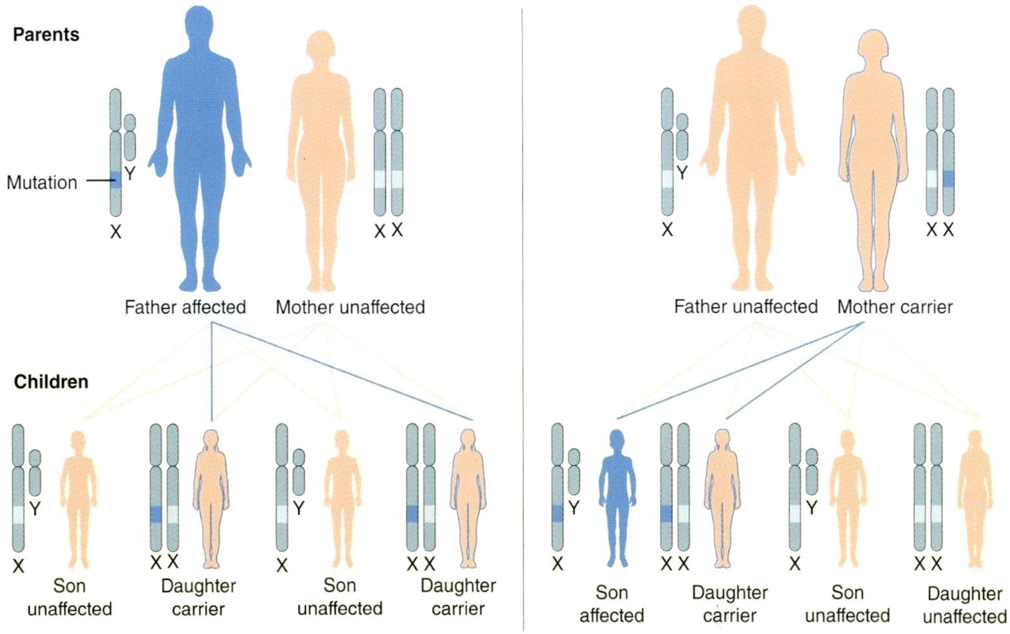

Fig. 28.14 X-linked recessive.

- For example, **Vitamin D-resistant rickets (X-linked hypophosphataemia), X-linked form of Charcot-Marie-Tooth disease.**
- **Criteria for X-linked dominant:**
  - Males and females affected but **females** are more affected than males though less severely.
  - Affected **males** transmit the disorder to their **daughters** but cannot transmit to sons.
  - Every person who is affected has **one parent** with the trait.

Y-Linked Inheritance (Holandric Inheritance)

- In this, **only males** are affected (Fig. 28.16).

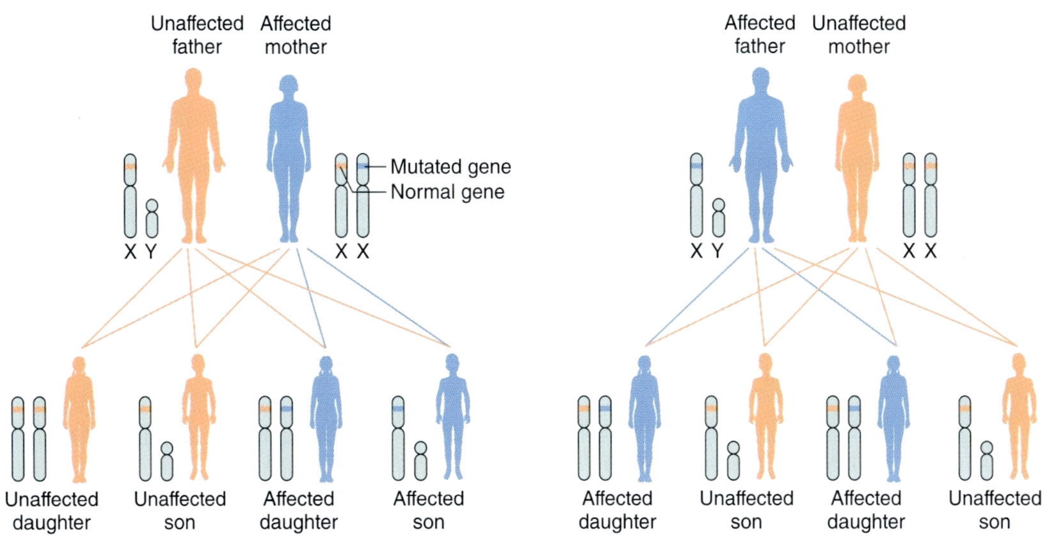

Fig. 28.15 X-linked dominant inheritance.

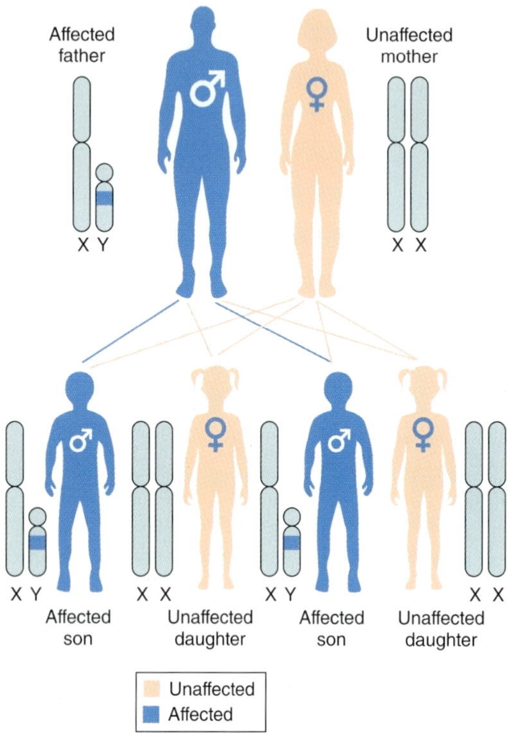

Fig. 28.16 Y-linked inheritance.

- An affected male can transmit the trait to **all his sons** but not to his daughters.
- For example, genes involved in **spermatogenesis** and **hairy ears** are carried on the Y chromosome.
- **Criteria for Y-linked inheritance:**
  - **Only males** are affected.
  - Males will transmit it to their **sons**.

MULTIFACTORIAL INHERITANCE (AN 74.3)

- Some of the common congenital and acquired disorders show **non-Mendelian** form of inheritance.
- These disorders are thought to be as a result of the interaction of **genetic** and **environmental factors**.
- Common birth defects like **neural tube defects, congenital heart disease, cleft lip and club foot** are believed to be inherited in a multifactorial fashion as threshold traits.
- These threshold traits are present only if a certain level of genetic liability and environmental exposure is reached.
- **Recurrence risks** in families are based on:
  - The disease **severity** (risk is higher for bilateral cleft lip than unilateral cleft lip).
  - The **degree of relationship** with the affected person.
  - The number of **close relatives** affected.
  - The **sex** of the affected case, if in case one sex is more commonly affected.
- These types of multifactorial disorders are **familial,** but pattern of inheritance is not clear.
- **Risk to first-degree relatives** is the square root of the population risk and risk is decreased for second-degree relatives.
- Some of the diseases with multifactorial inheritance are **diabetes mellitus, essential hypertension, coronary heart disease, cancer, cleft lip/palate, neural tube defects** and **congenital heart disease.**

ACHONDROPLASIA (AN 74.4)

- It arises from mutations which are **Autosomal dominant** (Fig. 28.12).
- Hence, if an individual with achondroplasia has a partner of average stature, there is **50% risk** for their offspring. But 80% of cases arise from **spontaneous mutations**.
- The mutations are seen in the fibroblast growth factor receptor type 3 **(FGFR3)** gene, and they tend to occur in offspring with **older fathers** (paternal origin),
- Achondroplasia is considered as one of the **RAMP** disorders: Recurrent, Autosomal dominant, Male biased, Paternal age effect disorders.
- **Assortative mating** means having a partner of same phenotype. In such cases, a **'double dose'** of the achondroplasia-causing mutation results in a severe condition.
- **Homozygous achondroplasia** is more **lethal** than heterozygous in the newborn period due to restrictive pulmonary disease and craniocervical junction constriction.
- If **both parents** have achondroplasia, offspring will be as follows:
  - Homozygous achondroplasia in **25%**.
  - Heterozygous achondroplasia in **50%**.
  - Normal stature in **25%**.
- Preimplantation diagnosis or prenatal diagnosis can rule out homozygosity.
- **Clinical features** include:
  - Small stature.
  - **Short limbs** with proximal shortening.

- **Macrocephaly** at birth.
- The anterior fontanelle persists to **5 or 6 years** of age.
- **Flattening** of the midface region—a flat nasal bridge, a short nasal spine due to defects in development of cartilaginous bone.
- Lumbar lordosis.
- Stiff elbow with limited extension.
- Short fingers.
- Hypermobile hips and knees.
- Hypotonia.

- Diagnostic confirmation is by **radiological assessment**.
- **SADDAN syndrome** is severe achondroplasia with developmental delay and acanthosis nigricans.

CYSTIC FIBROSIS

- It is caused by mutations in the gene encoding the cystic fibrosis transmembrane conductance regulator **(CFTR) on chromosome 7**.
- It is an **autosomal recessive** disorder.
- If two carrier parents conceive, the chance of homozygous child with cystic fibrosis is **1 in 4** for each pregnancy.
- **CFTR gene** regulates the transport of chloride ions across epithelial cell membranes in the lungs, gut, pancreas, etc.
- **Defective chloride transport** leads to the accumulation of mucus which in turn result in blockages and infections.
- Dehydration and mineral imbalances due to excess chloride output result in poor nutrition and growth.
- Antenatal foetal genetic testing by **Amniocentesis** or **Chorionic villus sampling** helps to determine whether the foetus is affected with 100% accuracy.

VITAMIN D RESISTANT RICKETS

- It is an **autosomal recessive** disorder.
- There is early onset of severe rickets with a triad of **clinical, skeletal and biochemical abnormalities**.
- Mutations in the **vitamin D receptor (VDR)** gene leads to partial or complete resistance to the action vitamin D3.
- **Vitamin D3** is the major stimulator for calcium absorption from intestine.
- Due to the lack of VDR signalling in the intestine, calcium absorption capacity is restricted and **Hypocalcaemia, Secondary hyperparathyroidism** and **Hypophosphataemia** develop.
- The clinical manifestations are similar to vitamin D deficiency rickets. Both types begin within the first year.
- The first symptom is **bowing** of the legs with shortening of stature.
- Cranial bossing and beading of the ribs may also be present.

HAEMOPHILIA

- Haemophilia A (classic haemophilia) is an X-linked bleeding disorder (Fig. 28.17).
- It is due to a mutation in the **Factor VIII gene** which is essential in the intrinsic coagulation pathway.
- It is the **most common** inherited bleeding disorders, with more incidence in **men**.
- Haemophilia B (Christmas disease) is due to deficiency in **Factor IX**.
- **Clinical conditions** have a wide range of presentation:
    - Haemarthrosis.
    - Intracranial bleeding with no major trauma.
    - Prolonged oozing of blood after tooth extractions or injury.
    - Unexplained GI bleeding or haematuria.
- **Haemophilia** can be classified as follows:
    - **Severe:**
        - Spontaneous bleeding occurs in first year of life.
    - **Moderately severe:**
        - Occasional spontaneous bleeding or severe bleeding with trauma before 5–6 years of age.
    - **Mild:**
        - Severe bleeding with major trauma or surgery usually presents later in life.
- **Prenatal diagnosis** of haemophilia A can be done by:
    - **Molecular genetic testing** by chorionic villus sampling or amniocentesis.
    - Percutaneous umbilical blood sampling **(PUBS)**.
    - Preimplantation genetic diagnosis **(PGD)**.
- **Gene therapy** can be platelet-based aiming at transport of clotting factors to vessel injury sites by platelets or intraarticular gene therapy in affected haemophilic joints.

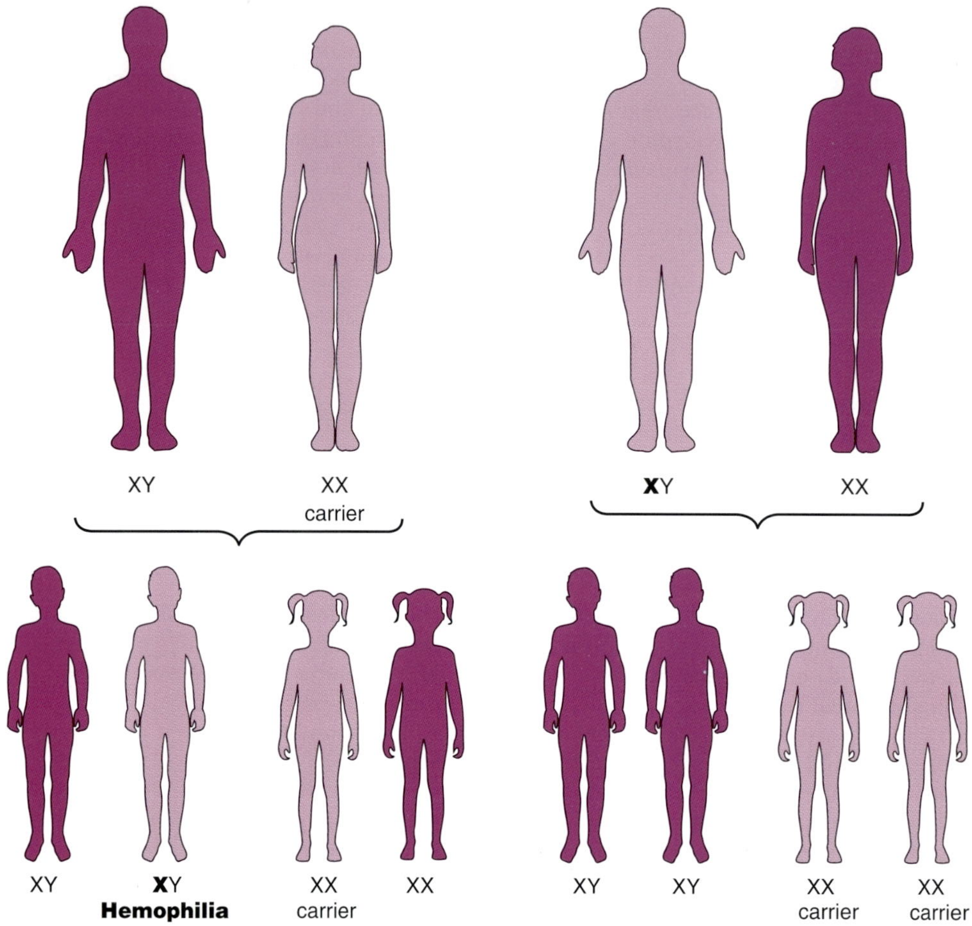

Fig. 28.17 Haemophilia inheritance. (Source: Atlas of Diagnostic Hematology: Marina Kremyanskaya, Mohamed Salama, Julie Teruya-Feldstein, Fig. 18.4, Elsevier Inc, 2021.)

DUCHENNE'S MUSCULAR DYSTROPHY

- DMD is an **X-linked recessive** disorder.
- It is caused by mutations in the dystrophin-encoding **DMD gene (largest known human gene)**.
- As a result of mutation, there is loss of function of dystrophin which is essential for proper **muscle contraction.** Thus, muscle fibres are easily damaged, leading to chronic muscle damage, inflammation and fibrosis.
- Young boys usually present with impaired muscle function, frequent falls and **Gower's sign**.
- Since it is a **progressive disease** and muscle loss is irreversible, disease-modifying treatments should be started as early as possible.

SICKLE CELL ANAEMIA

- Sickle cell anaemia is a **monogenic** disorder.
- It is caused by a **point mutation** in the **β-globin gene** (single base substitution A-T (β6Glu→Val)) that produces abnormal **haemoglobin S (Hb S)**.
- Homozygous individuals have the **Classical Sickle cell disease (SCD)** genotype.
- HbS polymerizes in the deoxygenated state causing sickling of erythrocytes which leads to vaso-occlusion and haemolysis.
- Sickle cell anaemia is an **Autosomal recessive** disease.
- If an individual gets only one copy of the defective gene, they do not have the disease but is called **'Sickle cell trait'**.

- Sickle cell trait usually do not present with any symptoms but they can pass the mutated gene onto their offspring.
- Three inheritance scenarios are as follows:
  - **Both parents** have sickle cell trait:
    - **25%** will have sickle cell anaemia.
    - **50%** may have sickle cell trait.
    - **25%** will not inherit the mutated gene.
  - **One parent has sickle cell anaemia** and the other has sickle cell trait:
    - **50%** will have sickle cell anaemia.
    - **50%** will have sickle cell trait.
  - **Both parents** have sickle cell anaemia:
    - Their children will definitely have the disease.
- Patients are present with severe pain, susceptibility to infection, end-organ damage and early mortality.
- **Allogeneic** haematopoietic **stem cell (HSC)** transplantation is considered as a curative treatment.
- **Diagnosis** is by:
  - **Electrophoresis** of haemoglobin.
  - Demonstration of **red cell sickling** at low-oxygen tensions.
  - **DNA tests.**

CHROMOSOMAL ABERRATIONS (AN 75.1)

- Chromosomal abnormalities can be classified as follows based on the abnormalities in number or structure of the chromosomes:
  - **Numerical:**
    i. Aneuploidy—Monosomy and Trisomy.
    ii. Polyploidy—Triploidy and Tetraploidy.
  - **Structural:**
    i. Translocations—Reciprocal and Robertsonian.
    ii. Deletions.
    iii. Insertions.
    iv. Inversions—Paracentric and Pericentric.
    v. Ring chromosomes.
    vi. Isochromosomes.
  - **Mixoploidy** (different cell lines)—Mosaicism and Chimerism.

NUMERICAL

i. **Aneuploidy**—It means the loss or gain of one or more chromosomes (Fig. 28.18).
  - **Monosomy**—a single chromosome is absent:
    - Monosomy for an **autosome** is incompatible with life.

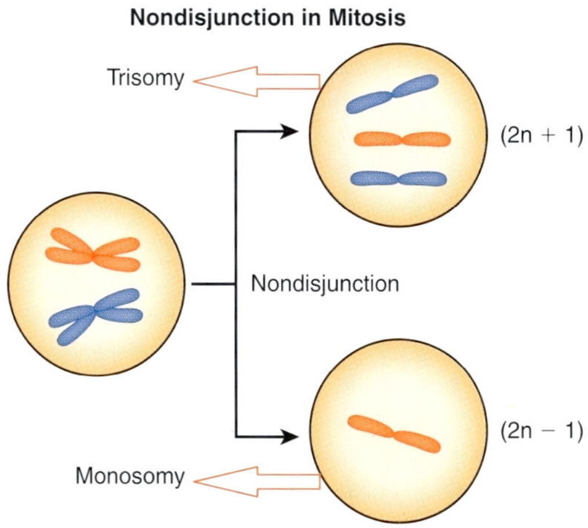

Fig. 28.18 Aneuploidy.

    - Absent X or Y chromosome results in a 45, X karyotype (**Turner** syndrome).
    - Monosomy can result from **nondisjunction** during meiosis.
    - As a result, one gamete receives two chromosomes **(disomy)** and the other receives none **(nullisomy).**
  - **Trisomy:**
    - In this condition, there will be an extra chromosome in addition to the normal number.
    - **Trisomy 21** means an additional number 21 chromosome due to nondisjunction and that condition is known as **Down syndrome**.
    - **Patau syndrome** is trisomy 13.
    - **Edwards syndrome** is trisomy 18.

ii. **Polyploidy**—it means having multiples of the haploid number of chromosomes:
  - In **triploidy** there will be **69 chromosomes** and they usually would not survive beyond second trimester.
  - Triploidy can be due to retention of a **polar body** or due to formation of a **diploid sperm.**
  - It can also be caused by fertilization of an ovum by **two sperms** in case of dispermy.
  - In tetraploidy there will be **92 chromosomes**.

STRUCTURAL

i. **Translocations**—It refers to the transfer of genetic material from one chromosome to another (Fig. 28.19).
  - **Reciprocal translocation**—when a break occurs in two chromosomes, the segments are exchanged between them to form new

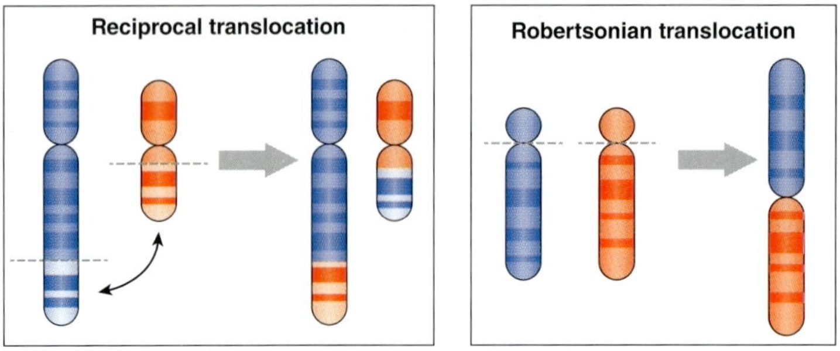

Fig. 28.19 Translocation.

chromosomes. Translocation between **11 and 22** is commonly seen.

- **Robertsonian translocation**—it is a type of reciprocal translocation where breakpoints are seen close to the centromeres of two **acrocentric** chromosomes **(13, 14, 15, 21 and 22)**.
  - ➢ As a result, the long arm of chromosomes fuse and short arms of each chromosomes are lost.
  - ➢ The chromosome number is reduced to **45** but since there is no loss or gain of important genetic material, hence it is functionally normal.
  - ➢ The most common Robertsonian translocation is between the long arms of **chromosomes 13** and **14**.
- **Translocation Down syndrome:**
  - ➢ Occurs as a result of the embryo inheriting two normal number of 21 chromosomes from each parent along with a translocation chromosome involving a number 21 chromosome.
  - ➢ It is a case of **Robertsonian** translocation.
  - ➢ There is no difference in the pattern of clinical presentation compared to pure trisomy 21.
  - ➢ But if the parents carry the balanced translocation, there is high risk of having further affected children.
  - ➢ Hence translocation tracing is done to identify **adult translocation carriers** in a family to avoid risks to future offspring.

ii. **Deletions**—this involves loss of part of a chromosome (Fig. 28.20).

- Large deletions are incompatible with life and can be visualized under light microscope.

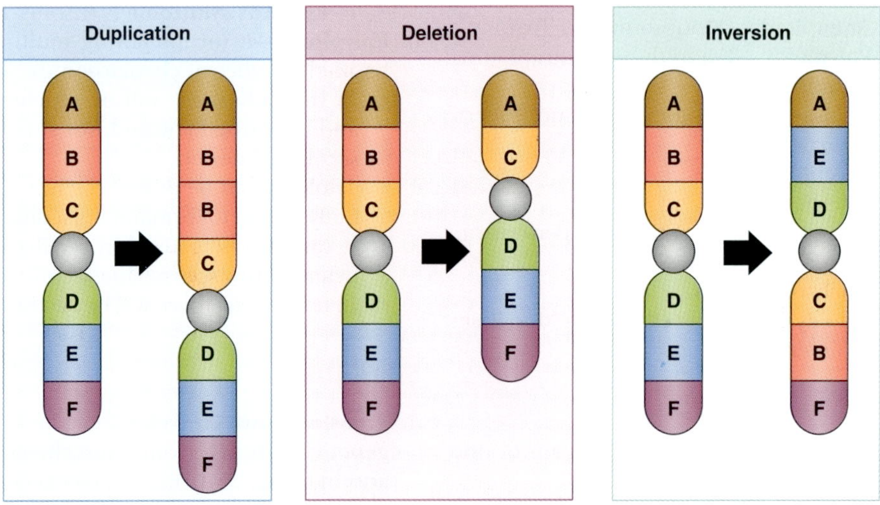

Fig. 28.20 Deletion, duplication, inversion.

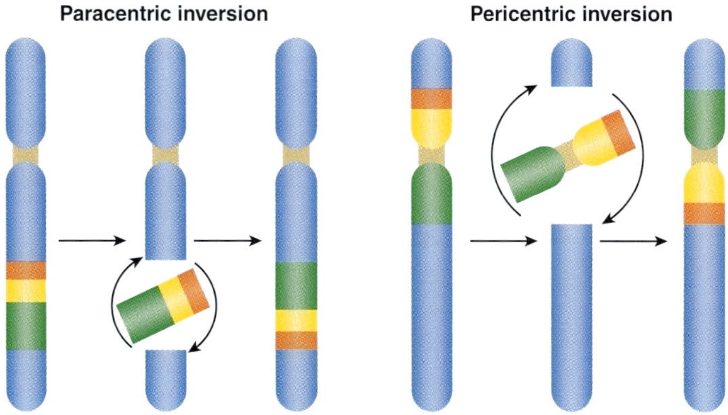

Fig. 28.21 Inversion.

- For example, in **Cri-du chat syndrome**, the short arm of **chromosome 5** is lost.
- Submicroscopic microdeletions include **Angelman syndrome** and **Prader-Willi syndrome.**

iii. **Insertion**—in this, a segment of one chromosome becomes inserted into another chromosome.

iv. **Inversion**—it involves a single chromosome in which a segment is reversed in position (Fig. 28.20).
- In **Pericentric inversion,** the inversion segment involves the centromere (Fig. 28.21).
- In **Paracentric inversion,** only one arm of the chromosome is involved.
- Since inversions are usually balanced rearrangements not involving any important genes, they rarely cause problems.

v. **Ring chromosomes**—when a break occurs on each arm of a chromosome, the two **'sticky'** ends reunite as a ring.
- The distal chromosomal fragments are lost and hence dangerous if autosomes are involved chromosome (Fig. 28.22).

vi. **Isochromosome**—in this type, there is duplication of one arm with the loss of the other.
- This happens when the centromere has divided **transversely** rather than the usual longitudinal division (Fig. 28.23).
- In **Turners syndrome,** isochromosome consists of two long arms of the X chromosome.

vii. **Duplication.**
- Chromosome duplications result in extra copies of a chromosomal region, which leads to different copies of genes within that area of the chromosome.
- Distal trisomy 14q is an example of duplication.

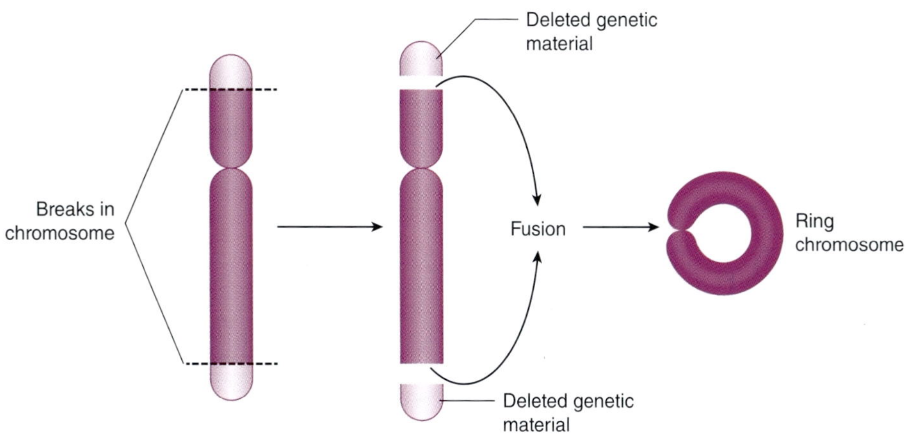

Fig. 28.22 Ring chromosome.

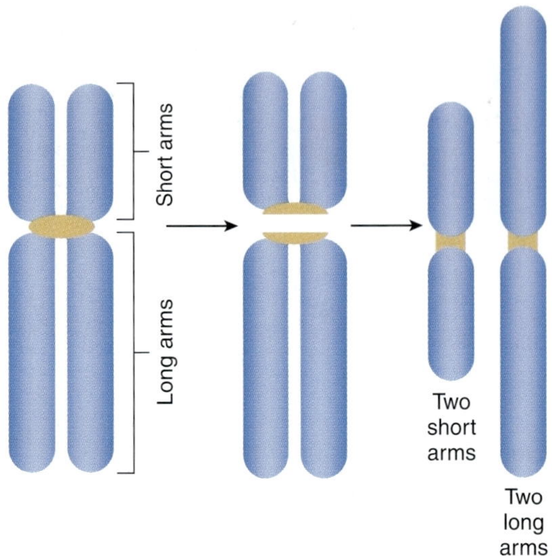

Fig. 28.23 Isochromosomes.

MIXOPLOIDY (AN 75.2)

Mosaicism:

- In this, a zygote gives rise to two or more cell lines that differ in their genetic constitution.
- It usually results from nondisjunction during embryonic mitotic division.
- In mosaic **Down** syndrome, some cells have two 21 chromosomes where as others have three.

Chimerism:

- In this type, an individual possesses two or more **genetically dissimilar cell lines** from more than one zygote.
- There are two types of human chimeras:
  - **Dispermic chimeras** are born when **two different sperms fertilize two ova.** The two zygotes thus formed fuse to form an embryo. If the zygotes are of different sex, it results in **true hermaphroditism**.
  - **Blood chimeras** occur as a result of exchange of cells between nonidentical twins through placenta in utero. As a result, **90%** of cells of **one twin** will have **blood group B,** whereas **90%** of the cells of the **other twin** will have blood **group A**.

CLINICAL NUGGETS

Klinefelter syndrome

- Men are born with an extra chromosome **(47,XXY).**
- The characteristic features are:
  - Tall with long arms and legs.
  - Poor muscle tone.
  - Reduced facial and body hair.
  - Small penis and testes.
  - Enlarged breasts (gynaecomastia).
  - Infertility.

GENOMIC IMPRINTING

- It is an epigenetic phenomenon. It was originally thought that the genes on chromosomes were equally expressed.
- But now it is recognized that different clinical features can result depending on whether a gene is inherited from the **father or the mother**. This happens due to **methylation of DNA** and this process is known as genomic imprinting.
- **Prader-Willi** and **Angelman syndromes (Chromosome 15q)** and **Beckwith-Wiedemann** and **Russel-Silver syndromes** are examples for genomic imprinting.

PRADER-WILLI SYNDROME (AN 75.3)

- Prader-Willi syndrome is caused by an absence of expression of imprinted genes in the **paternally derived region (i.e. 15q11.2-q13)** of chromosome 15 by one of several genetic mechanisms (paternal deletion, maternal uniparental disomy 15 and rarely an imprinting defect) (Fig. 28.24).
- Prader-Willi syndrome present with (code-**HHOS**):
  - **H**ypotonia.
  - **H**ypogonadism.
  - **O**besity.
  - **S**evere intellectual disability.

ANGELMAN SYNDROME

- Angelman syndrome results from deletion or mutation within **maternal chromosome 15q11-q13**.
- Angelman syndrome present with (code-**SAPI**) (Fig. 28.24):
  - **S**eizures.
  - **A**phasia.
  - **P**aroxysms of laughter.
  - **I**ntellectual disability.

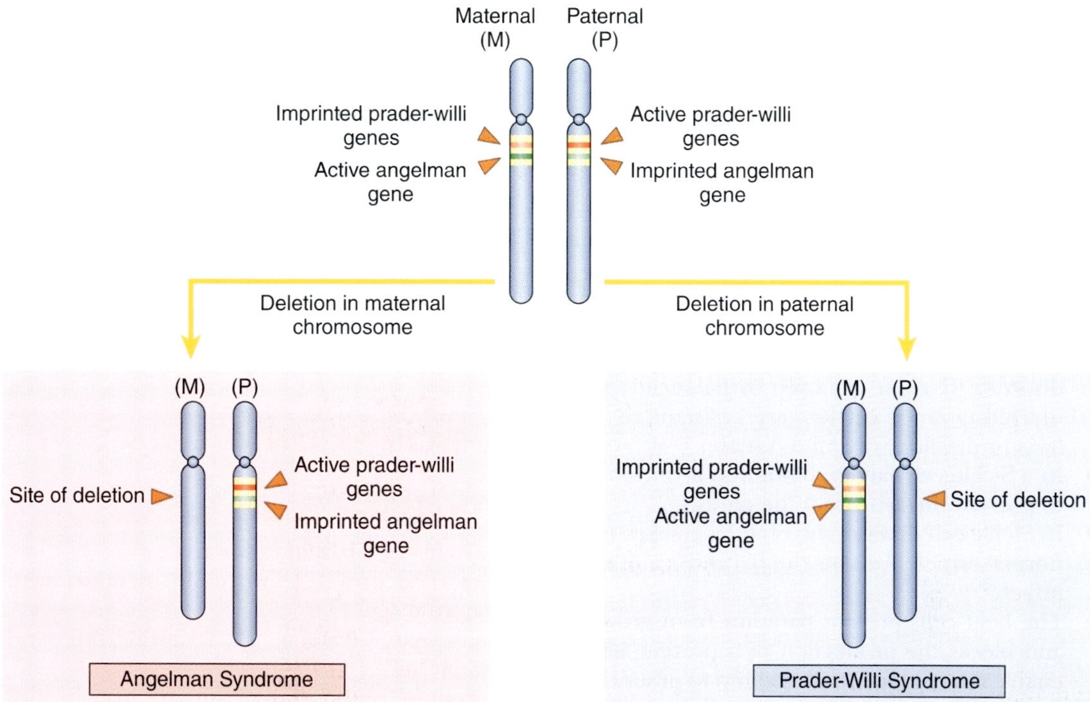

Fig. 28.24 Genomic imprinting. (Source: Robbins & Kumar Basic Pathology, 11th ed.: Abhijit Das, Abul K. Abbas, Andrea T. Deyrup, et. al., Fig. 4.24, Elsevier Inc. 2023.)

CLINICAL NUGGETS

Edwards syndrome

- Edwards syndrome is due to **trisomy 18** and the karyotype will be either **47,XX, + 18 or 47,XY, + 18**.
- The clinical conditions will be very severe with poor prognosis.
- There will be **severe learning difficulties** and **cardiac abnormalities** in the long run though death ensues before **1 year** of age in more than 50% of cases.
- Main reason is **advanced maternal age,** the additional chromosome usually of maternal origin.
- Microcephaly, elongated skull with prominent occiput, low-set ears, micrognathia, **rocker bottom feet** and prenatal growth deficiency are usually seen associated with this syndrome.
- Diaphragmatic hernia, omphalocele, spina bifida requires immediate attention.

Patau syndrome

- Patau syndrome is due to **trisomy 13** and the karyotype is either **47,XX, + 13 or 47,XY, + 13**.
- The clinical conditions will be very severe with poor prognosis as in case of Edwards syndrome.
- There will be severe learning difficulties and cardiac abnormalities in the long run but death ensues before **3 years of age** in more than 50% of cases.
- Main reason is advanced maternal age, the additional chromosome usually of **maternal origin**.
- Microcephaly, micrognathia, microphthalmia, polydactyly, rocker bottom feet, midline malformations and seizures are the usual presentations.
- All boys present with **undescended testis**.

POLYMORPHISM AND MUTATION (AN 75.4)

POLYMORPHISM

- This refers to a group of genetic variants like **blood groups** which occur in the population without causing any major health concerns.
- Genetic polymorphism means multiple **alleles at a locus** and at least two occurs at greater frequencies.
- Polymorphisms provide **markers** for diseases.

- For example, Single nucleotide polymorphisms **(SNPs),** microsatellites, Restriction fragment length polymorphisms **(RFLPs)** and minisatellites.

BALANCED POLYMORPHISM

- Means the protective effect of noninherited condition counters the negative effect of the deleterious allele.
- It generally refers to **maintaining heterozygotes** in a population.
- **Sickle cell disease** is an autosomal recessive disorder. It is an example of balanced polymorphism since carriers are resistant to **Malaria** or develop very mild disease.
- In a **Sickle cell carrier,** blood has atypical cells to prevent the actions of the parasite.
- In **Sickle cell disease,** the blood is thicker than normal, which prevents the parasite's ability to infect.
- The bent cells prevent parasites from growing and blocks the production of a protein which enable the red blood cells to bind to other cells, resulting in the spreading of the infection.

MUTATION

- DNA will be subjected to a variety of changes on exposure to harmful agents like X-rays and this process we call as mutation.
- Steps in the transmission of genetic information include:
  - **Replication** (DNA makes DNA).
  - **Transcription** (DNA makes RNA).
  - **RNA processing**.
  - **Translation** (RNA makes protein).
  - **Protein transport** and incorporation.
- If the DNA sequence is mutated, subsequent replications reproduce the mutation.
- The mechanisms causing mutations range from a single nucleotide alteration to the loss or rearrangement of chromosomes.
- Some mutations will cause proliferations of cells and ultimately result in cancer. If such mutations run in families, they are at higher risk of having the disease.
- The different methods to detect mutation are:
  - **Cytogenetics**—Karyotyping, FISH (fluorescence in situ hybridization), CGH (comparative genomic hybridization).
  - **Molecular genetics**—RFLP (restriction fragment length polymorphism), PCR (polymerase chain reaction), RT (reverse transcriptase), OLA (oligonucleotide ligation assay).

KLINISCHE PERLEN

DOWN SYNDROME

- It occurs in **1 in 800** newborns.
- The chance of a Down child increases with **maternal age**.
- Causes are **Trisomy 21, Translocation** and **Mosaicism**.
- Trisomy 21 and mosaicism are usually not inherited but **translocation** Down syndrome can be **inherited**.
- The clinical features include low muscle tone, short stature, a flat nasal bridge, a protruding tongue and learning disability.
- There is **increased risk** of developing Alzheimer's disease, congenital heart disease, childhood leukaemia, etc.
- **Screening tests done are:**
  1) **Nuchal translucency testing:** Ultrasound at 11–14 weeks.
  2) **Triple screen or quadruple screen:** at 15–18 weeks.
- **Diagnostic tests include:**
  1) **Chorionic villus sampling:** at 8–12 weeks.
  2) **Amniocentesis:** at 15–20 weeks.
  3) **Percutaneous umbilical blood sampling:** after 20 weeks (Fig. 28.25).

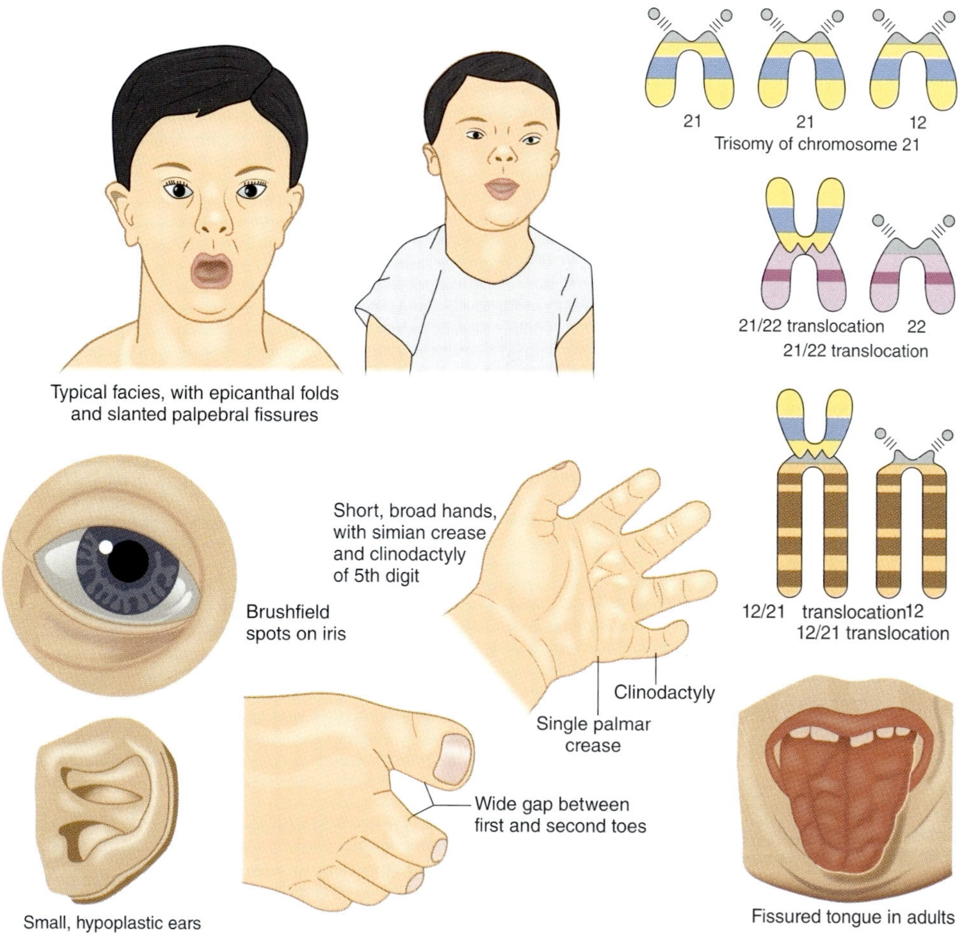

Fig. 28.25 Down syndrome.

BRAIN TEASERS

1. What is the genetic material transferred from one generation to another?
   A. Ribonucleic acid (RNA)
   B. Deoxyribonucleic acid (DNA)
   C. Histones
   D. Chromosomes
2. What are the two parts into which a chromosome is divided?
   A. Helices
   B. Strands
   C. Arms
   D. Fibres
3. What is the short arm of a chromosome called?
   A. q arm
   B. p arm
   C. Centromere
   D. Telomere
4. Which chromosomes have centromere at the extreme end?
   A. Metacentric
   B. Submetacentric
   C. Acrocentric
   D. Telocentric
5. What is the technique used to examine chromosomes in a given sample of cells?
   A. Gene mapping
   B. Chromosome pairing
   C. Karyotyping
   D. Chromatography
6. Which staining technique is used conventionally to classify chromosomes?
   A. C-banding
   B. G-banding
   C. R-banding
   D. Q-banding

7. In karyotyping, which group includes chromosomes 1 to 3?
   A. Group A
   B. Group B
   C. Group C
   D. Group D
8. What is the purpose of adding colchicine in chromosome preparation?
   A. Stain chromosomes
   B. Arrest cell division
   C. Induce cell division
   D. Enhance chromosome visibility
9. In autosomal dominant inheritance, which criteria are true?
   A. Males and females can be affected equally.
   B. Male-to-male transmission can occur.
   C. Successive generations are affected.
   D. All of the above.
10. Which trait has a 25% risk for each child in autosomal recessive inheritance?
    A. Huntington disease
    B. Thalassaemia
    C. Marfan syndrome
    D. Achondroplasia
11. What is the purpose of a pedigree in genetics?
    A. Stain chromosomes
    B. Arrest cell division
    C. Visualize modes of inheritance
    D. Enhance chromosome visibility
12. What is the primary cause of Angelman syndrome?
    A. Deletion or mutation within paternal chromosome 15q11-q13.
    B. Deletion or mutation within maternal chromosome 15q11-q13.
    C. Trisomy 21.
    D. Autosomal recessive mutation.
13. Which of the following is not a characteristic feature of Angelman syndrome?
    A. Seizures
    B. Aphasia
    C. Paroxysms of laughter
    D. Hemiplegia
14. Which syndrome is associated with microcephaly, elongated skull, low-set ears and rocker bottom feet?
    A. Angelman syndrome
    B. Edwards syndrome
    C. Patau syndrome
    D. Down syndrome
15. Which genetic variant occurs in the population without causing major health concerns?
    A. Mutation
    B. Monomorphism
    C. Polymorphism
    D. Trisomy
16. What does SNP stand for in genetic polymorphism?
    A. Single nucleotide polarity
    B. Single nucleotide polymorphism
    C. Simple nucleotide polymer
    D. Systematic nucleotide pool
17. What is the term for multiple alleles at a locus occurring at greater frequencies in the population?
    A. Monomorphism
    B. Polymorphism
    C. Mutation
    D. Hybridization
18. Which of the following is an example of genetic polymorphism?
    A. Haemophilia
    B. Sickle cell anaemia
    C. Blood groups
    D. Cystic fibrosis
19. What type of polymorphism provides markers for diseases?
    A. RFLPs
    B. Monosomy
    C. Aneuploidy
    D. Trisomy

Answers

1. (B); 2. (C); 3. (B); 4. (D); 5. (C); 6. (B); 7. (A); 8. (B); 9. (D); 10. (B); 11. (C); 12. (B); 13. (D); 14. (B); 15. (C); 16. (B); 17. (B); 18. (C); 19. (A).

FURTHER READINGS

Nicolescu RC, Lombet J, Cavalier E. Vitamin D-resistant rickets and cinacalcet—one more favorable experience. *Front Pediatr.* 2018;6:376. doi:10.3389/fped.2018.00376.

Aartsma-Rus A, Ginjaar IB, Bushby K. The importance of genetic diagnosis for Duchenne muscular dystrophy. *J Med Genet.* 2016;53:145-151.

Awa AA. *Biodosimetry of Human Exposure to Radiation: A Manual for Detecting Stable Chromosome Aberrations by the Conventional Giemsa Staining Method.* RERF; 2019.

Hoban MD, Orkin SH, Bauer DE. Genetic treatment of a molecular disorder: gene therapy approaches to sickle cell disease. *Blood.* 2016;127(7):839-848. doi:10.1182/blood-2015-09-618587.

Konkle BA, Huston H, Fletcher NS. Hemophilia B. In: Adam MP, Ardinger HH, Pagon RA, et al., eds. *GeneReviews®.* Seattle, WA: University of Washington; 1993–2019. https://www.ncbi.nlm.nih.gov/books/NBK1495/.

Pauli RM. Achondroplasia: a comprehensive clinical review. *Orphanet J Rare Dis.* 2019;14:1. doi:10.1186/s13023-018-0972-6.

Genetic Counselling

29

AN 75.5 Describe the principles of genetic counselling.

ANAMNESE

A couple, both carriers of an autosomal recessive genetic disorder, sought genetic counselling due to concerns about the potential risk to their offspring. Through karyotyping and genetic testing, it was confirmed that they both carried a mutation associated with the disorder. The genetic counsellor explained the 25% risk of having an affected child with each pregnancy. They were also informed about the option of prenatal testing for early diagnosis if they chose to conceive. The counsellor addressed their emotional concerns, provided information on available support groups and discussed alternative family planning options. This case scenario depicts the importance of genetic counselling while dealing with genetic disorders.

GENETIC COUNSELLING (AN 75.5)

- **Genetic diseases** often exhibit a familial tendency.
- The role of **family history** is crucial for diagnosis and risk assessment.
- **Mendelian inheritance** pattern allows the geneticist to evaluate the risk for disease in relatives of affected individuals.
- Family members contribute information about shared genes and environmental factors, influencing genetically complex diseases.
- Having a first-degree relative with a common disease raises an individual's risk for the disease two to threefold relative to the general population.

GENETIC COUNSELLING PROCESS

- Genetic counselling focuses on the patient and their family, addressing concerns about disease progression and transmission. Thus, it is a process of communication that addresses the concerns related to the progress and transmission of a hereditary disorder.
- **Consultand** is an individual who seeks genetic counselling.
- Responsibilities of a **genetic counsellor** are:
  - **Inform** other family members of their potential risk.
  - **Offer tests** for risk assessments for other family members.
  - **Explain** what approaches are available to the patient and family members to modify these risks.

Calculating Recurrence Risks Involve the Following Parameters

- **Numerical value of risk/quantification of risk**—where they predict the risk in percentage or odds ratio.
- **Nature of the risk/qualification**—where they educate the consultands about the long-term burden associated with the risk.
- Placing the risk in the present situation—where the counsellor enables consultands to place their risk as high or low.
- Those who are at **high risk** include:
  - **Early age** of onset of a disease in a first-degree relative.

  - Two affected **first-degree** relatives.
  - Two second-degree relatives with at least one having early onset of disease.
  - Presence of a **'moderate-risk'** family history in either paternal or maternal pedigree.
- **Clinical genetics** deals with the diagnosis and management of the medical and psychological aspects of hereditary disease which involves:
  - Making a correct diagnosis with laboratory investigations, which include genetic testing to find the mutations responsible.
  - Helping the affected person and family members understand the nature and consequences of the disorder.
  - Providing appropriate treatment and management.
- The **purpose** of genetic counselling is to:
  - Provide information and support to families at risk of having birth defects or genetic disorders.
  - Understand the medical facts and the available management.
  - Know the way heredity contributes to the disorder.
  - Understand the options for dealing with the recurrence of disease.

Problems Encountered in Genetic Counselling

i. **Consanguinity**—Relationships where they share at least one common ancestor not remote than a great-great-grandparent.

ii. **Incest**—Relationships which occur between first degree relatives, for example brother sister/parent child.

iii. **Disputed paternity**—Paternity could never be proved with absolute certainty. The development of genetic fingerprinting using **minisatellite repeat sequence probes** and **single nucleotide polymorphism** have overcome the difficulties to a great extent.

iv. **Adoption and genetic disorders**—As per the guidelines of **American College of Medical Genetics**, genetic testing in children for adoption can be done only if the tests undertaken are for disorders that manifest during childhood and preventive measures are available.
  - Genetic counselling is not limited to identification of individuals at risk for disease but also provides psychologically oriented counselling to help individuals adapt to the impact of the disorder in the family.

BRAIN TEASERS

1. What role does family history play in genetic counselling?
   A. Minimal significance
   B. Primary factor in diagnosis and risk assessment
   C. Solely environmental factors
   D. No impact on risk evaluation
2. How does Mendelian inheritance pattern aid geneticists in risk evaluation?
   A. It is irrelevant in risk assessment.
   B. Provides information about shared genes only.
   C. Helps evaluate the risk for disease in relatives.
   D. Focuses on environmental factors exclusively.
3. What is the impact of having a first-degree relative with a common disease on an individual's risk?
   A. No impact
   B. Decreases risk
   C. Raises risk two to threefold
   D. Raises risk fivefold
4. Which of the following is NOT a responsibility of a genetic counsellor?
   A. Informing family members of potential risk.
   B. Offering risk assessment tests for family members.
   C. Modifying risks for the patient.
   D. Providing emotional support.
5. Who is considered at high risk for genetic disorders?
   A. Individuals with late-onset diseases.
   B. Those with only one affected first-degree relative.
   C. Individuals with a moderate-risk family history.
   D. Those with no family history.
6. What does clinical genetics primarily deal with?
   A. Surgery
   B. Medication management
   C. Psychological aspects of hereditary disease
   D. Physiotherapy
7. What is one of the responsibilities of clinical genetics in genetic counselling?
   A. Providing inappropriate treatment.
   B. Disregarding laboratory investigations.
   C. Incorrect diagnosis.
   D. Making a correct diagnosis with genetic testing.
8. What is the purpose of genetic counselling?
   A. Only to provide information.
   B. Offering treatment options.
   C. Understanding the environmental factors.
   D. Providing information and support to families at risk.

9. What does genetic counselling aim to help individuals understand?
   A. Only the medical facts.
   B. Only the psychological aspects.
   C. How heredity contributes to the disorder.
   D. Environmental factors exclusively.
10. Is genetic counselling limited to identifying individuals at risk for disease?
    A. Yes
    B. No
11. What is one of the responsibilities of genetic counselling beyond risk identification?
    A. Providing laboratory tests
    B. Offering psychological counselling
    C. Disregarding family history
    D. Recommending surgeries
12. Which is NOT a purpose of genetic counselling?
    A. Providing information and support.
    B. Understanding medical facts only.
    C. Knowing how heredity contributes to the disorder.
    D. Recommending surgical interventions.
13. Who does genetic counselling aim to support and inform?
    A. Only the patient.
    B. Only the patient's immediate family.
    C. Both the patient and family members.
    D. Only healthcare professionals.

Answers

1. (B); 2. (C); 3. (C); 4. (C); 5. (C); 6. (C); 7. (D); 8. (D); 9. (C); 10. (B); 11. (B); 12. (D); 13. (C);

FURTHER READINGS

Biesecker B. Genetic counseling and the central tenets of practice. *Cold Spring Harb Perspect Med.* 2020; 10(3):a038968. https://doi.org/10.1101/cshperspect.a038968.

Abacan M, Alsubaie L, Barlow-Stewart K, et al. The global state of the genetic counseling profession. *Eur J Human Genet.* 2019;27(2):183-197. https://doi.org/10.1038/s41431-018-0252-x.

Jamal L, Schupmann W, Berkman BE. An ethical framework for genetic counseling in the genomic era. *J Genet Counsel.* 2020;29(5):718-727. https://doi.org/10.1002/jgc4.1207.

Lilienthal D, Cahr M. Genetic counseling and assisted reproductive technologies. *Cold Spring Harb Perspect Med.* 2020;10(11):a036566. https://doi.org/10.1101/cshperspect.a036566.

Goldman JS. Predictive genetic counseling for neurodegenerative diseases: past, present, and future. *Cold Spring Harb Perspect Med.* 2020;10(7):a036525. https://doi.org/10.1101/cshperspect.a036525.

30 Recent Advances in Genetics

ANAMNESE

A 32-year-old patient diagnosed with **Attention deficit hyperactivity disorder (ADHD)** faced challenges in finding an effective medication due to adverse reactions and inadequate response. Opting for pharmacogenomic testing, recent advancements in this field shed light on the individual's genetic variations influencing drug metabolism. The analysis pinpointed specific markers related to the **CYP2D6** gene, affecting the metabolism of commonly prescribed ADHD medications like **Methylphenidate**. With this insight, the healthcare team adjusted the treatment plan, opting for an alternative medication that better aligned with the patient's pharmacogenomic profile. The result was a significant improvement in symptom control with fewer side effects, emphasizing the value of pharmacogenomics in optimizing drug selection and enhancing patient outcomes.

PRECISION MEDICINE

The integration of genomic information into clinical care has advanced personalized or precision medicine. Tailoring treatments based on an individual's genetic makeup allows for more effective and targeted therapies, minimizing adverse effects. The **Trans-Omics for Precision Medicine (TOPMED)** Initiative of the NHLBI (National Heart, Lung and Blood Institute) is one example of a large-scale effort that is beginning to generate more comprehensive omics data for a wide range of study cohorts, based on already existing studies and sample material.

CRISPR TECHNOLOGY

The **CRISPR-Cas9 gene**-editing tool has revolutionized genetic research and holds promise for treating genetic disorders. It allows for precise modification of DNA, potentially correcting or mitigating disease-causing genetic mutations. Clustered regularly interspaced short palindromic repeats (CRISPR) technology is a novel therapeutic intervention which can help us edit the genome of patients with genetic aetiology, for example dilated cardiomyopathy (**DCM**) and potentially cure them permanently (Fig. 30.1).

POLYGENIC RISK SCORES (PRS)

Researchers have developed more sophisticated methods for calculating polygenic risk scores, which consider multiple genetic variants to predict an individual's risk for certain diseases. PRSs constitute a composite genomic biomarker, and potential applications for PRSs in clinical practice consists of risk prediction and disease screening, early diagnosis, prognostication and drug stratification to improve efficacy or reduce adverse drug reactions.

NONINVASIVE PRENATAL TESTING (NIPT)

Advances in NIPT have improved the accuracy of detecting genetic abnormalities in foetuses using a simple blood test, reducing the need for more invasive procedures. Compared to traditional prenatal screening, NIPT was more accurate in detecting **trisomies 21, 18** and **13** and decreased the need for diagnostic testing.

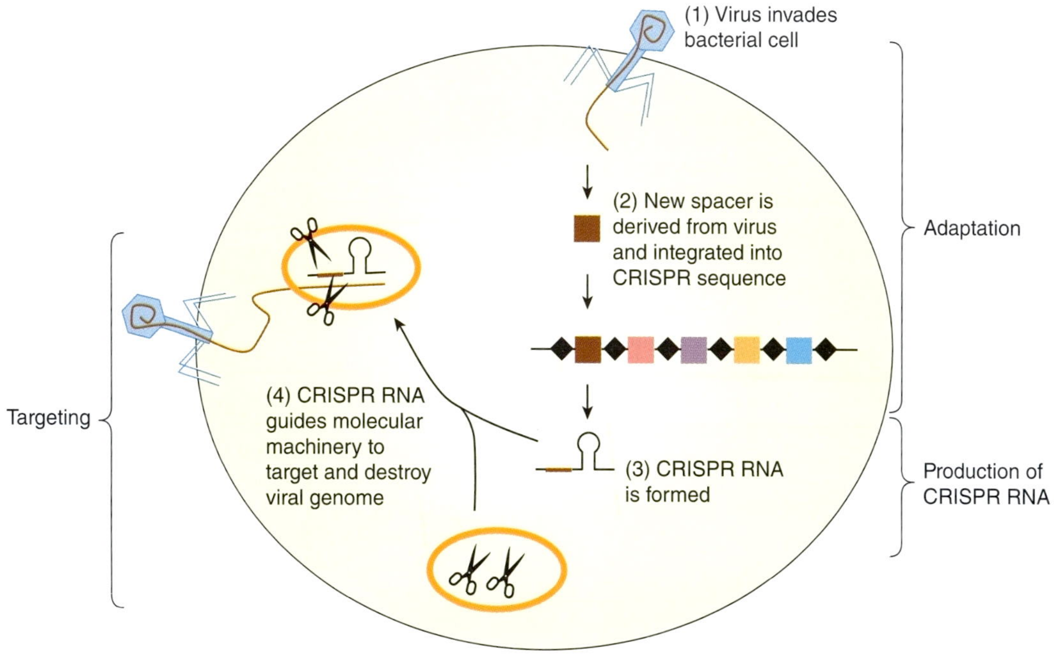

Fig. 30.1 CRISPR.

EPIGENETICS RESEARCH

Understanding how gene expression is regulated beyond the DNA sequence itself has expanded with epigenetics research. This field explores modifications to DNA that can influence gene activity, providing insights into the interaction between genetics and environmental factors. It is recognized that environmental exposures and nutritional disturbances during critical developmental windows can shape long-term disease risk through the modification of the epigenome. The precise regulation of gene expression during normal human development, largely governed by epigenetic mechanisms, involves critical processes such as DNA methylation at **CpG dinucleotides**, playing key roles in tissue-specific gene expression, regulation of imprinted genes, maintenance of genome stability and silencing of transposable elements.

SINGLE-CELL SEQUENCING

Traditional genetic sequencing often involves analysing bulk samples of cells. Single-cell sequencing allows researchers to study individual cells, providing a more detailed understanding of cellular heterogeneity and contributing to personalized medicine. A significant application of **scRNA-seq** technology is to construct a more refined and high-resolution catalogue of cells across diverse living organisms, often referred to as an atlas. This comprehensive resource serves as a tool for enhancing our understanding of diseases and facilitating the development of effective solutions.

PHARMACOGENOMICS

Advances in pharmacogenomics have improved our understanding of how individual genetic variations influence responses to medications. This information helps optimize drug selection and dosages for better treatment outcomes. Utilizing pharmacogenomic testing proves to be a valuable strategy in improving both the safety and effectiveness of medications. A majority of individuals, around 90%–95%, possess an actionable genotype for at least one pharmacogene associated with commonly used pharmacogenomically actionable medications. To maximize the impact on medication safety and clinical care, it is crucial to make genetic information accessible at the time of prescribing, emphasizing the importance of preemptive testing.

LIQUID BIOPSIES

Liquid biopsy techniques, such as analysing circulating **free DNA** in the blood, have gained prominence in cancer research. These noninvasive tests can provide information about tumour genetics, aiding in cancer diagnosis and monitoring treatment response. Liquid biopsies can sample numerous molecular entities within the blood, including free nucleic acids, such as cell-free nuclear DNA (**cfDNA**), cell-free mitochondrial DNA (**cf-mtDNA**), circulating tumour DNA (**ctDNA**) and cell-free RNA (**cfRNA**); extracellular vesicles, often containing nucleic acid components; proteins and metabolites.

FURTHER READINGS

Olivier M, Asmis R, Hawkins GA, Howard TD, Cox LA. The need for multi-omics biomarker signatures in precision medicine. *Int J Mol Sci.* 2019;20(19):4781. doi:10.3390/ijms20194781.

Ganipineni VDP, Gutlapalli SD, Danda S, et al. Clustered regularly interspaced short palindromic repeats (CRISPR) in cardiovascular disease: a comprehensive clinical review on dilated cardiomyopathy. *Cureus.* 2023; 15(3):e35774. doi:10.7759/cureus.35774.

Cross B, Turner R, Pirmohamed M. Polygenic risk scores: an overview from bench to bedside for personalised medicine. *Front Genet.* 2022;13:1000667. doi:10.3389/fgene.2022.1000667.

Health Quality Ontario. Noninvasive prenatal testing for trisomies 21, 18, and 13, sex chromosome aneuploidies, and microdeletions: a health technology assessment. *Ont Health Technol Assess Ser.* 2019; 19(4):1-166.

Svoboda LK, Neier K, Wang K, et al. Tissue and sex-specific programming of DNA methylation by perinatal lead exposure: implications for environmental epigenetics studies. *Epigenetics.* 2021;16(10):1102-1122. doi:10.1080/15592294.2020.1841872.

Jovic D, Liang X, Zeng H, Lin L, Xu F, Luo Y. Single-cell RNA sequencing technologies and applications: a brief overview. *Clin Transl Med.* 2022;12(3):e694. doi:10.1002/ctm2.694.

Haidar CE, Crews KR, Hoffman JM, Relling MV, Caudle KE. Advancing pharmacogenomics from single-gene to preemptive testing. *Annu Rev Genomics Hum Genet.* 2022;23:449-473. doi:10.1146/annurev-genom-111621-102737.

Gaitsch H, Franklin RJM, Reich DS. Cell-free DNA-based liquid biopsies in neurology. *Brain.* 2023; 146(5):1758-1774. doi:10.1093/brain/awac438.

Embryology and Genetics: FAQs from Previous Years University Papers

Question	Max Marks	Year
	Embryology	
Development and descent of testis	2, 3, 7	2013, 2017, 2021, 2023
Development of pituitary gland	2	2014, 2018, 2020
Somites	2, 3	2015, 2016, 2017, 2018
Derivatives of midgut	2	2013
Placenta—formation and developmental anomalies	1, 5, 8	2010, 2014, 2015, 2021, 2022
Development of kidney	1, 2, 3	2012, 2015, 2016, 2022
Development and congenital anomalies of face	5	2016, 2018
Development of portal vein	3	2014
Derivatives of mesonephric ducts in males	2	2017
Derivatives of the components of the first pharyngeal arch	5, 3	2012, 2016
Neural crest derivatives	1, 2, 3, 4	2012, 2016, 2017, 2021, 2022
Oogenesis	3	2016, 2021
Right atrium development	3, 5	2013, 2016, 2020, 2022
Dizygotic twins	3	2014
Development of lungs, stages	1, 3	2014, 2023
Intraembryonic mesoderm formation, parts and derivatives	5, 8	2013, 2020, 2022
Effects of fertilization, stages and consequences	3, 8	2013, 2021
Derivatives of prearterial segment of midgut loop	2	2012
Development of pancreas	3, 5	2013, 2019

Continued on following page

Question	Max Marks	Year
Development of spleen	5	2012
Neural tube—subdivisions and derivatives	3, 4	2012, 2023
Development of interventricular septum	2, 3	2016, 2018
Spermatogenesis	3, 4	2017, 2018, 2022
Development of anal canal	2	2011, 2015
Paramesonephric duct—formation and fate	2	2018, 2020, 2022
Yolk sac and its fate in humans	3	2012, 2019
Development of thyroid gland and the embryological basis of abnormal locations	2, 3, 5	2010, 2015, 2023
Meckel's diverticulum	2	2015
Chorionic villi	2	2018
Development of lips	1, 3	2011, 2022
Implantation, clinical aspects	3, 5, 8	2011, 2022, 2023
Spermiogenesis	2	2011
Cleft palate	3	2019
Derivatives of pharyngeal pouches	3	2019
Formation and fate of notochord	5, 8	2022, 2023
Formation and structure of umbilical cord	4	2023
Stage of meiosis 1 at which oogenesis is arrested	1	2023
Developmental sources of interatrial septum	1, 3	2019, 2022
Sites of ectopic pregnancy	1	2022
First pharyngeal pouch	2	2010
Graafian follicle	2, 5	2019, 2023
Development of second part of duodenum	4	2021
Name the nerve and muscle of third pharyngeal arch	1	2021
Decidua	2, 3	2020
Hindgut derivatives	1	2021
Derivatives of diencephalon	1	2021
Derivatives of second pharyngeal pouch	1	2021
Developmental source of diaphragm	1	2021
Two derivatives of second pharyngeal arch cartilage	1	2023
Embryological basis of nerve supply of tongue	3, 8	2022, 2023

Question	Max Marks	Year
Midgut—derivatives, rotation and associated anomalies	8	2022
Zona pellucida	2	2019
Two derivatives of first pharyngeal arch cartilage	1	2023
Formation and fate of primitive streak	4	2021
Two developmental sources of arch of aorta	1	2021
Derivatives of intraembryonic coelom	1	2021
Name two foetal membranes	1	2022
Structures present in the tertiary villus of placenta	1	2022
Derivatives of first pharyngeal pouch	1	2022
Developmental sources of ductus deferens	1	2022
Embryological basis of twinning	4	2023
16 Celled stage of embryo	1	2023
Structure which develops from the left horn of sinus venosus	1	2023
Maternal and foetal contribution to the development of placenta	1	2023
Development of breast and the associated anomalies	3	2020
	Genetics	
Barr body	2, 3	2014, 2015, 2017, 2021
Down syndrome/Trisomy 21	2, 3, 5	2015, 2016, 2017, 2022, 2023
Reciprocal translocation	2	2014
Klinefelter syndrome	2	2013
Turner's syndrome	1, 2, 3	2011, 2012, 2013, 2016, 2019, 2022
Numerical chromosomal abnormalities	3, 8	2018, 2023
Genetic counselling	3	2010
Mendelian inheritance	8	2021
Technique of karyotyping with its applications	3, 8	2020, 2023
Chromosomal aberrations	3, 8	2019, 2022
Chromosomes—structure and its classification	3, 4	2022
Structural abnormalities of chromosomes	3	2021
Various modes of inheritance with examples	8	2021
Name two autosomal recessive disorders	1	2022
Two examples for autosomal dominant inheritance	1	2023

Embryology Charts for Practical Examination

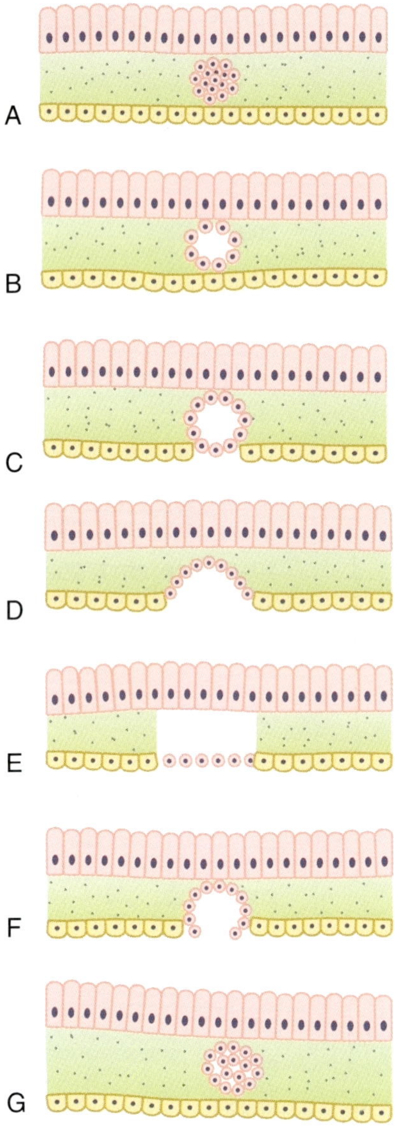

Fig. 1 Formation of notochord.

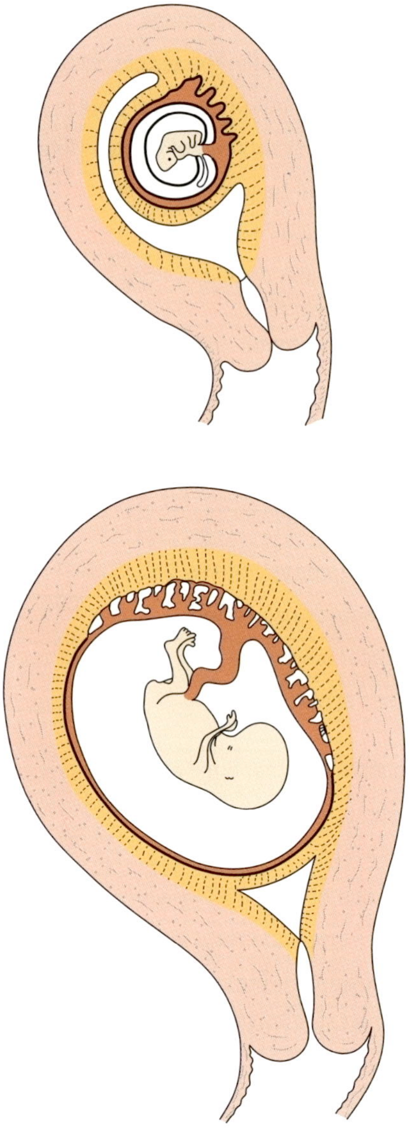

Fig. 2 Decidua.

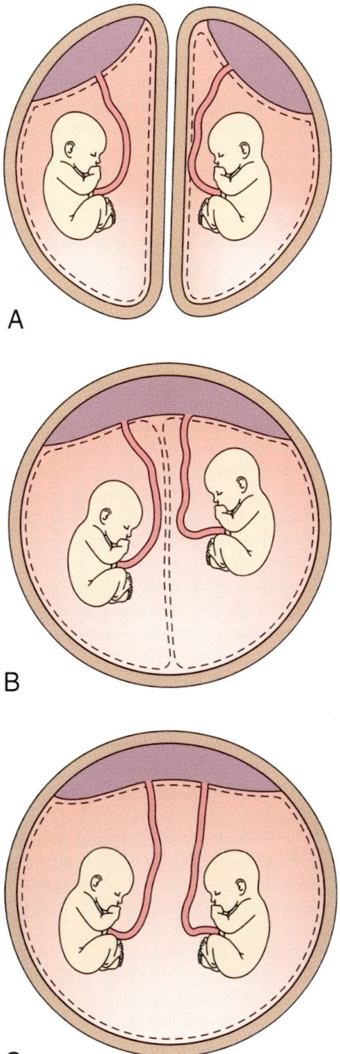
A
B
C

Fig. 3 Monozygotic twins.

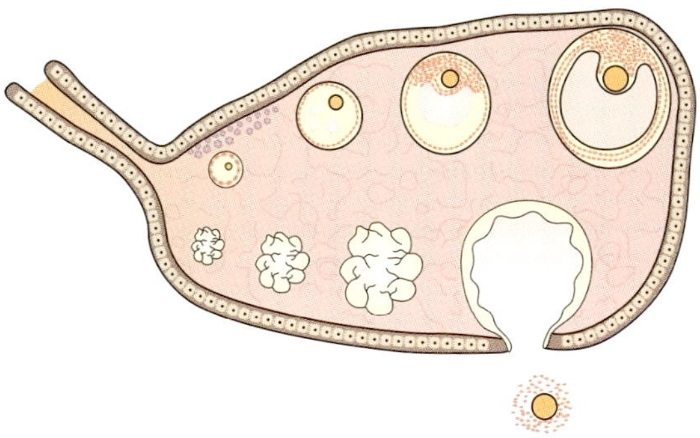

Fig. 4 Oogenesis.

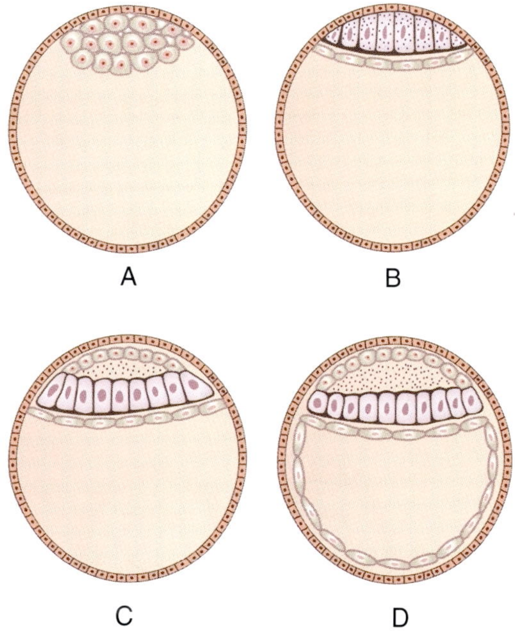
A B C D

Fig. 5 Events occurring in second week of development.

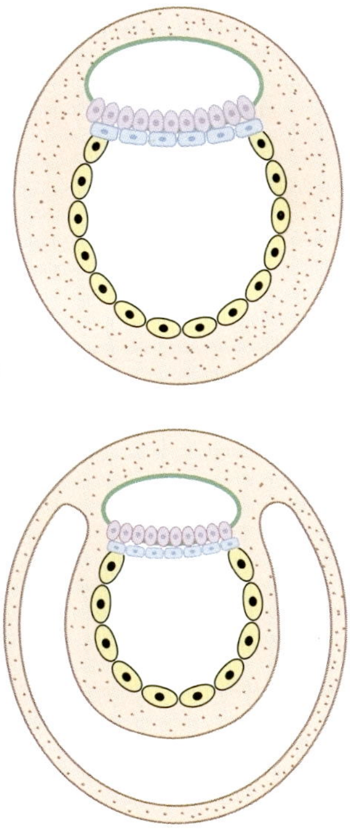
A
B

Fig. 6 Extraembryonic coelom.

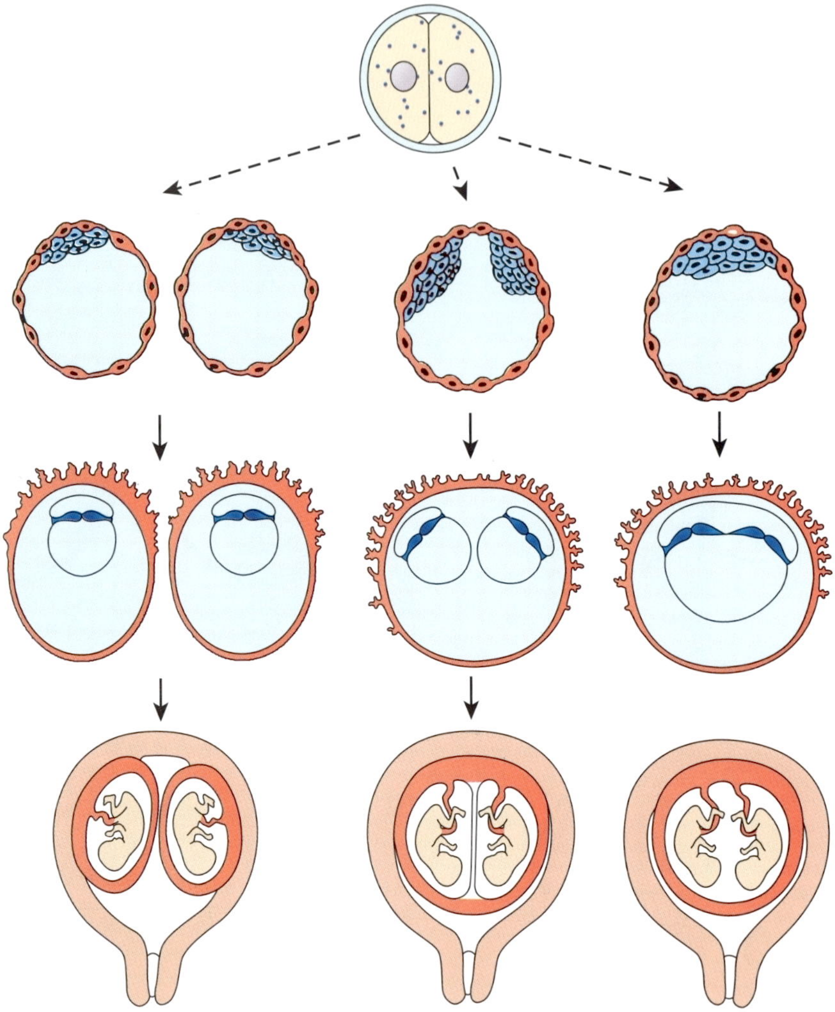

Fig. 7 Twinning.

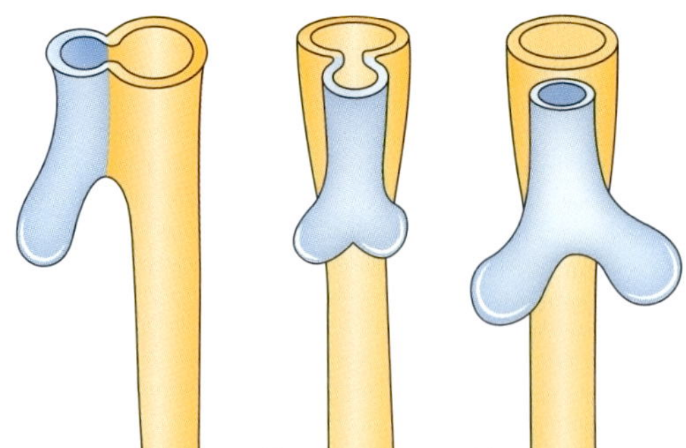

Fig. 8 Development of lung.

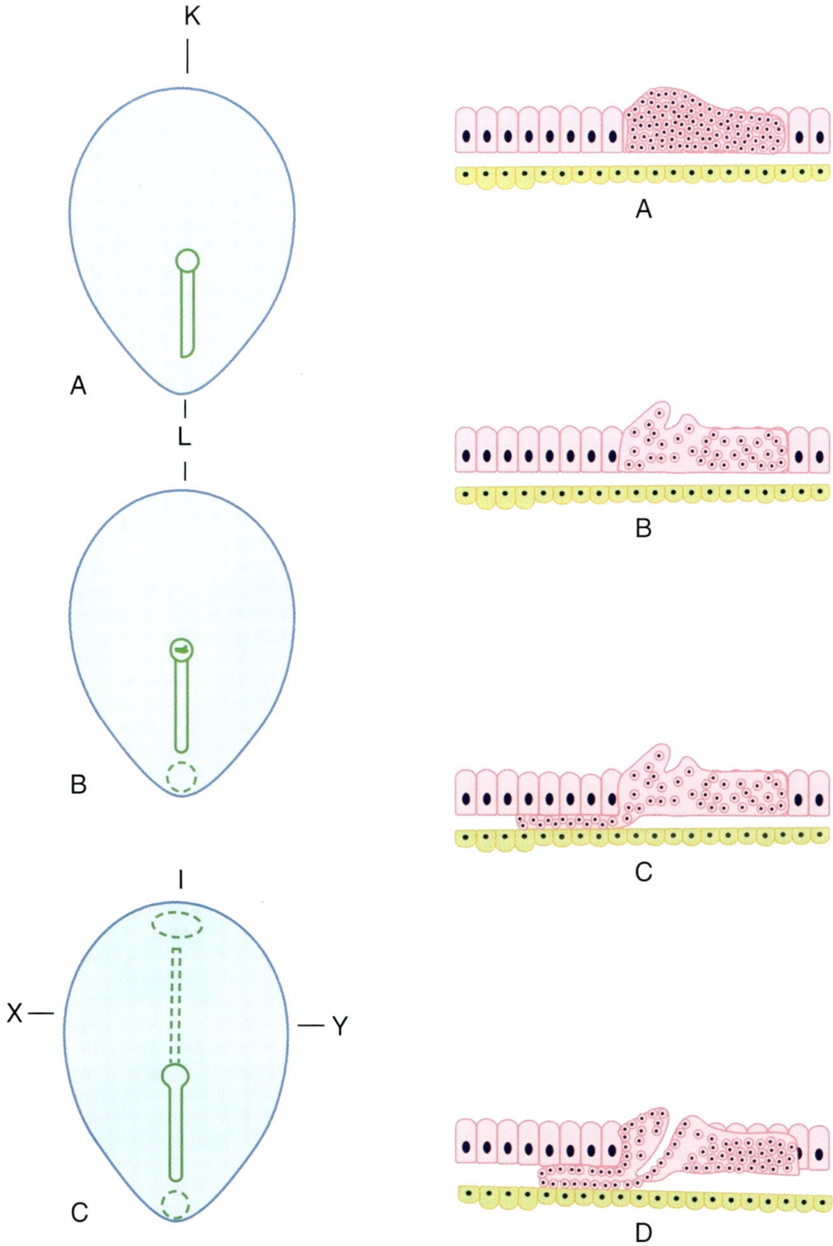

Fig. 9 Primitive streak.

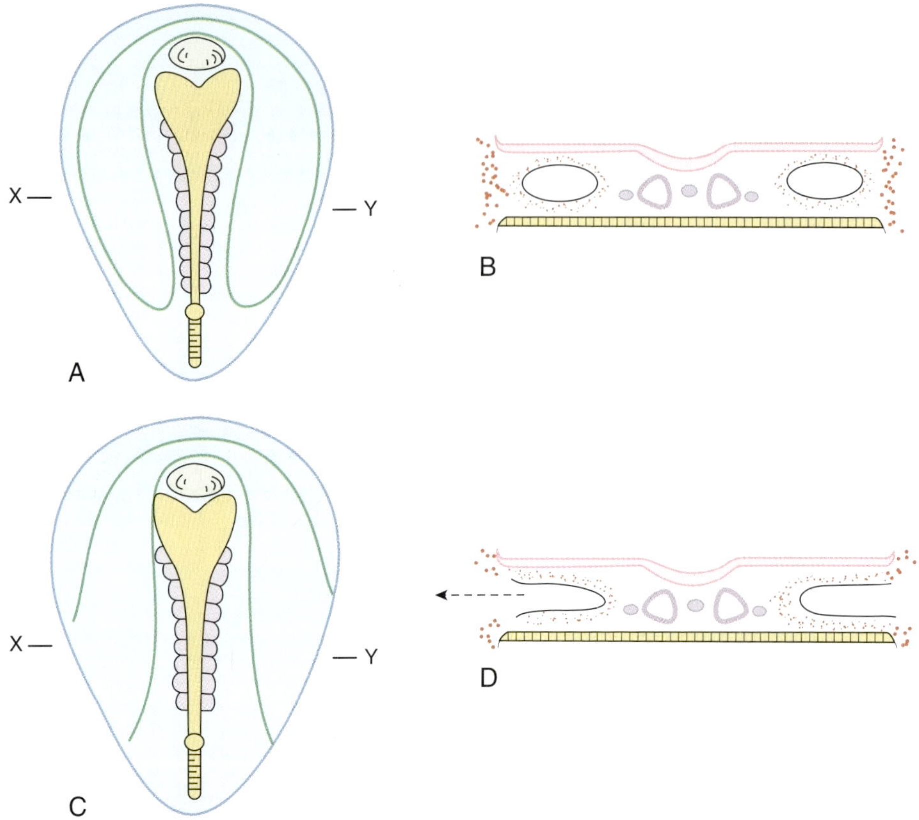

Fig. 10 Intraembryonic mesoderm.

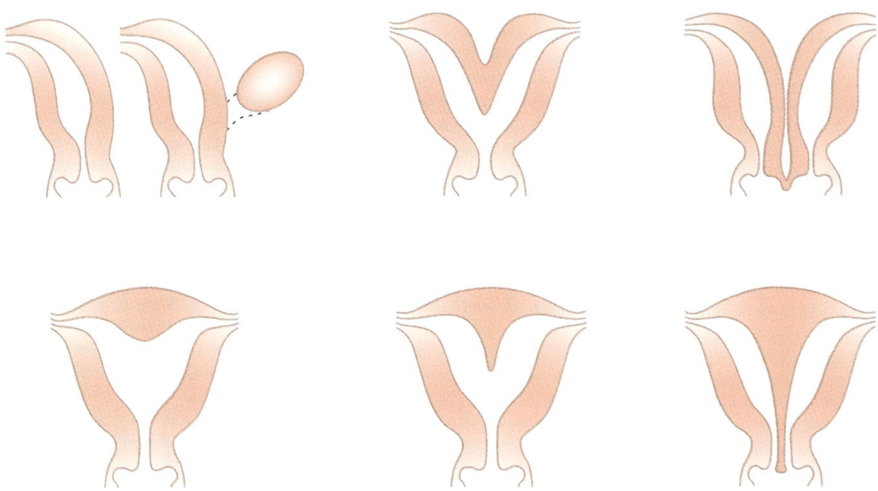

Fig. 11 Uterine anomalies.

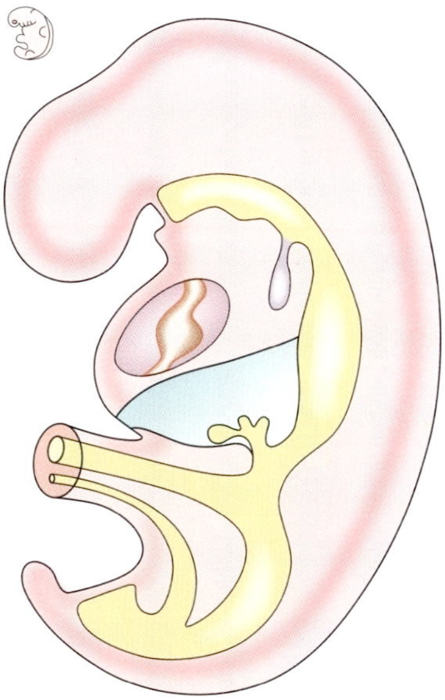

Fig. 12 Gut tube.

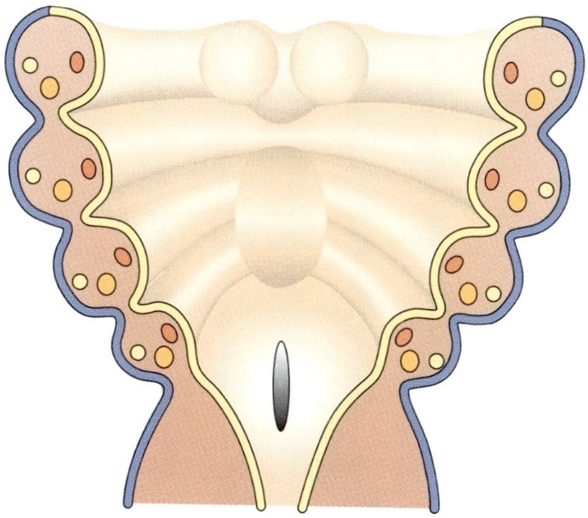

Fig. 14 Pharyngeal apparatus.

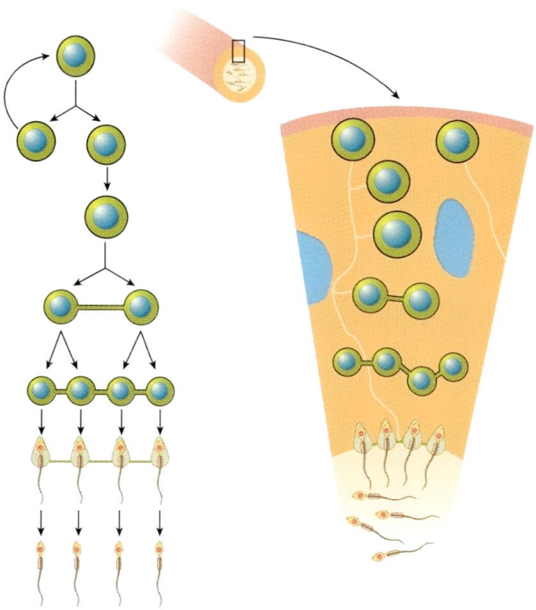

Fig. 13 Spermatogenesis.

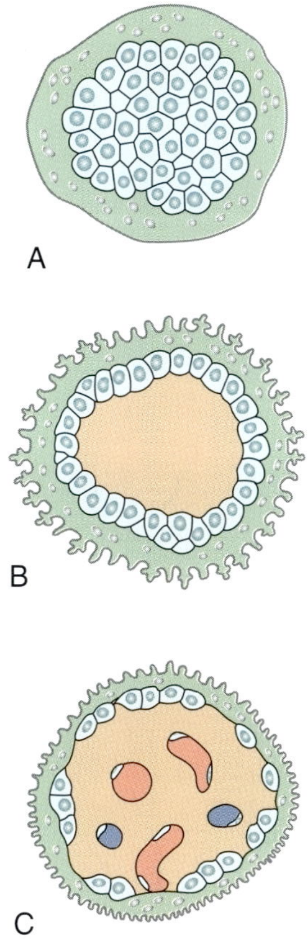

Fig. 15 Placenta—three types of villi.

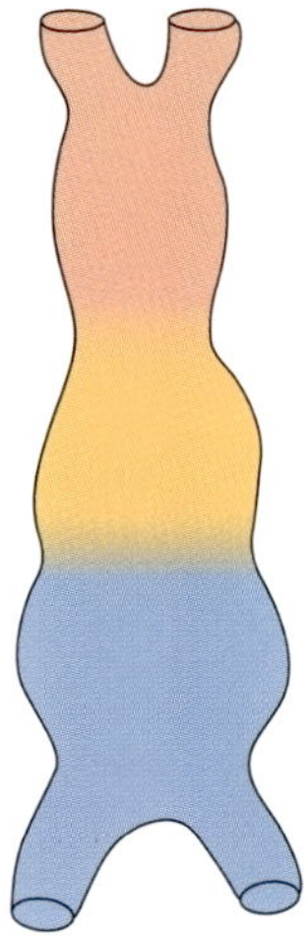

Fig. 16 Heart tube.

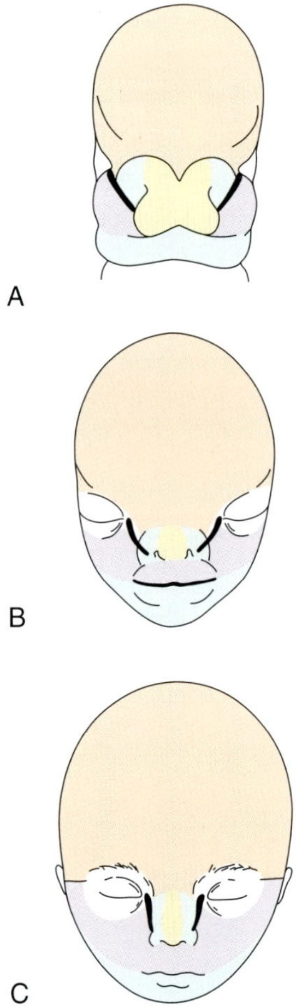

Fig. 17 Development of face.

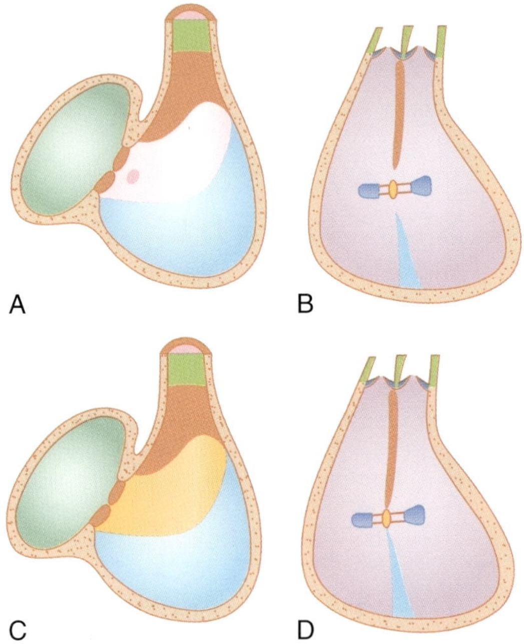

Fig. 18 Development of interventricular septum.

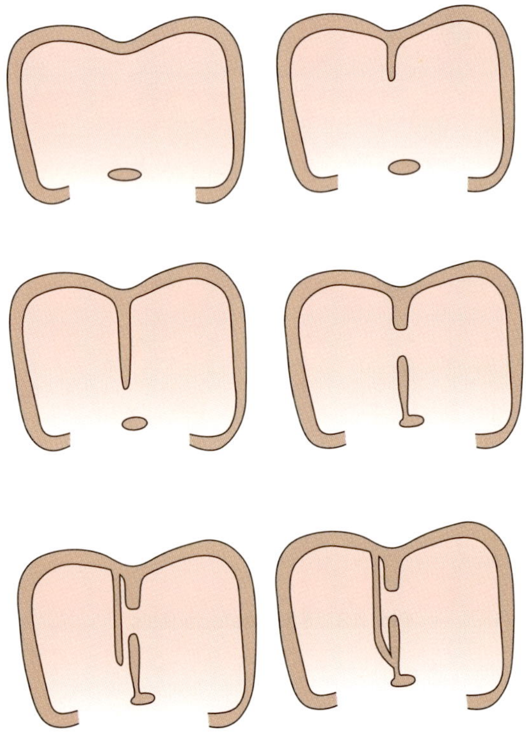

Fig. 19 Development of interatrial septum.

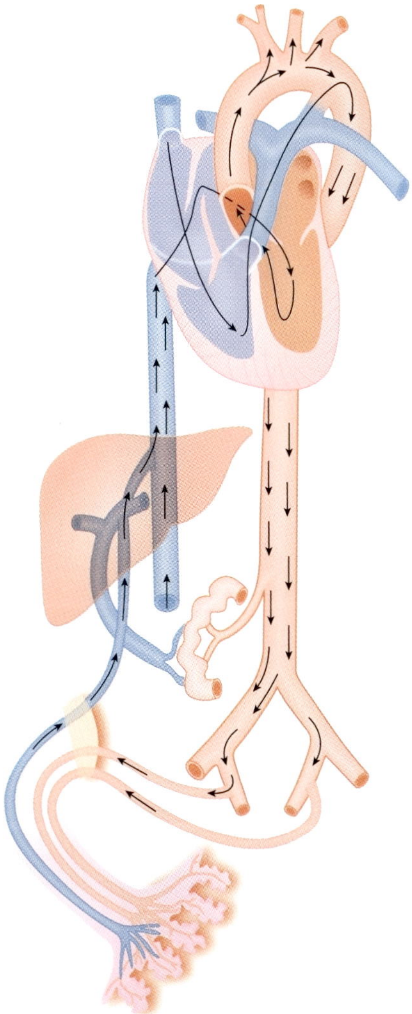

Fig. 20 Foetal circulation.

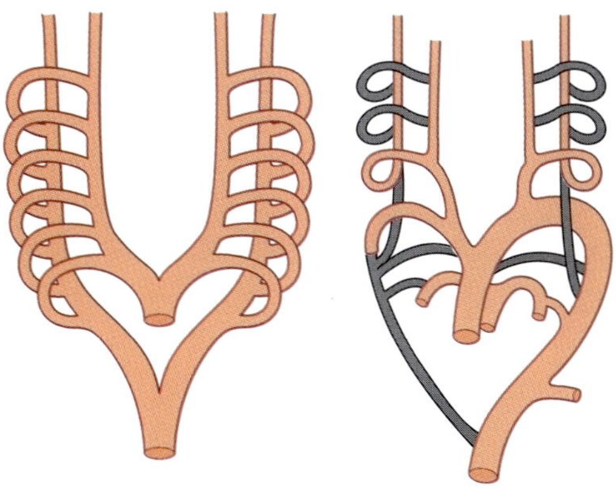

Fig. 21 Aortic arches.

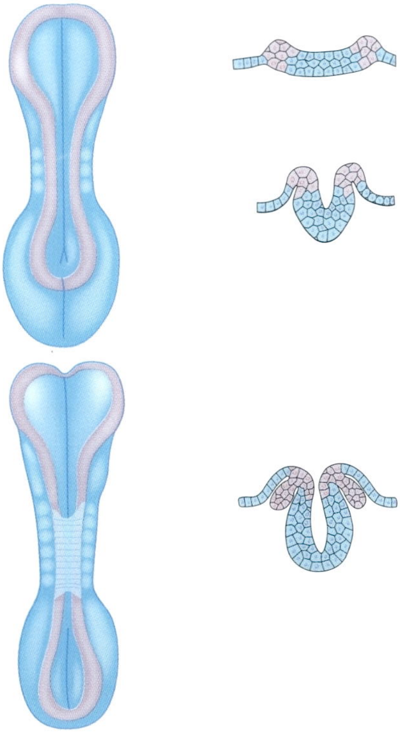

Fig. 22 Neurulation.

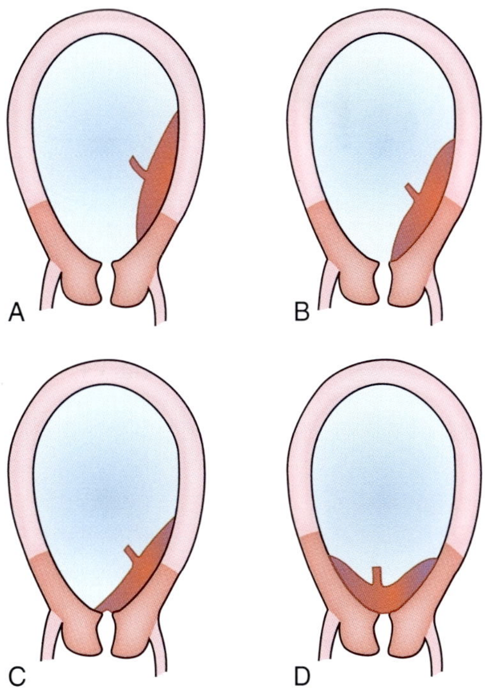

Fig. 23 Placenta praevia.

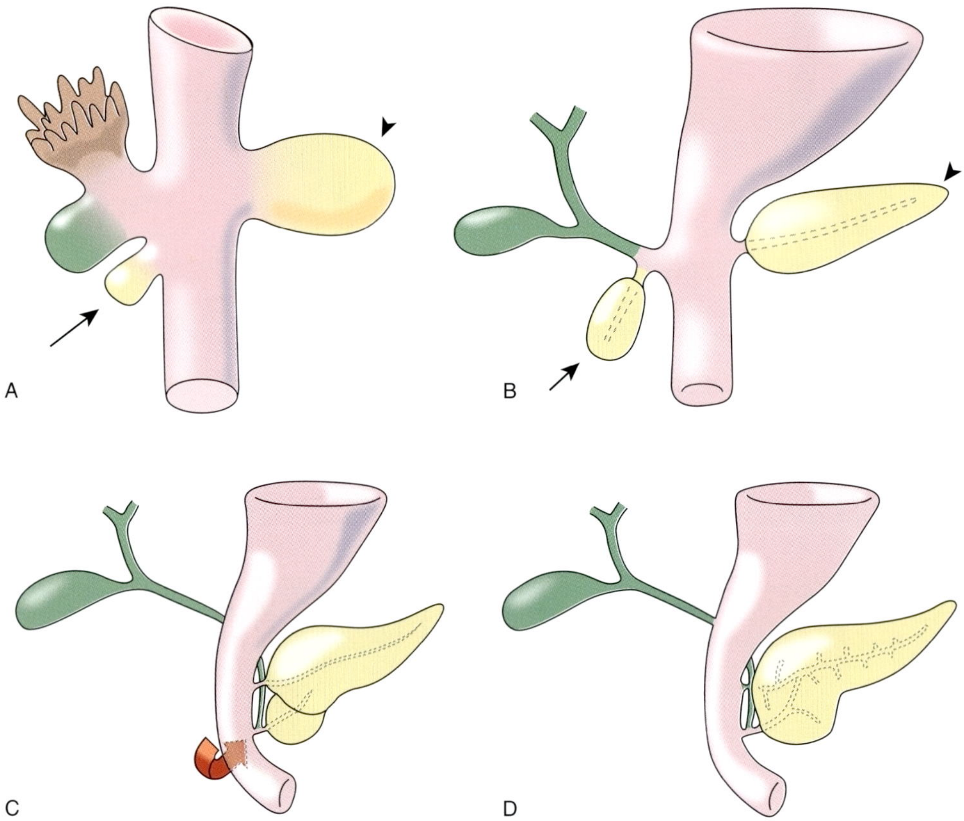

Fig. 24 Development of pancreas.

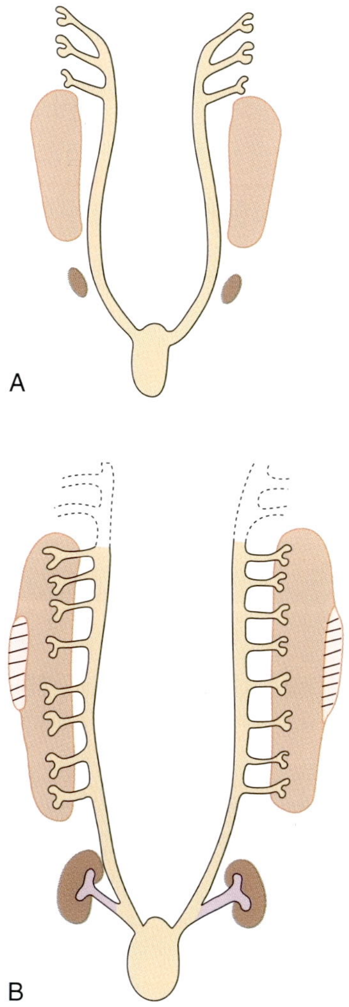

Fig. 25 Development of kidney.

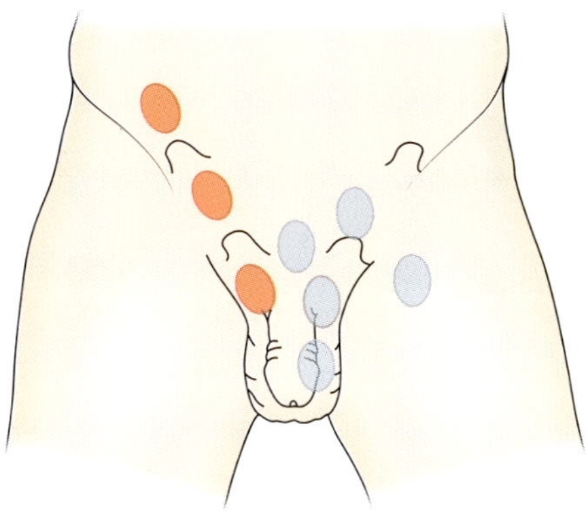

Fig. 26 Descent of testis and anomalies associated with it.

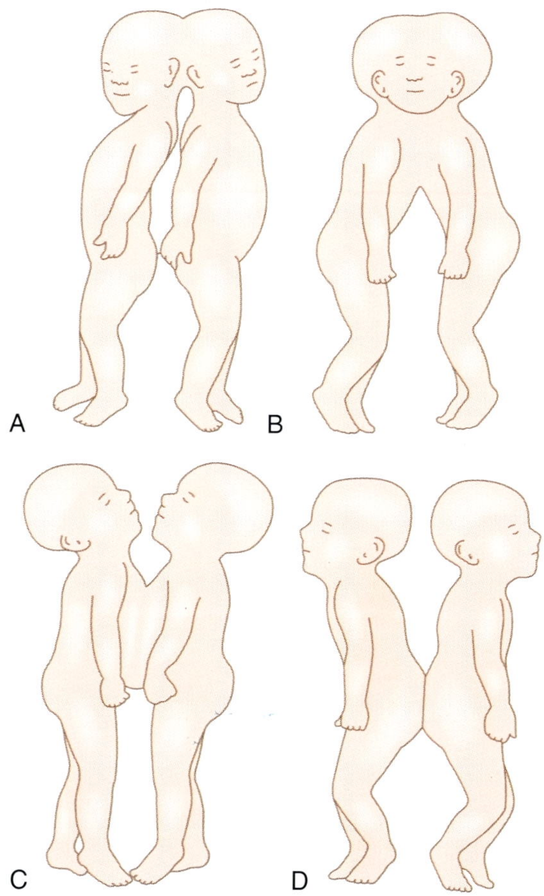

Fig. 27 Conjoined twins.

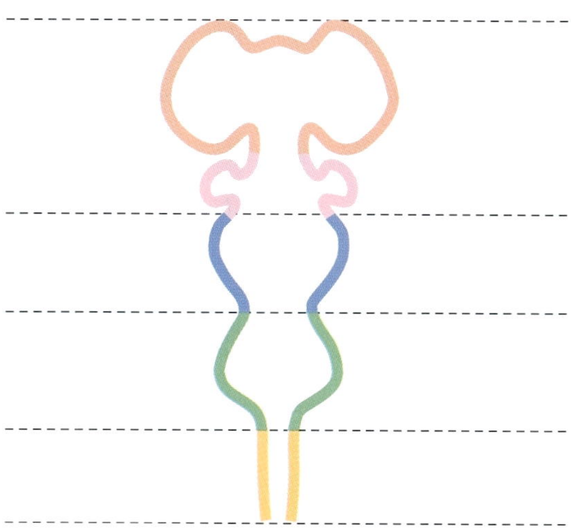

Fig. 28 Development of CNS.

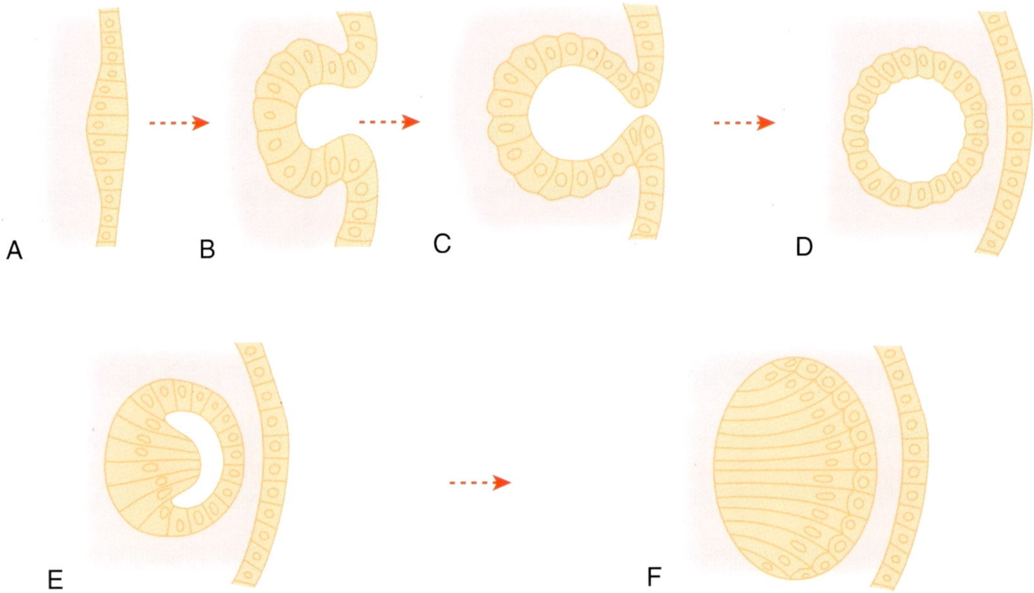

Fig. 29 Development of eye.

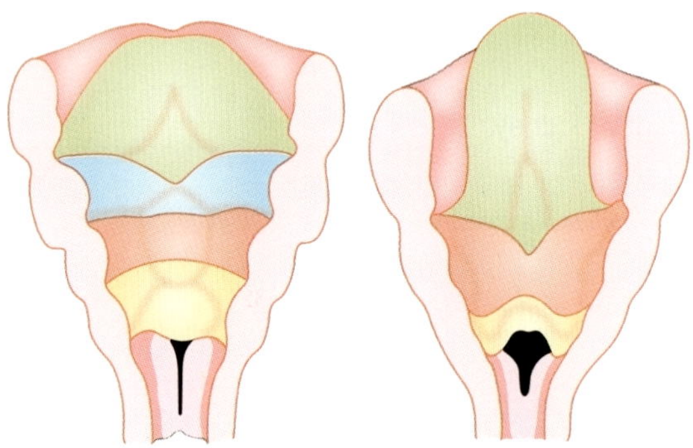

Fig. 30 Development of tongue.

Index

H

I

J

Q

R

S